Novel Treatment Strategies for Glioblastoma

Novel Treatment Strategies for Glioblastoma

Editor

Stanley Stylli

MDPI • Basel • Beijing • Wuhan • Barcelona • Belgrade • Manchester • Tokyo • Cluj • Tianjin

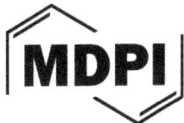

Editor
Stanley Stylli
Surgery (RMH)
The University of Melbourne
Parkville
Australia

Editorial Office
MDPI
St. Alban-Anlage 66
4052 Basel, Switzerland

This is a reprint of articles from the Special Issue published online in the open access journal *Cancers* (ISSN 2072-6694) (available at: www.mdpi.com/journal/cancers/special_issues/Novel_Treatment_Glioblastoma).

For citation purposes, cite each article independently as indicated on the article page online and as indicated below:

LastName, A.A.; LastName, B.B.; LastName, C.C. Article Title. *Journal Name* **Year**, *Volume Number*, Page Range.

ISBN 978-3-0365-2599-0 (Hbk)
ISBN 978-3-0365-2598-3 (PDF)

© 2021 by the authors. Articles in this book are Open Access and distributed under the Creative Commons Attribution (CC BY) license, which allows users to download, copy and build upon published articles, as long as the author and publisher are properly credited, which ensures maximum dissemination and a wider impact of our publications.
The book as a whole is distributed by MDPI under the terms and conditions of the Creative Commons license CC BY-NC-ND.

Contents

About the Editor vii

Preface to "Novel Treatment Strategies for Glioblastoma" ix

Stanley S. Stylli
Novel Treatment Strategies for Glioblastoma—A Summary
Reprinted from: *Cancers* **2021**, *13*, 5868, doi:10.3390/cancers13225868 1

Marija Dinevska, Natalia Gazibegovic, Andrew P. Morokoff, Andrew H. Kaye, Katharine J. Drummond, Theo Mantamadiotis and Stanley S. Stylli
Inhibition of Radiation and Temozolomide-Induced Glioblastoma Invadopodia Activity Using Ion Channel Drugs
Reprinted from: *Cancers* **2020**, *12*, 2888, doi:10.3390/cancers12102888 7

Michael O'Rawe, Ethan J. Kilmister, Theo Mantamadiotis, Andrew H. Kaye, Swee T. Tan and Agadha C. Wickremesekera
The Renin–Angiotensin System in the Tumor Microenvironment of Glioblastoma
Reprinted from: *Cancers* **2021**, *13*, 4004, doi:10.3390/cancers13164004 29

Vladimir Shapovalov, Liliya Kopanitsa, Lavinia-Lorena Pruteanu, Graham Ladds and David S. Bailey
Transcriptomics-Based Phenotypic Screening Supports Drug Discovery in Human Glioblastoma Cells
Reprinted from: *Cancers* **2021**, *13*, 3780, doi:10.3390/cancers13153780 47

Stanley S. Stylli
Novel Treatment Strategies for Glioblastoma
Reprinted from: *Cancers* **2020**, *12*, 2883, doi:10.3390/cancers12102883 83

Sarah Adriana Scuderi, Giovanna Casili, Alessio Ardizzone, Stefano Forte, Lorenzo Colarossi, Serena Sava, Irene Paterniti, Emanuela Esposito, Salvatore Cuzzocrea and Michela Campolo
KYP-2047, an Inhibitor of Prolyl-Oligopeptidase, Reduces GlioBlastoma Proliferation through Angiogenesis and Apoptosis Modulation
Reprinted from: *Cancers* **2021**, *13*, 3444, doi:10.3390/cancers13143444 95

Nguyen Thi Thanh Ho, Chinmay Satish Rahane, Subrata Pramanik, Pok-Son Kim, Arne Kutzner and Klaus Heese
FAM72, Glioblastoma Multiforme (GBM) and Beyond
Reprinted from: *Cancers* **2021**, *13*, 1025, doi:10.3390/cancers13051025 113

Vincenzo Di Nunno, Enrico Franceschi, Alicia Tosoni, Lidia Gatto, Raffaele Lodi, Stefania Bartolini and Alba Ariela Brandes
Glioblastoma: Emerging Treatments and Novel Trial Designs
Reprinted from: *Cancers* **2021**, *13*, 3750, doi:10.3390/cancers13153750 141

Chirayu R. Chokshi, Benjamin A. Brakel, Nazanin Tatari, Neil Savage, Sabra K. Salim, Chitra Venugopal and Sheila K. Singh
Advances in Immunotherapy for Adult Glioblastoma
Reprinted from: *Cancers* **2021**, *13*, 3400, doi:10.3390/cancers13143400 159

Kavitha Godugu, Mehdi Rajabi and Shaker A. Mousa
Anti-Cancer Activities of Thyrointegrin $\alpha_v\beta_3$ Antagonist Mono- and Bis-Triazole Tetraiodothyroacetic Acid Conjugated via Polyethylene Glycols in Glioblastoma
Reprinted from: *Cancers* **2021**, *13*, 2780, doi:10.3390/cancers13112780 . . . . **181**

Beate M. Schmitt, Anne S. Boewe, Claudia Götz, Stephan E. Philipp, Steffi Urbschat, Joachim Oertel, Michael D. Menger, Matthias W. Laschke and Emmanuel Ampofo
CK2 Activity Mediates the Aggressive Molecular Signature of Glioblastoma Multiforme by Inducing Nerve/Glial Antigen (NG)2 Expression
Reprinted from: *Cancers* **2021**, *13*, 1678, doi:10.3390/cancers13071678 . . . . **195**

Oleg Mozhei, Anja G. Teschemacher and Sergey Kasparov
Viral Vectors as Gene Therapy Agents for Treatment of Glioblastoma
Reprinted from: *Cancers* **2020**, *12*, 3724, doi:10.3390/cancers12123724 . . . . **213**

Elia Bozzato, Chiara Bastiancich and Véronique Préat
Nanomedicine: A Useful Tool against Glioma Stem Cells
Reprinted from: *Cancers* **2020**, *13*, 9, doi:10.3390/cancers13010009 . . . . **237**

Kimia Ghannad-Zadeh and Sunit Das
One-Carbon Metabolism Associated Vulnerabilities in Glioblastoma: A Review
Reprinted from: *Cancers* **2021**, *13*, 3067, doi:10.3390/cancers13123067 . . . . **255**

About the Editor

Stanley Stylli

Stanley Stylli completed his PhD in 2013 at The University of Melbourne. He is a researcher within the Department of Neurosurgery at The Royal Melbourne Hospital and an Honorary Fellow of the Department of Surgery (RMH) at The University of Melbourne. He has a background in glioblastoma research and focuses on invasion, with a particular emphasis on invadopodia and more recently extracellular vesicles. He also has a strong interest in the repurposing of drugs for the treatment of glioblastoma aimed at disrupting invadopodia and exosome-related processes to form the basis of novel anti-invasive therapies that can be utilized in the clinic. He is a member of The Invadosome Consortium, which is an international, open network of laboratories interested in tissue invasion, invadopodia and podosomes.

Preface to "Novel Treatment Strategies for Glioblastoma"

Glioblastoma is the most common and deadliest primary central nervous system tumor in adults. Glioblastomas diffusely invade into the surrounding normal brain tissue, resulting in a local neurologically destructive impact on the brain tissue and function. The extensive intra- and intertumoral heterogeneity displayed by glioblastoma cells and its tumor microenvironment give rise to a cancer that is extremely difficult to treat. Since the introduction of the Stupp protocol in 2005, there has not been a significant increase in the survival of patients with glioblastoma and prognosis continues to be poor with an approximate median survival of 12–15 months from diagnosis, despite ongoing improvements in surgical techniques, disease monitoring and systemic therapies. Despite the slow, incremental increase in glioblastoma patient survival, clinicians and researchers have maintained their motivation to make important gains in the understanding and management of glioblastoma. Chemotherapy-based approaches remain an essential part in the treatment of glioblastoma, and this area continues to evolve as we attempt to overcome the challenges of treatment resistance, efficient drug delivery to the tumor to limit off-target toxic side effects, drug efflux and blood–brain barrier permeability. The design of novel clinical trial strategies, the use of immunotherapeutic approaches, viral vectors used as cytotoxic agent or gene delivery tools, drug repurposing, nanomedicines and genomic based studies mapping this heterogeneous disease to define a cellular drug response are just some of the areas that signify that the management of glioblastoma is entering a new era, with an increasing number of potential treatments being made available to improve the survival outcome of glioblastoma patients.

Stanley Stylli
Editor

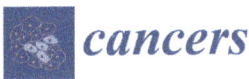

Editorial

Novel Treatment Strategies for Glioblastoma—A Summary

Stanley S. Stylli [1,2]

1 Department of Surgery, The University of Melbourne, The Royal Melbourne Hospital, Parkville, VIC 3050, Australia; sstylli@unimelb.edu.au or stanley.stylli@mh.org.au
2 Department of Neurosurgery, The Royal Melbourne Hospital, Parkville, VIC 3050, Australia

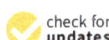

Citation: Stylli, S.S. Novel Treatment Strategies for Glioblastoma—A Summary. *Cancers* **2021**, *13*, 5868. https://doi.org/10.3390/cancers13225868

Received: 8 November 2021
Accepted: 18 November 2021
Published: 22 November 2021

Publisher's Note: MDPI stays neutral with regard to jurisdictional claims in published maps and institutional affiliations.

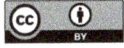

Copyright: © 2021 by the author. Licensee MDPI, Basel, Switzerland. This article is an open access article distributed under the terms and conditions of the Creative Commons Attribution (CC BY) license (https://creativecommons.org/licenses/by/4.0/).

Glioblastoma (GBM) is the most common primary central nervous system tumor in adults, accounting for approximately 80% of all brain-related malignancies [1]. It is a highly invasive disease and a paradigm of extensive intra- and intertumoral heterogeneity, presenting critical barriers to current therapies and invariably leading to treatment resistance as well as disease relapse. The current standard of care for GBM patients, involving maximal safe resection, radiotherapy and concomitant temozolomide (Stupp protocol) [2], has only provided a modest increase of 2.5 months in survival since its introduction in 2005. GBM patients have a poor prognosis, with a median survival of 12–15 months after diagnosis and a 5-year survival rate of less than 5%. Even though there have been limited advances in the progression of GBM therapeutics to significantly increase patient survival compared to other cancers, this has not dampened the motivation of researchers and clinicians to investigate novel treatment strategies for combating this disease. The Special Issue, 'Novel Treatment Strategies for Glioblastoma' [3], contains twelve articles (five original research articles and seven reviews) that explore a range of novel and strategic approaches for improving the treatment of GBM [4–15]. This editorial aims to briefly summarize the content of these articles.

The seven review articles focus on topics of great interest. O'Rawe et al. [9] highlight the dynamic relationship between the renin–angiotensin system (RAS), the GBM cancer stem cell niche and the tumor microenvironment (TME), and how it contributes to driving tumorigenesis and treatment resistance. They provide a concise overview on the effect of the RAS and its convergent signaling pathways on the TME, directly influencing various factors of cancer progression, including proliferation, invasion and survival. Importantly, they present data from observational and epidemiological cancer studies that involve the use of RAS inhibitors. Although the data remain inconclusive, RAS inhibitors appear to potentially be protective against cancer. They propose that existing commonly available medications can be repurposed as RAS-modulating drugs to therapeutically target the RAS in GBM, either as an alternative treatment or as an adjunct to the current standard of care.

Di Nunno et al. [10] review promising ongoing clinical trials for the treatment of primary and recurrent GBM, with a focus on novel trial design strategies. They discuss how these can be further developed in the future to streamline the testing of an ever-expanding cohort of innovative drugs to provide a tailored treatment approach for patients based on both molecular and clinical parameters. There are a number of biological obstacles that can hinder any therapeutic improvement in GBM treatment protocols, some of which are outlined in the review, including the (i) blood–brain and blood–tumor–brain barriers that impede the effective passage of therapeutic compounds to the tumor, (ii) the extensive heterogeneity of the tumor and (iii) the ability to develop/activate compensatory mechanisms to promote treatment resistance. The authors provide a summary of a number of trials for primary and recurrent GBM, but none to date have shown significant therapeutic improvements, even though there has been an increase in the molecular and biological understanding of the disease. Critical evaluation of the published results of clinical trial surveys has identified that there are well-known issues with GBM interventional trials that are terminated. These include a lack of accrual, funding problems, the absence of reliable surrogate endpoints and unbalanced patient distribution (higher numbers enrolled in the phase III component), which ultimately leads to an unpowered early efficacy study. Improvements for GBM interventional clinical trials design are presented, such as the use of 'phase 0' studies, which aim to target tumors with investigational agents based on the molecular profiling of the tumor coupled with an early assessment of these drugs to penetrate the blood–brain barrier.

As current treatment strategies have not delivered significant improvements in GBM patient survival, some emerging therapeutics have redirected their efforts towards reprogramming the patient's immune system to generate an anti-tumor response. The review by Chokshi et al. [11] focuses on evaluating several immunotherapeutic approaches that have been trialed for the treatment of GBM, including various vaccination strategies, immune checkpoint inhibitors (ICIs) and chimeric antigen receptor (CAR) T cells. The exposure of tumor-associated antigens to antigen-presenting cells, which activate immune effector cells to achieve an anti-cancer immune response, form the framework of cancer vaccine functionality. Single- and multiple-antigen vaccines are presented in this review, but as they have displayed varying degrees of response, none are currently listed as being integrated into a standard of care. Immune checkpoints exist as part of a complex system of stimulatory and inhibitory regulators, with immune cells upregulating these immune checkpoints to maintain immune homeostasis and avoid autoimmunity; however, it has been determined that cancer cells can also express immune checkpoint proteins to suppress the anti-cancer immune response. Antibodies against these checkpoints, acting as ICIs, have shown great progress against melanoma and non-small-cell lung cancer, especially in blocking programmed cell death protein 1 (PD-1), which is being tested against GBM.

One of the hallmarks of cancer cell biology is an altered cell metabolism, with metabolic reprogramming occurring in cancer cells to facilitate an increase in cell proliferation, maintain self-renewal and develop treatment resistance. The review by Ghannad-Zadeh et al. [12] focuses on a one-carbon mediated de novo purine-synthesis-based metabolic pathway, summarizing the evidence supporting its role in GBM cell proliferation and tumorigenesis, as well as proposing how it can be utilized as a therapeutic modality. Alterations of this pathway have been identified in brain-tumor-initiating cells, and therefore may serve as a phenotypic marker of tumor recurrence, especially as they have a higher mitochondrial reserve than differentiated glioma cells, allowing them to use adaptive metabolic strategies to resist therapeutic stress, leading to treatment resistance. In addition, purine nucleotide synthesis has been shown to regulate DNA repair and therapeutic resistance in GBM, with increased rates of de novo nucleotide synthesis providing GBM cells with the enhanced ability to repair temozolomide (TMZ)-mediated DNA damage. As studies have demonstrated a correlation between treatment resistance and purine metabolism in GBM, the direct inhibition of purine synthesis in GBM has fueled interest in the therapeutic efficacy of this approach, including a current on-going phase 0/I trial of mycophenolate mofetil (inhibitor of IMPDH1 and GTP synthesis) in primary and recurrent GBM. Although the research is in its infancy, targeting metabolic vulnerabilities in GBM may offer an attractive strategy to overcome treatment resistance and recurrence.

Ho et al. [13] discuss the role of the gene pair |-SRGAP2–FAM72-| in the cell cycle and GBM, with the possibility of defining new therapeutic possibilities for GBM. Endogenous FAM72 expression has been detected in the hippocampal dentate gyrus, where the |-SRGAP2–FAM72-| master gene pair regulates neural stem cell (NSC) renewal, neurogenesis and brain plasticity. Alterations in the intergenic region of the two sub-gene units (gene transcription control unit) can lead to dysregulated gene expression, which may transform NSCs into cancer stem cells, leading to GBM. Through the use of gene expression data of GBM patient tumor biopsies deposited within cBioportal, the authors have demonstrated that a strong correlation exists between high FAM72 expression and the highly mutated gene signatures (EGFR, TP53, NF1, SPTA1, PIK3CA or SCN9A, MXRA5, ADAM29, KDR, PIK3C2G and LRP1B), which can lead to cell cycle activation, cell transformation and proliferation. They propose that FAM72 is an attractive target for therapy, as it is a proliferative marker expressed in the late G2M phase of the cell cycle and exhibits low expression in normal, non-neuronal tissue.

Bozzato et al. [14] highlight how nanomedicines are being investigated as an alternative treatment approach for GBM in an attempt to overcome the limitations of conventional chemotherapies, such as the lack of tumor cell specificity, toxic side effects and low biological stability. Nanomedicines can bypass some of these limitations through the encapsulation of drugs in nanosized carriers (protecting them from degradation and reducing off-target side effects in the patient) and the ability to modify the surface of the nanocarrier with targeting moieties, allowing for easy transport through the BBB or the recognition of GBM or glioma stem cells. Importantly, the use of nanocarriers as a drug delivery system can also reduce the efflux of free drugs, as the nanomedicines enter the tumor cells through the process of endocytosis via endo-lysosomal trafficking, whereas free drugs enter through diffusion, which can be located near efflux pumps.

The manuscript by Mozhei et al. [15] reviews the idea of using viral vectors either as cytotoxic agents or gene delivery tools for the treatment of GBM and provides a concise summary of molecular strategies and current clinical trials, concluding that approaches based upon targeting a specific biochemical pathway or mutation will ultimately lead to failure due to the high genomic instability and clonal selection characteristics of GBM. However, they do suggest that engaging the immune system to induce an anti-tumor response should be explored further, or alternatively that a system should be designed which irreversibly targets dividing tumor cells and not quiescent brain cells. They present an extensive list of viral vector types that have been used in gene-therapy-based clinical trials for GBM and an overview of studies that have investigated vectors based on viral backgrounds, such as adenovirus, herpes simplex, reovirus, parvovirus and poliovirus. Importantly, they indicate that a major factor which will determine the success of viral gene therapy is the physical access of the virus to the GBM cells.

The five original articles in this Special Issue outline the innovative approaches and methodologies that research groups are utilizing to uncover novel treatment strategies for the treatment of GBM. Shapovalov et al. [8] used a genome-wide drug-induced gene expression (DIGEX) approach to define the cellular drug response phenotypes of two drugs, Mardepodect and Regorafenib, with three human GBM cell lines—U87MG, A172 and T98G. Employing a DIGEX approach allowed them to reposition the schizophrenia drug, Mardepodect, as a possible antiproliferative candidate for GBM, against Regorafenib, a drug which is already in clinical trials for GBM. The study was performed with a Clariom S Human Array, yielding more than 20,000 genes, which were linked to 18,316 identifiable protein-coding genes after being mapped to their Entrez IDs. They employed a dedicated analysis pipeline using UniProt, Entrez, Gene Ontology, the Pharos database, Reactome pathway and gene network analysis, focusing on the 200 genes with the most elevated or lowered gene expression levels and their corresponding subsets. They observed that both drugs upregulated genes encoding for specific growth factors, transcription factors, cellular signaling molecules and cell surface proteins, in addition to downregulating a broad range of targetable cell-cycle- and apoptosis-associated genes. The significant outcome of this approach is that it allowed for the detection of upregulated genes encoding for therapeutic targets of existing FDA-approved drugs, but also uncovered targets for which there are no approved drugs that may be future novel druggable targets as part of a chemistry-led discovery campaign. This approach provides a comprehensive phenotypic landscape for visualizing complex drug responses following the treatment of GBM cells, and shows that diagnosing and targeting GBM cellular phenotypes before and after drug treatment should be adopted as part of a personalized therapy program, given the pharmacological plasticity displayed by such an extremely heterogeneous disease as GBM.

As angiogenesis and apoptosis play key roles in the development of GBM, the study by Scuderi et al. [7] focused on the modulation of these two processes as a possible strategy to combat GBM progression. They used an inhibitor of the prolyl-oligopeptidase KYP-2047, which is known to modulate angiogenesis, in a series of in vitro experiments with various human GBM cell lines and in vivo experiments with a subcutaneous U87 xenograft model. They demonstrated that KYP-2047 treatment of the mice resulted in a reduced tumor burden, and that immunohistochemical studies of tumor sections revealed reduced expression of vascular endothelial growth factor, angiopoietins and endothelial-nitric-oxide synthase. The in vitro studies showed that KYP-2047 treatment was able to reduce GBM cell viability, which was coupled with an increased expression of the pro-apoptotic protein, Bax, p53 and caspase-3, and a reduction in Bcl-2.

Integrin $\alpha v \beta 3$ receptors are overexpressed in a number of different cancers, including GBM, especially at the tumor margins (invasive regions) and blood vessels within the tumor, facilitating tumor cell motility and invasion through interactions with the extracellular matrix. It is known that the extracellular domain of integrin $\alpha v \beta 3$ contains a novel small-molecule binding site, and the authors in the study by Godugu et al. [5] synthesized a number of high-affinity thyrointegrin $\alpha v \beta 3$ antagonists to investigate their therapeutic efficacy against primary human GBM cell lines and the commercially available U87 cell line, using both in vitro experiments and a subcutaneous xenograft model. They observed that all antagonists were able to reduce GBM cell viability, in addition to driving a decrease in angiogenesis. Importantly, treatment with the antagonists resulted in the reduced growth of subcutaneous tumors in a U87 xenograft model, as determined by tumor volume and weight.

Schmitt et al. [6] undertook a study investigating the impact of CK2 (a ubiquitously expressed, constitutively active serine/threonine kinase) on nerve/glial antigen (NG)2 in GBM, as both have been shown to be highly expressed in GBM, determined by examination of TCGA glioma datasets. Inhibition of CK2 via a CRISPR/Cas9-mediated knockout approach or the use of a pharmacological compound, CX-4945, significantly reduced NG2 gene and protein expression in GBM cells, but also resulted in a decrease in cell proliferation and migration. Notably, they also demonstrated that CX-4945 reduced NG2 expression in patient-derived GBM cells, indicating that CX-4945 should be investigated further in preclinical studies.

Finally, as there has been evidence linking ion channels in cancer cells to a pro-invasive phenotype, and also that invadopodia as cancer-cell-based structures function to degrade the ECM and facilitate the invasive capacity of the cells, Dinevska et al. [4] performed a screening of FDA-approved ion channel drugs (that have not been previously used for the treatment of GBM patients) for their ability to have a dual impact on GBM cells; firstly, by reducing cell viability (cytotoxic effect), and secondly, by diminishing their invasive capacity (by eliciting an anti-invadopodia effect). The initial screening examining the impact of FDA-approved ion channel drugs on cell viability resulted in three drugs, flunarizine dihydrochloride, econazole nitrate and quinine hydrochloride dihydrate, being explored further for their impact on invadopodia activity. Treatment of the GBM cell lines with the three drugs demonstrated a reduction in MMP-2 secretion and invadopodia activity in comparison to the untreated GBM cells. However, the most significant observation was the reduction in radiation/temozolomide-induced invadopodia activity in the GBM cells, as radiation and temozolomide treatment forms part of the standard of care for GBM patients [2], indicating that these drugs could potentially be incorporated into current treatment to target the enhanced invasive ability of GBM cells that survive this treatment.

In summary, this Special Issue contains a set of multidisciplinary contributions that utilize various techniques and methodologies to investigate novel treatment strategies for GBM. As Guest Editor, I wish to thank all of the authors for their involvement in the Special Issue, but more importantly for tackling this challenging disease with the intention of potentially providing alternative therapeutic strategies for GBM patients in the future, which could significantly improve patient outcome.

Funding: This research received no external funding.

Conflicts of Interest: The author declares no conflict of interest.

References

1. Ostrom, Q.T.; Cioffi, G.; Gittleman, H.; Patil, N.; Waite, K.; Kruchko, C.; Barnholtz-Sloan, J.S. CBTRUS Statistical Report: Primary Brain and Other Central Nervous System Tumors Diagnosed in the United States in 2012–2016. *Neuro Oncol.* **2019**, *21*, v1–v100. [CrossRef] [PubMed]
2. Stupp, R.; Mason, W.P.; van den Bent, M.J.; Weller, M.; Fisher, B.; Taphoorn, M.J.; Belanger, K.; Brandes, A.A.; Marosi, C.; Bogdahn, U.; et al. Radiotherapy plus concomitant and adjuvant temozolomide for glioblastoma. *N. Engl. J. Med.* **2005**, *352*, 987–996. [CrossRef] [PubMed]
3. Stylli, S.S. Novel Treatment Strategies for Glioblastoma. *Cancers* **2020**, *12*, 2883. [CrossRef] [PubMed]
4. Dinevska, M.; Gazibegovic, N.; Morokoff, A.P.; Kaye, A.H.; Drummond, K.J.; Mantamadiotis, T.; Stylli, S.S. Inhibition of Radiation and Temozolomide-Induced Glioblastoma Invadopodia Activity Using Ion Channel Drugs. *Cancers* **2020**, *12*, 2888. [CrossRef] [PubMed]
5. Godugu, K.; Rajabi, M.; Mousa, S.A. Anti-Cancer Activities of Thyrointegrin alphavbeta3 Antagonist Mono- and Bis-Triazole Tetraiodothyroacetic Acid Conjugated via Polyethylene Glycols in Glioblastoma. *Cancers* **2021**, *13*, 2780. [CrossRef] [PubMed]
6. Schmitt, B.M.; Boewe, A.S.; Gotz, C.; Philipp, S.E.; Urbschat, S.; Oertel, J.; Menger, M.D.; Laschke, M.W.; Ampofo, E. CK2 Activity Mediates the Aggressive Molecular Signature of Glioblastoma Multiforme by Inducing Nerve/Glial Antigen (NG)2 Expression. *Cancers* **2021**, *13*, 1678. [CrossRef] [PubMed]
7. Scuderi, S.A.; Casili, G.; Ardizzone, A.; Forte, S.; Colarossi, L.; Sava, S.; Paterniti, I.; Esposito, E.; Cuzzocrea, S.; Campolo, M. KYP-2047, an Inhibitor of Prolyl-Oligopeptidase, Reduces GlioBlastoma Proliferation through Angiogenesis and Apoptosis Modulation. *Cancers* **2021**, *13*, 3444. [CrossRef] [PubMed]
8. Shapovalov, V.; Kopanitsa, L.; Pruteanu, L.L.; Ladds, G.; Bailey, D.S. Transcriptomics-Based Phenotypic Screening Supports Drug Discovery in Human Glioblastoma Cells. *Cancers* **2021**, *13*, 3780. [CrossRef] [PubMed]
9. O'Rawe, M.; Kilmister, E.J.; Mantamadiotis, T.; Kaye, A.H.; Tan, S.T.; Wickremesekera, A.C. The Renin-Angiotensin System in the Tumor Microenvironment of Glioblastoma. *Cancers* **2021**, *13*, 4004. [CrossRef] [PubMed]
10. Di Nunno, V.; Franceschi, E.; Tosoni, A.; Gatto, L.; Lodi, R.; Bartolini, S.; Brandes, A.A. Glioblastoma: Emerging Treatments and Novel Trial Designs. *Cancers* **2021**, *13*, 3750. [CrossRef] [PubMed]
11. Chokshi, C.R.; Brakel, B.A.; Tatari, N.; Savage, N.; Salim, S.K.; Venugopal, C.; Singh, S.K. Advances in Immunotherapy for Adult Glioblastoma. *Cancers* **2021**, *13*, 3400. [CrossRef] [PubMed]
12. Ghannad-Zadeh, K.; Das, S. One-Carbon Metabolism Associated Vulnerabilities in Glioblastoma: A Review. *Cancers* **2021**, *13*, 3067. [CrossRef] [PubMed]
13. Ho, N.T.T.; Rahane, C.S.; Pramanik, S.; Kim, P.S.; Kutzner, A.; Heese, K. FAM72, Glioblastoma Multiforme (GBM) and Beyond. *Cancers* **2021**, *13*, 1025. [CrossRef] [PubMed]
14. Bozzato, E.; Bastiancich, C.; Preat, V. Nanomedicine: A Useful Tool against Glioma Stem Cells. *Cancers* **2020**, *13*, 9. [CrossRef] [PubMed]
15. Mozhei, O.; Teschemacher, A.G.; Kasparov, S. Viral Vectors as Gene Therapy Agents for Treatment of Glioblastoma. *Cancers* **2020**, *12*, 3724. [CrossRef] [PubMed]

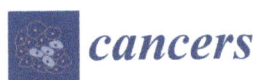

Article

Inhibition of Radiation and Temozolomide-Induced Glioblastoma Invadopodia Activity Using Ion Channel Drugs

Marija Dinevska [1], Natalia Gazibegovic [2], Andrew P. Morokoff [1,3], Andrew H. Kaye [1,4], Katharine J. Drummond [1,3], Theo Mantamadiotis [1,5] and Stanley S. Stylli [1,3,*]

1. Department of Surgery, The University of Melbourne, The Royal Melbourne Hospital, Parkville 3050, Victoria, Australia; mdinevska@student.unimelb.edu.au (M.D.); morokoff@unimelb.edu.au (A.P.M.); a.kaye@unimelb.edu.au (A.H.K.); kjd@unimelb.edu.au (K.J.D.); theo.mantamadiotis@unimelb.edu.au (T.M.)
2. Victoria University, St. Albans 3021, Victoria, Australia; natalia.gazibegovic@outlook.com
3. Department of Neurosurgery, The Royal Melbourne Hospital, Parkville 3050, Victoria, Australia
4. Hadassah University Medical Centre, Jerusalem 91120, Israel
5. Department of Microbiology & Immunology, School of Biomedical Sciences, The University of Melbourne, Parkville 3010, Victoria, Australia
* Correspondence: stanley.stylli@mh.org.au or sstylli@unimelb.edu.au

Received: 8 September 2020; Accepted: 30 September 2020; Published: 8 October 2020

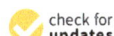

Simple Summary: Glioblastoma accounts for approximately 40–50% of all primary brain cancers and is a highly aggressive cancer that rapidly disseminates within the surrounding normal brain. Dynamic actin-rich protrusions known as invadopodia facilitate this invasive process. Ion channels have also been linked to a pro-invasive phenotype and may contribute to facilitating invadopodia activity in cancer cells. The aim of our study was to screen ion channel-targeting drugs for their cytotoxic efficacy and potential anti-invadopodia properties in glioblastoma cells. We demonstrated that the targeting of ion channels in glioblastoma cells can lead to a reduction in invadopodia activity and protease secretion. Importantly, the candidate drugs exhibited a significant reduction in radiation and temozolomide-induced glioblastoma cell invadopodia activity. These findings support the proposed pro-invasive role of ion channels via invadopodia in glioblastoma, which may be ideal therapeutic targets for the treatment of glioblastoma patients.

Abstract: Glioblastoma (GBM) is the most prevalent and malignant type of primary brain cancer. The rapid invasion and dissemination of tumor cells into the surrounding normal brain is a major driver of tumor recurrence, and long-term survival of GBM patients is extremely rare. Actin-rich cell membrane protrusions known as invadopodia can facilitate the highly invasive properties of GBM cells. Ion channels have been proposed to contribute to a pro-invasive phenotype in cancer cells and may also be involved in the invadopodia activity of GBM cells. GBM cell cytotoxicity screening of several ion channel drugs identified three drugs with potent cell killing efficacy: flunarizine dihydrochloride, econazole nitrate, and quinine hydrochloride dihydrate. These drugs demonstrated a reduction in GBM cell invadopodia activity and matrix metalloproteinase-2 (MMP-2) secretion. Importantly, the treatment of GBM cells with these drugs led to a significant reduction in radiation/temozolomide-induced invadopodia activity. The dual cytotoxic and anti-invasive efficacy of these agents merits further research into targeting ion channels to reduce GBM malignancy, with a potential for future clinical translation in combination with the standard therapy.

Keywords: glioma; glioblastoma; invasion; invadopodia; ion channels; drug repurposing

1. Introduction

Malignant brain tumors are among the most aggressive cancers, resulting in impaired health-related quality of life and survival measured in months or a few years [1]. As classified by the World Health Organization (WHO), glioblastoma (GBM) is a highly malignant grade IV astrocytoma accounting for approximately 50% of all gliomas [2–4]. Although GBM has an incidence of less than 10 per 100,000, it is incurable; thus, the burden of disease on patients and carers remains significant, resulting in an average loss of 12 years of life [5].

The current therapeutic regime for GBM patients follows the "Stupp Protocol", which involves maximal safe surgical resection of the tumor followed by radiotherapy (RT) and concomitant chemotherapy with temozolomide (TMZ), an oral DNA alkylating agent and subsequent adjuvant TMZ for 6–12 months [6]. Despite a modest increase in survival since the introduction of TMZ (14.6 month median survival), 50% of GBM patients do not respond to TMZ, developing resistance to both RT and TMZ [7]. In addition, GBM widely infiltrates the surrounding brain parenchyma [8]. This invasive capacity hinders surgical resection, making gross tumor debulking impossible with inevitable tumor recurrence within 1–2 cm of the resection cavity [8,9].

Cancer cell invasion is a multi-step process orchestrated by tumor cell interactions with the tumor microenvironment [10]. This process is initiated by cell polarization and adhesion to the extracellular matrix (ECM), which is followed by acquired cancer cell mobility and ECM degradation [8]. More specifically, research has indicated that dynamic actin-rich subcellular protrusions known as invadopodia are integral in facilitating cancer cell invasion [11]. These structures serve to proteolytically degrade the ECM through the complex interactions within a network of signaling molecules and proteins [12,13]. Invadopodia can extend up to 8 µm into the surrounding environment and have a diameter ranging from 0.1 to 0.8 µm [12]. The physical force generated by actin polymerization and the action of transmembrane and secreted matrix metalloproteinases (MMP-2 and -9) in ECM degradation are integral to the invadopodia-mediated invasion of malignant cells [14]. Numerous proteins, including Tks5 (Tyrosine Kinase substrate with 5 SH3 domains) and cortactin, are involved in the processes required for the biogenesis of invadopodia, which include cell signaling, adhesion, and actin remodeling [15]. Our laboratory has previously demonstrated that expression levels of the invadopodia regulator Tks5 in human glioma biopsies are related to prognosis [16]. Importantly, the amplification of the cortactin gene (CTTN) is evident in a number of cancers, correlating with enhanced tumor invasiveness and poor prognosis [17,18].

Ion channels regulate several cancer promoting processes, including tumor cell invasion [19,20]. Under physiological conditions, potassium, sodium, and calcium channels are responsible for maintaining intracellular ionic balance, cell shape, and cell volume [21]. However, during tumorigenesis, the altered expression of ion channel genes can lead to the dysregulation of normal cellular functions, including proliferation, migration, and apoptosis [22]. For example, potassium channels, such as calcium-activated potassium channels (that is, KCa3.1), have been linked to enhanced invasion via the regulation of cellular ionic balance [19,23–25]. The gene encoding KCa3.1, KCNN4, is overexpressed in 32% of gliomas and correlates with shorter survival [26]. Additionally, potassium channels have been described to contribute to cancer cell invasion via their interaction with molecules associated with invadopodia formation, such as focal adhesion kinase (FAK), integrins, and cortactin [25]. Likewise, voltage-gated calcium channels (VGCCs) and non-voltage activated calcium permeable channels are associated with malignant transformations in a number of cancers, including glioma [27]. A study by Zhang et al. [28] demonstrated a decrease in cell migration in human GBM cell lines following the inhibition of T-type Ca^{2+} channels (low-voltage activated channels). Under resting membrane conditions, these ion channels play an integral role in the maintenance of intracellular Ca^{2+} and have been linked to tumor cell migration and invasion in GBM cells [29]. In the context of tumor cell invasion, the role of ion channels is only beginning to be understood [19]. The proposed influence of ion channels on actin cytoskeletal rearrangement and various proteins including cortactin and integrins may contribute to mechanisms mediating invadopodia formation and activity in cancer cells [30,31]. This highlights the potential for ion channel blockers to target invadopodia and inhibit GBM cell invasion.

Over the past decade, the standard of care for GBM has remained unchanged, emphasizing the urgent need for drug discovery and development. This process requires high-throughput screening of candidate compounds, followed by extensive pre-clinical and clinical studies [32]. However, major limitations with this approach include both the time from the initial studies to clinical implementation (ranging from 11.4 to 13.5 years) and the associated costs ($161 million to $1.8 billion) [32]. For this reason, drug repurposing has become an increasingly attractive option. This is advantageous as it offers a reduction in the time required for pre-clinical and clinical studies and the associated costs, as drug toxicity, pharmacokinetics, dosage, and safety are already understood [33].

In this study, we investigated the cytotoxicity and anti-invasion activity of a panel of ion channel-binding drugs on GBM cells. The aim of this work was to screen a panel of 20 ion channel-targeting drugs for their ability to inhibit GBM cell viability and invadopodia activity.

2. Results

2.1. GBM Tissue Exhibits Increased Invadopodia Regulator and Ion Channel Gene Expression

To investigate the clinical relevance of invadopodia regulator (Table 1) and ion channel (Table 2) genes in glioma, we used the online database, Oncomine^{TM}. The expression levels of the pro-invadopodia regulators cortactin, MMP-2, Src, NWASP (Neural Wiskott-Aldrich syndrome protein), Tks4 (Tyrosine Kinase substrate with 4 SH3 domains), Tks5, and Nck (non-catalytic region of tyrosine kinase adaptor protein), and ion channel (calcium, sodium, and potassium) genes in GBM and non-tumor brain tissue were examined. MMP-2 and Nck1 (non-catalytic region of tyrosine kinase adaptor protein 1) were the most frequently overexpressed invadopodia regulators in GBM compared to non-tumor brain tissue (Table 1).

The data presented in Table 2 demonstrate that the potassium and calcium ion channels, KCNH2 and CACNA1C, were most frequently overexpressed in GBM tissue compared to normal tissue. Subsequently, the SurvExpress online database for cancer gene expression data was used to examine the clinical relevance of invadopodia regulators and ion channel gene expression in GBM.

Figure 1 demonstrates poorer survival outcomes for high gene expression of the pro-invadopodia regulator, CTTN, or ion channel, CACNA1F. The co-expression of CTTN and CACNA1F reveals a further impact on survival, and additional combinations are listed in Table 3. Together, these data suggests a role for ion channels in the process of glioma cell invasion mediated by invadopodia.

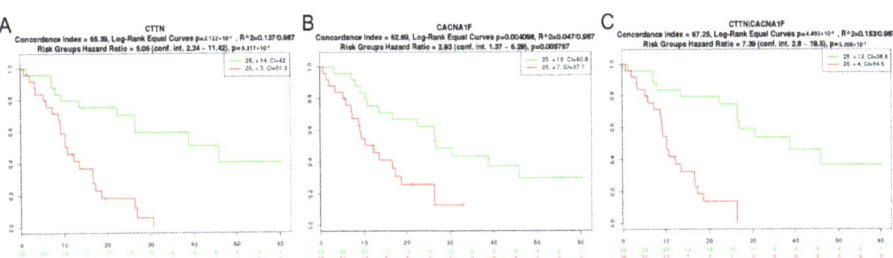

Figure 1. Co-expression of invadopodia regulator and ion channel genes correlates with poor GBM patient survival. (**A**) High invadopodia regulator (cortactin gene, CTTN), (**B**) ion channel (CACNA1S), and (**C**) combined gene expression indicates significantly poorer survival outcomes in GBM patients from the Nutt Louis dataset (deposited within the SurvExpress database). The Kaplan–Meier plots show the two risk groups, the log-rank test of differences between risk groups, the hazard ratio estimate, and the concordance indices.

Table 1. Invadopodia regulator genes are overexpressed in glioblastoma (GBM) tissue compared to normal brain tissue.

Invadopodia Marker	Number of GBM Tissue Samples	Number of Normal Tissue Samples	Total Measured Genes	Mean Fold Change (Log2)	p Value	Sample Type	Platform	Study
CTTN	542	10	12,624	1.353	3×10^{-3}	mRNA	Human Genome U2A	TCGA
MMP2	27	4	14,836	6.426	5.00×10^{-4}	mRNA	ND	Bredel Brain 2 [34]
MMP2	30	3	9957	4.537	3.00×10^{-3}	mRNA	ND	Liang [35]
MMP2	80	4	19,574	2.92	2.98×10^{-4}	mRNA	Human Genome U2A	Murat [36]
MMP2	81	23	19,574	3.548	7.99×10^{-16}	mRNA	Human Genome U2A	Sun [37]
MMP2	542	10	12,624	4.818	4.06×10^{-10}	mRNA	Human Genome U2A	TCGA
Nck1	27	4	14,836	1.717	1.00×10^{-2}	mRNA	ND	Bredel Brain 2 [34]
Nck1	30	3	9957	1.626	1.90×10^{-2}	mRNA	ND	Liang [35]
Nck1	80	4	19,574	1.885	5.00×10^{-3}	mRNA	Human Genome U2A	Murat [36]
Nck1	81	23	19,574	1.305	5.41×10^{-7}	mRNA	Human Genome U2A	Sun [37]
Nck1	542	10	12,624	2.056	4.06×10^{-9}	mRNA	Human Genome U2A	TCGA
Nck2	80	4	19,574	1.135	2.00×10^{-3}	mRNA	Human Genome U2A	Murat [36]
NWASP	81	23	19,574	1.338	1.10×10^{-2}	mRNA	Human Genome U2A	Sun [37]
Src	80	4	19,574	1.035	4.50×10^{-2}	mRNA	Human Genome U2A	Murat [36]
Src	81	23	19,574	1.601	2.00×10^{-3}	mRNA	Human Genome U2A	Sun [37]
Tks4	27	4	14,836	3.257	1.12×10^{-4}	mRNA	ND	Bredel Brain 2 [34]
Tks4	30	3	9957	1.492	1.40×10^{-2}	mRNA	ND	Liang [35]
Tks4	80	4	19,574	2.241	1.32×10^{-6}	mRNA	Human Genome U2A	Murat [36]
Tks4	81	23	19,574	2.194	2.50×10^{-4}	mRNA	Human Genome U2A	Sun [37]
Tks5	27	4	14,836	1.399	4.80×10^{-2}	mRNA	ND	Bredel Brain 2 [34]
Tks5	22	7	7689	1.263	5.00×10^{-3}	mRNA	ND	Yamanaka [38]

mRNA expression levels of invadopodia regulators in GBM and normal brain tissue were retrieved from the Oncomine database (mean fold change versus normal brain and overall p value in that dataset are displayed. The Student t-test is used to generate the p value). Gene expression data have been log transformed and normalized. Not defined (ND); Human Genome U2A—Human Genome U133 Plus 2.0 Array; TCGA—The Cancer Genome Atlas; MMP2—matrix metalloproteinase-2; NWASP—Neural Wiskott–Aldrich syndrome protein; Tks4—tyrosine kinase substrate with 4 SH3 domains; Tks5—tyrosine kinase substrate with 5 SH3 domains; Nck—non-catalytic region of tyrosine kinase adaptor protein; mRNA—messenger RNA; RNA—ribonucleic acid.

Table 2. Ion channel genes are overexpressed in GBM tissue compared to normal brain tissue.

Ion Channel Gene	Number of GBM Tissue Samples	Number of Normal Tissue Samples	Total Measured Genes	Mean Fold Change (Log2)	p Value	Sample Type	Platform	Study
KCNH2	106	32	18,823	1.175	3.49×10^{-13}	DNA	RefSeq Genes	Beroukhim Brain [39]
KCNA5	107	32	18,823	1.054	2.15×10^{-4}	DNA	RefSeq Genes	Beroukhim Brain [39]
KCNJ10	107	33	18,823	1.041	2.00×10^{-3}	DNA	RefSeq Genes	Beroukhim Brain [39]
KCNB1	107	33	18,823	1.064	2.00×10^{-3}	DNA	RefSeq Genes	Beroukhim Brain [39]
CACNA1S	107	33	18,823	1.041	3.20×10^{-2}	DNA	RefSeq Genes	Beroukhim Brain [39]
CACNA1C	107	33	18,823	1.041	1.20×10^{-2}	DNA	RefSeq Genes	Beroukhim Brain [39]
KCNN4	21	3	14,836	2.219	1.40×10^{-2}	mRNA	ND	Bredel Brain 2 [34]
CACNA1D	27	4	14,836	1.377	6.00×10^{-3}	mRNA	ND	Bredel Brain 2 [34]
CACNA1C	22	3	19,574	8.62	6.00×10^{-3}	mRNA	Human Genome U2A	Lee Brain [40]
KCNH2	22	3	19,574	1.869	1.00×10^{-3}	mRNA	Human Genome U2A	Lee Brain [40]
KCNB1	22	3	19,574	2.325	2.10×10^{-2}	mRNA	Human Genome U2A	Lee Brain [40]
CACNA1D	22	3	19,574	3.293	3.85×10^{-4}	mRNA	Human Genome U2A	Lee Brain [40]
KCNH2	80	4	19,574	1.252	5.00×10^{-3}	mRNA	Human Genome U2A	Murat Brain [36]
KCNH2	27	7	8603	1.101	1.20×10^{-2}	mRNA	Human Genome U95A	Shai Brain [41]
KCNH2	81	23	19,574	2.142	1.70×10^{-2}	mRNA	Human Genome U2A	Sun Brain [37]
KCNH2	542	10	12,624	1.094	1.20×10^{-2}	mRNA	Human Genome U2A	TCGA
KCNH2	582	37	18,823	1.320	4.80×10^{-169}	DNA	RefSeq Genes	TCGA 2
KCNA5	582	37	18,823	1.034	5.75×10^{-8}	DNA	RefSeq Genes	TCGA 2
KCNJ10	582	37	18,823	1.061	1.65×10^{-46}	DNA	RefSeq Genes	TCGA 2
KCNB1	582	37	18,823	1.126	3.54×10^{-68}	DNA	RefSeq Genes	TCGA 2
KCNN4	582	37	18,823	1.046	6.02×10^{-10}	DNA	RefSeq Genes	TCGA 2
SCN5A	582	37	18,823	1.019	6.64×10^{-5}	DNA	RefSeq Genes	TCGA 2
SCN8A	582	37	18,823	1.012	1.60×10^{-2}	DNA	RefSeq Genes	TCGA 2

Table 2. Cont.

Ion Channel Gene	Number of GBM Tissue Samples	Number of Normal Tissue Samples	Total Measured Genes	Mean Fold Change (Log2)	p Value	Sample Type	Platform	Study
CACNA1S	582	37	18,823	1.055	2.28×10^{-30}	DNA	RefSeq Genes	TCGA 2
CACNA1C	582	37	18,823	1.032	1.11×10^{-7}	DNA	RefSeq Genes	TCGA 2
CACNA1D	582	37	18,823	1.013	7.00×10^{-3}	DNA	RefSeq Genes	TCGA 2
CACNA1B	582	37	18,823	1.019	1.00×10^{-3}	DNA	RefSeq Genes	TCGA 2
CACNA1G	582	37	18,823	1.027	4.56×10^{-16}	DNA	RefSeq Genes	TCGA 2

mRNA and DNA expression levels of ion channels in GBM and normal brain tissue were retrieved from the Oncomine database (mean fold change versus normal brain and overall p value in that dataset are displayed. The Student t-test is used to generate the p value.). Gene expression data have been log transformed and normalized. Not defined (ND); Human Genome U2A—Human Genome U133 Plus 2.0 Array; Human Genome U95A—Human Genome U95A-Av2 Array; DNA—deoxyribonucleic acid; mRNA—messenger RNA; RNA—ribonucleic acid; TCGA—The Cancer Genome Atlas; KCNH2—hERG (the human Ether-à-go-go-Related Gene); KCNA5—Potassium voltage-gated channel, shaker-related subfamily, member 5; KCNJ10—Potassium Inwardly Rectifying Channel Subfamily J Member 10; KCNB1—Potassium Voltage-Gated Channel Subfamily B Member 1; CACNA1S—Calcium Voltage-Gated Channel Subunit Alpha1 S; CACNA1C—Calcium Voltage-Gated Channel Subunit Alpha1 C; KCNN4—Potassium Calcium-Activated Channel Subfamily N Member 4; CACNA1D—Calcium Voltage-Gated Channel Subunit Alpha1 D; CACNA1G—Calcium Voltage-Gated Channel Subunit Alpha1 G; SCN5A—Sodium Voltage-Gated Channel Alpha Subunit 5; SCN8A—Sodium Voltage-Gated Channel Alpha Subunit 8; RefSeq—Reference Sequence.

Table 3. Pro-invadopodia regulator and ion channel gene co-expression correlates with shorter survival in GBM patients.

Gene	Study Dataset	Number of Patients	p-Value	Concordance Index
CTTN	Nutt Louis [42]	50	2.12×10^{-5}	65.39
CTTN+CACNA1F	Nutt Louis [42]	50	4.49×10^{-6}	67.25
MMP2	Freije Nelson GPL96 [43]	85	5.95×10^{-3}	59.74
MMP2+CACNA1B	Freije Nelson GPL96 [43]	85	1.71×10^{-3}	62.46
MMP2+CACNA1F	Freije Nelson GPL96 [43]	85	5.05×10^{-3}	60.94
MMP2+CACNA1S	Freije Nelson GPL96 [43]	85	1.87×10^{-3}	62.04
MMP2+KCNH2	Freije Nelson GPL96 [43]	85	4.28×10^{-4}	64.08
MMP2+KCNJ10	Freije Nelson GPL96 [43]	85	1.32×10^{-3}	61.17
MMP2+KCNN4	Freije Nelson GPL96 [43]	85	2.51×10^{-3}	61.97
MMP2+SCN8A	Freije Nelson GPL96 [43]	85	1.90×10^{-3}	61.26
MMP9	Freije Nelson GPL96 [43]	85	2.18×10^{-3}	59.84
MMP9+CACNA1B	Freije Nelson GPL96 [43]	85	1.36×10^{-3}	63.62
MMP9+CACNA1G	Freije Nelson GPL96 [43]	85	4.06×10^{-5}	65.92
MMP9+KCN5A	Freije Nelson GPL96 [43]	85	1.31×10^{-4}	63.24
Nck	Freije Nelson GPL96 [43]	85	1.05×10^{-3}	62.01
Nck+CACNA1C	Freije Nelson GPL96 [43]	85	3.55×10^{-4}	62.17
Nck+CACNA1G	Freije Nelson GPL96 [43]	85	5.06×10^{-4}	62.94
Nck+CACNA1I	Freije Nelson GPL96 [43]	85	1.61×10^{-5}	64.53
Nck+CACNA1S	Freije Nelson GPL96 [43]	85	2.50×10^{-4}	63.33
Nck+KCNA5	Freije Nelson GPL96 [43]	85	4.68×10^{-4}	62.1
Nck+KCNH2	Freije Nelson GPL96 [43]	85	2.27×10^{-4}	63.92
Nck+KCNJ10	Freije Nelson GPL96 [43]	85	1.35×10^{-4}	62.56
SH3PXD2A	Yamanaka Nishio [38]	29	3.80×10^{-2}	77.89
SH3PXD2A+KCNA5	Yamanaka Nishio [38]	29	1.49×10^{-2}	84.21
SH3PXD2A+KCNJ10	Yamanaka Nishio [38]	29	1.04×10^{-3}	84.21
SH3PXD2A+SCN5A	Yamanaka Nishio [38]	29	7.27×10^{-3}	85.26
Src	Lee Nelson GPL570 [40]	27	3.80×10^{-2}	62.36
Src+CACNA1D	Lee Nelson GPL570 [40]	27	2.10×10^{-2}	64.94
Src+CACNA1G	Lee Nelson GPL570 [40]	27	3.04×10^{-2}	58.91
Src+CACNA1S	Lee Nelson GPL570 [40]	27	3.39×10^{-2}	61.21
Src+KCNB1	Lee Nelson GPL570 [40]	27	3.39×10^{-2}	61.78
Src+SCN8A	Lee Nelson GPL570 [40]	27	2.10×10^{-2}	60.92
Src	Nutt Louis [42]	50	1.10×10^{-2}	56.48
Src+CACNA1F	Nutt Louis [42]	50	4.10×10^{-3}	62.49
Src+CACNA1H	Nutt Louis [42]	50	6.58×10^{-3}	65.8
Src	GBM TCGA	538	5.76×10^{-3}	54.65
Src+CACNA1C	GBM TCGA	538	6.60×10^{-3}	54.68
Src+CACNA1G	GBM TCGA	538	7.24×10^{-3}	54.67
Src+CACNA1H	GBM TCGA	538	7.75×10^{-3}	54.59
Src+KCNA5	GBM TCGA	538	7.48×10^{-3}	54.59
Src+KCNN4	GBM TCGA	538	7.03×10^{-3}	54.82

Co-expression of pro-invadopodia regulator and ion channel genes correlates with poorer GBM patient outcome as determined by analysis of GBM-derived datasets in the SurvExpress online database for cancer gene expression (the log-rank test was used to generate the p value).

2.2. GBM Cells Form Functional Invadopodia and Express Invadopodia Regulator Proteins

Invadopodia are actin-rich protrusions that facilitate the invasion of tumor cells from the tumor bulk into the surrounding healthy parenchyma [12,13]. MMPs (specifically MMP-2 and MMP-9) are enriched and secreted at the tips of invadopodia, thus mediating the proteolytic degradation of the ECM [11]. We utilized gelatin-based zymography to examine the conditioned medium isolated from three GBM cell lines and determine the extracellular secreted levels of MMP-2 and MMP-9. Analysis of the conditioned media of the LN229, U87MG, and MU41 GBM cell lines revealed the presence of pro-MMP-2 (72 kDa) and active-MMP-2 (65 kDa). The LN229 cell line displayed the highest level of MMP-2 secretion, while the U87MG cell line showed the least (Figure 2A).

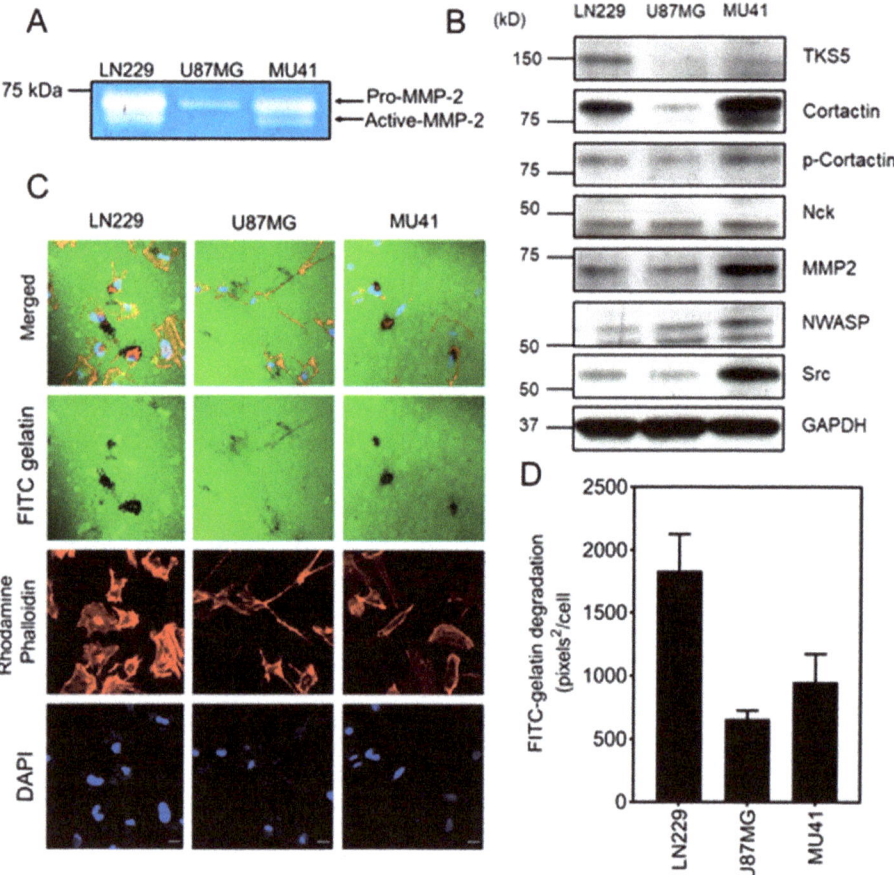

Figure 2. GBM cell lines secrete MMP-2 and form functional fluorescein isothiocyanate (FITC)–gelatin degrading invadopodia. (A) Gelatin-based zymogram analysis of LN229, U87MG, and MU41 cells cultured in serum-free conditioned media for 24 h showing MMP-2 activity. (B) Western blot analysis of GBM cell lines for a range of pro-invadopodia regulator proteins (Src, NWASP, MMP-2, Nck, phospho-cortactin, cortactin, and TKS5), the uncropped Western Blot figure is in Figure S2 (C) LN229, U87MG, and MU41 cells were plated on a thin film of cross-linked FITC-labeled gelatin for 24 h. Cells were stained with rhodamine phalloidin (red) to visualize actin filaments and DAPI (4′,6-diamidino-2-phenylindole) (blue) for cell nuclei. FITC–gelatin degradation is evident as black areas devoid of FITC-labeled gelatin. Images were acquired with a 60× oil immersion lens using a Nikon A1 confocal system. (D) Quantification of the basal invadopodia-mediated FITC–gelatin degradation. Representative of $n = 3$ independent experiments, error bars represent SEM. Scale bar = 20 μm.

Several invadopodia regulator proteins, including Tks5, Src, and cortactin, participate in the formation and matrix-degrading activity of invadopodia. Therefore, we next examined the expression of these proteins in the LN229, U87MG, and MU41 cell lines (Figure 2B). The protein expression profile of these regulators varied across cell lines, with Tks5 highly expressed in LN229 cells. Cortactin was highly expressed in the MU41 and LN229 cell lines. Notably, Src, MMP-2, and NWASP were detected at higher levels in the MU41 cell line.

As the GBM cells secreted MMP-2 and expressed a range of invadopodia regulator proteins, we next used a fluorescent gelatin matrix degradation assay to determine whether the GBM cell lines could form functional invadopodia. This assay, which measures MMP-2-mediated invasion by determining the clearance of fluorescein isothiocyanate (FITC)-labeled gelatin (absence of green) colocalized with rhodamine phalloidin actin-stained puncta, showed activity in the three GBM cell lines (Figure 2C). LN229 cells exhibited the highest FITC–gelatin degrading activity, followed by MU41 and U87MG cells (Figure 2D). This observation was consistent with the levels of MMP-2 secreted by each cell line (Figure 2A).

To further verify the presence of invadopodia, we co-stained GBM cells for Tks5 and cortactin as they colocalize with invadopodia and are integral for invadopodia formation and activity. As demonstrated in Figure 3, the co-localization of Tks5/cortactin with actin puncta validated the presence of invadopodia in the LN229, U87MG, and MU41 GBM cell lines.

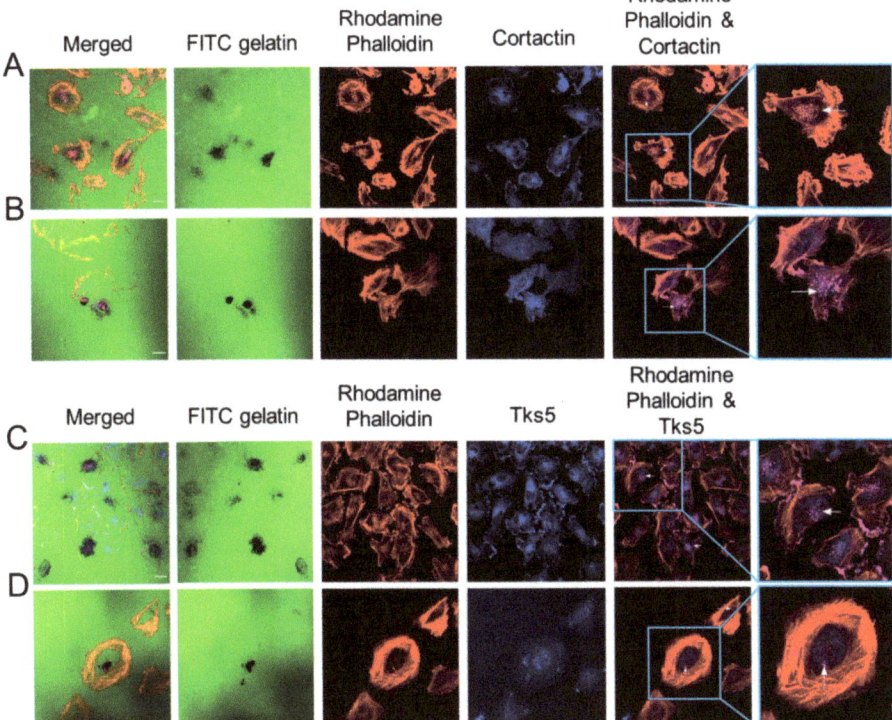

Figure 3. Cortactin and Tks5 co-localize with actin in GBM cell invadopodia. LN229 and MU41cells were seeded on FITC-labeled gelatin coverslips for 24 h prior to fixing and staining for rhodamine phalloidin to probe for F-actin filaments, cortactin, and Tks5 primary antibodies and an Alexa 405 secondary antibody (blue). Images were acquired with a 60× oil immersion lens using a Nikon A1 confocal system. Images displayed co-localization with actin puncta as follows: LN229 ((**A**)-cortactin), MU41 ((**B**)-cortactin), LN229 ((**C**)-Tks5), and MU41 ((**D**)-Tks5). White arrows denote co-localization with cortactin or Tks5 and actin puncta. Figure is representative of $n = 3$ experiments. Scale bar = 20 μm.

2.3. Ion Channel-Targeting Drugs Reduce GBM Cell Viability

The current standard of care for GBM patients is inadequate, and there is an urgent need to develop additional treatment options to target tumor cells that survive radiotherapy and chemotherapy. To identify ion channel-binding drugs that can kill GBM cells, we screened 20 drugs (Table 4) that inhibit ion channels (It must be noted that flunarizine dihydrochloride is the only ion channel drug in the list that is not currently FDA (Food and Drug Administration)-approved for clinical use in the USA). The drugs were first screened for their ability to reduce GBM cell viability using an MTT (3-(4,5-dimethylthiazol-2-yl)-2,5-diphenyltetrazolium bromide) cell proliferation assay and then screened for their anti-invasive properties and regulation of invadopodia activity. The cytotoxicity of the 20 ion channel drugs was assessed across a range of concentrations (0.01, 0.1, 1, and 10 µM) in the three GBM cell lines (Figure S1).

Table 4. Ion channel drugs used in this study.

Drug	Indication	Ion Channel
Amiloride hydrochloride dihydrate	Cardiovascular disease	Sodium
Ouabain	Neurological disease	Sodium
Oxcarbazepine	Neurological disease	Sodium
Primidone	Neurological disease	Sodium
Procaine hydrochloride	Neurological disease	Sodium
Zonisamide	Neurological disease	Sodium
Azelnidipine	Neurological disease	Calcium
Cinepazide maleate	Inflammation	Calcium
Diltiazem hydrochloride	Cardiovascular disease	Calcium
Econazole nitrate	Neurological disease	Calcium
Flunarizine dihydrochloride	Neurological disease	Calcium
Nicardipine hydrochloride	Neurological disease	Calcium
Nilvadipine	Cardiovascular disease	Calcium
Glimepiride	Type 2 diabetes mellitus	Potassium
Glyburide	Endocrinology	Potassium
Nateglinide	Immunology	Potassium
Quinine hydrochloride dihydrate	Cardiovascular disease	Potassium
Repaglinide	Endocrinology	Potassium
Tolbutamide	Type 2 diabetes mellitus	Potassium

The degree of cytotoxicity varied amongst the cell lines and drugs. To rank the drugs based on cytotoxic efficacy, a 20–30% threshold reduction in cell viability across the concentrations was applied. This identified the three most potent drugs: flunarizine dihydrochloride, econazole nitrate, and quinine hydrochloride dihydrate, which we further investigated.

2.4. Ion Channel Drugs Reduce MMP-2 Secretion and Invasion

Following the shortlisting of ion channel drugs based on their cytotoxicity profiles, we examined the impact of the drugs on MMP-2 secretion. LN229 and MU41 cells were investigated further, as they had the highest MMP-2 secretion and invadopodia activity (Figure 2). Econazole nitrate and quinine hydrochloride dihydrate-treated LN229 and MU41 cells showed a decrease in MMP-2 secretion, while flunarizine dihydrochloride led to a reduction of MMP-2 secretion in MU41 cells only (Figure 4A,B). Subsequently, we investigated the ability of these drugs to reduce invadopodia-mediated FITC–gelatin degradation (Figure 4C–F). All three drugs resulted in reduced invadopodia-mediated gelatin-degradation activity in both GBM cells lines. Quinine hydrochloride dihydrate treatment resulted in the greatest reduction in FITC–gelatin degradation in both cell lines. This is consistent with the reduced level of MMP-2 secretion following quinine hydrochloride dihydrate treatment. Interestingly, the level of MMP-2 secretion in flunarizine dihydrochloride-treated LN229 cells (Figure 4A) did not correspond to the inhibitory effect seen in the invadopodia-mediated FITC–gelatin degradation assay, indicating that this drug may influence other factors regulating invadopodia biogenesis.

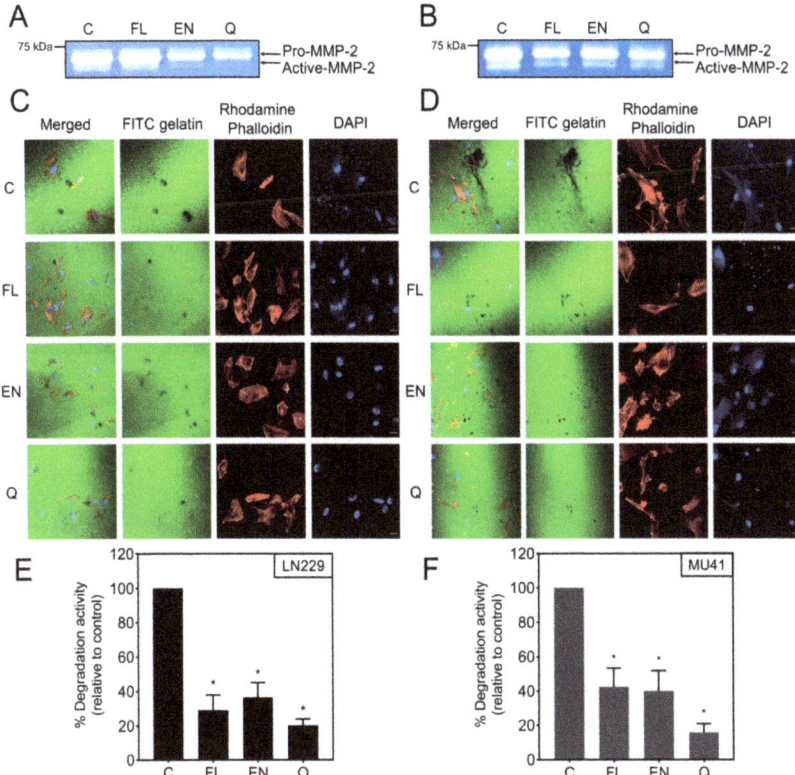

Figure 4. Ion channel drugs inhibit MMP-2 secretion and invadopodia activity in GBM cells. Gelatin-based zymogram analysis of (**A**) LN229 and (**B**) MU41 GBM cells in serum-free conditioned media treated with 10 µM flunarizine dihydrochloride (FL), econazole nitrate (EN), and quinine hydrochloride dihydrate (Q) for 72 h. Representative of $n = 2$ experiments. (**C**) LN229 and (**D**) MU41 GBM cells were seeded on coverslips coated with a thin film of cross-linked FITC-labeled gelatin following 72-h treatment with 10 µM of FL, EN, and Q. Following a 24-h incubation, cells were fixed and stained with rhodamine phalloidin (red) to probe for actin filaments and DAPI (blue) for nuclear staining. Black areas devoid of FITC-labeled gelatin represent areas of gelatin degradation. Graphical representation of (**E**) LN229 and (**F**) MU41 invadopodia mediated FITC–gelatin degradative activity (relative to untreated control). Mean of $n = 3$ independent experiments, error bars represent SEM, * $p < 0.05$. Scale bar = 20 µm.

2.5. MMP-2 Secretion and Invadopodia Gelatin Degradation Is Enhanced Following Radiation and Temozolomide Treatment

To investigate the impact of RT and TMZ on invadopodia-mediated invasion, GBM cells were treated with 2 Gy RT and 50 µM TMZ. Zymographic analysis of conditioned GBM cell medium highlighted an increase in pro-MMP-2 secretion in both LN229 and MU41 cell lines, while an increase in active-MMP-2 was seen in the LN229 cell line only (Figure 5C). As MMP-2 secretion increased following RT/TMZ treatment, we next examined the effect of RT/TMZ treatment on the ability of GBM cells to form functional FITC–gelatin-degrading invadopodia. The GBM cell lines showed an increase in the level of invadopodia-mediated FITC–gelatin degradation post-RT/TMZ treatment (Figure 5A,B). The increase in MMP-2 secretion and invadopodia-mediated FITC–gelatin degradation suggests that cells that survive RT/TMZ treatment may acquire a more pro-invasive phenotype.

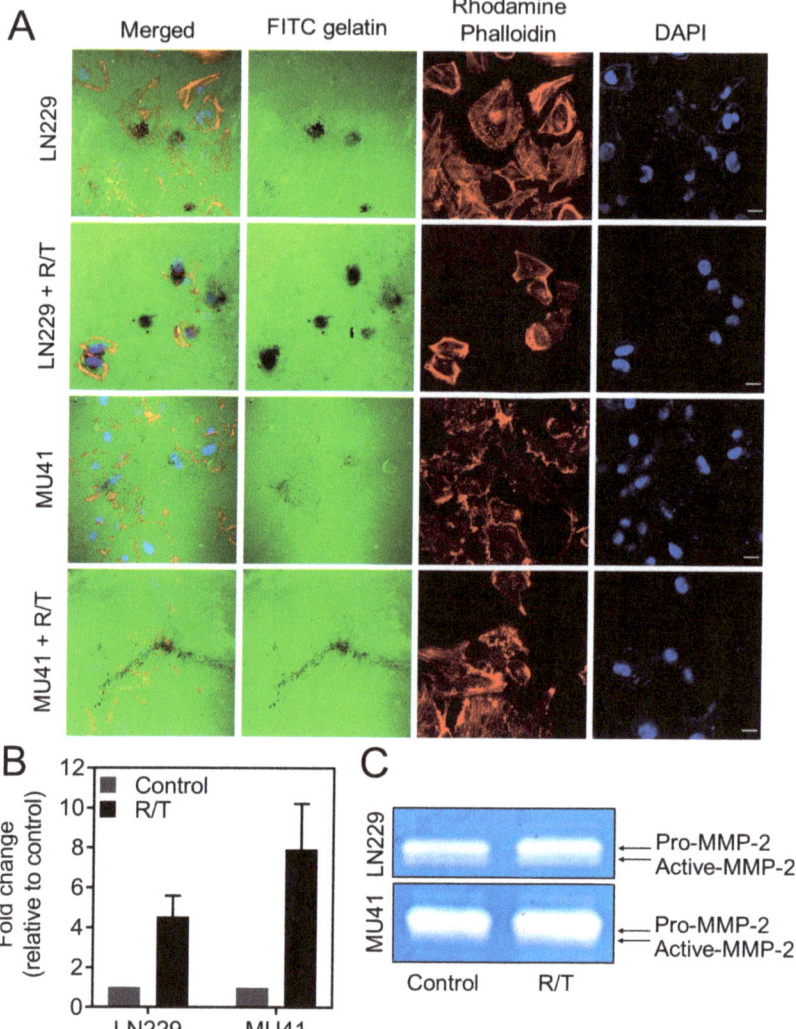

Figure 5. Radiation/temozolomide (R/T) treatment enhances MMP-2 secretion and invadopodia activity in GBM cells (**A**) LN229 and MU41 GBM cells were seeded and incubated for 24 h on coverslips coated with a thin film of cross-linked FITC-labeled gelatin 24 h post-treatment with R/T (2 Gy/50 µM). Then, the cells were stained with rhodamine–phalloidin (red) for actin filaments and DAPI for nuclei labelling (blue). FITC–gelatin degradation is evident as black areas devoid of FITC-labeled gelatin. (**B**) Fold change of FITC–gelatin degradation per GBM cell relative to the corresponding untreated cells for each

cell line. Mean of $n = 3$ independent experiments, error bars represent SEM. Scale bar = 20 µm, applicable to all images in the panel. (**C**) LN229 and MU41 GBM cells were treated with R/T (2 Gy/50 µM) for 24 h and incubated in serum-free Optimem before conditioned medium was analyzed via gelatin-based zymography. Representative of $n = 2$ independent experiments.

2.6. Inhibition of RT/TMZ-Induced Invadopodia Activity

We next examined the ability of the selected candidate drugs to reduce RT/TMZ-induced invadopodia activity in the GBM cells. Here, we demonstrate that treatment with flunarizine dihydrochloride, econazole nitrate, and quinine hydrochloride dihydrate resulted in a significant decrease in RT/TMZ induced invadopodia activity in both the LN229 and MU41 GBM cells (Figure 6). The greatest reduction in invadopodia-mediated FITC–gelatin degradation was noted with quinine hydrochloride dihydrate in the MU41 cell line and flunarizine dihydrochloride in the LN229 cell line.

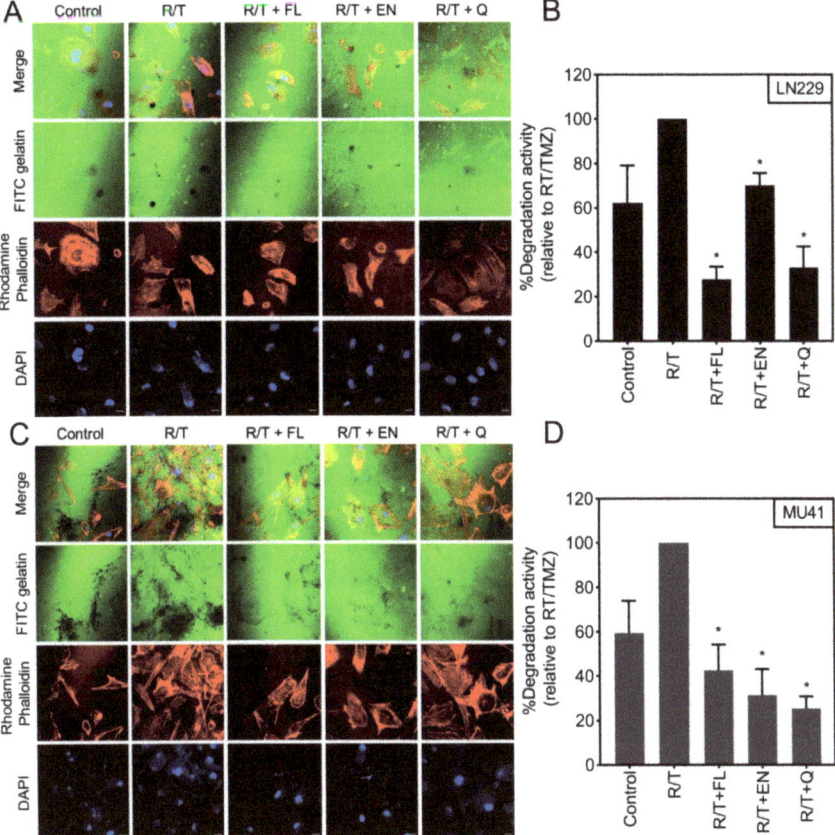

Figure 6. Ion channel-targeting drugs reduce radiation and temozolomide enhanced invadopodia activity. (**A**) LN229 and (**B**) MU41 GBM cells were subjected to R/T (2 Gy/50 µM) and 10 µM treatment of flunarizine dihydrochloride (FL), econazole nitrate (EN), or quinine hydrochloride dihydrate (Q) for 72 h prior to being seeded a thin film of cross-linked FITC-labeled gelatin. Cells were stained with rhodamine phalloidin (red) to visualize actin filaments and DAPI (blue) for cell nuclei. FITC–gelatin degradation is evident as black areas devoid of FITC-labeled gelatin. Graphical representation of (**C**) LN229 and (**D**) MU41 invadopodia-mediated FITC–gelatin degradative activity per GBM cell (relative to R/T treated groups). Mean of $n = 3$ independent experiments, error bars represent SEM, * $p < 0.05$. Scale bar = 20 µm.

With a focus on identifying drugs with dual "anti-invasive" and "cytotoxic" activity on RT/TMZ-resistant GBM cells, we also examined cell viability with the three candidate drugs in RT/TMZ pre-treated cells. While these drugs led to a reduction in cell viability in most cell lines when compared to the RT/TMZ-only treated, only econazole nitrate in conjunction with RT/TMZ significantly reduced the cell viability of LN229 and U87MG cells when compared to RT/TMZ-only treated cells (Figure 7).

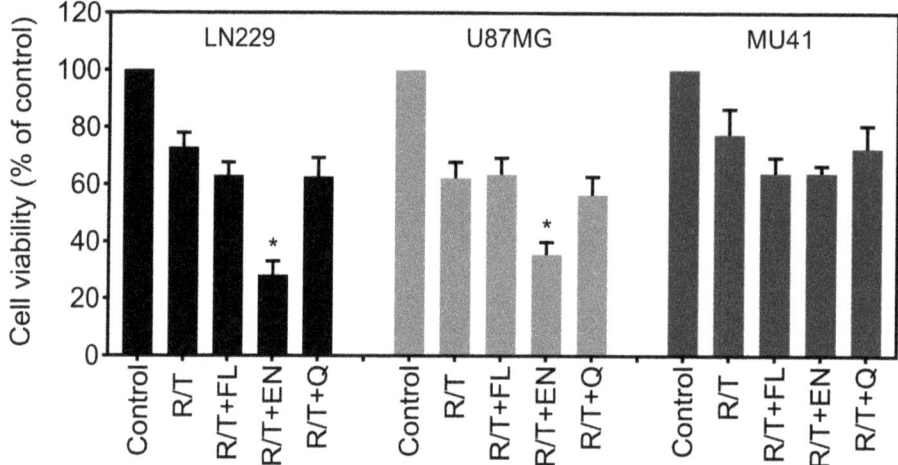

Figure 7. Econazole nitrate can further reduce cell viability following R/T treatment. LN229, U87MG and MU41 GBM cells were treated R/T (2 Gy/50 µM) and 10 µM of each candidate drug: flunarizine dihydrochloride (FL), econazole nitrate (EN), and quinine hydrochloride dihydrate (Q) for 7 days. Subsequently, cell viability was determined using an MTT (3-(4,5-dimethylthiazol-2-yl)-2,5-diphenyltetrazolium bromide) cell proliferation assay. Cell viability is represented as a percentage relative to the control cells. Mean of $n = 3$ experiments, error bars represent SEM, * $p < 0.05$ (relative to R/T).

3. Discussion

Despite a multi-modal treatment approach involving maximal-safe surgical resection, adjuvant radiotherapy, and chemotherapy, GBM remains invariably fatal, which is facilitated by infiltrative growth into the surrounding healthy brain tissue [44]. Tumor cell invasion is a complex process involving cancer cell cytoskeletal changes and remodeling of the ECM mediated by invadopodia [14,45–47]. Ion channels have been shown to facilitate various aspects of cancer progression, including invasion [48]. Koltai [49] has proposed a role for sodium ion channels in protease secretion, while potassium channels can contribute to an invasive phenotype through the altered regulation of intracellular Ca^{2+} levels, leading to cytoskeletal changes [19,49]. Importantly, the relevance of invadopodia and ion channels in GBM can be highlighted by the overexpression of key invadopodia regulators (Table 1) and ion channels in GBM tissue (Table 2) and their impact on glioma patient survival (Figure 1).

The aim of this work was to screen a panel of 20 ion channel-targeting drugs for their ability to select candidate drugs that inhibit GBM cell viability and invadopodia activity. This study identified three drugs that behaved in a "dualistic" manner, reducing both cell viability and invadopodia activity. The shortlisted drugs were flunarizine dihydrochloride (a calcium antagonist approved for use for the prevention of migraines) [50,51], econazole nitrate (an anti-fungal calcium antagonist) [52], and quinine hydrochloride dihydrate (an anti-malarial potassium channel blocker) [53]. A decrease in MMP-2 secretion (Figure 4A,B) was observed with econazole nitrate and quinine hydrochloride dihydrate in both the LN229 and MU41 GBM cell lines, while flunarizine dihydrochloride resulted in reduced MMP-2 secretion only in the MU41 cell line.

Furthermore, treatment with the three shortlisted ion channel drugs revealed a statistically significant reduction in the level of invadopodia-mediated FITC–gelatin degradation activity in the GBM cell lines (Figure 4C–F), suggesting that all three drugs exhibit an "anti-invadopodia" effect. These findings were consistent with the trend seen in the reduced level of MMP-2 secretion following treatment with econazole nitrate and quinine hydrochloride dihydrate (Figure 4A,B). This w–s not observed with flunarizine dihydrochloride treatment of the LN229 GBM cell line. Although flunarizine dihydrochloride led to a decrease in invadopodia-mediated FITC–gelatin degradation, the secreted levels of MMP-2 were not significantly altered, indicating that flunarizine dihydrochloride may exert its action on the dynamics of actin cytoskeletal reorganization and subsequent invadopodia formation and not on the secretion of proteases (Figure 4A). Studies have proposed that Ca^{2+} oscillations are required for the initiation of invadopodia formation [48,54]. Flunarizine dihydrochloride, as a calcium channel antagonist, may reduce Ca^{2+} oscillations and interfere with the assembly of invadopodia. An impact on the dynamics of invadopodia could lead to a reduction in the number and size of invadopodia (less invadopodia/smaller invadopodia leading to reduced focal FITC–gelatin degradation) [55,56].

Several studies have shown that radiotherapy promotes an invasive and pro-migratory phenotype in GBM [57,58]. Trog et al. [59] showed that RT and TMZ promote the upregulation of pro-invasive proteins such as MMP-2 and MT1-MMP (Membrane type 1-matrix metalloproteinase) in vitro. Consistent with these findings, we demonstrated that clinically relevant doses of RT and TMZ not only led to an increase in the level of MMP-2 secretion but also an increase in invadopodia-mediated FITC–gelatin degradation activity (Figure 5) in GBM cells. Such findings suggest that RT/TMZ treatment promotes an invasive phenotype through invadopodia via the upregulated expression and secretion of MMP-2 in cells that survive treatment [59].

Considering the increase in invasion following RT and TMZ treatment and the "anti-invadopodia" activity of the ion channel drugs, we sought to examine whether treatment with these agents could inhibit treatment-induced enhanced invadopodia activity. While econazole nitrate was the only drug to result in a significant reduction in cell viability following RT/TMZ treatment (Figure 7), all three drugs led to a significant reduction in RT/TMZ-induced invadopodia activity (Figure 6). These results suggest that targeting ion channels can overcome the infiltrative and invasive properties of GBM cells by interfering with invadopodia activity. Flunarizine dihydrochloride and econazole nitrate both block calcium channels and may promote anti-invasive activity. This may occur via the inhibition of the Ca^{2+} influx required for the activation of other ion channels, such as potassium and chloride channels, which are known to enhance cell migration and invasion [60]. Alternatively, these agents may also act to reduce the invadopodia-mediated focal ECM degradation by blocking the Ca^{2+} signaling required for the upregulation of proteolytic enzymes such as MMPs and cathepsins [54,60]. As a potassium channel blocker, quinine hydrochloride dihydrate may act by antagonizing potassium channels such as KCa3.1. These channels are involved in mediating cell volume changes required for the reorganization of the actin cytoskeleton and promoting an invasive phenotype in cancer cells [23,24,61].

After identifying drugs that complement the current recommended therapy for GBM patients, one must also consider drug delivery and blood–brain barrier (BBB) penetrance. This is a significant challenge in the use of small molecule compounds in the clinical treatment of GBM where the penetrance of the BBB is limited [62]. Flunarizine dihydrochloride has been shown to have a concentration in the brain that is 10 times higher than in the plasma [50,51,63], whilst quinine has been used for the treatment of malarial-causing parasites in the central nervous system [53,64]. Furthermore, econazole nitrate has also been patented as a neuroprotective agent (US 2010/0298394A1) [52]. This suggests that these drugs can cross the BBB. The predicted BBB penetrance of the candidate ion channel drugs is presented in Table S2. Plasma levels that have been achieved for the candidate agents are listed in Table S3. Therefore, we propose that flunarizine dihydrochloride, econazole nitrate, and quinine hydrochloride dihydrate demonstrate the potential for clinical applicability as an adjuvant treatment, in combination with the current standard of care for GBM patients. Furthermore, we posit that targeting ion channels to regulate invadopodia activity and inhibit GBM cell invasion is a promising therapeutic avenue that merits further investigation.

4. Materials and Methods

4.1. Ion Channel Drugs

The ion channel drugs used in this study were supplied by Selleckchem, (Selleckchem, Houston, TX, USA) at a concentration of 10 mM in DMSO and were stored at −80 °C until use. The ion channel drugs utilized in this study were included within a larger commercial library supplied by Selleckchem and were screened to provide preliminary data examining their impact on invadopodia activity in GBM cells, as there is evidence that ion channels can regulate tumor cell invasion [19,20].

4.2. Cell Lines and Cell Culture

LN229, U87MG, and MU41 human GBM cell lines were maintained in Dulbecco's Modified Eagle's Medium (Life Technologies, Carlsbad, CA, USA) supplemented with 10% heat-inactivated fetal bovine serum (HyClone, Global Life Sciences Solutions, Parramatta, Australia) and 1% antibiotic-antimycotic (Life Technologies). All cell lines were incubated at 37 °C in a 10% CO2 humidified atmosphere. LN229 and U87MG human GBM cell lines were obtained from the ATCC Biological material repository. The MU41 human GBM cell line was harvested from a GBM patient biopsy sample at the Royal Melbourne Hospital (Melbourne Health Research Ethics Approval Number HREC 2009.116).

4.3. Zymographic Analysis

LN229 and MU41 GBM cells were seeded in 6-well plates and allowed to adhere for 24 h. Cells were washed with sterile phosphate-buffered saline (PBS) before a further 24-h incubation in 2 mL serum-free Optimem® (Thermo Fisher Scientific, Waltham, MA, USA). Then, 200 µL aliquots of the conditioned Optimem® medium were sampled and stored at −80 °C until further use. Optimem® media samples were normalized based on the GBM cell protein concentration using a BCA (bicinchoninic acid) protein assay (Pierce, ThermoFisher Scientific) and by performing densitometry of GAPDH bands in corresponding Western blots. The conditioned medium samples were diluted 1:1 with 2× Novex tris-glycine SDS sample buffer (Invitrogen, Thermo Fisher Scientific, Waltham, MA, USA) prior to being loaded in 10% gelatin substrate zymogram NuPAGE 10 well pre-cast gels (Novex, Invitrogen, Thermo Fisher Scientific, Waltham, MA, USA) and separated at 125 V for 90 min in 1× Novex tris-glycine SDS running buffer. The gels were incubated in 1× Novex zymogram renaturing buffer for 30 min and subsequently incubated in 1× Novex zymogram developing buffer for 30 min. Then, they were incubated overnight at 37 °C with fresh 1× Novex zymogram developing buffer. Following incubation, the gels were washed in distilled water before being stained in SimplyBlue SafeStain (Life Technologies) for 1 h. The gels were washed with distilled water until clear bands (representing gelatinolytic activity) against the undigested blue-stained gel were visible; then, gels were scanned using a flatbed scanner, and image files were used for analysis.

4.4. Invadopodia Degradation Assay

Fluorescein isothiocyanate (FITC)-conjugated gelatin prepared as per previously established protocol [65] was used to coat 25 mm round coverslips. LN229 and MU41 GBM cells were pre-treated with either 2 Gy radiation and 50 µM of temozolomide, or 10 µM of FL, EN, and Q. Following a 72-h incubation, cells were trypsinised and seeded at a density of 1×10^5 cells per FITC-conjugated gelatin coverslip and incubated for a further 24 h. The cells were washed with PBS, fixed in 4% paraformaldehyde, and then permeabilized using with 0.2% Triton-X-100. Subsequently, they were stained with rhodamine phalloidin (actin filaments and invadopodia puncta) and DAPI (nuclei), and the coverslips mounted on glass slides with VectaShield (Vector Laboratories, Burlingame, CA, USA) mounting medium. Images were acquired using a Nikon A1+ confocal microscope system with a Plan Apo VC 60× Oil DIC N2 immersion objective. A total of 10–15 images were acquired for each experimental condition. Image J (Version 1.52e) was used for the analysis of the confocal images. The region and threshold tools were used to define the total area of FITC–gelatin degradation in an image field, while the particle counter macro was used to determine the area of degradation, which was normalized with respect to the number of cells (DAPI-positive nuclei).

4.5. Cell Viability

LN229, U87MG, and MU41 GBM cells were seeded (1×10^4 cells /100μl) in 96-well plates and allowed to adhere for 24 h. Initially, the cells were treated with the 20 ion channel drugs over a concentration range (0.01, 0.1, 1, and 10 μM) (Table 1) for 7 days. Further experiments examining the effect of the shortlisted ion channel agents on cell viability in conjunction with RT and TMZ involved 2 Gy RT and 50 μM of TMZ pre-treatment 4 h prior to the addition of the ion channel drugs (10 μM). A CellTiter 96 Non-Radioactive Cell Proliferation Assay (MTT) (Promega, Alexandria, Australia) was used as per the manufacturer's instructions to assess cell viability post-treatment.

4.6. Western Blot Analysis

Western blot analysis of GBM cell protein lysates (20 μg) was performed using NuPAGE 4–12% Bis-Tris pre-cast gels (Invitrogen) and transferred onto a 0.45 μm nitrocellulose blotting membrane (GE Healthsciences, Parramatta, Australia). The membrane was blocked in 3% bovine serum albumin in 1% TBST (Tris-buffered saline with Tween) for 1 h prior to overnight incubation with a primary antibody, including GAPDH, NWASP, Nck-1, phospho-cortactin (1:1000, Cell Signalling Technologies, Danvers, MA, USA), MMP-2, c-Src, cortactin, and Tks5 (1:1000, Santa Cruz Biotechnology). The membrane was subsequently incubated with the appropriate secondary antibody and developed using enhanced chemiluminescence reagent (GE Healthcare, Melbourne, Australia) and exposure onto Fujifilm Super RX film.

4.7. Oncomine Data Mining

Differential mRNA and DNA expression levels of invadopodia regulators and ion channels in GBM tissue were retrieved from the Oncomine™ v4.5 (www.oncomine.org Compendia Bioscience™, Ann Arbor, MI, USA, part of Life Technologies) database. Oncomine™ is an online cancer microarray database containing 715 datasets (86,733 samples) compiled from various studies. The threshold for inclusion for data analysis was set to $p < 0.05$ for significance and an mRNA expression fold difference of >2. All data are log transformed, and the standard deviation is normalized to one per array studied. A list of all analyzed genes is provided in Table S1. Further details regarding the Oncomine™ analyses are provided in the Supplementary Methods.

4.8. SurvExpress

Glioma patient survival analysis was conducted using gene expression datasets deposited in the SurvExpress (http://bioinformatica.mty.itesm.mx/SurvExpress) database [66]. SurvExpress is an online database for evaluating cancer gene expression data using survival analysis. Data sourced from the SurvExpress platform was used for the survival analysis of invadopodia regulator and ion channel gene co-expression in glioma patients. Further details regarding the SurvExpress analyses are provided in the Supplementary Methods.

4.9. Statistical Analysis

Statistical significance was determined using an unpaired, unequal variance, two-tailed t-test with the use of GraphPad Prism 7 (Prism 7.00 for Windows, GraphPad Software, La Jolla, CA, USA, www.graphpad.com). Values were considered statistically significant if the $p < 0.05$. In all figures * denotes $p < 0.05$ and error bars represent the standard error of the mean (SEM).

5. Conclusions

During recent years, studies have been investigating the role of invadopodia in mediating cancer invasion. GBM, the most common primary brain tumor, is a highly proliferative and invasive cancer, and the current standard therapy involving surgical resection, radiotherapy, and chemotherapy (temozolomide) is insufficient to eradicate the tumor. Therefore, new therapies are required to not only reduce the number of cells surviving the current therapy but also to reduce the neurologically destructive invasive ability of the GBM cells. Ion channels have emerged as contributors to tumor pathophysiology in the various hallmarks of cancer including cell proliferation, migration, and invasion via their capacity in cell volume regulation. The data from our current study demonstrates that there is potential for repurposing ion channel agents with ion channel targets as novel prospective therapeutic agents to be utilized in targeting the invasive GBM cells that survive the current treatment for GBM patients.

Supplementary Materials: The following are available online at http://www.mdpi.com/2072-6694/12/10/2888/s1, Figure S1: Cell viability profile of GBM cells (LN229, U87MG, MU41) following treatment with ion channel drugs, Table S1: Invadopodia regulator genes and ion channel genes utilized in the analyses of online gene expression GBM datasets deposited within the Oncomine® and SurvExpress databases, Figure S2: The uncropped Western Blot figure, Table S2: Candidate drug predicted blood–brain barrier penetrance properties. We examined information on the three candidate drugs, flunarazine dihydrochloride, quinine hydrochloride dihydrate, and econazole nitrate present in the online database, 'DrugBank'(go.drugbank.com), Table S3: Clinically achievable plasma levels of candidate ion channel drugs.

Author Contributions: Conceptualization, S.S.S.; Methodology, S.S.S.; Formal analysis, M.D.; Investigation, M.D. and N.G.; Data Curation, M.D. and N.G.; writing—original draft preparation, M.D., T.M. and S.S.S.; writing—review and editing, M.D., N.G., A.P.M., A.H.K., K.J.D., T.M., and S.S.S.; Supervision, S.S.S.; Project administration, S.S.S.; Funding Acquisition, S.S.S., A.H.K. and K.J.D. All authors have read and agreed to the published version of the manuscript.

Funding: This work was supported by the following funding sources: Perpetual IMPACT Philanthropy Grant IPAP2017/0766 and The Royal Melbourne Hospital Neuroscience Foundation.

Conflicts of Interest: The authors declare no conflict of interest.

References

1. Ellor, S.V.; Pagano-Young, T.A.; Avgeropoulos, N.G. Glioblastoma: Background, standard treatment paradigms, and supportive care considerations. *J. Law Med. Ethic.* **2014**, *42*, 171–182. [CrossRef] [PubMed]
2. Delgado-López, P.D.; Corrales-García, E.M. Survival in glioblastoma: A review on the impact of treatment modalities. *Clin. Transl. Oncol.* **2016**, *18*, 1062–1071. [CrossRef] [PubMed]
3. Zygogianni, A.; Protopapa, M.; Kougioumtzopoulou, A.; Simopoulou, F.; Nikoloudi, S.; Kouloulias, V. From imaging to biology of glioblastoma: New clinical oncology perspectives to the problem of local recurrence. *Clin. Transl. Oncol.* **2018**, *20*, 989–1003. [CrossRef] [PubMed]
4. Goodenberger, M.L.; Jenkins, R.B. Genetics of adult glioma. *Cancer Genet.* **2012**, *205*, 613–621. [CrossRef]
5. Taylor, O.G.; Brzozowski, J.S.; Skelding, K.A. Glioblastoma Multiforme: An Overview of Emerging Therapeutic Targets. *Front. Oncol.* **2019**, *9*, 1–11. [CrossRef]
6. Stupp, R.; Mason, W.P.; van den Bent, M.J.; Weller, M.; Fisher, B.; Taphoorn, M.J.; Belanger, K.; Brandes, A.A.; Marosi, C.; Bogdahn, U.; et al. Radiotherapy plus Concomitant and Adjuvant Temozolomide for Glioblastoma. *N. Engl. J. Med.* **2005**, *352*, 987–996. [CrossRef] [PubMed]
7. Lee, S.Y. Temozolomide resistance in glioblastoma multiforme. *Gene Funct. Dis.* **2016**, *3*, 198–210. [CrossRef] [PubMed]
8. Paw, I.; Carpenter, R.C.; Watabe, K.; Debinski, W.; Lo, H.-W. Mechanisms regulating glioma invasion. *Cancer Lett.* **2015**, *362*, 1–7. [CrossRef] [PubMed]
9. Nakada, M.; Nakada, S.; DeMuth, T.; Tran, N.L.; Hoelzinger, D.B.; Berens, M.E. Molecular targets of glioma invasion. *Cell. Mol. Life Sci.* **2007**, *64*, 458–478. [CrossRef] [PubMed]

10. De Gooijer, M.C.; Navarro, M.G.; Bernards, R.; Wurdinger, T.; Van Tellingen, O. An Experimenter's Guide to Glioblastoma Invasion Pathways. *Trends Mol. Med.* **2018**, *24*, 763–780. [CrossRef]
11. Brown, G.T.; Murray, G.I. Current mechanistic insights into the roles of matrix metalloproteinases in tumour invasion and metastasis. *J. Pathol.* **2015**, *237*, 273–281. [CrossRef] [PubMed]
12. Artym, V.V.; Zhang, Y.; Seillier-Moiseiwitsch, F.; Yamada, K.M.; Mueller, S.C. Dynamic Interactions of Cortactin and Membrane Type 1 Matrix Metalloproteinase at Invadopodia: Defining the Stages of Invadopodia Formation and Function. *Cancer Res.* **2006**, *66*, 3034–3043. [CrossRef] [PubMed]
13. Paz, H.; Pathak, N.; Yang, J. Invading one step at a time: The role of invadopodia in tumor metastasis. *Oncogene* **2013**, *33*, 4193–4202. [CrossRef] [PubMed]
14. Sibony-Benyamini, H.; Gil-Henn, H. Invadopodia: The leading force. *Eur. J. Cell Biol.* **2012**, *91*, 896–901. [CrossRef] [PubMed]
15. Yamaguchi, H.; Pixley, F.; Condeelis, J. Invadopodia and podosomes in tumor invasion. *Eur. J. Cell Biol.* **2006**, *85*, 213–218. [CrossRef] [PubMed]
16. Stylli, S.S.; Stacey, T.T.; Kaye, A.H.; Lock, P. Prognostic significance of Tks5 expression in gliomas. *J. Clin. Neurosci.* **2012**, *19*, 436–442. [CrossRef]
17. Stylli, S.S.; Kaye, A.H.; Lock, P. Invadopodia: At the cutting edge of tumour invasion. *J. Clin. Neurosci.* **2008**, *15*, 725–737. [CrossRef]
18. Buccione, R.; Caldieri, G.; Ayala, I. Invadopodia: Specialized tumor cell structures for the focal degradation of the extracellular matrix. *Cancer Metastasis Rev.* **2009**, *28*, 137–149. [CrossRef]
19. Prevarskaya, N.; Skryma, R.; Shuba, Y. Ion channels and the hallmarks of cancer. *Trends Mol. Med.* **2010**, *16*, 107–121. [CrossRef]
20. Hanahan, D.; Weinberg, R.A. Hallmarks of Cancer: The Next Generation. *Cell* **2011**, *144*, 646–674. [CrossRef]
21. Joshi, A.D.; Parsons, D.W.; Velculescu, V.E.; Riggins, G.J. Sodium ion channel mutations in glioblastoma patients correlate with shorter survival. *Mol. Cancer* **2011**, *10*, 17. [CrossRef] [PubMed]
22. Pollak, J.; Rai, K.G.; Funk, C.C.; Arora, S.; Lee, E.; Zhu, J.; Price, N.D.; Paddison, P.J.; Ramirez, J.-M.; Rostomily, R.C. Ion channel expression patterns in glioblastoma stem cells with functional and therapeutic implications for malignancy. *PLoS ONE* **2017**, *12*, e0172884. [CrossRef] [PubMed]
23. Cuddapah, V.A.; Robel, S.; Watkins, S.; Sontheimer, H. A neurocentric perspective on glioma invasion. *Nat. Rev. Neurosci.* **2014**, *15*, 455–465. [CrossRef] [PubMed]
24. Cuddapah, V.A.; Turner, K.L.; Seifert, S.; Sontheimer, H. Bradykinin-induced chemotaxis of human gliomas requires the activation of KCa3.1 and ClC-3. *J. Neurosci.* **2013**, *33*, 1427–1440. [CrossRef] [PubMed]
25. D'Alessandro, G.; Ecatalano, M.; Sciaccaluga, M.; Chece, G.; Cipriani, R.; Rosito, M.; Grimaldi, A.; Lauro, C.; Cantore, G.; Santoro, A.; et al. KCa3.1 channels are involved in the infiltrative behavior of glioblastoma in vivo. *Cell Death Dis.* **2013**, *4*, e773. [CrossRef]
26. Turner, K.L.; Honasoge, A.; Robert, S.M.; McFerrin, M.M.; Sontheimer, H. A proinvasive role for the Ca(2+)-activated K(+) channel KCa3.1 in malignant glioma. *Glia* **2014**, *62*, 971–981. [CrossRef]
27. Deliot, N.; Constantin, B. Plasma membrane calcium channels in cancer: Alterations and consequences for cell proliferation and migration. *Biochim. Biophys. Acta. (BBA)-Biomembr.* **2015**, *1848*, 2512–2522. [CrossRef]
28. Zhang, Y.; Zhang, J.; Jiang, D.; Zhang, N.; Qian, Z.; Liu, C.; Tao, J. Inhibition of T-type Ca2+ channels by endostatin attenuates human glioblastoma cell proliferation and migration. *Br. J. Pharmacol.* **2012**, *166*, 1247–1260. [CrossRef]
29. Simon, O.J.; Müntefering, T.; Grauer, O.M.; Meuth, S.G. The role of ion channels in malignant brain tumors. *J. Neuro-Oncol.* **2015**, *125*, 225–235. [CrossRef]
30. Stock, C.; Ludwig, F.T.; Hanley, P.J.; Schwab, A. Roles of Ion Transport in Control of Cell Motility. *Compr. Physiol.* **2013**, *3*, 59–119. [CrossRef]
31. Molenaar, R.J. Ion Channels in Glioblastoma. *ISRN Neurol.* **2011**, *2011*, 1–7. [CrossRef] [PubMed]
32. Sleire, L.; Førde, H.E.; Netland, I.A.; Leiss, L.; Skeie, B.S.; Enger, P. Øyvind Drug repurposing in cancer. *Pharmacol. Res.* **2017**, *124*, 74–91. [CrossRef] [PubMed]
33. Pushpakom, S.; Iorio, F.; Eyers, P.A.; Escott, K.J.; Hopper, S.; Wells, A.; Doig, A.J.; Guilliams, T.; Latimer, J.; McNamee, C.; et al. Drug repurposing: Progress, challenges and recommendations. *Nat. Rev. Drug Discov.* **2018**, *18*, 41–58. [CrossRef] [PubMed]

34. Bredel, M.; Bredel, C.; Juric, D.; Harsh, G.R.; Vogel, H.; Recht, L.D.; Sikic, B.I. Functional network analysis reveals extended gliomagenesis pathway maps and three novel MYC-interacting genes in human gliomas. *Cancer Res.* **2005**, *65*, 8679–8689. [CrossRef]
35. Liang, Y.; Diehn, M.; Watson, N.P.; Bollen, A.W.; Aldape, K.D.; Nicholas, M.K.; Lamborn, K.R.; Berger, M.S.; Botstein, D.; Brown, P.O.; et al. Gene expression profiling reveals molecularly and clinically distinct subtypes of glioblastoma multiforme. *Proc. Natl. Acad. Sci. USA* **2005**, *102*, 5814–5819. [CrossRef]
36. Murat, A.; Migliavacca, E.; Gorlia, T.; Lambiv, W.L.; Shay, T.; Hamou, M.-F.; De Tribolet, N.; Regli, L.; Wick, W.; Kouwenhoven, M.C.; et al. Stem Cell–Related "Self-Renewal" Signature and High Epidermal Growth Factor Receptor Expression Associated with Resistance to Concomitant Chemoradiotherapy in Glioblastoma. *J. Clin. Oncol.* **2008**, *26*, 3015–3024. [CrossRef]
37. Sun, L.; Hui, A.-M.; Su, Q.; Vortmeyer, A.; Kotliarov, Y.; Pastorino, S.; Passaniti, A.; Menon, J.; Walling, J.; Bailey, R.; et al. Neuronal and glioma-derived stem cell factor induces angiogenesis within the brain. *Cancer Cell* **2006**, *9*, 287–300. [CrossRef]
38. Yamanaka, R.; Arao, T.; Yajima, N.; Tsuchiya, N.; Homma, J.; Tanaka, R.; Sano, M.; Oide, A.; Sekijima, M.; Nishio, K. Identification of expressed genes characterizing long-term survival in malignant glioma patients. *Oncogene* **2006**, *25*, 5994–6002. [CrossRef]
39. Beroukhim, R.; Getz, G.; Nghiemphu, L.; Barretina, J.; Hsueh, T.; Linhart, D.; Vivanco, I.; Lee, J.C.; Huang, J.H.; Alexander, S.; et al. Assessing the significance of chromosomal aberrations in cancer: Methodology and application to glioma. *Proc. Natl. Acad. Sci. USA* **2007**, *104*, 20007–20012. [CrossRef]
40. Lee, Y.; Scheck, A.C.; Cloughesy, T.; Lai, A.; Dong, J.; Farooqi, H.K.; Liau, L.M.; Horvath, S.; Mischel, P.S.; Nelson, S. Gene expression analysis of glioblastomas identifies the major molecular basis for the prognostic benefit of younger age. *BMC Med. Genom.* **2008**, *1*, 52. [CrossRef]
41. Shai, R.; Shi, T.; Kremen, T.J.; Horvath, S.; Liau, L.M.; Cloughesy, T.F.; Mischel, P.S.; Nelson, S.F. Gene expression profiling identifies molecular subtypes of gliomas. *Oncogene* **2003**, *22*, 4918–4923. [CrossRef] [PubMed]
42. Nutt, C.L.; Mani, D.R.; Betensky, R.A.; Tamayo, P.; Cairncross, J.G.; Ladd, C.; Pohl, U.; Hartmann, C.; McLaughlin, M.E.; Batchelor, T.; et al. Gene expression-based classification of malignant gliomas correlates better with survival than histological classification. *Cancer Res.* **2003**, *63*, 1602–1607. [PubMed]
43. Freije, W.A.; Castro-Vargas, F.E.; Fang, Z.; Horvath, S.; Cloughesy, T.; Liau, L.M.; Mischel, P.S.; Nelson, S. Gene Expression Profiling of Gliomas Strongly Predicts Survival. *Cancer Res.* **2004**, *64*, 6503–6510. [CrossRef] [PubMed]
44. Olar, A.; Aldape, K.D. Using the molecular classification of glioblastoma to inform personalized treatment. *J. Pathol.* **2014**, *232*, 165–177. [CrossRef]
45. Saykali, B.A.; El-Sibai, M. Invadopodia, Regulation, and Assembly in Cancer Cell Invasion. *Cell Commun. Adhes.* **2014**, *21*, 207–212. [CrossRef]
46. Mao, L.; Whitehead, C.A.; Paradiso, L.; Kaye, A.H.; Morokoff, A.P.; Luwor, R.B.; Stylli, S.S. Enhancement of invadopodia activity in glioma cells by sublethal doses of irradiation and temozolomide. *J. Neurosurg.* **2018**, *129*, 598–610. [CrossRef]
47. Whitehead, C.A.; Nguyen, H.P.; Morokoff, A.P.; Luwor, R.B.; Paradiso, L.; Kaye, A.H.; Mantamadiotis, T.; Stylli, S.S. Inhibition of Radiation and Temozolomide-Induced Invadopodia Activity in Glioma Cells Using FDA-Approved Drugs. *Transl. Oncol.* **2018**, *11*, 1406–1418. [CrossRef]
48. Prevarskaya, N.; Skryma, R.; Shuba, Y. Ion Channels in Cancer: Are Cancer Hallmarks Oncochannelopathies? *Physiol. Rev.* **2018**, *98*, 559–621. [CrossRef]
49. Koltai, T. Voltage-gated sodium channel as a target for metastatic risk reduction with re-purposed drugs. *F1000Research* **2015**, *4*, 297. [CrossRef]
50. Kataki, M.; T Mani Senthil Kumar, K.; Rajkumari, A. Neuropsychopharmacological profiling of flunarizine: A calcium channel blocker. *Int. J. Pharmatech Res.* **2010**, *2*, 1703–1713.
51. Fischer, W.; Kittner, H.; Regenthal, R.; De Sarro, G. Anticonvulsant profile of flunarizine and relation to Na(+) channel blocking effects. *Basic Clin. Pharmacol. Toxicol.* **2004**, *94*, 79–88. [CrossRef] [PubMed]
52. Steiner, J.P.; Nath, A.; Haughey, N. Antifungal Agents as Neuroprotectants. US Patent 2010/0298394A1, 25 November 2010.
53. Golden, E.B.; Cho, H.-Y.; Hofman, F.M.; Louie, S.G.; Schönthal, A.H.; Chen, T.C. Quinoline-based antimalarial drugs: A novel class of autophagy inhibitors. *Neurosurg. Focus* **2015**, *38*, E12. [CrossRef] [PubMed]

54. Iamshanova, O.; Pla, A.F.; Prevarskaya, N. Molecular mechanisms of tumour invasion: Regulation by calcium signals. *J. Physiol.* **2017**, *595*, 3063–3075. [CrossRef] [PubMed]
55. Hoskin, V.; Szeto, A.; Ghaffari, A.; Greer, P.A.; Côté, G.P.; Elliott, B.E. Ezrin regulates focal adhesion and invadopodia dynamics by altering calpain activity to promote breast cancer cell invasion. *Mol. Biol. Cell* **2015**, *26*, 3464–3479. [CrossRef] [PubMed]
56. Brisson, L.; Alfarouk, K.; Goré, J.; Roger, S. pH regulators in invadosomal functioning: Proton delivery for matrix tasting. *Eur. J. Cell Biol.* **2012**, *91*, 847–860. [CrossRef] [PubMed]
57. Wild-Bode, C.; Weller, M.; Rimner, A.; Dichgans, J.; Wick, W. Sublethal irradiation promotes migration and invasiveness of glioma cells: Implications for radiotherapy of human glioblastoma. *Cancer Res.* **2001**, *61*, 2744–2750. [PubMed]
58. Wang, S.-C.; Yu, C.-F.; Hong, J.-H.; Tsai, C.-S.; Chiang, C.-S. Radiation Therapy-Induced Tumor Invasiveness Is Associated with SDF-1-Regulated Macrophage Mobilization and Vasculogenesis. *PLoS ONE* **2013**, *8*, e69182. [CrossRef]
59. Trog, D.; Yeghiazaryan, K.; Fountoulakis, M.; Friedlein, A.; Moenkemann, H.; Haertel, N.; Schueller, H.; Breipohl, W.; Schild, H.; Leppert, D.; et al. Pro-invasive gene regulating effect of irradiation and combined temozolomide-radiation treatment on surviving human malignant glioma cells. *Eur. J. Pharmacol.* **2006**, *542*, 8–15. [CrossRef]
60. Schwab, A.; Stock, C. Ion channels and transporters in tumour cell migration and invasion. *Philos. Trans. R. Soc. B Biol. Sci.* **2014**, *369*, 20130102. [CrossRef]
61. Thompson, E.G.; Sontheimer, H. A role for ion channels in perivascular glioma invasion. *Eur. Biophys. J.* **2016**, *45*, 635–648. [CrossRef]
62. Munson, J.M.; Bonner, M.Y.; Fried, L.; Hofmekler, J.; Arbiser, J.L.; Bellamkonda, R.V. Identifying new small molecule anti-invasive compounds for glioma treatment. *Cell Cycle* **2013**, *12*, 2200–2209. [CrossRef] [PubMed]
63. Ciancarelli, I.; Tozzi-Ciancarelli, M.G.; Di Massimo, C.; Marini, C.; Carolei, A. Flunarizine Effects on Oxidative Stress in Migraine Patients. *Cephalalgia* **2004**, *24*, 528–532. [CrossRef] [PubMed]
64. Bebin, M.; Bleck, T.P. New Anticonvulsant Drugs. *Drugs* **1994**, *48*, 153–171. [CrossRef] [PubMed]
65. Stylli, S.S.; Stacey, T.T.I.; Verhagen, A.M.; Xu, S.S.; Pass, I.; Courtneidge, S.A.; Lock, P.; I, S.T.T. Nck adaptor proteins link Tks5 to invadopodia actin regulation and ECM degradation. *J. Cell Sci.* **2009**, *122*, 2727–2740. [CrossRef]
66. Aguirre-Gamboa, R.; Gomez-Rueda, H.; Martinez-Ledesma, E.; Martinez-Torteya, A.; Chacolla-Huaringa, R.; Rodriguez-Barrientos, A.; Tamez-Peña, J.G.; Trevino, V. SurvExpress: An Online Biomarker Validation Tool and Database for Cancer Gene Expression Data Using Survival Analysis. *PLoS ONE* **2013**, *8*, e74250. [CrossRef]

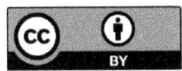

© 2020 by the authors. Licensee MDPI, Basel, Switzerland. This article is an open access article distributed under the terms and conditions of the Creative Commons Attribution (CC BY) license (http://creativecommons.org/licenses/by/4.0/).

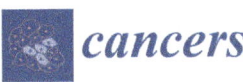

Review

The Renin–Angiotensin System in the Tumor Microenvironment of Glioblastoma

Michael O'Rawe [1,†], Ethan J. Kilmister [2,†], Theo Mantamadiotis [3], Andrew H. Kaye [4], Swee T. Tan [2,3,5,*] and Agadha C. Wickremesekera [1,2,3,*]

1. Department of Neurosurgery, Wellington Regional Hospital, Wellington 6021, New Zealand; michael.orawe@ccdhb.org.nz
2. Gillies McIndoe Research Institute, Wellington 6021, New Zealand; ethankilmister467@gmail.com
3. Department of Surgery, The Royal Melbourne Hospital, The University of Melbourne, Parkville, VIC 3000, Australia; theo.mantamadiotis@unimelb.edu.au
4. Department of Neurosurgery, Hadassah Hebrew University Medical Centre, Jerusalem 91000, Israel; andrewk@hadassah.org.il
5. Wellington Regional Plastic, Maxillofacial & Burns Unit, Hutt Hospital, Lower Hutt 5040, New Zealand
* Correspondence: swee.tan@gmri.org.nz (S.T.T.); agadha.wickremesekera@ccdhb.org.nz (A.C.W.)
† Equal first authors.

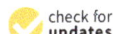

Citation: O'Rawe, M.; Kilmister, E.J.; Mantamadiotis, T.; Kaye, A.H.; Tan, S.T.; Wickremesekera, A.C. The Renin–Angiotensin System in the Tumor Microenvironment of Glioblastoma. *Cancers* **2021**, *13*, 4004. https://doi.org/10.3390/cancers13164004

Academic Editor: Sheila K. Singh

Received: 17 July 2021
Accepted: 6 August 2021
Published: 9 August 2021

Publisher's Note: MDPI stays neutral with regard to jurisdictional claims in published maps and institutional affiliations.

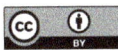

Copyright: © 2021 by the authors. Licensee MDPI, Basel, Switzerland. This article is an open access article distributed under the terms and conditions of the Creative Commons Attribution (CC BY) license (https://creativecommons.org/licenses/by/4.0/).

Simple Summary: Glioblastoma (GB) is the most aggressive brain cancer in humans. Patient survival outcomes have remained dismal despite intensive research over the past 50 years, with a median overall survival of only 14.6 months. We highlight the critical role of the renin–angiotensin system (RAS) on GB cancer stem cells and the tumor microenvironment which, in turn, influences cancer stem cells in driving tumorigenesis and treatment resistance. We present recent developments and underscore the need for further research into the GB tumor microenvironment. We discuss the novel therapeutic targeting of the RAS using existing commonly available medications and utilizing model systems to further this critical investigation.

Abstract: Glioblastoma (GB) is an aggressive primary brain tumor. Despite intensive research over the past 50 years, little advance has been made to improve the poor outcome, with an overall median survival of 14.6 months following standard treatment. Local recurrence is inevitable due to the quiescent cancer stem cells (CSCs) in GB that co-express stemness-associated markers and components of the renin–angiotensin system (RAS). The dynamic and heterogeneous tumor microenvironment (TME) plays a fundamental role in tumor development, progression, invasiveness, and therapy resistance. There is increasing evidence showing the critical role of the RAS in the TME influencing CSCs via its upstream and downstream pathways. Drugs that alter the hallmarks of cancer by modulating the RAS present a potential new therapeutic alternative or adjunct to conventional treatment of GB. Cerebral and GB organoids may offer a cost-effective method for evaluating the efficacy of RAS-modulating drugs on GB. We review the nexus between the GB TME, CSC niche, and the RAS, and propose re-purposed RAS-modulating drugs as a potential therapeutic alternative or adjunct to current standard therapy for GB.

Keywords: glioblastoma; renin–angiotensin system; pluripotent stem cells; organoids; cancer stem cells; cancer stem cell niche; tumor microenvironment

1. Introduction

Glioblastoma (GB), the most common and most aggressive primary brain cancer in humans, is classified as a WHO grade IV astrocytoma, and is characterized by microvascular proliferation and central necrosis [1]. Primary GB arises de novo and accounts for 90% of cases with a predilection for older individuals, while secondary GB arises from low-grade astrocytoma and affects younger patients [2]. GB has been categorized into four distinct molecular subtypes: classical, mesenchymal, neural, and proneural [3], although other studies have only identified classical, mesenchymal, and proneural subtypes [4]. The classical subtype includes amplification or mutation of epidermal growth factor receptor (EGFR), the mesenchymal subtype includes deletions of the 17q11.2 region containing the gene *NF1*, and the proneural subtype is characterized by high levels of platelet-derived growth factor receptor α (PDGFRα) expression and point mutations in *isocitrate dehydrogenase 1* (*IDH1*) and *p53* [3].

Various genetic or epigenetic changes may affect the prognosis of GB patients including *IDH* mutations and O6-methylguanine-DNA methyltransferase (MGMT) methylation status. GB may be divided into IDH-wild-type and IDH-mutant tumors. IDH is an enzyme that catalyzes oxidative decarboxylation of isocitrate to 2-oxoglutarate. The most common mutation in GB affects *IDH1* with a single amino acid missense mutation at arginine 132 which is replaced by histidine [5]. IDH-wild-type GB is more common, tends to arise de novo, and is generally more aggressive with a worse prognosis than IDH-mutant GB. By contrast, IDH-mutant GB is predominantly observed in secondary GB and is associated with a better prognosis [6]. The current standard treatment for GB involves maximal safe surgical resection with adjuvant chemotherapy and radiotherapy, known as the Stupp protocol [7]. Temozolomide, an alkylating agent, is used as first-line chemotherapy for GB with its efficacy related to the methylation status of the *MGMT* promoter [8]. *MGMT* methylation is associated with an improved overall survival in GB patients [9]. Despite this intensive treatment, tumor recurrence in GB patients is inevitable with an overall median survival time of 14.6 months with a range of 12–14 months which has not changed since the introduction of the Stupp protocol in 2005 [10,11].

We reviewed the dynamic relationship between the tumor microenvironment (TME), the RAS, and cancer stem cells (CSCs) in GB. We speculate that RAS-modulating drugs may offer a potential therapeutic alternative or adjunct to current standard therapy. Further functional and epidemiological studies are required to investigate the efficacy of RAS-targeting drugs in the treatment of GB.

2. GB Tumor Microenvironment

The GB tumor microenvironment (TME) is highly heterogeneous and consists of cancer cells and non-cancer cells. Non-cancer cell types include immune cells, such as tumor-associated macrophages (TAMs), resident glial cells, peripheral macrophages, endothelial cells, pericytes, astrocytes, CSCs, fibroblasts, and other components such as the extracellular matrix (ECM) [12]. Given the rarity of extracranial metastasis from GB [13], it appears that GB development requires the unique intracerebral microenvironment inclusive of the blood–brain barrier (BBB) [14]. The TME, with emphasis on glioma-associated microglia/macrophages, pericytes, and reactive astrocytes, is increasingly recognized to play a critical role in GB development and progression [15]. The idea that cytokines, growth factors, chemokines, inflammatory mediators, and remodeling enzymes are involved in intra- and inter-cellular communications within the TME is not novel [16]. Additionally, constant communication between GB cells and the surrounding TME [14] is facilitated by extracellular vesicles that expedite bi-directional cross-talk within the TME [12,17].

Anatomically distinct regions of the TME, known as tumor niches, are thought to contain CSCs and play a fundamental role in the regulation of metabolism, immune surveillance, survival, invasion, and self-maintenance with the renin–angiotensin system (RAS) playing a critical role [15,18,19]. The GB TME may consist of several distinct tumor niches including the hypoxic tumor niche, the perivascular or angiogenic tumor niche, and the vascular-invasive tumor niche. The perivascular niche contains CSCs in close juxtaposition with the abnormal angiogenic vasculature and provides a supportive environment for CSC growth, maintenance, and survival. The vasculature in the hypoxic tumor niche is either non-functional or has regressed, leading to areas of necrosis that are surrounded by rows of hypoxic palisading tumor cells [20]. The vascular-invasive tumor niche contains tumor cells co-opted with normal blood vessels that migrate deep into the brain parenchyma [20].

GB is highly vascular and is characterized by extensive neovascularization and pathological angiogenesis predominantly induced by vascular endothelial growth factor (VEGF), which is produced by tumor cells, CSCs, and immune cells [21,22]. Other angiogenic factors, such as transforming growth factor-β_1 (TGF-β_1), platelet-derived growth factor-BB, and fibroblast growth factor-2, may also play a role in the pathological angiogenesis [23,24]. In addition to endothelial proliferation, bone marrow-derived endothelial and pericyte progenitor cells may be recruited and incorporated into the growing vessels [25]. There is also evidence that CSCs may be involved in neovascularization by differentiating into endothelial cells or pericytes in GB [26–28]. Increased VEGF expression also fosters an immunosuppressive microenvironment that enables tumors, including GB, to evade host immune surveillance [29]. The abnormal vasculature in GB includes dilated and leaky vessels and glomeruloid microvascular proliferation in which endothelial cells and pericytes form poorly organized vascular structures, which effectively disrupt the BBB, leading to cerebral edema. In addition, the blood–brain tumor barrier (BBTB) hinders drug delivery to the tumor [30].

The BBB is a highly specialized, selectively permeable barrier between the brain and the systemic blood supply that helps to maintain homeostasis of the cerebral microenvironment. The structure of the BBB includes endothelial cells with tight junctions, adherens junctions, astrocytes, pericytes, and the basement membrane [31]. The BBB plays several fundamental roles, including supplying the brain with essential nutrients, such as oxygen and glucose, mediating the efflux of waste products, facilitating the movement of nutrients and plasma proteins, and restricting toxins into the central nervous system (CNS) [32]. Disruption of the BBB and its tight regulation of the cerebral microenvironment leads to increased blood vessel permeability with plasma and fluid leakage into the tumor tissue causing cerebral edema and raised interstitial and intracranial pressure [33]. The combination of abnormal vasculature in GB and the disruption of the BBB leads to impaired blood flow and reduced oxygen delivery within the tumor [34]. Microvascular thrombosis may also occur causing occlusion of the blood vessels, further promoting intra-tumoral hypoxia, leading to pseudo-palisading necrosis [35]. Hypoxia is also a consequence of increased oxygen diffusion distance due to the fact that of tumor growth and expansion [34], which may, in and of itself, be a key regulator of tumor cell survival, stemness, and immune surveillance in the TME [36–38]. Hypoxia also sustains tumor cell proliferation, invasiveness, and contributes to chemotherapy and radiotherapy resistance. This occurs via inhibition of free radicals, which reduces the efficacy of radiotherapy [39], and through upregulation of the multi-drug resistance gene, *MDR1/ABCB1*, which reduces chemotherapy effectiveness. Hypoxia-inducible factor-1 (HIF-1) and HIF-2 mediate the response to hypoxia on a molecular level in GB [40] and may potentially modify CSCs [41]. The GB microenvironmental niche also consists of pseudo-palisading glioma cells that upregulate HIF proteins, inducing expression of factors, such as VEGF and interleukin 8 (IL-8), which are implicated in tumor cell survival, metabolism, invasion, and angiogenesis. The resultant cross-talk releases pro-inflammatory signals from the areas of necrosis in the hypoxic tumor niche into the surrounding TME, promoting immunosuppression, and angiogenesis [42].

Immune cells, including circulating monocytes, neutrophils, and myeloid-derived suppressor cells (MDSCs), are another source of angiogenic factors. In ovarian cancer, MDSCs increase CSC characteristics by increasing microRNA-101 expression, which induces the expression of stemness genes [43]. It is interesting to speculate that MDSCs also regulate the stemness of CSCs within the GB TME via this mechanism (Figure 1). These cells may enter the brain as a result of breakdown of the BBB in GB and the production of tumor-derived chemokines and cytokines, contributing to the immunosuppressive GB TME [44–46]. TAMs are the dominant immune cell population in GB and may include resident microglial cells and peripheral macrophages [47,48]. Traditionally, TAMs have been defined as either anti-tumoral M1/Th1 (classical-activated macrophages) or pro-tumoral M2/Th2 (alternative-activated macrophages) phenotypes. M1 macrophages foster the inflammatory response by secreting pro-inflammatory cytokines such as IL-12, tumor necrosis factor-α (TNF-α), CXCL-10, and interferon-γ (IFN-γ) and produce high levels of nitric oxide synthase to exert anti-tumor cell activity (Figure 1). M2 macrophages, on the other hand, play a key immunosuppressive function by secreting anti-inflammatory cytokines, such as IL-10, IL-13, and IL-4, and express abundant arginase-1, mannose receptor CD206, and scavenger receptors to promote tumor progression [49–51]. The release of TGF-β by TAMs has been shown to induce matrix metalloproteinase 9 (MMP9) and, thus, increase CSC invasiveness [52]. A more recent study has demonstrated that the TAM population is in a constant state of transition or plasticity between the two phenotypes and that M1 phenotype expression may be enhanced by TME changes or therapeutic interventions [51]. Resident microglia are present within the brain, but it is the recruitment of peripheral macrophages to the GB TAM pool, in particular, that may mediate tumor phagocytosis with disruption of the signal regulatory protein α receptor (SIRP-α)–CD47 axis. This facilitates immune evasion because the antiphagocytic "don't eat me" surface protein CD47 is upregulated, which binds to SIRP-α on phagocytic cells to inhibit phagocytosis [53]. However, even in the absence of macrophages, resident microglia may be transformed into effector cells of tumor cell phagocytosis, in response to anti-CD47 blockade [54]. In models of pancreatic ductal adenocarcinoma, for example, RP-182 may selectively induce conformational switching of the mannose receptor CD206, which is expressed on the M2 TAM phenotype, ultimately reprogramming M2-like TAMs into an anti-tumor M1-like phenotype [55]. The immunosuppressive phenotype of TAMs may be controlled by long-chain fatty acid metabolism, and chemical inhibitors targeting this metabolic pathway may block TAM polarization in vitro and tumor growth in vivo [56]. GB-derived exosomes may reprogram M1 macrophages to M2 macrophages and condition M2 macrophages to become strongly immunosuppressive TAMs [57].

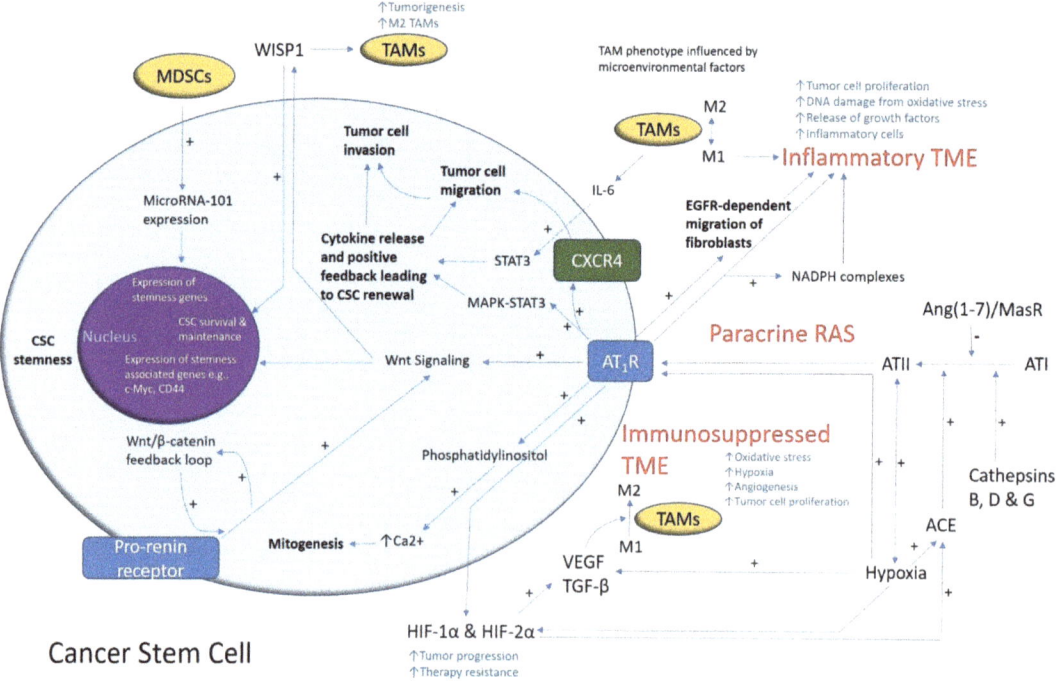

Figure 1. A schema demonstrating the role of the renin–angiotensin system (RAS) and its convergent signaling pathways in the glioblastoma tumor microenvironment (TME) and cancer stem cells (CSCs). A cancer stem cell (with the cytoplasm depicted in light blue and the nucleus in purple) residing within the glioblastoma TME. Angiotensin II (ATII), the physiologically active

end-product of the paracrine RAS, activates ATII receptor 1 (AT_1R) leading to increased tumor cell proliferation, oxidative stress, hypoxia and angiogenesis, and inflammation—the hallmarks of cancer. This contributes to an inflammatory TME by increasing the number of inflammatory cells, partly by increasing the number of NADPH complexes, leading to tumor cell proliferation, DNA damage from oxidative stress, and release of growth factors. AT_1R also activates phosphatidylinositol signaling, which increases cytosolic Ca^{2+} to promote mitogenesis. Hypoxia increases paracrine RAS activity by upregulating angiotensin-converting enzyme (ACE) and the expression of hypoxia-inducible factor 1α (HIF-1α) and HIF-2α, which increase tumor progression and treatment resistance. HIF-1α, HIF-2α, and hypoxia increase the expression of vascular endothelial growth factor (VEGF) which increases angiogenesis. AT_1R, via MAPK-STAT3 signaling, contributes to a cytokine release that leads to CSC renewal. C-X-C chemokine receptor type 4 (CXCR4) promotes tumor cell migration and invasion. AT_1R signaling and the prorenin receptor, which act in a feedback loop with Wnt/β-catenin, increase Wnt signaling which promotes CSC stemness by upregulating stemness-associated markers. Myeloid-derived suppressor cells (MDSCs) promote CSC characteristics by increasing microRNA-101 expression that induces expression of stemness-related genes in CSCs. The Ang(1–7)/MasR axis opposes the ACE/ATII/AT_1R axis. Cathepsins B, D, and G act as bypass loops for the RAS. Under the influence of the TME, polarization of tumor-associated macrophages (TAMs)—immune cells that are located within the TME—changes from the M1 to M2 phenotype. M2 TAMs induce the proliferation of CSCs via interleukin 6 (IL-6)-induced activation of STAT3, leading to cytokine release and positive feedback contributing to CSC renewal. Glioblastoma CSCs secrete Wnt-induced signaling protein 1 (WISP1), which facilitates a pro-tumor TME by promoting the survival of CSCs and M2 TAMs, and also promotes CSC maintenance. Abbreviations: ATI, angiotensin I; AT_2R, ATII receptor 2; Ang(1–7), angiotensin 1–7; ATIII, angiotensin III; MAPK, mitogen-activated protein kinase. Figure modified and reproduced with permission from the *J Histochem Cytochem* [19].

3. Glioblastoma Cancer Stem Cells

The CSC concept proposes that a small distinct population of cells within a tumor with self-renewal capability are responsible for driving tumorigenesis [58,59]. These CSCs may be defined as stem cell-like cells within a tumor that also have the capacity for proliferation and multi-potency. This may be regarded as a functional definition insofar as CSCs may be characterized through the generation of serially transplantable tumors that faithfully recapitulate the parent tumor [60]. There is marked intra- and inter-tumoral heterogeneity including, differing numbers of highly tumorigenic CSCs [61]. Such heterogeneity may be best explained by a combination of different models of cancer, including the stochastic model (also known as the clonal evolution model), the CSC concept of cancer (also known as the hierarchical model of cancer), and the concept of plasticity [62,63].

The traditional model of cancer is predicated on the stochastic model of carcinogenesis which proposes that cancer cells are derived from normal cells that acquire genetic and/or epigenetic mutations resulting in typically unidirectional transitions from benign to malignant cells. These malignant tumor cells have unrestricted division capacities and their high mutation rates increase the likelihood of successive generations of cloned cells being adapted to the selection pressures of the tumor site. However, the stochastic model does not fully account for all aspects of cancer biology including tumor recurrence following treatment [64].

In contrast, the CSC concept of cancer proposes that CSCs contribute to carcinogenesis, invasion, metastasis, therapy resistance, and recurrence [65,66]. CSCs divide asymmetrically into non-tumorigenic cancer cells, which form the bulk of a tumor, and identical highly tumorigenic but less abundant CSCs, which sit at the apex of the cellular hierarchy [67]. CSCs have been postulated to originate from non-malignant stem cells or progenitor cells [66] or dedifferentiated cancer cells [68]. The overlap between the stochastic model and the CSC concept may be explained by the concept of cellular plasticity whereby cancer cells may reversibly transition between stem-like and non-stem-like cell states [69]. This process of transition may be driven by embryonic stem cell (ESC)-associated regulatory networks and may be affected by the dynamic TME including the CSC niche [70]. Moreover, certain cancer cells may de-differentiate and re-enter the CSC pool, thus regaining the capacity for tumorigenesis and clonal expansion [71].

CSCs have been found in many different cancer types, including myeloid leukemia [72], pancreatic cancer [73], breast cancer [74], oral cavity squamous cell carcinoma (SCC) [75–77], primary [78] and metastatic [79] cutaneous SCC, primary [80] and metastatic [81] colon adenocarcinoma, metastatic malignant melanoma [82,83], and GB [84]. The aggressive nature of GB and its resistance to conventional therapy has been attributed to the presence of CSCs [85] that were first postulated in human brain tumors, identified by their expression of the neural stem cell surface marker CD133 [86]. Stem-like neural precursor cells responsible for the growth and recurrence in serial transplantations were identified in GB [87]. The presence of such quiescent CSCs is well-supported in the literature and the interaction of such cells with the ECM and TME factors, including TGF-β and hypoxia, may contribute to their resistance to conventional therapy [88] (Figure 1). There is evidence that CSCs may be stimulated to differentiate into endothelial cells by activating Notch1 signaling [89] and may be associated with induction of cytokines, MMPs, and adhesion proteins in the TME [90].

A crucial function of stem cells is self-renewal, for which the Notch, Sonic hedgehog, and Wnt signaling pathways may be essential [91] (Figure 1). GB expresses a number of stemness-associated markers including cell surface markers (CD133, CD15, A2B5, and L1CAM), cytoskeletal proteins (nestin), transcription factors (SOX2, NANOG, and OCT4), post-transcriptional factors (Musashi1), and polycomb transcriptional suppressors (Bmi1 and Ezh2) [85]. There is also evidence of plasticity and bi-directional interconversion between CSCs and cancer cells [92]. In a landmark study, pluripotent stem cells were formed from reprogrammed mouse embryonic and adult fibroblasts by the addition of transcription factors OCT4, SOX2, c-MYC, and KLF4 [93]. These factors, in addition to NANOG, which are expressed by ESCs, have been identified in GB [84]. The capacity of GB cells for perpetual self-renewal may rely on the contribution from transcription factors such as OCT4 and SOX2 [85]. SOX2 is highly expressed in GB [84] and may play a key role in maintaining plasticity for bi-directional cellular conversion in GB [94]. Moreover, silencing of SOX2 inhibits tumor proliferation in GB [95] and, thus, it may be a potential therapeutic target in the treatment of GB [96]. Another potential therapeutic target involves the JAK–STAT3 signaling pathway which is also associated with the self-renewal capacity of GB. Inhibition of this pathway may impede the migratory and invasive potential of GB by decreasing activation of the transcription factor STAT3 and, thus, reducing the levels of MMPs and associated invadopodia activity [97]. In addition, STAT3 binding to the *Notch1* promoter inhibits this signaling pathway and may impede the maintenance of glioma stem-like cells while reducing the expression of glioma stem cell markers CD133, SOX2, and nestin [98] (Figure 1).

4. The Renin–Angiotensin System and Convergent Signaling Pathways in Glioblastoma

The RAS has been proposed to play an important role in the TME [19] in various cancer types, including lung cancer, through its effect on tumor cells, non-malignant cells, hypoxia, angiogenesis, and the inflammatory response [99]. The RAS is a complex physiological system and has a multitude of interactions with many different convergent signaling pathways that operate in carcinogenesis, some of which lie outside the scope of this article.

Classically, the RAS regulates blood pressure and electrolyte and fluid homeostasis involving primarily the renal, cardiovascular, and endocrine systems [100]. The RAS pathway is composed of multiple steps culminating in the formation of the main effector hormone, angiotensin II (ATII) [101]. Activity of this key homeostatic system in the CNS is well documented [102]. In this review article, RAS inhibition broadly refers to inhibition of any of the components of the RAS, reducing its downstream effects.

Angiotensinogen, primarily synthesized in the liver by hepatocytes, is cleaved by renin, to form angiotensin I (AT1) [103]. Angiotensinogen is synthesized and secreted by astrocytes and is converted to several neuroactive peptides [104,105]. Angiotensinogen is also produced within neurons, which can secrete or retain it intracellularly. These neuroactive peptides bind their respective receptors within the local microenvironment to induce receptor signaling by different cell types [104,105]. Renin is physiologically derived from the juxtaglomerular apparatus in the kidneys and its release is tightly regulated by macula densa and local baroreceptors [106]. Renin is formed by the binding of prorenin to the prorenin receptor (PRR) [107] and is also catalyzed by enzymes such as cathepsins B, D, and G [108–111]. ATI is converted to ATII by angiotensin-converting enzyme (ACE), also known as ACE1, which is primarily found in the lungs [112]. ATII binds to ATII receptor 1 (AT_1R) and ATII receptor 2 (AT_2R) [113]. ATII binding to AT_1R causes MAPK–STAT3 activation [114] and phosphatidylinositol signaling, which increases cytosolic Ca^{2+} and effects mitogenesis [115]. AT_1R signaling increases RAS activity in the TME, and the formation of NF-κB and TGF-$β_1$ which promotes cellular proliferation, inflammation, and angiogenesis [116]. AT_2R activation by ATII inhibits cellular growth and enhances apoptosis [116]. ATII can be further converted into angiotensin III (ATIII), and then angiotensin IV (ATIV) by aminopeptidase-A (AP-A) and aminopeptidase-N (AP-N), respectively. ATIV binds to ATII receptor 4 (AT_4R), and in high concentrations, may bind to AT_1R. Angiotensin (1–7) (Ang(1–7)) is produced by the cleavage of either ATI by neutral endopeptidase (NEP) or ATII by ACE2, an isoform of ACE. Ang(1–7) binds to Mas receptors (MasRs) [117,118]. ATI may also be cleaved by ACE2 to form Ang(1–9), which can be cleaved by ACE1 and is converted to Ang(1–7), which in addition to binding to MasRs, can also bind to AT_2R with low affinity, and Mas-related-G protein coupled receptors (MrgDs) [119]. MrgDs are a recently discovered component of the RAS [102], and their role in the GB TME is yet to be defined. Lastly, the primary ligand for MrgDs is almandine, an Ang(1–7) analog formed by decarboxylation of Ang(1–7) [102] (Figure 2).

Key components of the RAS are also activated in CNS diseases [101]. Renin, and its precursor prorenin, are expressed variably in neurons, astrocytes, oligodendrocytes, and microglia in different regions of the brain [120,121]. PRR is widely distributed in different organs throughout the body including the brain, eyes, and immune system [122]. ACE1 is expressed in areas of the brain involved in blood pressure control and homeostasis including the choroid plexus, organum vasculosum of the lamina terminalis, subfornical organ, and area postrema [104]. ACE2 is found in the endothelium of the brain in various regions including the cortex and brainstem [123]. ACE2 contributes to the neuroprotective ACE2/Ang(1–7)MasR signaling axis by converting ATII to Ang(1–7) which is a ligand for MasR [124].

The RAS, as a constituent of the TME, is involved in several hallmarks of cancer, including angiogenesis, hypoxia, and tumor cell proliferation [125]. Components of the RAS are expressed in different types of cancer including colon adenocarcinoma [126] and malignant melanoma [127]. RAS components are also expressed by CSCs in oral cavity SCC [128,129], renal clear cell carcinoma [130], primary [131], and metastatic [132], cutaneous SCC, metastatic colon adenocarcinoma [133], metastatic malignant melanoma [82,83], and GB [134]. In GB, PRR, AT_1R, and AT_2R are co-expressed with stemness-associated markers [134]. PRR is highly expressed in GB compared with lower-grade gliomas; this higher expression of PRR in higher-grade glioma is notable as the Wnt/β-catenin signaling pathway is implicated in the self-renewal of stem cells [135] (Figure 1).

The Wnt/β-catenin signaling pathway, which sits downstream of the RAS, is implicated in tumor initiation in several cancer types [136]. In brief, this pathway results in active β-catenin translocating into the nucleus, upregulating the expression of oncogenes such as c-Myc, AXIN2, and CCND1 [136]. PRR is a component of the Wnt receptor complex and acts as an adapter between vacuolar H^+-adenosine triphosphate (V-ATPase) and low-density lipoprotein receptor-related protein 6. V-ATPase, a proton pump, is essential for cellular acidification and is involved in the mechanism for β-catenin activation [137]. This process facilitates binding of Wnts to their respective Wnt receptor complex [138]. Further, PRR promotes brain cancers via the Wnt/β-catenin signaling pathway, and in addition to being a membrane receptor, exists in the cytoplasm and increases the protein expression of Wnt2 within glioma cells [135]. This evidence underscores the PRR as a potential oncoprotein via Wnt/β-catenin pathway-related carcinogenesis [136], which influences cell stemness [139], tumorigenesis, and cellular proliferation [140,141]. Renin is expressed in GB and may contribute to the mechanisms of neovascularization in GB [142].

Furthermore, downregulation of the Ang(1–7)/MAS signaling axis by podocalyxin results in enhanced GB cell invasion and proliferation [143]. Finally, bypass loops of the RAS involving various cathepsins that may also contribute to the proliferative activity in GB, for example, cathepsin G coverts ATI to AII and from AGT directly to ATII, which binds to AT_1R, to promote cancer progression [144–146]. GB CSCs have been shown to secrete Wnt-induced signaling protein 1 (WISP1) that promotes the survival of both the CSCs and M2 TAMs to promote a pro-TME [147] (Figure 1).

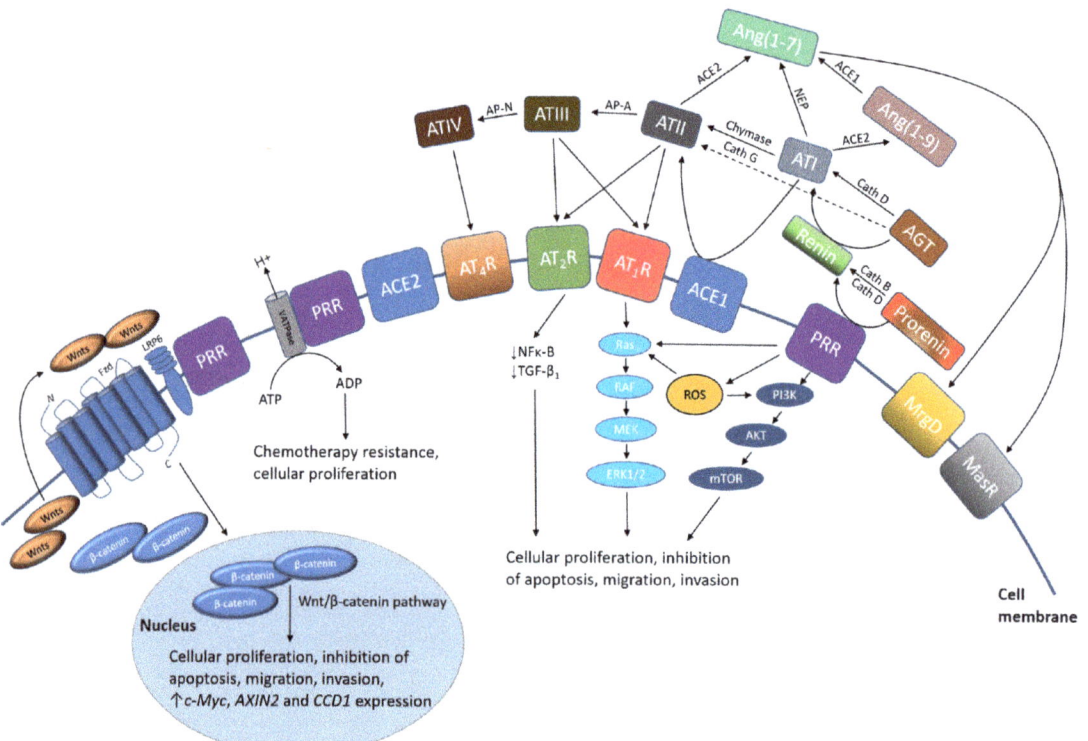

Figure 2. A schema showing the effect of the renin–angiotensin system (RAS) and its convergent signaling pathways on the tumor microenvironment to influence cellular proliferation, invasiveness, and cell survival in cancer development. The RAS interacts with downstream pathways, such as the Ras/RAF/MEK/ERK (light blue) pathway and the PI3K/AKT/mTOR (dark blue) pathway, and the upstream Wnt/β-catenin pathway (intermediate blue) that influence cellular proliferation, migration, inhibition of apoptosis, migration, and invasion (see text). PRR, pro-renin receptor; LRP6, low-density lipoprotein receptor-related protein; Fzd, frizzled receptor; Cath G, cathepsin G; Cath B, cathepsin B; Cath D, cathepsin D; ACE1, angiotensin-converting enzyme 1; ACE2, angiotensin-converting enzyme 2; ADP, adenosine diphosphate; AGT, angiotensinogen; ATP, adenosine triphosphate; Ang(1–7), angiotensin (1–7); Ang(1–9), angiotensin (1–9); AP-A, aminopeptidase-A; NEP, neutral endopeptidase; AP-N, aminopeptidase-N; ATI, angiotensin I; ATII, angiotensin II; ATIII, angiotensin III; ATIV, angiotensin IV; AT_1R, angiotensin II receptor 1; AT_2R, angiotensin II receptor 2; AT_4R, angiotensin II receptor 4; MrgD, Mas-related-G protein coupled receptor; MasR, Mas receptor; mTOR, mammalian target of rapamycin; NF-κB, nuclear factor kappa B; TGF-$β_1$, transforming growth factor-$β_1$; V-ATPase, vacuolar H^+-adenosine triphosphate.

Other related signaling pathways, such as the PI3K/AKT/mammalian target of rapamycin (mTOR) and Ras/RAF/MEK/ERK pathways within the GB TME, downstream to the RAS, are activated via AT_1R and PRR signal transduction. MAPK/ERK signaling is activated upon binding of renin or prorenin to PRR, and this upregulates ERK1/2 in various cell types including neurons [148]. ERK1/2 activation induces TGF-$β_1$ formation and cellular proliferation, both of which influence cancer development [136]. Supporting this is the fact that silencing of PRR downregulates expression of ERK1/2, AKT, and NF-κB [149]. Additionally, PRR activation leads to the production of reactive oxygen species, which activates both the PI3K/AKT/mTOR and Ras/RAF/MEK/ERK pathways (Figure 2). It is interesting to speculate that both pathways operate in conjunction with the RAS and Wnt/β-catenin to influence proliferation, survival, stemness, and invasiveness of CSCs within the GB TME.

The use of RAS inhibitors (RASis) in the treatment of cancer may mitigate the cytotoxic treatment-related adverse effects experienced by cancer patients to improve their overall quality of life [150]. A meta-analysis of 17 observational studies by Shen et al. [123] show RASis are associated with a reduced risk of cancer [151]. A prospective population-based study also shows long-term (>3 years) administration of RASis is associated with a decreased risk of cancer in patients with a DD genotype, which is associated with high levels of ACE and, thus, increased RAS activity. This is relevant as increased levels of ATII caused by elevated RAS activity promotes cancer progression by its actions on AT_1R [152]. Other epidemiological studies have shown a protective benefit of RASis against colorectal cancer [153,154] and an overall reduced risk of cancer [155]. RASis have also been shown to improve the overall survival of patients with aggressive non-metastatic pancreatic ductal adenocarcinoma [156]. Although current data remain inconclusive, RASis appear to be broadly protective against cancer [157].

A retrospective study analyzing clinical data from 810 patients enrolled in two large multicenter studies investigating the role of two drugs targeting the RAS combined with statins in GB, shows no benefit in overall survival [158]. A recent trial on repurposing multiple drugs in combination with temozolomide, including two drugs that affect the RAS (i.e., captopril and celecoxib) for patients with GB, observed maintenance of good quality of life [159]. Captopril, an ACE inhibitor, and celecoxib, which inhibits cyclocoxygenase-2, reduce RAS activity [19]. In addition, RASis, in combination with bevacizumab, improve survival in patients with GB [160], although there is no overall survival benefit of this VEGF inhibitor as a monotherapy for de novo or recurrent GB [161]. PRR may be a critical biomarker and a therapeutic target for the treatment of GB with its connections to V-ATPase function [162], and the Wnt/β-catenin, MAPK/ERK, and PI3K/AKT/mTOR pathways [135,136,149,163] (Figure 1). Several other steps of the RAS pathway can potentially be targeted [164]. The effects of a novel approach, targeting the RAS, its bypass loops, and converging pathways simultaneously using multiple repurposed drugs on the quality of life and progression-free survival in GB patients are currently being investigated in a clinical trial [165]. Therapeutic options may be facilitated by augmenting the compensatory mechanisms of the RAS [136,164–166].

5. Recent Developments

Recent technological breakthroughs in generating human cerebral organoids [167] from pluripotent cells, combined with genetic engineering [168], mass spectroscopic proteomics [169], and next generation gene sequencing tools [170], allow more detailed investigation into the GB TME, and the role of the RAS in this *niche*. Cerebral organoids have been shown to more faithfully recapitulate the temporal and spatial aspects of the developing brain [171,172]. Vascularized cerebral organoids have been developed by utilizing ectopic expression of human ETS variant 2 in engineered ESCs to form a vascular-like network in organoids akin to endothelial cells [173]. In addition, VEGF has been used to induce blood vessel-like structures in cerebral organoids expressing markers associated with the BBB, namely, CD31 and claudin-5 [174]. In addition, human umbilical vein endothelial cells have been used to develop cerebral organoids with a well-developed tubular vascular structure. In another notable development, choroid plexus-like organoids modeled cerebrospinal fluid production with a selective barrier akin to the BBB, which may be used to model the BBTB in the GB TME [175–177]. Using RNA sequencing, moreover, GB cerebral organoid models have been shown to best mimic the cellular states and plasticity found in the GB TME compared to gliospheres, tumor organoids, and orthotopic patient-derived xenografts [177].

6. Conclusions

Despite intensive research into the biology and treatment of GB, the prognosis of patients with GB remains dismal. Understanding the heterogeneity of the tumor–host microenvironment in GB, the role of RAS and CSCs, and mapping salient interactions on a cellular level employing techniques, such as single-cell RNA sequencing, may lead to the discovery of potential therapeutic targets [178]. Cerebral and GB organoids represent an exciting yet relatively cost-effective way to delineate relevant signaling pathways within the GB TME, including the RAS, and provide models for developing and testing drug screening and therapeutic targets including RASis [179].

Author Contributions: M.O. and E.J.K. drafted the manuscript. T.M., A.H.K., S.T.T. and A.C.W. critically revised the manuscript. All authors commented on and approved the manuscript.

Funding: This research received no external funding.

Conflicts of Interest: The authors declare that the research was conducted in the absence of any commercial or financial relationships that could be construed as a potential conflict of interest. S.T.T. is an inventor of the patents Cancer Diagnosis and Therapy (PCT/NZ2015/050108; AUS/2012302419; JAP/2017528398; US/0281472), Cancer Therapeutic (PCT/NZ2018/050006), and Novel Pharmaceutical Compositions for Cancer Therapy (PCT/NZ2019/050087).

References

1. Louis, D.N.; Perry, A.; Reifenberger, G.; Von Deimling, A.; Figarella-Branger, D.; Cavenee, W.K.; Ohgaki, H.; Wiestler, O.D.; Kleihues, P.; Ellison, D.W. The 2016 World Health Organization Classification of Tumors of the Central Nervous System: A summary. *Acta Neuropathol.* **2016**, *131*, 803–820. [CrossRef]
2. Crespo, I.; Vital, A.L.; Gonzalez-Tablas, M.; Patino Mdel, C.; Otero, A.; Lopes, M.C.; De Oliveira, C.; Domingues, P.; Orfao, A.; Tabernero, M.D. Molecular and Genomic Alterations in Glioblastoma Multiforme. *Am. J. Pathol.* **2015**, *185*, 1820–1833. [CrossRef] [PubMed]
3. Verhaak, R.G.; Hoadley, K.A.; Purdom, E.; Wang, V.; Qi, Y.; Wilkerson, M.D.; Miller, C.R.; Ding, L.; Golub, T.; Mesirov, J.P.; et al. Integrated genomic analysis identifies clinically relevant subtypes of glioblastoma characterized by abnormalities in PDGFRA, IDH1, EGFR, and NF1. *Cancer Cell* **2010**, *17*, 98–110. [CrossRef] [PubMed]
4. Wang, Q.; Hu, B.; Hu, X.; Kim, H.; Squatrito, M.; Scarpace, L.; DeCarvalho, A.C.; Lyu, S.; Li, P.; Li, Y.; et al. Tumor Evolution of Glioma-Intrinsic Gene Expression Subtypes Associates with Immunological Changes in the Microenvironment. *Cancer Cell* **2017**, *32*, 42–56.e46. [CrossRef] [PubMed]
5. Capper, D.; Zentgraf, H.; Balss, J.; Hartmann, C.; Von Deimling, A. Monoclonal antibody specific for IDH1 R132H mutation. *Acta Neuropathol.* **2009**, *118*, 599–601. [CrossRef] [PubMed]
6. Garrett, M.; Fujii, Y.; Osaka, N.; Ito, D.; Hirota, Y.; Sasaki, A.T. Emerging Roles of Wild-type and Mutant IDH1 in Growth, Metabolism and Therapeutics of Glioma. In *Gliomas*; Debinski, W., Ed.; Exon Publications: Brisbane, Australia, 2021. [CrossRef]
7. Stupp, R.; Mason, W.P.; Van den Bent, M.J.; Weller, M.; Fisher, B.; Taphoorn, M.J.; Belanger, K.; Brandes, A.A.; Marosi, C.; Bogdahn, U.; et al. Radiotherapy plus concomitant and adjuvant temozolomide for glioblastoma. *N. Engl. J. Med.* **2005**, *352*, 987–996. [CrossRef]
8. Hegi, M.E.; Diserens, A.C.; Gorlia, T.; Hamou, M.F.; De Tribolet, N.; Weller, M.; Kros, J.M.; Hainfellner, J.A.; Mason, W.; Mariani, L.; et al. MGMT gene silencing and benefit from temozolomide in glioblastoma. *N. Engl. J. Med.* **2005**, *352*, 997–1003. [CrossRef]
9. Binabaj, M.M.; Bahrami, A.; ShahidSales, S.; Joodi, M.; Joudi Mashhad, M.; Hassanian, S.M.; Anvari, K.; Avan, A. The prognostic value of MGMT promoter methylation in glioblastoma: A meta-analysis of clinical trials. *J. Cell Physiol.* **2018**, *233*, 378–386. [CrossRef]
10. Das, S.; Marsden, P.A. Angiogenesis in glioblastoma. *N. Engl. J. Med.* **2013**, *369*, 1561–1563. [CrossRef]
11. Gately, L.; McLachlan, S.A.; Dowling, A.; Philip, J. Life beyond a diagnosis of glioblastoma: A systematic review of the literature. *J. Cancer Surviv.* **2017**, *11*, 447–452. [CrossRef]
12. Simon, T.; Jackson, E.; Giamas, G. Breaking through the glioblastoma micro-environment via extracellular vesicles. *Oncogene* **2020**, *39*, 4477–4490. [CrossRef] [PubMed]
13. Awan, M.; Liu, S.; Sahgal, A.; Das, S.; Chao, S.T.; Chang, E.L.; Knisely, J.P.; Redmond, K.; Sohn, J.W.; Machtay, M.; et al. Extra-CNS metastasis from glioblastoma: A rare clinical entity. *Expert Rev. Anticancer Ther.* **2015**, *15*, 545–552. [CrossRef] [PubMed]
14. Da Ros, M.; De Gregorio, V.; Iorio, A.L.; Giunti, L.; Guidi, M.; De Martino, M.; Genitori, L.; Sardi, I. Glioblastoma Chemoresistance: The Double Play by Microenvironment and Blood-Brain Barrier. *Int. J. Mol. Sci.* **2018**, *19*, 2879. [CrossRef] [PubMed]

15. Schiffer, D.; Annovazzi, L.; Casalone, C.; Corona, C.; Mellai, M. Glioblastoma: Microenvironment and Niche Concept. *Cancers* **2018**, *11*, 5. [CrossRef]
16. Balkwill, F.R.; Capasso, M.; Hagemann, T. The tumor microenvironment at a glance. *J. Cell Sci.* **2012**, *125*, 5591–5596. [CrossRef]
17. Sullivan, R.; Maresh, G.; Zhang, X.; Salomon, C.; Hooper, J.; Margolin, D.; Li, L. The Emerging Roles of Extracellular Vesicles As Communication Vehicles within the Tumor Microenvironment and Beyond. *Front. Endocrinol.* **2017**, *8*, 194. [CrossRef]
18. Haznedaroglu, I.C.; Malkan, U.Y. Local bone marrow renin-angiotensin system in the genesis of leukemia and other malignancies. *Eur. Rev. Med. Pharmacol. Sci.* **2016**, *20*, 4089–4111.
19. Kilmister, E.J.; Tan, S.T. The Role of the Renin-Angiotensin System in the Cancer Stem Cell Niche. *J. Histochem. Cytochem.* **2021**, 00221554211026295. [CrossRef]
20. Hambardzumyan, D.; Bergers, G. Glioblastoma: Defining Tumor Niches. *Trends Cancer* **2015**, *1*, 252–265. [CrossRef]
21. Bao, S.; Wu, Q.; Sathornsumetee, S.; Hao, Y.; Li, Z.; Hjelmeland, A.B.; Shi, Q.; McLendon, R.E.; Bigner, D.D.; Rich, J.N. Stem cell-like glioma cells promote tumor angiogenesis through vascular endothelial growth factor. *Cancer Res.* **2006**, *66*, 7843–7848. [CrossRef]
22. Calabrese, C.; Poppleton, H.; Kocak, M.; Hogg, T.L.; Fuller, C.; Hamner, B.; Oh, E.Y.; Gaber, M.W.; Finklestein, D.; Allen, M.; et al. A perivascular niche for brain tumor stem cells. *Cancer Cell* **2007**, *11*, 69–82. [CrossRef]
23. Zhang, Q.; Xiang, W.; Xue, B.Z.; Yi, D.Y.; Zhao, H.Y.; Fu, P. Growth factors contribute to the mediation of angiogenic capacity of glioma-associated mesenchymal stem cells. *Oncol. Lett.* **2021**, *21*, 215. [CrossRef] [PubMed]
24. Monteforte, A.; Lam, B.; Sherman, M.B.; Henderson, K.; Sligar, A.D.; Spencer, A.; Tang, B.; Dunn, A.K.; Baker, A.B. (*) Glioblastoma Exosomes for Therapeutic Angiogenesis in Peripheral Ischemia. *Tissue Eng. Part A* **2017**, *23*, 1251–1261. [CrossRef] [PubMed]
25. Du, R.; Lu, K.V.; Petritsch, C.; Liu, P.; Ganss, R.; Passegue, E.; Song, H.; Vandenberg, S.; Johnson, R.S.; Werb, Z.; et al. HIF1alpha induces the recruitment of bone marrow-derived vascular modulatory cells to regulate tumor angiogenesis and invasion. *Cancer Cell* **2008**, *13*, 206–220. [CrossRef] [PubMed]
26. Wang, R.; Chadalavada, K.; Wilshire, J.; Kowalik, U.; Hovinga, K.E.; Geber, A.; Fligelman, B.; Leversha, M.; Brennan, C.; Tabar, V. Glioblastoma stem-like cells give rise to tumour endothelium. *Nature* **2010**, *468*, 829–833. [CrossRef] [PubMed]
27. Ricci-Vitiani, L.; Pallini, R.; Biffoni, M.; Todaro, M.; Invernici, G.; Cenci, T.; Maira, G.; Parati, E.A.; Stassi, G.; Larocca, L.M.; et al. Tumour vascularization via endothelial differentiation of glioblastoma stem-like cells. *Nature* **2010**, *468*, 824–828. [CrossRef] [PubMed]
28. Cheng, L.; Huang, Z.; Zhou, W.; Wu, Q.; Donnola, S.; Liu, J.K.; Fang, X.; Sloan, A.E.; Mao, Y.; Lathia, J.D.; et al. Glioblastoma stem cells generate vascular pericytes to support vessel function and tumor growth. *Cell* **2013**, *153*, 139–152. [CrossRef]
29. Tamura, R.; Tanaka, T.; Akasaki, Y.; Murayama, Y.; Yoshida, K.; Sasaki, H. The role of vascular endothelial growth factor in the hypoxic and immunosuppressive tumor microenvironment: Perspectives for therapeutic implications. *Med. Oncol.* **2019**, *37*, 2. [CrossRef] [PubMed]
30. Van Tellingen, O.; Yetkin-Arik, B.; De Gooijer, M.C.; Wesseling, P.; Wurdinger, T.; De Vries, H.E. Overcoming the blood-brain tumor barrier for effective glioblastoma treatment. *Drug Resist. Updat.* **2015**, *19*, 1–12. [CrossRef] [PubMed]
31. Ballabh, P.; Braun, A.; Nedergaard, M. The blood-brain barrier: An overview: Structure, regulation, and clinical implications. *Neurobiol. Dis.* **2004**, *16*, 1–13. [CrossRef]
32. Abbott, N.J.; Patabendige, A.A.; Dolman, D.E.; Yusof, S.R.; Begley, D.J. Structure and function of the blood-brain barrier. *Neurobiol. Dis.* **2010**, *37*, 13–25. [CrossRef] [PubMed]
33. Bergers, G.; Song, S. The role of pericytes in blood-vessel formation and maintenance. *Neuro. Oncol.* **2005**, *7*, 452–464. [CrossRef] [PubMed]
34. Monteiro, A.R.; Hill, R.; Pilkington, G.J.; Madureira, P.A. The Role of Hypoxia in Glioblastoma Invasion. *Cells* **2017**, *6*, 45. [CrossRef]
35. Rong, Y.; Durden, D.L.; Van Meir, E.G.; Brat, D.J. 'Pseudopalisading' necrosis in glioblastoma: A familiar morphologic feature that links vascular pathology, hypoxia, and angiogenesis. *J. Neuropathol. Exp. Neurol.* **2006**, *65*, 529–539. [CrossRef]
36. Seidel, S.; Garvalov, B.K.; Wirta, V.; Von Stechow, L.; Schanzer, A.; Meletis, K.; Wolter, M.; Sommerlad, D.; Henze, A.T.; Nister, M.; et al. A hypoxic niche regulates glioblastoma stem cells through hypoxia inducible factor 2 alpha. *Brain* **2010**, *133*, 983–995. [CrossRef] [PubMed]
37. Soeda, A.; Park, M.; Lee, D.; Mintz, A.; Androutsellis-Theotokis, A.; McKay, R.D.; Engh, J.; Iwama, T.; Kunisada, T.; Kassam, A.B.; et al. Hypoxia promotes expansion of the CD133-positive glioma stem cells through activation of HIF-1alpha. *Oncogene* **2009**, *28*, 3949–3959. [CrossRef]
38. Bar, E.E.; Lin, A.; Mahairaki, V.; Matsui, W.; Eberhart, C.G. Hypoxia increases the expression of stem-cell markers and promotes clonogenicity in glioblastoma neurospheres. *Am. J. Pathol.* **2010**, *177*, 1491–1502. [CrossRef]
39. Guardia, G.D.A.; Correa, B.R.; Araujo, P.R.; Qiao, M.; Burns, S.; Penalva, L.O.F.; Galante, P.A.F. Proneural and mesenchymal glioma stem cells display major differences in splicing and lncRNA profiles. *NPJ Genom. Med.* **2020**, *5*, 2. [CrossRef] [PubMed]
40. Zagzag, D.; Lukyanov, Y.; Lan, L.; Ali, M.A.; Esencay, M.; Mendez, O.; Yee, H.; Voura, E.B.; Newcomb, E.W. Hypoxia-inducible factor 1 and VEGF upregulate CXCR4 in glioblastoma: Implications for angiogenesis and glioma cell invasion. *Lab. Investig.* **2006**, *86*, 1221–1232. [CrossRef]
41. Bar, E.E. Glioblastoma, cancer stem cells and hypoxia. *Brain Pathol.* **2011**, *21*, 119–129. [CrossRef]

42. Filatova, A.; Acker, T.; Garvalov, B.K. The cancer stem cell niche(s): The crosstalk between glioma stem cells and their microenvironment. *Biochim. Biophys. Acta* **2013**, *1830*, 2496–2508. [CrossRef]
43. Cui, T.X.; Kryczek, I.; Zhao, L.; Zhao, E.; Kuick, R.; Roh, M.H.; Vatan, L.; Szeliga, W.; Mao, Y.; Thomas, D.G.; et al. Myeloid-derived suppressor cells enhance stemness of cancer cells by inducing microRNA101 and suppressing the corepressor CtBP2. *Immunity* **2013**, *39*, 611–621. [CrossRef]
44. Feng, X.; Szulzewsky, F.; Yerevanian, A.; Chen, Z.; Heinzmann, D.; Rasmussen, R.D.; Alvarez-Garcia, V.; Kim, Y.; Wang, B.; Tamagno, I.; et al. Loss of CX3CR1 increases accumulation of inflammatory monocytes and promotes gliomagenesis. *Oncotarget* **2015**, *6*, 15077–15094. [CrossRef]
45. Liang, J.; Piao, Y.; Holmes, L.; Fuller, G.N.; Henry, V.; Tiao, N.; De Groot, J.F. Neutrophils promote the malignant glioma phenotype through S100A4. *Clin. Cancer Res.* **2014**, *20*, 187–198. [CrossRef]
46. Mi, Y.; Guo, N.; Luan, J.; Cheng, J.; Hu, Z.; Jiang, P.; Jin, W.; Gao, X. The Emerging Role of Myeloid-Derived Suppressor Cells in the Glioma Immune Suppressive Microenvironment. *Front. Immunol.* **2020**, *11*, 737. [CrossRef]
47. Charles, N.A.; Holland, E.C.; Gilbertson, R.; Glass, R.; Kettenmann, H. The brain tumor microenvironment. *Glia* **2011**, *59*, 1169–1180. [CrossRef]
48. Zhu, C.; Kros, J.M.; Cheng, C.; Mustafa, D. The contribution of tumor-associated macrophages in glioma neo-angiogenesis and implications for anti-angiogenic strategies. *Neuro. Oncol.* **2017**, *19*, 1435–1446. [CrossRef]
49. Jayasingam, S.D.; Citartan, M.; Thang, T.H.; Mat Zin, A.A.; Ang, K.C.; Ch'ng, E.S. Evaluating the Polarization of Tumor-Associated Macrophages Into M1 and M2 Phenotypes in Human Cancer Tissue: Technicalities and Challenges in Routine Clinical Practice. *Front. Oncol.* **2019**, *9*, 1512. [CrossRef] [PubMed]
50. Pires-Afonso, Y.; Niclou, S.P.; Michelucci, A. Revealing and Harnessing Tumour-Associated Microglia/Macrophage Heterogeneity in Glioblastoma. *Int. J. Mol. Sci.* **2020**, *21*, 689. [CrossRef]
51. Pan, Y.; Yu, Y.; Wang, X.; Zhang, T. Tumor-Associated Macrophages in Tumor Immunity. *Front. Immunol.* **2020**, *11*, 583084. [CrossRef]
52. Ye, X.Z.; Xu, S.L.; Xin, Y.H.; Yu, S.C.; Ping, Y.F.; Chen, L.; Xiao, H.L.; Wang, B.; Yi, L.; Wang, Q.L.; et al. Tumor-associated microglia/macrophages enhance the invasion of glioma stem-like cells via TGF-beta1 signaling pathway. *J. Immunol.* **2012**, *189*, 444–453. [CrossRef]
53. Jaiswal, S.; Jamieson, C.H.; Pang, W.W.; Park, C.Y.; Chao, M.P.; Majeti, R.; Traver, D.; Van Rooijen, N.; Weissman, I.L. CD47 is upregulated on circulating hematopoietic stem cells and leukemia cells to avoid phagocytosis. *Cell* **2009**, *138*, 271–285. [CrossRef]
54. Hutter, G.; Theruvath, J.; Graef, C.M.; Zhang, M.; Schoen, M.K.; Bennett, M.L.; Olson, A.; Azad, T.D.; Sinha, R.; et al. Microglia are effector cells of CD47-SIRPalpha antiphagocytic axis disruption against glioblastoma. *Proc. Natl. Acad. Sci. USA* **2019**, *116*, 997–1006. [CrossRef]
55. Jaynes, J.M.; Sable, R.; Ronzetti, M.; Bautista, W.; Knotts, Z.; Abisoye-Ogunniyan, A.; Li, D.; Calvo, R.; Dashnyam, M.; Singh, A.; et al. Mannose receptor (CD206) activation in tumor-associated macrophages enhances adaptive and innate antitumor immune responses. *Sci. Transl. Med.* **2020**, *12*, aax6337. [CrossRef]
56. Wu, H.; Han, Y.; Rodriguez Sillke, Y.; Deng, H.; Siddiqui, S.; Treese, C.; Schmidt, F.; Friedrich, M.; Keye, J.; Wan, J.; et al. Lipid droplet-dependent fatty acid metabolism controls the immune suppressive phenotype of tumor-associated macrophages. *EMBO Mol. Med.* **2019**, *11*, e10698. [CrossRef]
57. Azambuja, J.H.; Ludwig, N.; Yerneni, S.S.; Braganhol, E.; Whiteside, T.L. Arginase-1+ Exosomes from Reprogrammed Macrophages Promote Glioblastoma Progression. *Int. J. Mol. Sci.* **2020**, *21*, 3990. [CrossRef]
58. Reya, T.; Morrison, S.J.; Clarke, M.F.; Weissman, I.L. Stem cells, cancer, and cancer stem cells. *Nature* **2001**, *414*, 105–111. [CrossRef]
59. Clarke, M.F.; Dick, J.E.; Dirks, P.B.; Eaves, C.J.; Jamieson, C.H.; Jones, D.L.; Visvader, J.; Weissman, I.L.; Wahl, G.M. Cancer stem cells–perspectives on current status and future directions: AACR Workshop on cancer stem cells. *Cancer Res.* **2006**, *66*, 9339–9344. [CrossRef]
60. Tang, D.G. Understanding cancer stem cell heterogeneity and plasticity. *Cell Res.* **2012**, *22*, 457–472. [CrossRef]
61. Adams, J.M.; Strasser, A. Is tumor growth sustained by rare cancer stem cells or dominant clones? *Cancer Res.* **2008**, *68*, 4018–4021. [CrossRef]
62. Rich, J.N. Cancer stem cells: Understanding tumor hierarchy and heterogeneity. *Medecine* **2016**, *95*, S2–S7. [CrossRef]
63. Najafi, M.; Mortezaee, K.; Ahadi, R. Cancer stem cell (a)symmetry & plasticity: Tumorigenesis and therapy relevance. *Life Sci.* **2019**, *231*, 116520. [CrossRef]
64. Aponte, P.M.; Caicedo, A. Stemness in Cancer: Stem Cells, Cancer Stem Cells, and Their Microenvironment. *Stem Cells Int.* **2017**, *2017*, 5619472. [CrossRef]
65. Gurel, C.; Inetas, G.; Hortu, I.; Tunc, E.; Kuscu, G.C.; Dindaroglu, F.C.; Sahin, O.; Buhur, A.; Oktem, G. Cancer and Cancer Stem Cells: New Molecular Perspectives. *Crit. Rev. Oncog.* **2019**, *24*, 99–104. [CrossRef]
66. Clara, J.A.; Monge, C.; Yang, Y.; Takebe, N. Targeting signalling pathways and the immune microenvironment of cancer stem cells—A clinical update. *Nat. Rev. Clin. Oncol.* **2020**, *17*, 204–232. [CrossRef]
67. Bradshaw, A.; Wickremsekera, A.; Tan, S.T.; Peng, L.; Davis, P.F.; Itinteang, T. Cancer Stem Cell Hierarchy in Glioblastoma Multiforme. *Front. Surg.* **2016**, *3*, 21. [CrossRef]
68. Eun, K.; Ham, S.W.; Kim, H. Cancer stem cell heterogeneity: Origin and new perspectives on CSC targeting. *BMB Rep.* **2017**, *50*, 117–125. [CrossRef]

69. Plaks, V.; Kong, N.; Werb, Z. The cancer stem cell niche: How essential is the niche in regulating stemness of tumor cells? *Cell Stem Cell* **2015**, *16*, 225–238. [CrossRef]
70. Quail, D.F.; Taylor, M.J.; Postovit, L.M. Microenvironmental regulation of cancer stem cell phenotypes. *Curr. Stem Cell Res. Ther.* **2012**, *7*, 197–216. [CrossRef]
71. Chaffer, C.L.; Weinberg, R.A. How does multistep tumorigenesis really proceed? *Cancer Discov.* **2015**, *5*, 22–24. [CrossRef]
72. Zhao, C.; Chen, A.; Jamieson, C.H.; Fereshteh, M.; Abrahamsson, A.; Blum, J.; Kwon, H.Y.; Kim, J.; Chute, J.P.; Rizzieri, D.; et al. Hedgehog signalling is essential for maintenance of cancer stem cells in myeloid leukaemia. *Nature* **2009**, *458*, 776–779. [CrossRef]
73. Li, C.; Heidt, D.G.; Dalerba, P.; Burant, C.F.; Zhang, L.; Adsay, V.; Wicha, M.; Clarke, M.F.; Simeone, D.M. Identification of pancreatic cancer stem cells. *Cancer Res.* **2007**, *67*, 1030–1037. [CrossRef]
74. Al-Hajj, M.; Wicha, M.S.; Benito-Hernandez, A.; Morrison, S.J.; Clarke, M.F. Prospective identification of tumorigenic breast cancer cells. *Proc. Natl. Acad. Sci. USA* **2003**, *100*, 3983–3988. [CrossRef]
75. Baillie, R.; Itinteang, T.; Yu, H.H.; Brasch, H.D.; Davis, P.F.; Tan, S.T. Cancer stem cells in moderately differentiated oral tongue squamous cell carcinoma. *J. Clin. Pathol.* **2016**, *69*, 742–744. [CrossRef]
76. Yu, H.H.; Featherston, T.; Tan, S.T.; Chibnall, A.M.; Brasch, H.D.; Davis, P.F.; Itinteang, T. Characterization of cancer stem cells in moderately differentiated buccal mucosal squamous cell carcinoma. *Front. Surg.* **2016**, *3*, 46. [CrossRef] [PubMed]
77. Ram, R.; Brasch, H.D.; Dunne, J.C.; Davis, P.F.; Tan, S.T.; Itinteang, T. The identification of three cancer stem cell subpopulations within moderately differentiated lip squamous cell carcinoma. *Front. Surg.* **2017**, *4*, 12. [CrossRef]
78. Koh, S.P.; Brasch, H.D.; De Jongh, J.; Itinteang, T.; Tan, S.T. Cancer stem cell subpopulations in moderately differentiated head and neck cutaneous squamous cell carcinoma. *Heliyon* **2019**, *5*, e02257. [CrossRef]
79. Kilmister, E.J.; Patel, J.; Van Schaijik, B.; Bockett, N.; Brasch, H.D.; Paterson, E.; Sim, D.; Davis, P.F.; Roth, I.M.; Itinteang, T.; et al. Cancer Stem Cell Subpopulations Are Present Within Metastatic Head and Neck Cutaneous Squamous Cell Carcinoma. *Front. Oncol.* **2020**, *10*, 1091. [CrossRef]
80. Munro, M.J.; Wickremesekera, S.K.; Peng, L.; Marsh, R.W.; Itinteang, T.; Tan, S.T. Cancer stem cell subpopulations in primary colon adenocarcinoma. *PLoS ONE* **2019**, *14*, e0221963. [CrossRef]
81. Humphries, H.N.; Wickremesekera, S.K.; Marsh, R.W.; Brasch, H.D.; Mehrotra, S.; Tan, S.T.; Itinteang, T. Characterization of Cancer Stem Cells in Colon Adenocarcinoma Metastasis to the Liver. *Front. Surg.* **2018**, *4*, 76. [CrossRef]
82. Wickremesekera, A.C.; Brasch, H.D.; Lee, V.M.; Davis, P.F.; Parker, A.; Koeck, H.; Itinteang, T.; Tan, S.T. Cancer stem cell subpopulations in metastatic melanoma to the brain express components of the renin-angiotensin system. *J. Cancer Metastasis Treat.* **2019**, *5*, 62. [CrossRef]
83. Yoganandarajah, V.; Patel, J.; Van Schaijik, B.; Bockett, N.; Brasch, H.D.; Paterson, E.; Sim, D.; Davis, P.F.; Roth, I.M.; Itinteang, T.; et al. Identification of Cancer Stem Cell Subpopulations in Head and Neck Metastatic Malignant Melanoma. *Cells* **2020**, *9*, 324. [CrossRef] [PubMed]
84. Bradshaw, A.; Wickremesekera, A.; Brasch, H.D.; Chibnall, A.M.; Davis, P.F.; Tan, S.T.; Itinteang, T. Cancer Stem Cells in Glioblastoma Multiforme. *Front. Surg.* **2016**, *3*, 48. [CrossRef]
85. Kalkan, R. Glioblastoma Stem Cells as a New Therapeutic Target for Glioblastoma. *Clin. Med. Insights. Oncol.* **2015**, *9*, 95–103. [CrossRef]
86. Singh, S.K.; Clarke, I.D.; Terasaki, M.; Bonn, V.E.; Hawkins, C.; Squire, J.; Dirks, P.B. Identification of a cancer stem cell in human brain tumors. *Cancer Res.* **2003**, *63*, 5821–5828.
87. Galli, R.; Binda, E.; Orfanelli, U.; Cipelletti, B.; Gritti, A.; De Vitis, S.; Fiocco, R.; Foroni, C.; Dimeco, F.; Vescovi, A. Isolation and characterization of tumorigenic, stem-like neural precursors from human glioblastoma. *Cancer Res.* **2004**, *64*, 7011–7021. [CrossRef]
88. Tejero, R.; Huang, Y.; Katsyv, I.; Kluge, M.; Lin, J.Y.; Tome-Garcia, J.; Daviaud, N.; Wang, Y.; Zhang, B.; Tsankova, N.M.; et al. Gene signatures of quiescent glioblastoma cells reveal mesenchymal shift and interactions with niche microenvironment. *EBioMedicine* **2019**, *42*, 252–269. [CrossRef]
89. Cui, C.; Chen, X.; Liu, Y.; Cao, B.; Xing, Y.; Liu, C.; Yang, F.; Li, Y.; Yang, T.; Hua, L.; et al. beta1,4-Galactosyltransferase V activates Notch1 signaling in glioma stem-like cells and promotes their transdifferentiation into endothelial cells. *J. Biol. Chem.* **2018**, *293*, 2219–2230. [CrossRef] [PubMed]
90. Guichet, P.O.; Guelfi, S.; Teigell, M.; Hoppe, L.; Bakalara, N.; Bauchet, L.; Duffau, H.; Lamszus, K.; Rothhut, B.; Hugnot, J.P. Notch1 stimulation induces a vascularization switch with pericyte-like cell differentiation of glioblastoma stem cells. *Stem Cells* **2015**, *33*, 21–34. [CrossRef]
91. Iwadate, Y. Plasticity in Glioma Stem Cell Phenotype and Its Therapeutic Implication. *Neurol. Med. Chir.* **2018**, *58*, 61–70. [CrossRef]
92. Safa, A.R.; Saadatzadeh, M.R.; Cohen-Gadol, A.A.; Pollok, K.E.; Bijangi-Vishehsaraei, K. Glioblastoma stem cells (GSCs) epigenetic plasticity and interconversion between differentiated non-GSCs and GSCs. *Genes Dis.* **2015**, *2*, 152–163. [CrossRef] [PubMed]
93. Takahashi, K.; Yamanaka, S. Induction of pluripotent stem cells from mouse embryonic and adult fibroblast cultures by defined factors. *Cell* **2006**, *126*, 663–676. [CrossRef] [PubMed]
94. Berezovsky, A.D.; Poisson, L.M.; Cherba, D.; Webb, C.P.; Transou, A.D.; Lemke, N.W.; Hong, X.; Hasselbach, L.A.; Irtenkauf, S.M.; Mikkelsen, T.; et al. Sox2 promotes malignancy in glioblastoma by regulating plasticity and astrocytic differentiation. *Neoplasia* **2014**, *16*, 193–206.e25. [CrossRef]

95. Gangemi, R.M.; Griffero, F.; Marubbi, D.; Perera, M.; Capra, M.C.; Malatesta, P.; Ravetti, G.L.; Zona, G.L.; Daga, A.; Corte, G. SOX2 silencing in glioblastoma tumor-initiating cells causes stop of proliferation and loss of tumorigenicity. *Stem Cells* **2009**, *27*, 40–48. [CrossRef] [PubMed]
96. Garros-Regulez, L.; Garcia, I.; Carrasco-Garcia, E.; Lantero, A.; Aldaz, P.; Moreno-Cugnon, L.; Arrizabalaga, O.; Undabeitia, J.; Torres-Bayona, S.; Villanua, J.; et al. Targeting SOX2 as a Therapeutic Strategy in Glioblastoma. *Front. Oncol.* **2016**, *6*, 222. [CrossRef] [PubMed]
97. Senft, C.; Priester, M.; Polacin, M.; Schroder, K.; Seifert, V.; Kogel, D.; Weissenberger, J. Inhibition of the JAK-2/STAT3 signaling pathway impedes the migratory and invasive potential of human glioblastoma cells. *J. Neurooncol.* **2011**, *101*, 393–403. [CrossRef]
98. Yahyanejad, S.; King, H.; Iglesias, V.S.; Granton, P.V.; Barbeau, L.M.; Van Hoof, S.J.; Groot, A.J.; Habets, R.; Prickaerts, J.; Chalmers, A.J.; et al. NOTCH blockade combined with radiation therapy and temozolomide prolongs survival of orthotopic glioblastoma. *Oncotarget* **2016**, *7*, 41251–41264. [CrossRef]
99. Catarata, M.J.; Ribeiro, R.; Oliveira, M.J.; Robalo Cordeiro, C.; Medeiros, R. Renin-Angiotensin System in Lung Tumor and Microenvironment Interactions. *Cancers* **2020**, *12*, 1457. [CrossRef]
100. Sparks, M.A.; Crowley, S.D.; Gurley, S.B.; Mirotsou, M.; Coffman, T.M. Classical Renin-Angiotensin system in kidney physiology. *Compr. Physiol.* **2014**, *4*, 1201–1228. [CrossRef]
101. Nakagawa, P.; Gomez, J.; Grobe, J.L.; Sigmund, C.D. The Renin-Angiotensin System in the Central Nervous System and Its Role in Blood Pressure Regulation. *Curr. Hypertens. Rep.* **2020**, *22*, 7. [CrossRef]
102. Jackson, L.; Eldahshan, W.; Fagan, S.C.; Ergul, A. Within the Brain: The Renin Angiotensin System. *Int. J. Mol. Sci.* **2018**, *19*, 876. [CrossRef]
103. Cassis, L.A.; Saye, J.; Peach, M.J. Location and regulation of rat angiotensinogen messenger RNA. *Hypertension* **1988**, *11*, 591–596. [CrossRef]
104. Bodiga, V.L.; Bodiga, S. Renin Angiotensin System in Cognitive Function and Dementia. *Asian J. Neurosci.* **2013**, *2013*, 1–18. [CrossRef]
105. Grobe, J.L.; Xu, D.; Sigmund, C.D. An intracellular renin-angiotensin system in neurons: Fact, hypothesis, or fantasy. *Physiology* **2008**, *23*, 187–193. [CrossRef]
106. Kopp, U.C.; DiBona, G.F. Neural regulation of renin secretion. *Semin. Nephrol.* **1993**, *13*, 543–551. [PubMed]
107. Riquier-Brison, A.D.M.; Sipos, A.; Prokai, A.; Vargas, S.L.; Toma, L.; Meer, E.J.; Villanueva, K.G.; Chen, J.C.M.; Gyarmati, G.; Yih, C.; et al. The macula densa prorenin receptor is essential in renin release and blood pressure control. *Am. J. Physiol. Renal. Physiol.* **2018**, *315*, F521–F534. [CrossRef]
108. Jutras, I.; Reudelhuber, T.L. Prorenin processing by cathepsin B in vitro and in transfected cells. *FEBS Lett.* **1999**, *443*, 48–52. [CrossRef]
109. Neves, F.A.; Duncan, K.G.; Baxter, J.D. Cathepsin B is a prorenin processing enzyme. *Hypertension* **1996**, *27*, 514–517. [CrossRef]
110. Naseem, R.H.; Hedegard, W.; Henry, T.D.; Lessard, J.; Sutter, K.; Katz, S.A. Plasma cathepsin D isoforms and their active metabolites increase after myocardial infarction and contribute to plasma renin activity. *Basic Res. Cardiol.* **2005**, *100*, 139–146. [CrossRef]
111. Rykl, J.; Thiemann, J.; Kurzawski, S.; Pohl, T.; Gobom, J.; Zidek, W.; Schluter, H. Renal cathepsin G and angiotensin II generation. *J. Hypertens.* **2006**, *24*, 1797–1807. [CrossRef]
112. Balyasnikova, I.V.; Metzger, R.; Sun, Z.L.; Berestetskaya, Y.V.; Albrecht, R.F.; Danilov, S.M. Development and characterization of rat monoclonal antibodies to denatured mouse angiotensin-converting enzyme. *Tissue Antigens* **2005**, *65*, 240–251. [CrossRef]
113. Nakagawa, P.; Sigmund, C.D. How Is the Brain Renin-Angiotensin System Regulated? *Hypertension* **2017**, *70*, 10–18. [CrossRef]
114. Hashemzehi, M.; Beheshti, F.; Hassanian, S.M.; Ferns, G.A.; Khazaei, M.; Avan, A. Therapeutic potential of renin angiotensin system inhibitors in cancer cells metastasis. *Pathol. Res. Pract.* **2020**, *216*, 153010. [CrossRef]
115. Yu, C.; Tang, W.; Wang, Y.; Shen, Q.; Wang, B.; Cai, C.; Meng, X.; Zou, F. Downregulation of ACE2/Ang-(1-7)/Mas axis promotes breast cancer metastasis by enhancing store-operated calcium entry. *Cancer Lett.* **2016**, *376*, 268–277. [CrossRef]
116. Ziaja, M.; Urbanek, K.A.; Kowalska, K.; Piastowska-Ciesielska, A.W. Angiotensin II and Angiotensin Receptors 1 and 2-Multifunctional System in Cells Biology, What Do We Know? *Cells* **2021**, *10*, 381. [CrossRef]
117. Bernstein, K.E.; Koronyo, Y.; Salumbides, B.C.; Sheyn, J.; Pelissier, L.; Lopes, D.H.; Shah, K.H.; Bernstein, E.A.; Fuchs, D.T.; Yu, J.J.; et al. Angiotensin-converting enzyme overexpression in myelomonocytes prevents Alzheimer's-like cognitive decline. *J. Clin. Investig.* **2014**, *124*, 1000–1012. [CrossRef] [PubMed]
118. Elased, K.M.; Cunha, T.S.; Marcondes, F.K.; Morris, M. Brain angiotensin-converting enzymes: Role of angiotensin-converting enzyme 2 in processing angiotensin II in mice. *Exp. Physiol.* **2008**, *93*, 665–675. [CrossRef]
119. Tetzner, A.; Gebolys, K.; Meinert, C.; Klein, S.; Uhlich, A.; Trebicka, J.; Villacañas, Ó.; Walther, T. G-Protein–Coupled Receptor MrgD Is a Receptor for Angiotensin-(1–7) Involving Adenylyl Cyclase, cAMP, and Phosphokinase A. *Hypertension* **2016**, *68*, 185–194. [CrossRef]
120. Labandeira-Garcia, J.L.; Rodriguez-Perez, A.I.; Garrido-Gil, P.; Rodriguez-Pallares, J.; Lanciego, J.L.; Guerra, M.J. Brain Renin-Angiotensin System and Microglial Polarization: Implications for Aging and Neurodegeneration. *Front. Aging Neurosci.* **2017**, *9*, 129. [CrossRef]
121. Xu, Q.; Jensen, D.D.; Peng, H.; Feng, Y. The critical role of the central nervous system (pro)renin receptor in regulating systemic blood pressure. *Pharmacol. Ther.* **2016**, *164*, 126–134. [CrossRef] [PubMed]

122. Ichihara, A.; Yatabe, M.S. The (pro)renin receptor in health and disease. *Nat. Rev. Nephrol.* **2019**, *15*, 693–712. [CrossRef]
123. Hamming, I.; Timens, W.; Bulthuis, M.L.; Lely, A.T.; Navis, G.; Van Goor, H. Tissue distribution of ACE2 protein, the functional receptor for SARS coronavirus. A first step in understanding SARS pathogenesis. *J. Pathol.* **2004**, *203*, 631–637. [CrossRef] [PubMed]
124. Cui, C.; Xu, P.; Li, G.; Qiao, Y.; Han, W.; Geng, C.; Liao, D.; Yang, M.; Chen, D.; Jiang, P. Vitamin D receptor activation regulates microglia polarization and oxidative stress in spontaneously hypertensive rats and angiotensin II-exposed microglial cells: Role of renin-angiotensin system. *Redox Biol.* **2019**, *26*, 101295. [CrossRef] [PubMed]
125. Wegman-Ostrosky, T.; Soto-Reyes, E.; Vidal-Millan, S.; Sanchez-Corona, J. The renin-angiotensin system meets the hallmarks of cancer. *J. Renin Angiotensin Aldosterone Syst.* **2015**, *16*, 227–233. [CrossRef]
126. Beitia, M.; Solano-Iturri, J.D.; Errarte, P.; Sanz, B.; Perez, I.; Etxezarraga, M.C.; Loizate, A.; Asumendi, A.; Larrinaga, G. Altered expression of renin-angiotensin system receptors throughout colorectal adenoma-adenocarcinoma sequence. *Int. J. Med. Sci.* **2019**, *16*, 813–821. [CrossRef] [PubMed]
127. Renziehausen, A.; Wang, H.; Rao, B.; Weir, L.; Nigro, C.L.; Lattanzio, L.; Merlano, M.; Vega-Rioja, A.; Del Carmen Fernandez-Carranco, M.; Hajji, N.; et al. The renin angiotensin system (RAS) mediates bifunctional growth regulation in melanoma and is a novel target for therapeutic intervention. *Oncogene* **2019**, *38*, 2320–2336. [CrossRef]
128. Featherston, T.; Yu, H.H.; Dunne, J.C.; Chibnall, A.M.; Brasch, H.D.; Davis, P.F.; Tan, S.T.; Itinteang, T. Cancer Stem Cells in Moderately Differentiated Buccal Mucosal Squamous Cell Carcinoma Express Components of the Renin-Angiotensin System. *Front. Surg.* **2016**, *3*, 52. [CrossRef] [PubMed]
129. Itinteang, T.; Dunne, J.C.; Chibnall, A.M.; Brasch, H.D.; Davis, P.F.; Tan, S.T. Cancer stem cells in moderately differentiated oral tongue squamous cell carcinoma express components of the renin-angiotensin system. *J. Clin. Pathol.* **2016**, *69*, 942–945. [CrossRef]
130. Siljee, S.; Milne, B.; Brasch, H.D.; Bockett, N.; Patel, J.; Davis, P.F.; Kennedy-Smith, A.; Itinteang, T.; Tan, S.T. Expression of Components of the Renin-Angiotensin System by Cancer Stem Cells in Renal Clear Cell Carcinoma. *Biomolecules* **2021**, *11*, 537. [CrossRef]
131. Nallaiah, S.; Lee, V.M.Y.; Brasch, H.D.; De Jongh, J.; Schaijik, B.V.; Marsh, R.; Tan, S.T.; Itinteang, T. Cancer stem cells within moderately differentiated head and neck cutaneous squamous cell carcinoma express components of the renin-angiotensin system. *J. Plast. Reconstr. Aesthet. Surg.* **2019**, *72*, 1484–1493. [CrossRef]
132. Siljee, S.; Buchanan, O.; Brasch, H.D.; Bockett, N.; Patel, J.; Paterson, E.; Purdie, G.L.; Davis, P.F.; Itinteang, T.; Tan, S.T. Cancer Stem Cells in Metastatic Head and Neck Cutaneous Squamous Cell Carcinoma Express Components of the Renin-Angiotensin System. *Cells* **2021**, *10*, 243. [CrossRef]
133. Narayanan, A.; Wickremesekera, S.K.; Van Schaijik, B.; Marsh, R.W.; Brasch, H.D.; Tan, S.T.; Itinteang, T. Cancer stem cells in liver metastasis from colon adenocarcinoma express components of the renin-angiotensin system. *J. Cancer Metastasis Treat.* **2019**, *5*, 36. [CrossRef]
134. Bradshaw, A.R.; Wickremesekera, A.C.; Brasch, H.D.; Chibnall, A.M.; Davis, P.F.; Tan, S.T.; Itinteang, T. Glioblastoma Multiforme Cancer Stem Cells Express Components of the Renin-Angiotensin System. *Front. Surg.* **2016**, *3*, 51. [CrossRef]
135. Kouchi, M.; Shibayama, Y.; Ogawa, D.; Miyake, K.; Nishiyama, A.; Tamiya, T. (Pro)renin receptor is crucial for glioma development via the Wnt/beta-catenin signaling pathway. *J. Neurosurg.* **2017**, *127*, 819–828. [CrossRef]
136. Wang, J.; Nishiyama, A.; Matsuyama, M.; Wang, Z.; Yuan, Y. The (pro)renin receptor: A novel biomarker and potential therapeutic target for various cancers. *Cell Commun. Signal.* **2020**, *18*, 39. [CrossRef]
137. Nguyen, G. Renin, (pro)renin and receptor: An update. *Clin. Sci.* **2011**, *120*, 169–178. [CrossRef]
138. Cruciat, C.M.; Ohkawara, B.; Acebron, S.P.; Karaulanov, E.; Reinhard, C.; Ingelfinger, D.; Boutros, M.; Niehrs, C. Requirement of prorenin receptor and vacuolar H^+-ATPase-mediated acidification for Wnt signaling. *Science* **2010**, *327*, 459–463. [CrossRef] [PubMed]
139. Zheng, H.; Ying, H.; Wiedemeyer, R.; Yan, H.; Quayle, S.N.; Ivanova, E.V.; Paik, J.-H.; Zhang, H.; Xiao, Y.; Perry, S.R.; et al. PLAGL2 regulates Wnt signaling to impede differentiation in neural stem cells and gliomas. *Cancer Cell* **2010**, *17*, 497–509. [CrossRef] [PubMed]
140. Pu, P.; Zhang, Z.; Kang, C.; Jiang, R.; Jia, Z.; Wang, G.; Jiang, H. Downregulation of Wnt2 and beta-catenin by siRNA suppresses malignant glioma cell growth. *Cancer Gene Ther.* **2009**, *16*, 351–361. [CrossRef]
141. Pulvirenti, T.; Van Der Heijden, M.; Droms, L.A.; Huse, J.T.; Tabar, V.; Hall, A. Dishevelled 2 Signaling Promotes Self-Renewal and Tumorigenicity in Human Gliomas. *Cancer Res.* **2011**, *71*, 7280. [CrossRef] [PubMed]
142. Ariza, A.; Fernandez, L.A.; Inagami, T.; Kim, J.H.; Manuelidis, E.E. Renin in glioblastoma multiforme and its role in neovascularization. *Am. J. Clin. Pathol.* **1988**, *90*, 437–441. [CrossRef] [PubMed]
143. Liu, B.; Liu, Y.; Jiang, Y. Podocalyxin promotes glioblastoma multiforme cell invasion and proliferation by inhibiting angiotensin-(1-7)/Mas signaling. *Oncol. Rep.* **2015**, *33*, 2583–2591. [CrossRef] [PubMed]
144. Gopinath, S.; Malla, R.; Alapati, K.; Gorantla, B.; Gujrati, M.; Dinh, D.H.; Rao, J.S. Cathepsin B and uPAR regulate self-renewal of glioma-initiating cells through GLI-regulated Sox2 and Bmi1 expression. *Carcinogenesis* **2013**, *34*, 550–559. [CrossRef] [PubMed]
145. Cheng, Y.C.; Ding, Y.M.; Hueng, D.Y.; Chen, J.Y.; Chen, Y. Caffeine suppresses the progression of human glioblastoma via cathepsin B and MAPK signaling pathway. *J. Nutr. Biochem.* **2016**, *33*, 63–72. [CrossRef]

146. Koh, S.P.; Wickremesekera, A.C.; Brasch, H.D.; Marsh, R.; Tan, S.T.; Itinteang, T. Expression of Cathepsins B, D, and G in Isocitrate Dehydrogenase-Wildtype Glioblastoma. *Front. Surg.* **2017**, *4*, 28. [CrossRef]
147. Tao, W.; Chu, C.; Zhou, W.; Huang, Z.; Zhai, K.; Fang, X.; Huang, Q.; Zhang, A.; Wang, X.; Yu, X.; et al. Dual Role of WISP1 in maintaining glioma stem cells and tumor-supportive macrophages in glioblastoma. *Nat. Commun.* **2020**, *11*, 3015. [CrossRef]
148. Krop, M.; Lu, X.; Danser, A.H.; Meima, M.E. The (pro)renin receptor. A decade of research: What have we learned? *Pflugers Arch.* **2013**, *465*, 87–97. [CrossRef]
149. Arundhathi, A.; Chuang, W.H.; Chen, J.K.; Wang, S.E.; Shyr, Y.M.; Chen, J.Y.; Liao, W.N.; Chen, H.W.; Teng, Y.M.; Pai, C.C.; et al. Prorenin receptor acts as a potential molecular target for pancreatic ductal adenocarcinoma diagnosis. *Oncotarget* **2016**. [CrossRef]
150. Pinter, M.; Kwanten, W.J.; Jain, R.K. Renin-Angiotensin System Inhibitors to Mitigate Cancer Treatment-Related Adverse Events. *Clin. Cancer Res.* **2018**, *24*, 3803–3812. [CrossRef]
151. Shen, J.; Huang, Y.M.; Wang, M.; Hong, X.Z.; Song, X.N.; Zou, X.; Pan, Y.H.; Ling, W.; Zhu, M.H.; Zhang, X.X.; et al. Renin-angiotensin system blockade for the risk of cancer and death. *J. Renin Angiotensin Aldosterone Syst.* **2016**, *17*. [CrossRef]
152. Van der Knaap, R.; Siemes, C.; Coebergh, J.W.; Van Duijn, C.M.; Hofman, A.; Stricker, B.H. Renin-angiotensin system inhibitors, angiotensin I-converting enzyme gene insertion/deletion polymorphism, and cancer: The Rotterdam Study. *Cancer* **2008**, *112*, 748–757. [CrossRef] [PubMed]
153. Makar, G.A.; Holmes, J.H.; Yang, Y.X. Angiotensin-converting enzyme inhibitor therapy and colorectal cancer risk. *J. Natl. Cancer Inst.* **2014**, *106*, djt374. [CrossRef] [PubMed]
154. Dai, Y.N.; Wang, J.H.; Zhu, J.Z.; Lin, J.Q.; Yu, C.H.; Li, Y.M. Angiotensin-converting enzyme inhibitors/angiotensin receptor blockers therapy and colorectal cancer: A systematic review and meta-analysis. *Cancer Causes Control* **2015**, *26*, 1245–1255. [CrossRef] [PubMed]
155. Chiang, Y.Y.; Chen, K.B.; Tsai, T.H.; Tsai, W.C. Lowered cancer risk with ACE inhibitors/ARBs: A population-based cohort study. *J. Clin. Hypertens.* **2014**, *16*, 27–33. [CrossRef]
156. Liu, H.; Naxerova, K.; Pinter, M.; Incio, J.; Lee, H.; Shigeta, K.; Ho, W.W.; Crain, J.A.; Jacobson, A.; Michelakos, T.; et al. Use of Angiotensin System Inhibitors Is Associated with Immune Activation and Longer Survival in Nonmetastatic Pancreatic Ductal Adenocarcinoma. *Clin. Cancer Res.* **2017**, *23*, 5959–5969. [CrossRef]
157. Rosenthal, T.; Gavras, I. Renin-Angiotensin Inhibition in Combating Malignancy: A Review. *Anticancer Res.* **2019**, *39*, 4597–4602. [CrossRef]
158. Happold, C.; Gorlia, T.; Nabors, L.B.; Erridge, S.C.; Reardon, D.A.; Hicking, C.; Picard, M.; Stupp, R.; Weller, M.; Group, E.B.T.; et al. Do statins, ACE inhibitors or sartans improve outcome in primary glioblastoma? *J. Neurooncol.* **2018**, *138*, 163–171. [CrossRef]
159. Kast, R.E.; Karpel-Massler, G.; Halatsch, M.E. CUSP9* treatment protocol for recurrent glioblastoma: Aprepitant, artesunate, auranofin, captopril, celecoxib, disulfiram, itraconazole, ritonavir, sertraline augmenting continuous low dose temozolomide. *Oncotarget* **2014**, *5*, 8052–8082. [CrossRef]
160. Levin, V.A.; Chan, J.; Datta, M.; Yee, J.L.; Jain, R.K. Effect of angiotensin system inhibitors on survival in newly diagnosed glioma patients and recurrent glioblastoma patients receiving chemotherapy and/or bevacizumab. *J. Neurooncol.* **2017**, *134*, 325–330. [CrossRef] [PubMed]
161. Ameratunga, M.; Pavlakis, N.; Wheeler, H.; Grant, R.; Simes, J.; Khasraw, M. Anti-angiogenic therapy for high-grade glioma. *Cochrane Database Syst. Rev.* **2018**, *11*, CD008218. [CrossRef] [PubMed]
162. Burcklé, C.; Bader, M. Prorenin and its ancient receptor. *Hypertension* **2006**, *48*, 549–551. [CrossRef] [PubMed]
163. Juillerat-Jeanneret, L.; Celerier, J.; Chapuis Bernasconi, C.; Nguyen, G.; Wostl, W.; Maerki, H.P.; Janzer, R.C.; Corvol, P.; Gasc, J.M. Renin and angiotensinogen expression and functions in growth and apoptosis of human glioblastoma. *Br. J. Cancer* **2004**, *90*, 1059–1068. [CrossRef] [PubMed]
164. Roth, I.M.; Wickremesekera, A.C.; Wickremesekera, S.K.; Davis, P.F.; Tan, S.T. Therapeutic Targeting of Cancer Stem Cells via Modulation of the Renin-Angiotensin System. *Front. Oncol.* **2019**, *9*, 745. [CrossRef] [PubMed]
165. Tan, D.C.; Roth, I.M.; Wickremesekera, A.C.; Davis, P.F.; Kaye, A.H.; Mantamadiotis, T.; Stylli, S.S.; Tan, S.T. Therapeutic Targeting of Cancer Stem Cells in Human Glioblastoma by Manipulating the Renin-Angiotensin System. *Cells* **2019**, *8*, 1364. [CrossRef] [PubMed]
166. Abiodun, O.A.; Ola, M.S. Role of brain renin angiotensin system in neurodegeneration: An update. *Saudi J. Biol. Sci.* **2020**, *27*, 905–912. [CrossRef] [PubMed]
167. Di Lullo, E.; Kriegstein, A.R. The use of brain organoids to investigate neural development and disease. *Nat. Rev. Neurosci.* **2017**, *18*, 573–584. [CrossRef]
168. Li, Y.; Muffat, J.; Omer, A.; Bosch, I.; Lancaster, M.A.; Sur, M.; Gehrke, L.; Knoblich, J.A.; Jaenisch, R. Induction of Expansion and Folding in Human Cerebral Organoids. *Cell Stem Cell* **2017**, *20*, 385–396.e3. [CrossRef]
169. Pan, Y.; Lu, P.; Yin, L.; Chen, K.; He, Y. Effect of fluoride on the proteomic profile of the hippocampus in rats. *Z. Naturforsch. C. J. Biosci.* **2015**, *70*, 151–157. [CrossRef]
170. Adilijiang, A.; Hirano, M.; Okuno, Y.; Aoki, K.; Ohka, F.; Maeda, S.; Tanahashi, K.; Motomura, K.; Shimizu, H.; Yamaguchi, J.; et al. Next Generation Sequencing-Based Transcriptome Predicts Bevacizumab Efficacy in Combination with Temozolomide in Glioblastoma. *Molecules* **2019**, *24*, 3046. [CrossRef]
171. Velasco, S.; Kedaigle, A.J.; Simmons, S.K.; Nash, A.; Rocha, M.; Quadrato, G.; Paulsen, B.; Nguyen, L.; Adiconis, X.; Regev, A.; et al. Individual brain organoids reproducibly form cell diversity of the human cerebral cortex. *Nature* **2019**, *570*, 523–527. [CrossRef]

172. Blue, R.; Miranda, S.P.; Gu, B.J.; Chen, H.I. A Primer on Human Brain Organoids for the Neurosurgeon. *Neurosurgery* **2020**, *87*, 620–629. [CrossRef]
173. Cakir, B.; Xiang, Y.; Tanaka, Y.; Kural, M.H.; Parent, M.; Kang, Y.J.; Chapeton, K.; Patterson, B.; Yuan, Y.; He, C.S.; et al. Engineering of human brain organoids with a functional vascular-like system. *Nat. Methods* **2019**, *16*, 1169–1175. [CrossRef]
174. Ham, O.; Jin, Y.B.; Kim, J.; Lee, M.O. Blood vessel formation in cerebral organoids formed from human embryonic stem cells. *Biochem. Biophys. Res. Commun.* **2020**, *521*, 84–90. [CrossRef]
175. Pellegrini, L.; Bonfio, C.; Chadwick, J.; Begum, F.; Skehel, M.; Lancaster, M.A. Human CNS barrier-forming organoids with cerebrospinal fluid production. *Science* **2020**, *369*, aaz5626. [CrossRef]
176. Krieger, T.G.; Tirier, S.M.; Park, J.; Jechow, K.; Eisemann, T.; Peterziel, H.; Angel, P.; Eils, R.; Conrad, C. Modeling glioblastoma invasion using human brain organoids and single-cell transcriptomics. *Neuro. Oncol.* **2020**, *22*, 1138–1149. [CrossRef]
177. Pine, A.R.; Cirigliano, S.M.; Nicholson, J.G.; Hu, Y.; Linkous, A.; Miyaguchi, K.; Edwards, L.; Singhania, R.; Schwartz, T.H.; Ramakrishna, R.; et al. Tumor Microenvironment Is Critical for the Maintenance of Cellular States Found in Primary Glioblastomas. *Cancer Discov.* **2020**, *10*, 964–979. [CrossRef] [PubMed]
178. Caruso, F.P.; Garofano, L.; D'Angelo, F.; Yu, K.; Tang, F.; Yuan, J.; Zhang, J.; Cerulo, L.; Pagnotta, S.M.; Bedognetti, D.; et al. A map of tumor-host interactions in glioma at single-cell resolution. *Gigascience* **2020**, *9*, giaa109. [CrossRef] [PubMed]
179. Zhang, C.; Jin, M.; Zhao, J.; Chen, J.; Jin, W. Organoid models of glioblastoma: Advances, applications and challenges. *Am. J. Cancer Res.* **2020**, *10*, 2242–2257. [PubMed]

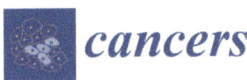

Article

Transcriptomics-Based Phenotypic Screening Supports Drug Discovery in Human Glioblastoma Cells

Vladimir Shapovalov [1], Liliya Kopanitsa [1], Lavinia-Lorena Pruteanu [1], Graham Ladds [2] and David S. Bailey [1,*]

1. IOTA Pharmaceuticals Ltd., St Johns Innovation Centre, Cowley Road, Cambridge CB4 0WS, UK; vladimir.shapovalov@iotapharma.com (V.S.); liliya.kopanitsa@iotapharma.com (L.K.); lavinia.pruteanu@iotapharma.com (L.-L.P.)
2. Department of Pharmacology, University of Cambridge, Tennis Court Road, Cambridge CB2 1PD, UK; grl30@cam.ac.uk
* Correspondence: david.bailey@iotapharma.com

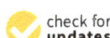

Citation: Shapovalov, V.; Kopanitsa, L.; Pruteanu, L.-L.; Ladds, G.; Bailey, D.S. Transcriptomics-Based Phenotypic Screening Supports Drug Discovery in Human Glioblastoma Cells. *Cancers* **2021**, *13*, 3780. https://doi.org/10.3390/cancers13153780

Academic Editor: Stanley Stylli

Received: 9 June 2021
Accepted: 20 July 2021
Published: 27 July 2021

Publisher's Note: MDPI stays neutral with regard to jurisdictional claims in published maps and institutional affiliations.

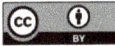

Copyright: © 2021 by the authors. Licensee MDPI, Basel, Switzerland. This article is an open access article distributed under the terms and conditions of the Creative Commons Attribution (CC BY) license (https://creativecommons.org/licenses/by/4.0/).

Simple Summary: Glioblastoma (GBM) remains a particularly challenging cancer, with an aggressive phenotype and few promising treatment options. Future therapy will rely heavily on diagnosing and targeting aggressive GBM cellular phenotypes, both before and after drug treatment, as part of personalized therapy programs. Here, we use a genome-wide drug-induced gene expression (DIGEX) approach to define the cellular drug response phenotypes associated with two clinical drug candidates, the phosphodiesterase 10A inhibitor Mardepodect and the multi-kinase inhibitor Regorafenib. We identify genes encoding specific drug targets, some of which we validate as effective antiproliferative agents and combination therapies in human GBM cell models, including HMGCoA reductase (*HMGCR*), salt-inducible kinase 1 (*SIK1*), bradykinin receptor subtype B2 (*BDKRB2*), and Janus kinase isoform 2 (*JAK2*). Individual, personalized treatments will be essential if we are to address and overcome the pharmacological plasticity that GBM exhibits, and DIGEX will play a central role in validating future drugs, diagnostics, and possibly vaccine candidates for this challenging cancer.

Abstract: We have used three established human glioblastoma (GBM) cell lines—U87MG, A172, and T98G—as cellular systems to examine the plasticity of the drug-induced GBM cell phenotype, focusing on two clinical drugs, the phosphodiesterase PDE10A inhibitor Mardepodect and the multi-kinase inhibitor Regorafenib, using genome-wide drug-induced gene expression (DIGEX) to examine the drug response. Both drugs upregulate genes encoding specific growth factors, transcription factors, cellular signaling molecules, and cell surface proteins, while downregulating a broad range of targetable cell cycle and apoptosis-associated genes. A few upregulated genes encode therapeutic targets already addressed by FDA approved drugs, but the majority encode targets for which there are no approved drugs. Amongst the latter, we identify many novel druggable targets that could qualify for chemistry-led drug discovery campaigns. We also observe several highly upregulated transmembrane proteins suitable for combined drug, immunotherapy, and RNA vaccine approaches. DIGEX is a powerful way of visualizing the complex drug response networks emerging during GBM drug treatment, defining a phenotypic landscape which offers many new diagnostic and therapeutic opportunities. Nevertheless, the extreme heterogeneity we observe within drug-treated cells using this technique suggests that effective pan-GBM drug treatment will remain a significant challenge for many years to come.

Keywords: glioblastoma; drug-inducible gene expression; Mardepodect; Regorafenib; drug targets; tumor antigens

1. Introduction

Glioblastoma (GBM) is characterized by pronounced cellular heterogeneity, with different glioblastoma cell lineages presumed to emanate from glioma stem cells (GSCs) within the same patient tumor [1]. GSCs often retain neural differentiation characteristics, although they do not terminally differentiate [2]. Transcriptomics studies have previously identified gene expression signatures that correlate with patient survival [3]. Using single-cell RNA sequencing, individual tumor cells can be positioned within a spectrum spanning proneural to mesenchymal cell types, with the mesenchymal phenotype correlating with significantly poorer patient survival [4]. Moreover, tumor-initiation studies with cell surface marker-enriched GBM populations, xenografted into immunodeficient mouse models, show that these cells retain their capability to re-form the full spectrum of proneural to mesenchymal phenotypes observed in the original patient tumors [5], emphasizing the phenotypic plasticity and stem-like characteristics of GBM tumor cells.

At a genetic level, attention has centered on the 'driver' mutations implicated in the development of GBM and other cancers, confirmed by sequencing at the single-cell level [6]. Nevertheless, despite an increasing understanding of the molecular evolution of such tumors, and the development of powerful new approaches such as immunotherapy to target them, GBM clinical outcomes remain poor [7]. New drug and vaccine targets which translate into effective therapies are urgently required.

One of the hallmarks of GBM is its extreme resistance to growth inhibition by traditional anti-proliferative drugs as monotherapies, such as EGFR inhibitors [8]. To address this challenge, several novel GBM treatment modalities, such as combination drug therapy [9], immunotherapy [10], and adjuvant-enabled CAR-T cell therapy [11] are being developed. Work in other cancers has highlighted the importance of phenotypic plasticity in cancer initiation, progression, and resistance to therapy [12], and progress in GBM treatment is likely to mirror that in other cancers, such as multiple myeloma and melanoma where phenotyping is central to therapy selection [13,14].

The last decade has seen a resurgence in phenotypic screening, largely due to the realization that sifting through the thousands of potential therapeutic targets delivered from genomics, one by one, is both time-consuming and expensive [15,16]. Building oncology drug discovery campaigns on mechanistically validated chemical compounds and relevant phenotypic screens is now an established route to accelerated drug discovery [17,18]. Moreover, rapidly repositioning existing drugs for use in GBM could provide radically new and effective GBM pipelines [19].

Drug-focused chemical biology has one further big advantage—it provides insights into the quality of drug candidates on their way to drug development. The genome-wide drug induced gene expression (DIGEX) techniques employed here provide a formidable platform for comparing drug action, using thousands of 'reporter' gene expression data points to tease apart drug properties. The approach can also provide new insights into the dynamics of the drug response, a feature that could prove invaluable in an adaptive clinical trial setting.

Previous work from our laboratory has used genome-wide DIGEX to define the GBM cell phenotype and its modulation by drugs. In that work, we focused on the prototypic PI3K growth inhibitor LY-294002 and the natural product Fucoxanthin as chemical probes [20]. In the current study, we extend these detailed observations to a suite of three well-characterized GBM cell lines—U87MG, A172, and T98G—and two further growth inhibitory drugs in the clinic, the phosphodiesterase 10A (PDE10A) inhibitor Mardepodect (PF-02545920) and the multi-protein kinase inhibitor Regorafenib (Stivarga, BAY 73-4506).

Mardepodect is a CNS penetrant PDE10A inhibitor [21,22], developed by Pfizer initially for schizophrenia [23] and later repositioned for Huntington's Chorea within the AMARYLLIS clinical trial [24]. Mardepodect is thought to increase cAMP/PKA signaling in medium spiny neurons of the human striatum, which in turn leads to potentiation of dopamine D1 receptor signaling with concomitant inhibition of dopamine D2 receptor signaling. However, although safe and well tolerated, and capable of crossing the blood–

brain barrier, Mardepodect failed to achieve satisfactory therapeutic endpoints in either schizophrenia or Huntington's chorea. Here, we show that Mardepodect potently inhibits the growth and proliferation of GBM cells, raising the new possibility of its repositioning in GBM.

Regorafenib was originally approved for patients with treatment-refractory metastatic colorectal cancer as an adjunct to sorafenib treatment [25]. Regorafenib has a radically different molecular mode of action to that of Mardepodect, promiscuously targeting many protein kinases including VEGFR-1, -2, -3, TIE 2, PDGFR, FGFR, KIT, RAF-1, RET, and BRAF [26]. Regorafenib has already been evaluated for its effects on GBM within the REGOMA clinical trial [27] and is currently a component of the ongoing GBM AGILE adaptive clinical trial [28].

Although to date no drug, including Regorafenib, has provided effective therapy for GBM, it is still important to define the GBM cell response to every FDA approved drug showing promise in GBM, since such drugs are valuable assets and may elicit responses that can be exploited in new ways, perhaps in combination therapy or phenotypic modulation.

Thus, in this study, we reposition the schizophrenia drug Mardepodect as a possible antiproliferative candidate in GBM. Using DIGEX we compare the effects of Mardepodect to those of Regorafenib, a drug already in clinical trials for GBM.

We chose to study Mardepodect and Regorafenib not only because the two drugs are clinical candidates, but also because they cover highly complementary pharmacological space and, in combination, might synergize in providing a novel way to address the pronounced drug resistance which characterizes GBM.

Previously, we have used a range of pharmacological probes, including PDE inhibitors, to show that raised cAMP levels are associated with growth inhibition in rat C6 glioma cells [29]. Here, we focus on human PDE10A, a dual specificity cyclic nucleotide phosphodiesterase that is expressed in GBM but has not previously been studied as a potential therapeutic target. Using DIGEX, we compare and contrast the transcription phenotypes accompanying growth inhibition by the PDE inhibitor Mardepodect with those of the kinase inhibitor Regorafenib, reasoning that this information might enable us to design new combination therapies targeting these two anti-proliferative signaling pathways.

2. Materials and Methods

2.1. Cells Used in This Study

Cell proliferation experiments were carried out in the well characterized established GBM cell lines U87MG, A172, and T98G. The human glioblastoma astrocytoma cell lines U87MG (ECACC 89081402) and A172 (ECACC 88062428) were obtained from the European Collection of Authenticated Cell Cultures. The T98G cell line was obtained from the American Type Culture Collection (ATCC® CRL1690™, Manassas, VA, USA). The mutational landscapes of all three cell lines have been archived within Expasy (www.expasy.org/cellosaurus accessed on 15 November 2020) as U-87MG ATCC (RRID:CVCL_0022), A-172 (RRID:CVCL_0131), and T98G (RRID:CVCL_0556).

All cell lines were maintained in Dulbecco's modified Eagle's medium: Nutrient Mixture F-12 (DMEM/F12, Gibco, ThermoFisher, Loughborough, UK) supplemented with 10% fetal bovine serum (FBS, Sigma, Dorset, UK) and 5% antibiotic antimycotic solution (10,000 units of penicillin, 10 mg streptomycin, and 25 µg/mL amphotericin B, Sigma, Dorset, UK) at 37 °C in humidified atmospheres of 95% air and 5% CO_2.

2.2. Compounds Used in This Study

The compounds LY-294002, Regorafenib, Mardepodect (PF-02545920), Atorvastatin, and Simvastatin were purchased from Sigma UK. AZD1480 and Ruxolitinib were purchased from Selleckchem (München, Germany). HG-9-91-01 and Icatibant were purchased from MedChemExpress (Insight Biotechnology Limited, Wembley, Middlesex, UK). WH-4-023 and WIN 64338 were purchased from Tocris (Bio-techne Ltd., Abingdon, UK). Stock solutions of all compounds, except Icatibant, were prepared in dimethyl sulfoxide (DMSO) before addition to culture medium for testing. Stock solutions of Icatibant were prepared in water.

2.3. Proliferation Assay

Inhibition of proliferation by compounds in the three glioblastoma cell lines was determined using the Cell Counting Kit-8 (CCK-8) assay (Sigma, UK), as described previously [20].

2.4. Drug Combination Assays and Their Analysis

To study the effects of combined treatments with Mardepodect, Regorafenib, LY-294002, and Fucoxanthin with inhibitors of JAK2 kinase, SIK1, and HMGCoA reductase, proliferation assays were performed, followed by an analysis of the observed combination effects with the additive Loewe synergy effect as a baseline model, using Combenefit software (version 2.021) [30] for analysis.

2.5. Microarray Analysis

Cells were seeded into T25 flasks at a density of 500,000 cells/flask and allowed to adhere and grow for 24 h. The culture medium was removed, and fresh medium containing test compound in 1% DMSO at the previously determined 72 h IC50 concentration was added to each flask. Control cells were treated with medium containing 1% DMSO alone. All experiments were performed in triplicate. The cells were visualized during culture using the EVOS Cell Imaging System (Thermo Fisher Scientific, UK).

After 24 h of treatment, the cells were trypsinized and total RNA was isolated using the RNeasy Mini kit (Qiagen, Manchester, UK) as described previously [20]. Expression analysis was performed on a Clariom S Human Array (Thermo Fisher Scientific, catalog number 902926) using a fixed number of probes per transcript and probe sets comprising a subset of 10 probes per gene, yielding >20,000 annotated genes, as documented by the NetAffx Analysis Center (www.affymetrix.com/analysis/netaffx/, accessed on 3 November 2020).

The raw data from all samples, in triplicate, were normalized taking average signal intensities, and an expression matrix was created by applying the Robust Multi-array Average (RMA) algorithm as a multi-chip model [31]. The control housekeeping gene intron/exon separation area under the receiving operating curve value threshold was selected as 0.8, ensuring high quality in all samples. Finally, the Clariom S chip probe sets were mapped to their Entrez IDs, resulting in a list of 18,316 identifiable protein-coding genes after exclusion of duplicate and non-coding gene sequence signals.

Specific genes were analyzed and annotated using the UniProt (www.uniprot.org accessed on 4 November 2020), Entrez (www.ncbi.nlm.nih.gov/gene accessed on 4 November 2020), and Gene Ontology (www.geneontology.org/ accessed on 5 November 2020) databases, together allowing identification of the putative function of particular genes, as well as the pathways in which they have been observed previously. In the analyses reported, UniProt protein entries are denoted in block capitals with NCBI Gene entries in italics. The Pharos database (www.pharos.nih.gov accessed on 9 June 2020) was used to identify potential drug targets based on their inherent druggability [32]. Color coding of these genes in the accompanying tables is based on the system used by the University of New Mexico (http://juniper.health.unm.edu/tcrd/ accessed on 9 June 2020). Principle component analysis (PCA) was used to study the reproducibility of gene expression among the different drug treatments. Reactome pathway analysis (https://www.reactome.org accessed on 3 June 2020) and gene network analysis (www.genenetwork.nl accessed on 4 January 2021) were also conducted, focusing on the 200 genes with most elevated, or lowered gene expression levels, and their subsets.

3. Results

3.1. Established Cell Lines Used in These Studies

Established cell lines, while possessing lengthy passage histories, provide well characterized, robust and relatively reproducible systems in which to compare drug responses, and studies with them have provided the bulk of the information we have on drug response in GBM. Well-adapted to large-scale tissue culture, established cell lines are also good starting points for dissecting the underlying biochemical and pharmacological processes governing the GBM drug response—and purifying the effectors involved. In this study, we have used the established cell lines U87MG, A172, and T98G to investigate drug-induced gene expression changes. All three cell lines have been completely sequenced and their mutational landscapes defined. They are also the three most highly represented GBM cell lines in more than 1000 studies reported in the GBM Drug Bank [33].

3.2. Compounds Used to Probe Drug-Induced Gene Expression

The primary focus of the current studies was to define the effects of the drug Mardepodect on GBM cell transcription. Mardepodect, a Phase 3 clinical candidate developed by Pfizer as PF-02545920 for schizophrenia and more recently repositioned for Huntington's Disease, is a potent PDE10A inhibitor with CNS penetrant properties that may make it suitable for repositioning in GBM.

A second objective was to compare the Mardepodect response to that of the Bayer drug Regorafenib, approved by the FDA for colorectal carcinoma and currently in clinical trials for GBM [27,28]. Regorafenib is a well characterized multi-kinase inhibitor [26].

In an earlier study [20], we characterized the DIGEX profiles of two additional growth inhibitors, the chemical probe LY-294002 (another well characterized multi-kinase inhibitor), and Fucoxanthin (a xanthophyll natural product). Here, we use the profiles of both LY-294002 and Fucoxanthin as benchmarks against which to compare the gene expression profiles of Mardepodect and Regorafenib.

3.3. Growth Inhibition Characteristics of the Compounds

Dose response relationships are shown for all four compounds—Mardepodect, Regorafenib, LY-294002, and Fucoxanthin—in a standardized 72 h proliferation assay, using the three human GBM cell lines—U87MG, T98G and A172—growing in serum-containing medium (Figure 1).

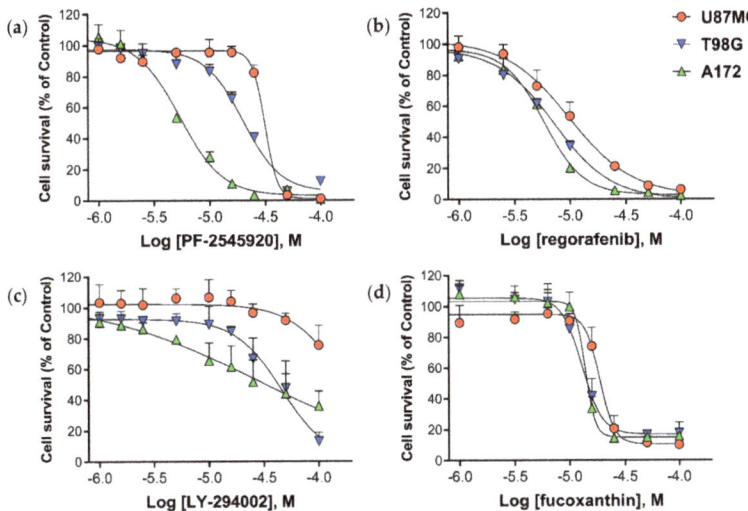

Figure 1. Survival of the three human GBM cell lines U87MG, A172, and T98G, treated with (**a**) Mardepodect (PF-02545920); (**b**) Regorafenib; (**c**) LY-294002; (**d**) Fucoxanthin. Data are presented as the mean ± standard error of the mean (SEM) (n = 6–10).

The IC50$_{72h}$ determined for Mardepodect varied from 32 μM for U87MG cells, to 5 μM for A172 cells, with T98G cells showing an intermediate IC50$_{72h}$ of approximately 16 μM. In contrast, the dose–response relationships observed for Regorafenib and Fucoxanthin were similar in all three cell lines, giving an IC50$_{72h}$ of approximately 10 μM.

3.4. DIGEX Profiles for the Four Treatments

Having determined the cellular IC50$_{72h}$ for Regorafenib, Mardepodect, LY-294002 and Fucoxanthin, we prepared RNA samples from batches of cells treated for 24 h with these compounds at their IC50$_{72h}$ concentrations, a standardized treatment protocol designed to capture significant DIGEX information under conditions of minimal toxicity. Twenty-four-hour dosing also mirrors a preferred clinical dosing regimen. The protocol gives highly reproducible DIGEX results, validated by PCA analysis (Supplementary Figure S1).

3.5. Upregulated Genes Accompanying Drug Treatments in U87MG Cells

In initial experiments, we focused on the human glioblastoma cell line U87MG. Treatment of U87MG cells under standardized conditions with any of the four proliferation inhibitors—Mardepodect, Regorafenib, LY-294002, or Fucoxanthin—upregulated many genes when compared to control cells grown under the same culture conditions but without inhibitors. The 200 genes with the most elevated expression levels in each drug treatment were identified and compared in a four-way Venn diagram (Figure 2). Amongst the 200 gene sets in U87MG cells, the genes partitioned between different drug treatments were identified (Table 1).

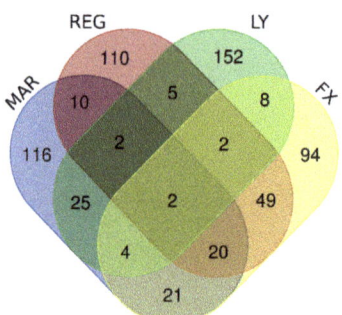

Figure 2. Four-way Venn diagram showing an analysis of the 200 genes with most elevated expression levels in U87MG cells treated with Mardepodect (MAR), Regorafenib (REG), LY-294002 (LY), and Fucoxanthin (FX).

Table 1. Genes, partitioned between the drug treatments, based on sets of 200 genes with most elevated expression levels in U87MG cells (shown in Figure 2).

Gene Group	Gene Number	Gene Names
Upregulated by Mardepodect, Regorafenib, LY-294002 and Fucoxanthin	2	PNLIPRP3, FAM49A
Upregulated by Mardepodect and Regorafenib	34	PNLIPRP3, FAM49A, PFKFB2, WDR78, GDF15, HMOX1, MSC, TRIB3, GPNMB, ERICH2, CRYM, SLC22A15, NUPR1, LURAP1L, ATP6V0D2, CLEC2D, GCNT3, SLIT3, IDH1, CTH, TM4SF19, RFTN2, KCP, RPS6KA2, KIF26B, UNC5B, PLK2, PLXDC2, FLYWCH1, THBS2, PPARGC1A, PLEKHF1, SLFN5, HECW1
Upregulated by the two multi-kinase inhibitors Regorafenib and LY-294002	11	ADARB1, SOD2, TTLL1, RSPO3, PPIL6, GPCPD1, H1F0, PFKFB2, WDR78, PNLIPRP3, FAM49A
Upregulated by Mardepodect only, not by Regorafenib, LY-294002 or Fucoxanthin	116	Gene names are found in Supplementary Table S1
Upregulated by Regorafenib only, not by Mardepodect, LY-294002 or Fucoxanthin	110	Gene names are found in Supplementary Table S1

3.6. Interpretation of the U87MG DIGEX Signatures

All four compounds produced richly complex DIGEX signatures in transcriptomic analyses of U87MG cells. However, relatively few genes were shared between treatments within the Top 200 upregulated genes (Figure 2 and Table 1). Concomitantly, many elevated genes were seen that were restricted to each treatment. These are documented in the Supplementary Materials (Supplementary Table S1). From these initial results we concluded that:

1. The DIGEX signature for each cell/treatment combination is reproducible and specific, confirmed by the PCA analysis (Supplementary Figure S1).
2. A GBM cell line such as U87MG, can radically change its DIGEX response when encountering different drug treatments, exhibiting considerable transcriptional plasticity.

We found the extreme diversity of gene expression produced within a single cell line by a single biological event—growth inhibition—somewhat surprising. However, the data show clearly that the U87MG cell line can deploy a vast range of specific drug-induced transcriptional responses when growth is inhibited under standardized conditions.

3.7. Two Genes Upregulated by All Four Drug Treatments in U87MG

We next examined more closely the few genes that were shared between treatments. Only two genes in the Top 200 upregulated set were upregulated by all four U87MG treatments: *PNLIPRP3* and *FAM49A*.

The *PNLIPRP3* gene encodes the protein Pancreatic Lipase Related Protein 3 (LIPR3), a rarely studied gene as judged by PubMed citation, previously observed as overexpressed in hepatocellular carcinoma [34]. We note from the literature that the peptide glioma growth inhibitor hHSS1/C19orf63/EMC10 also upregulates *PNLIPRP3* very highly in U87 cells [35]. From its entry in the Human Protein Atlas [36], *PNLIPRP3* has not been associated with either a favorable or unfavorable prognosis in glioma and is not expressed even at low levels in most normal human tissues.

The encoded LIPR3 protein bears a signal sequence and is most likely secreted from the cell, suggesting it might possibly represent an informative circulating biomarker for GBM. LIPR3 also possesses the catalytic triad characteristic of the esterase active site, and shares 47% overall homology to human pancreatic lipase (LIPP). LIPP is an important drug target upon which much medicinal chemistry has been undertaken, culminating in the development of the lipase inhibitor Xenical (otherwise known as Orlistat) approved for obesity management, reviewed in [37].

The *FAM49A* gene, also known as *CYRI-A*, encodes CYFIP-related Rac1 interactor A, a highly conserved regulator of the small GTPase RAC1, to which it binds [38]. *FAM49A* is expressed in the brain where the protein regulates chemotaxis, cell migration and epithelial polarization [39]. In contrast to LIPR3/*PNLIPRP3*, CYRIA/*FAM49A* is widely expressed in both normal and cancerous tissues and is a marker for unfavorable prognosis in both renal and urothelial cancer [40]. The X-ray structure of the closely related CYRIB protein has recently been solved [41], opening the way to homology modeling and structure-based drug design for CYRIA, if required.

3.8. Which U87MG Genes Are Upregulated in Mardepodect and Regorafenib Treatments?

As mentioned previously, we were especially interested in comparing the drug responses of GBM cells to the two clinical compounds Mardepodect and Regorafenib.

Including *PNLIPRP3* and *FAM49A*, U87MG cells treated with these compounds share 34 of their top set of 200 upregulated genes (Table 1). This set of 34 genes is particularly striking, encoding several cell membrane-associated proteins (GPNMB, CLC2D/*CLEC2D*, GCNT3, T4S19/*TM4SF19*, UNC5B, RFTN2, PXDC2/*PLXDC2*), cytoplasmic metabolism-related proteins (F262/*PFKFB2*, IDHC/*IDH1*, CGL/*CTH*), and transcription regulators (CRYM, MUSC/*MSC*, NUPR1, FWCH1/*FLYWCH1*, PRGC1/*PPARGC1A*), as well as secreted growth and cell guidance factors (GDF15, SLIT3, KCP, TSP2/*THBS2*). Several kinases associated with cancer cell survival, including KS6A2/*RPS6KA2* and PLK2, are also amongst this gene set.

We also see upregulation of the gene encoding growth/differentiation factor GDF15 in both Mardepodect and Regorafenib treated U87MG cells. GDF15 is of potential diagnostic and therapeutic significance in GBM, since elevated levels of GDF15 in the cerebrospinal fluid are associated with worse GBM outcome [42,43]. Conversely, downregulation of GDF15 increases T-cell infiltration into GBM tumors, improves immune responses and prolongs survival [44]. Reducing GDF-15 production and signaling have been proposed as ways of improving outcomes more generally in immunotherapy [45].

Also of potential clinical importance is the upregulation of the gene encoding the pseudokinase Tribbles homolog 3 (TRIB3). Like GDF-15, TRIB3 upregulation is associated with poor prognosis in GBM [46]. In ovarian cancer, TRIB3 downregulation inhibits progression via the MEK/ERK signaling pathway [47]. TRIB3 has also been reported to facilitate GBM progression, both by suppressing autophagy [46], and enhancing stemness [48].

3.9. Pathway Enrichment Analysis for the Upregulated U87MG Gene Sets

To gain further insight into the possible functional significance of the DIGEX data, pathway enrichment analyses were performed on the Top 200 upregulated gene sets accompanying individual drug treatments, using the Reactome database (Supplementary Tables S2 and S3). Although mainly based on studies in non-GBM cell systems, such pathway enrichment analyses can highlight important gene networks that are shared by GBM cells.

Several distinctive genes characterized the Mardepodect-upregulated pathway signature "PIP3 activates AKT signaling" in U87MG cells, including those encoding the EMT-promoting transcription factors SNAI1 (Snail) and SNAI2 (Slug), which have key roles in tumor growth, invasion, and metastasis in GBM [49,50]. Again, highlighted within this signature is the pseudokinase *TRIB3* (Tribbles homolog 3), discussed previously in the context of the upregulated genes shared by Mardepodect and Regorafenib. All three members of the NR4A nuclear receptor gene family (*NR4A1*, *NR4A2*, and *NR4A3*) are also present within the Mardepodect "generic transcription" pathway signature, together with two members of the Ras related GTP binding (RRAG) gene family (*RRAGC* and *RRAGD*).

In contrast, Regorafenib-treated U87MG cells show prominent pathways for the "Response of EIF2AK1 (HRI) to heme deficiency", "Netrin-1 signaling", "Serine biosynthesis", and "Transcriptional activation of mitochondrial biogenesis" pathways (Table S2). The "Response of EIF2AK1 (HRI) to heme deficiency" pathway signature contains the component genes *DDIT3*, *TRIB3*, *ATF3*, and *ASNS*, a grouping associated with endoplasmic reticulum (ER) stress, and characteristic of genotoxic agents [51]. DDIT3 is a member of the CCAAT/enhancer-binding protein (C/EBP) family of transcription factors. It also features prominently amongst the most highly upregulated pathways in Fucoxanthin treated U87MG cells. Importantly, in glioblastoma the ATF4-ATF3-DDIT3 axis also triggers G2/M arrest [52].

Targeting energy metabolism has been suggested as a fruitful therapeutic strategy in GBM [53]. *PPARGC1A*, the gene encoding PRGC1, a transcriptional coactivator regulating energy metabolism via multiple transcription factor interactions, including the cAMP response element binding (CREB) protein and nuclear respiratory factors (NRFs), is a component of the "mitochondrial biogenesis" pathway. This pathway also contains TBL1X, an F-box-like protein involved in the recruitment of the ubiquitin/19S proteasome complex to nuclear receptor-regulated transcription units [54].

The "netrin signaling" pathway includes Netrin-4 (NET4/*NTN4*), a specific netrin family member previously reported to promote GBM proliferation through ITB4/*ITGB4* signaling [55]. Netrins are laminin-related proteins that function in axon guidance and neurite growth and migration, tumorigenesis, angiogenesis and neural cell adhesion to endothelial cells, processes that are known to occur in GBM [56].

Upregulated alongside Netrin-4 is *UNC5B*, the gene which encodes the netrin receptor. In the absence of netrin, UNC5B triggers apoptosis, but an excess of netrin promotes cell survival, inducing interaction of UNC5B with the brain specific GTPase PIKE-L which opposes apoptosis by activating nuclear PI3K [56]. This interaction triggers activation of PI3K-signaling, prevents UNC5B's pro-apoptotic activity and enhances neuronal survival. Studies of cell survival in glioma show that netrin acts as a pro-survival ligand for UNC5B in glioma as well [57], while also promoting invasion and angiogenesis of GBM cells by activating RhoA, cathepsin B, cAMP response element binding protein, and Notch signaling [58,59]. The genes encoding the secreted proteins ABLM1, ABLM3, and SLIT3, implicated in cell guidance and migration, are found within the same netrin cluster.

Taken together, the upregulation of these pathways by Regorafenib treatment indicates a delicately balanced network of cell proliferation and invasion.

Inspection of the pathways upregulated by LY-294002 and Fucoxanthin show the emergence of several new themes, including 'signaling by interleukins'. In LY-294002-treated U87MG cells, we see upregulation of the interleukin pathway genes *RPS6KA5, IL36B, DUSP4, GAB2, FOS, PELI2, PTGS2, STX3, CCL20, IRS2, MAP3K8, SQSTM1, FOXO1, MMP1,* and *SOD2*, while the secretory chemokines *CCL20, CXCL8, CXCL1,* and *CXCL2*, component genes of the "Interleukin-10 signaling" pathway, show enhanced upregulation in Fucoxanthin-treated U87MG cells.

3.10. Downregulated Genes Revealed by DIGEX

Amongst the genes in U87MG downregulated by the four growth inhibitory compounds, 36 are shared within the top set of 200 most highly downregulated genes in each treatment (Figure 3 and Table 2). This is in sharp contrast to the upregulated genes, where only two genes were upregulated by all four treatments (Figure 2). The majority of the U87MG downregulated genes shared between treatments are associated with cell division, suggesting a coordinated and specific downregulation of the transcription of cell division genes in response to growth inhibition by these four compounds.

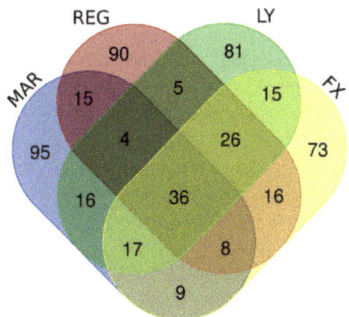

Figure 3. Four-way Venn diagram showing an analysis of the 200 genes with most lowered expression levels in U87MG cells treated with Mardepodect (MAR), Regorafenib (REG), LY-294002 (LY), and Fucoxanthin (FX).

Amongst the most downregulated U87MG genes in all treatments is that encoding the transcription factor E2F8, the master regulator of the cell cycle [60]. Downregulation of E2F8 has been reported as a driver for prostate cancer growth suppression [61], and if cancer selectivity could be obtained, might represent a good target for stabilizing growth inhibition in GBM.

Other prominently downregulated genes which might encode good drug targets include RIR2/*RRM2*, which encodes the regulatory subunit M2 of ribonucleotide reductase, the enzyme that catalyzes the biosynthesis of deoxyribonucleotides for DNA synthesis. RIR2 is specifically inhibited by hydroxyurea and has been suggested as a combination therapy with temozolomide for GBM [62].

Table 2. Genes, partitioned between the drug treatments, based on sets of 200 genes with most elevated expression levels in U87MG cells (shown in Figure 3).

Gene Group	Gene Number	Gene Names
Downregulated by Mardepodect, Regorafenib, LY-294002, and Fucoxanthin	36	KIAA1524, ESCO2, E2F8, HIST1H1B, LMNB1, HIST1H2BB, CDCA3, HIST2H3A, HIST1H2BM, TCF19, FBXO5, HIST1H3B, TYMS, DNA2, ORC1, HIST1H2BI, FAM111B, RRM2, ZWINT, HIST1H3A, ASF1B, HIST1H2BH, GPR19, HELLS, PLK4, HIST1H2AG, RAD54L, CDC45, HIST1H3F, HIST1H2AI, SPC25, KIFC1, KIF15, GINS2, UBE2T, HJURP
Downregulated by Mardepodect and Regorafenib	63	ARL14EPL, HIST1H4D, PBK, HIST1H2AB, RFC3, ATAD2, BARD1, KIF20A, MCM7, KIF11, HIST1H2BJ, TRMU, MKI67, CENPE, ASPM, SPAG5, KIF4A ANGPTL4, ANLN, TACC3, HIST2H4A, HIST2H4B, CPA4, PLEKHG4B, H2AFX, GTSE1, NCAPG, KIAA1524, ESCO2, E2F8, HIST1H1B, LMNB1, HIST1H2BB, CDCA3, HIST2H3A, HIST1H2BM, TCF19, FBXO5, HIST1H3B, TYMS, DNA2, ORC1, HIST1H2BI, FAM111B, RRM2, ZWINT, HIST1H3A, ASF1B, HIST1H2BH, GPR19, HELLS, PLK4, HIST1H2AG, RAD54L, CDC45, HIST1H3F, HIST1H2AI, SPC25, KIFC1, KIF15, GINS2, UBE2T, HJURP
Downregulated by Mardepodect only, not Regorafenib, LY-294002, or Fucoxanthin	95	Gene names are found in Supplementary Table S4
Downregulated by Regorafenib only, not Mardepodect, LY-294002, or Fucoxanthin	90	Gene names are found in Supplementary Table S4

Further substantially downregulated genes include those encoding the transcription factor TCF19, which is associated with cancer cell survival and proliferation [63], and FAM111B, which encodes the DNA replication-associated serine protease F111B associated with both proliferation and cell cycle control [64,65]. Many genes encoding histones, important in maintaining nuclear and chromosome structure during cell cycling and division, are also significantly downregulated.

The mechanism controlling such a marked downregulation of genes encoding nuclear structural proteins after drug treatment is unclear. It is possible that mRNAs encoding nuclear components are no longer required in non-proliferating GBM cells and simply decay. Alternatively, the cells may be undergoing a controlled program of transcriptional and translational rebalancing, in which survival processes predominate and translation of cell division genes is specifically downregulated. Such dysregulation and restoration of translational homeostasis has been reported in fragile X syndrome where mRNA stability is thought to play a central role [66]. In either case, a new transcriptional equilibrium is being established, influenced by the presence of Mardepodect within the cells.

3.11. Pathway Analysis for the U87MG Downregulated Gene Sets

Pathway analyses were also performed for the U87MG downregulated gene sets, shown in Supplementary Tables S5 and S6. These confirmed that all four compounds exerted anti-mitotic effects in U87MG cells, but also highlighted specific genes within these pathways. For example, members of the MCM (mini-chromosome maintenance) gene family are broadly downregulated within cells treated with all four compounds, while pathways downregulated by Fucoxanthin often include SKP2 as a prominent component. SKP2 is a member of the F-box family of SCF ubiquitin ligases, pointing to reprogramming of the ubiquitin system during Fucoxanthin treatment.

3.12. Summary of the U87MG Results

Taken together, these DIGEX and pathway analyses highlight the considerable transcriptional plasticity of U87MG cells, with the upregulation of specific tumor cell survival pathways accompanying the downregulation of genes controlling mitosis and cell division.

This pattern is consistent with transcriptional reprograming leading to a quiescent and/or drug resistant tumor cell population, a previously recognized mode of targeted therapy evasion [14,67].

3.13. Which DIGEX Genes Are Shared between Mardepodect Treated U87MG, T98G, and A172 Cells?

The U87MG DIGEX profiles for Mardepodect were then compared to those identified in T98G and A172 cells, to search for common targets (and identify specific differences) between the three cell lines. An overview of the Top 200 most highly induced genes within each cell type is shown in Figure 4, with individual genes listed in Table 3.

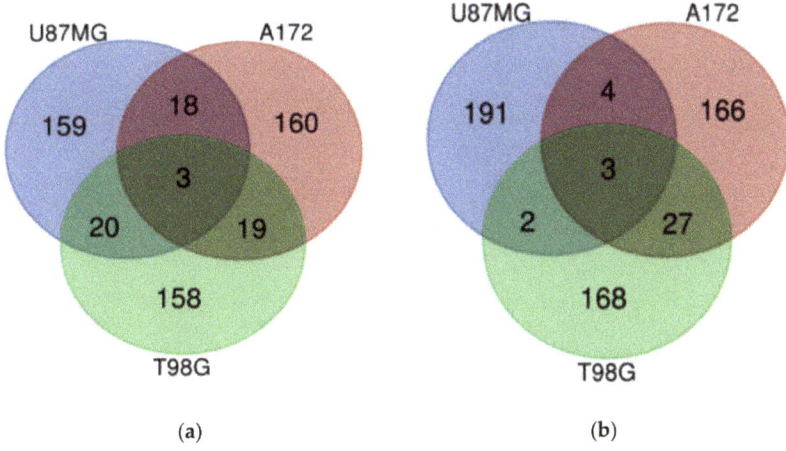

Figure 4. Venn diagrams showing the partitioning of the 200 genes most significantly modulated by Mardepodect in U87MG, A172, and T98G cells; (**a**) upregulated genes; (**b**) downregulated genes.

Table 3. Genes modulated by Mardepodect, shared between U87MG, A172, and T98G cells.

Sharing Groups	Upregulated	Downregulated
U87MG, A172, and T98G	GDF15, DUSP1, SIK1	CPA4, FAM111B, CCL2
U87MG and A172	HMOX1, SLC11A2, GPNMB, GPR183, UAP1L1, PLEKHO1, DUSP4, LIPG, NUPR1, PPARGC1A, LURAP1L, AK5, FAM49A, RRAGD, RRAGC, TM4SF19, FBXO32, RFTN2	E2F8, TNFRSF11B, PI3, TXNIP
U87MG and T98G	NR4A2, CD55, HES1, SLC16A6, S1PR1, NR4A1, C8orf4, CEMIP, DNAJB9, TNFAIP6, SNAI1, SGK1, ITGB3, RND3, TRIB1, GRAMD4, NR4A3, ZCWPW2, IL6, RPS6KA2	CD84, HIST1H2BM
A172 and T98G	HMGCR, DDIT4, FASN, CLCN5, SLC2A3, JAKMIP2, IDI1, AGT, CYP51A1, HLA-DMA, SCD, FDFT1, MVD, HMGCS1, ST3GAL5, DHCR7, ZBED8, RELL2, INSIG1	EDN1, IRF1, PLXNA2, TRIM22, SERTAD4, TNFRSF9, TNFSF10, RARRES3, LGALS9, CCNE2, KRT18, IL7R, VCAM1, TNFAIP2, ENC1, RNF150, ANKRD1, ROR1, APOL3, CYR61, GBP4, CTGF, PRDM1, ALPK2, LYPD1, BIRC3, IL2RG

3.13.1. Upregulated Genes

Our first observation was that over 75% of the Mardepodect upregulated genes in the three cell lines were cell-specific, suggesting that each GBM cell line responds in a unique way to Mardepodect treatment. A complete list of cell-specific genes is provided in Supplementary Table S7.

In contrast, very few upregulated genes were shared between the three Mardepodect-treated cell lines. Only three genes were expressed in common within the Top 200 upregulated gene sets: *GDF15*, *DUSP1*, and *SIK1*, all of which encode proteins that are involved in important growth-related processes.

- GDF15 is a secreted growth factor, reportedly overexpressed in the cerebrospinal fluid (CSF) of GBM patients with poor treatment outcomes [42]. GDF15 binds to the GFRAL/RET receptor complex, stimulating cell growth through the ERK and AKT signaling pathways [68]. GDF15 has been suggested as a tumor-associated clinical biomarker suitable for liquid biopsy detection [69].
- DUS1/*DUSP1* is a dual specificity phosphatase which dephosphorylates and inactivates the MAP kinase MAPK1/ERK2, leading amongst other effects to aberrant regulation of the cell cycle. DUS1 plays important roles in the initiation, progression, and recurrence of GBM [70].
- SIK1 is a serine/threonine protein kinase that regulates transcription by phosphorylating transcriptional coactivators such as the CRTCs and HDACs. When cAMP levels increase, SIKs are phosphorylated by activated PKA and sequestered by phosphorylated 14-3-3 proteins as inactive complexes in the cytoplasm [71]. Increased *SIK1* transcription in Mardepodect-treated GBM cells may reflect changes in these cAMP-driven processes.

When the three Mardepodect-treated cell types were analyzed pair-wise, more extensive correlations were revealed.

Strikingly, both A172 and T98G cells upregulated many genes associated with the cholesterol/isoprenoid biosynthesis pathway, including *HMGCR*, *IDI1*, *CYP51A1*, *FDFT1*, *MVD*, *HMGCS1*, *DHCR7*, and *INSIG1*. In parallel, but at a lower abundance, several genes involved in fatty acid metabolism were also upregulated, namely *DDIT4*, *FASN*, and *SCD*. These changes in lipid biosynthesis and metabolism are consistent with enhanced sterol and fatty acid biosynthesis, perhaps associated with autophagy [72].

Upregulated gene expression in T98G and U87MG cells showed many commonalities. Most noticeably, all members of the NR4 nuclear receptor transcription factor family—*NR4A1*, *NR4A2*, and *NR4A3*—were upregulated in both T98G and U87MG by Mardepodect treatment, as were the transcriptional repressor *HES1*, the epithelial to mesenchymal (EMT) transactivator *SNAI1*, and the histone methylation reader *ZCWPW2*. Several genes encoding members of the MAPK-signaling system were also upregulated in T98G and U87MG cells, including: the transcriptional and immune response regulator *TCIM (C8orf4)* which positively regulates G1-to-S-phase transition in the cell cycle, and promotes cell proliferation and inhibits apoptosis in thyroid and lung cancer [73,74]; the serine/threonine-protein kinase *SGK1* which also regulates cell growth, proliferation, survival, migration, and apoptosis through phosphorylation of MAPK1/ERK2, and interaction with MAP2K1/MEK1 and MAP2K2/MEK2; and the adapter protein TRIB1 which regulates COP1 ubiquitin ligase and MAP kinase signaling.

Genes controlling other processes such as complement decay (*CD55*), as well as cell adhesion, migration and hyaluronan degradation (*ITGB3*, *CEMIP*, *TNFAIP6*), were also upregulated.

Levels of the genes encoding 2 well-characterized druggable targets, KS6A2/*RPS6KA2* and the G-protein coupled receptor (GPCR) S1PR1, were also elevated.

- KS6A2/*RPS6KA2*, also known as RSK/RSK3, is a member of the RSK serine/threonine-protein kinase family that acts as a downstream effector of ERK in the MAPK1/ERK2 and MAPK3/ERK1 signaling pathway, mediating cellular proliferation and survival in prostate cancer [75]. The related RSK kinase, KS6A3/RSK2, encoded by *RPS6KA3*, has been reported to regulate growth and invasion in GBM [76].
- S1PR1 is the GPCR for the bioactive lyso-sphingolipid sphingosine 1-phosphate (S1P) which is coupled to the G_i subclass of heteromeric G proteins. In cancer cells, signaling

through S1PR1 leads to the activation of RAC1, SRC, PTK2/FAK1, as well as MAP kinases, and influences cell proliferation and survival in GBM [77].

Three further upregulated genes encode functionally relevant proteins: the small GTPase RND3; the mediator of E2F1-induced apoptosis, GRAM4/*GRAMD4*; and the interleukin IL6, which participates in an important axis for intrinsic VEGF production [78].

Comparison of the Mardepodect-upregulated genes shared in U87MG and A172 reveals further new signatures, with genes encoding the key glioma-associated cell surface proteins GPNMB and T4S19 (*TM4SF19*) being upregulated in concert with the anti-apoptotic heme-degrading enzyme HMOX1, reported to facilitate glioma survival and progression [79].

Interestingly, while the *FAM49A* gene is induced in the Top 200 genes expressed in Mardepodect-treated U87MG and A172 cells, the other gene induced by all four compounds in U87MG cells, namely *PNLIPRP3*, is notably absent. *PNLIPRP3* appears to be specifically induced in drug-treated U87MG cells.

3.13.2. Downregulated Genes Shared between Cells

Cell-specific gene signatures are also seen within the Mardepodect downregulated genes (Supplementary Table S8), with a small number of highly downregulated genes occurring in all three cell lines, namely those encoding the nuclear serine protease F111B/*FAM111B*, the chemokine CCR2 receptor ligand CCL2 and the secreted carboxypeptidase CBPA4/*CPA4*. As proteases, both F111B and CBPA4 are druggable targets. CBPA4 is secreted as a zymogen, raising the further possibility of multi-level targeting during its maturation. The CCL2/CCR2 signaling axis is particularly relevant as a therapeutic target since its downregulation inhibits glioma development [80,81].

3.14. Differential Gene Expression Is Recapitulated in the Corresponding Pathway Analyses

Pathway analyses using the Reactome database were then undertaken to further examine the changes in individual gene expression profiles observed between the cell lines. They confirmed the striking divergence in signaling between U87MG and the other two cell lines.

In Mardepodect-treated U87MG cells, PIP3/AKT- and PTEN-driven signaling pathways were highly upregulated (Supplementary Tables S9 and S10), reflected in upregulation of genes encoding the transcription regulators RRAGC/RRAGD and SNAI1/SNAI2 associated with these pathways. Enhanced PI3K signaling has previously been reported in this cell line [82].

In contrast, in both T98G and A172 cells, Mardepodect treatment prominently upregulated sterol biosynthesis pathways. Although these pathways are driven by the Sterol Response Element-Binding Proteins (SREBPs/SREBFs) [83], levels of the genes for the transcription factors SRBP1 (*SREBF1*) and SRBP2 (*SREBF2*) themselves were not elevated upon Mardepodect treatment, consistent with the post-translational regulation of these proteins by protein processing [84].

Differences in pathway upregulation in the U87MG compared to the T98G and A172 cell lines most likely reflects both their origins and stage of differentiation, as well as the more generally heightened transcriptional plasticity of U87MG cells. These pathway profiles may be useful diagnostics for analyzing GBM drug-response phenotypes in the clinic.

Cell-specific differences are also seen amongst the pathways downregulated by Mardepodect (Supplementary Tables S11 and S12). The prominent cell cycle and cell division pathways characteristically downregulated in U87MG cells, are replaced in both T98G and A172 cells by immune-type cytokine signaling. Further downregulation of these pathways (and genes expressed within them) could be fruitful therapeutic targets.

To visualize functional connectivities within cell-specific DIGEX signatures, network analysis was undertaken for each signature. Again, highly significant differences between the cell lines were seen (Supplementary Figures S2 and S3).

Taken together, these results demonstrate that a single drug treatment (in this case Mardepodect) elicits quite different gene expression responses in specific GBM cell lines. If these DIGEX signatures translate to freshly isolated patient-derived GBM cells, both the signatures themselves as well as the component drug targets within them, could form the basis for new personalized GBM treatment strategies.

3.15. How Do the DIGEX Signatures of Mardepodect-Treated Cells Compare to Those Seen in Regorafenib-Treated Cells?

An analysis of the Top 200 genes upregulated by Mardepodect in the three cell lines has been shown in Figure 4 and Table 3—only *GDF15*, *DUSP1*, and *SIK1* were coordinately upregulated in all three cell lines. Likewise, only three downregulated genes were shared in Mardepodect treated cells—*CPA4*, *FAM111B*, and *CCL2*. The small number of shared genes suggests that the drug response elicited by Mardepodect in the three cell lines is pleiotropic, involving the expression and recruitment of a wide variety of downstream signaling effectors, an observation confirmed by pathway analysis (Supplementary Tables S9–S12).

In sharp contrast, there was extensive overlap in both upregulated and downregulated gene expression profiles in the three cell lines treated with Regorafenib, with 30 upregulated genes and 41 downregulated genes shared within the Top 200 expressed genes (Figure 5 and Table 4).

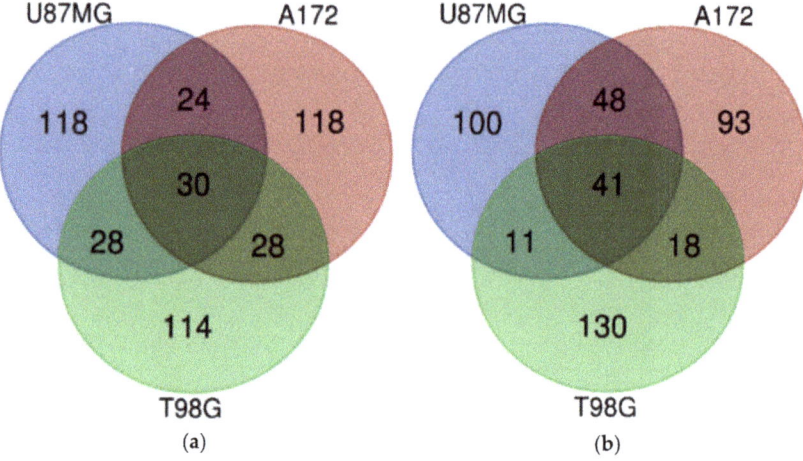

Figure 5. Venn diagrams showing the 200 most significantly modulated genes in Regorafenib-treated U87MG, A172, and T98G cells; (**a**) elevated genes; (**b**) downregulated genes.

Only *GDF15* was shared within the upregulated gene sets in Mardepodect and Regorafenib treated cells; the genes *DUSP1* and *SIK1*, seen previously in cells treated with Mardepodect alone, were absent, even within pairwise cell line comparisons.

Similar disparities were noted amongst the gene sets downregulated by Mardepodect and Regorafenib. Three genes—*CPA4*, *FAM111B*, and *CCL2*—were observed as downregulated in all three Mardepodect-treated cell lines (Figure 4), but only one of these, *FAM111B*, was seen in the Top 200 downregulated genes in Regorafenib-treated cells. *CPA4* was entirely absent from any of the Top 200 gene sets downregulated by Regorafenib, and *CCL2* was only downregulated in the A172/T98G pairwise comparison.

To summarize, the three GBM cell types differ markedly in their DIGEX profiles when growth is inhibited by Mardepodect and Regorafenib under standardized conditions, yielding highly informative and distinctive drug response signatures.

Table 4. Genes modulated by Regorafenib, shared between U87MG, A172, and T98G cells.

Cell Line Groups	Upregulated Genes	Downregulated Genes
U87MG, A172, and T98G	TUBE1, GDF15, TRIB3, PTPDC1, WARS, ERICH2, SLC22A18, SLC6A9, CD22, ATF3, FAM49A, CBS, SLFN5, TMEM159, DDIT3, PSAT1, IL20RB, SOHLH2, TTLL1, PCK2, P2RX7, ASNS, NUPR1, DFNA5, AARS, CCDC169, GTPBP2, PPIL6, RAB39B, KCNH1	IL7R, ESCO2, E2F8, MCM3, CLSPN, DTL, HIST1H1B, LMNB1, PCNA, EXO1, GINS1, MCM6, ATAD2, BARD1, HIST1H2BM, SERTAD4, MCM10, FBXO5, POLE2, TYMS, DNA2, MCM5, F3, ORC1, UHRF1, FAM111B, RRM2, HIST1H3A, ATAD5, HELLS, E2F1, H2AFX, CCNE2, SPC25, MCM2, MCM4, FANCB, GINS2, WDR76, HIST1H2AB, CDC25A
U87MG and A172	ESRP1, PKD1L2, HMOX1, TBL1X, KCNT2, MSC, LURAP1L, ANK2, UNC5B, GPNMB, STK32A, PHGDH, IDH1, PIP5KL1, THBS4, PLPPR4, SLC43A1, HKDC1, TPK1, TM4SF19, MOCOS, PTPN13, SCN9A, CLIP4	TMPO, KIAA1524, MKI67, TGFBR2, KIF20B, ZGRF1, RAD51, ASPM, LDLR, SPAG5, RFC3, DUSP6, CDCA3, HIST2H3A, LRR1, CENPI, BRIP1, TACC3, TCF19, SGOL2, STIL, MCM7, CASC5, HIST1H3B, STARD13, KIF11, ZWINT, ASF1B, FEN1, HIST1H2BO, PLK4, RAD54L, ZNF367, CDC45, NCAPD2, POLQ, PBK, NCAPG, CDC6, HIST1H2BJ, POLA2, KIFC1, ARL6IP6, CDCA5, UBE2T, LIN9, HJURP, XRCC2
U87MG and T98G	TSPAN1, PRELID3A, DUS4L, PPARGC1A, TSLP, UHRF1BP1, STAT2, CCDC113, TUFT1, RCAN1, GADD45A, SH3BGR, CLDN1, C6orf48, GARNL3, TNFRSF9, ABI3BP, CTH, DDR2, SLC22A15, CCPG1, GPR1, CCNB1IP1, DMGDH, GPCPD1, ERN1, CYP2R1, ACAD11	STC1, MEST, CCNF, EGLN3, SPRY1, HIST1H4D, HIST1H2BI, FAM20C, HIST1H2BH, EGR1, CDK2
A172 and T98G	GRB10, FYN, PCDH1, PPP1R3B, HOXB9, FAM129A, SYCP2L, SYT14, SEL1L3, S1PR1, SLC1A4, THBS3, VEGFA, OSBPL6, ULBP1, ARHGEF2, SESN2, AGT, DTNA, MAP2, CHAC1, C10orf107, LCA5L, CREB5, STEAP1, CYP4V2, ADGRG1, AFF3	EDN1, MMP13, HIST1H3H, MYCBP, HIST1H4L, GMNN, CCND1, CENPW, TNFRSF11B, HIST1H4A, MIS18BP1, CCL2, TRIB2, CDC7, PRDM1, CSNK1G1, MYB, HIST1H2BF

3.16. What Can Be Inferred from the Cell-Specific DIGEX Signatures?

Finally, we examined the cell line-specific gene sets from each treatment. Results obtained by treating U87MG cells with all four inhibitors showed many compound-specific genes (Figure 2 and Table 1), with the two clinical candidates Mardepodect and Regorafenib each showing over 100 compound-specific genes amongst the Top 200 examined.

Extending these observations to all three GBM cell lines, we again see expression of a high level of cell-specific genes (Supplementary Tables S7 and S8 for Mardepodect; Supplementary Tables S13 and S14 for Regorafenib). Network analysis confirmed the marked differences in DIGEX profiles between treated cell lines (Supplementary Figure S4).

In summary, taking the Top 200 genes in each DIGEX profile operationally defines a distinctive drug 'fingerprint', specific to each cell line, from which much underlying biological information can be retrieved.

3.17. Which Genes Encode Proteins That Could Be Viable Drug Targets in GBM?

The development of new GBM therapies requires target validation to be coupled to effective drug and vaccine production. In this study, we have used genome-wide gene expression analysis of drug-treated cells to reveal subsets of genes which are characteristic of the underlying cell biology of the GBM cells. These DIGEX signatures are powerful diagnostics—but how many of the genes thus identified represent viable drug targets?

Complete profiles of the Top 200 differentially expressed genes drawn from the set of 18,316 tracked in all three GBM cell lines studied, are shown for all treatments in Supplementary Table S15. These gene sets contain many biological targets that have not previously been directly associated with GBM, including specific adhesion molecules, transcription factors, protein kinases, and glycosyltransferases. We used the Pharos, NCBI Gene, and UniProt databases to identify, classify, and annotate all the likely drug and vaccine targets present in the three cell lines. In the analysis below, UniProt protein entries are denoted in block capitals with corresponding NCBI Gene entries in italics.

The Pharos database is a chemical biology resource that allows rapid association of genes encoding proteins with potential chemical modulators, including both approved drugs and exploratory compounds. We use the database as part of a drug target triage strategy, separating the Top 200 gene sets into groups encoding (1) proteins with associated FDA approved drug modulators; (2) proteins with chemical modulators that can be used as starting points for drug discovery; and (3) proteins which merit further biological study.

3.17.1. U87MG Cells Treated with Mardepodect

To illustrate this process, focusing on the cell line U87MG treated with Mardepodect, we see that one of the most highly upregulated genes is *PNLIPRP3*, encoding the lipase LIPR3, previously seen as one of only two genes that are shared within the Top 200 most highly upregulated genes in all four initial drug treatments in this cell line (Figure 2).

The *PNLIPRP3* gene encodes a novel druggable protein, with a well-defined Lipase domain harboring the active site, sandwiched between an N-terminal signal peptide and a hydrophobic PLAT domain—a structure the gene shares with pancreatic lipase (LIPP/*PNLIP*) and the other members of this gene family (LIPR1/*PNLIPRP1* and LIPR2/*PNLIPRP2*). However, LIPR3 has no specific FDA-approved or exploratory chemical leads associated with it, and is therefore annotated by Pharos as Tdark, implying a protein without well-defined biological precedent as a drug target and without chemical leads [85].

Although no drug discovery campaigns have been reported for LIPR3, the pancreatic lipase gene family of which LIPR3 is a member has been the subject of considerable medicinal chemistry attention due to the role of the closely related LIPP protein in obesity, for which there is an FDA-approved drug (Orlistat) with an associated X-ray co-crystal structure [37].

PNLIPRP3 is highly induced only in drug treated U87MG cells and is not highly upregulated by Mardepodect in either T98G or A172 cells (Supplementary Table S15). It is not even modestly expressed in normal tissues [36]. We classify LIPR3/*PNLIPRP3* as a novel druggable GBM target in cells with the U87MG phenotype.

Using Pharos classification alone as a benchmark, amongst the Top 200 U87MG genes upregulated by Mardepodect, we identify 36 (18%) as encoding potential targets with currently unexplored biology; 118 (59%) as target genes corresponding to proteins for which biological targeting rationales exist but which have no associated chemical modulators; 36 genes (18%) encoding proteins with exploratory chemical leads; and only 7 genes encoding proteins with corresponding FDA-approved drugs.

The FDA-approved target class is important, since drugs targeting these proteins could be repositioned immediately within clinical trials in GBM. The relative paucity of validated FDA-approved drugs for the targets we reveal by DIGEX suggests that target validation remains a key challenge for GBM drug discovery.

For Mardepodect-treated U87MG cells, the 7 upregulated FDA-approved targets as classified by Pharos comprise: the Vitamin D-binding nuclear receptor VDR; the secreted cytokine IL6; the Thioredoxin Reductase TRXR1/*TXNRD1*; the kinase-insert domain receptor VGFR2 (known variously as *KDR*, *FLK1*, *CD309*, *VEGFR*, or *VEGFR2*), the integrin beta chain ITB3/*ITGB3*, and the GPCRs S1PR1 and EDNRA.

3.17.2. T98G and A172 Cells Treated with Mardepodect

Broadening this analysis from U87MG to the other two GBM cells T98G and A172, we see that very few of the U87MG Pharos-annotated FDA-approved drug target genes are replicated within the Top 200 genes upregulated by Mardepodect, translating into a gene signature with a radically different FDA-approved drug profile.

For T98G cells, 12 genes form the 'FDA signature', comprising the two interleukins *IL1B* and *IL6*; five G-protein coupled receptors (the dopamine receptor *DRD2*, the adrenoceptor *ADRB2*, the adenosine receptor *ADORA1*, the sphingosine-1-phosphate receptor *S1PR1*, and the bradykinin receptor *BDKRB2*); the heparin-binding growth factor *VEGFA*; two cholesterol biosynthesis enzymes *HMGCR* and *HSD11B1*; the phosphodiesterase *PDE4D*; and, as in U87MG cells, the integrin beta chain *ITGB3*. Except for *ITGB3* upregulation, the U87MG and T98G FDA drug signatures are mutually exclusive.

For A172 cells, the FDA signature includes nine components: the two cholesterol biosynthesis enzymes *HMGCR* and *FDPS*; the phosphodiesterase *PDE7B*; the somatostatin receptor *SSTR2*; the androgen receptor *AR* (also known as the nuclear receptor *NR3C4*); the NMDA receptor *GRIN2A*; the carbonic anhydrase isozyme *CA12*; the thyroid hormone receptor *THRA*; and the lipase *LIPF*. Again, the U87MG and A172 FDA drug signatures are mutually exclusive. T98G and A172 cells notably share *HMGCR* expression.

Turning our attention from FDA targets to the more extensive Exploratory drug target class exemplified within Pharos, we find many attractive, chemistry-led drug discovery targets.

For U87MG, these include the GPCRs T2R14/*TAS2R14*, C3AR/*C3AR1*, C5AR1, GPR84, and GP183/*GPR183*; the kinases SIK1, PDK4, ACKR3, PLK2, KS6A2/*RPS6KA2*, F262/*PFKFB2*, SGK1, KITM/*TK2*, and CHKA; the interleukin IL1A; the metalloproteinases ATS5/*ADAMTS5* and MMP14; the nuclear receptor NR4A2; the asparagine N-linked glycosyltransferase TUSC3; the cell adhesion molecule KIAA1462/*JCAD*; the transporters ACATN/*SLC33A1*, XCT/*SLC7A11*, NRAM2/*SLC11A2*, and CLCN7; the lipases LIPE/*LIPG* and LIPR/*PNLIPRP3*; the enzymes CGL/*CTH*, DHB14/*HSD17B14*, HMOX1, OGT1/*OGT*, AK1C1/*AKR1C1*, FHIT, and IDHC/*IDH1*; the dual specificity phosphatase DUS1/*DUSP1*; the ligand-gated chloride channel GBRR1/*GABRR1* (otherwise known as the GABA(C) receptor); the G-protein linked potassium channel KCNJ3; and the phosphocholine/phosphoethanolamine phosphatase PHOP1/*PHOSPHO1*.

Several previously validated anti-proliferative targets are contained within this U87MG Exploratory target set, including:

1. The atypical chemokine GPCR ACKR3/CXCR7, which in glioma cells transduces signals via the MEK/ERK pathway, mediating resistance to apoptosis and promoting cell growth and survival [86]; and
2. The nuclear receptor NR4A2, previously validated as a drug target in glioblastoma [87].

Mardepodect-inhibited A172 and U87MG cells share some of these Exploratory targets, including LIPE/*LIPG*, HMOX1, GP183/*GPR183*, DUS1/*DUSP1*, NRAM2/*SLC11A2*, and the serine/threonine protein kinase SIK1. Druggable components of the cholesterol/fatty acid biosynthesis pathways are also prominent within the A172 Exploratory target set (DHCR7; HMCS1/*HMGCS1*; FDFT/*FDFT1*; KIME/*MVK*; MVD1/*MVD*; IDI1; DHB7/*HSD17B7*; CP51A/*CYP51A1*; ACACA; SCD; ELOV6/*ELOVL6*; FAS/*FASN*; ABHD6; FABPH/*FABP3*), together with more established anticancer drug discovery targets such as the PI3-kinase P3C2B/*PIK3C2B* and the lysine-specific demethylase KDM4D. We also see unique targets, such as the small GTPase RAB7L/*RAB29* (involved with LRRK2 in vesicle trafficking); the P2X receptor P2RX7; the cell adhesion protein VITRN/*VIT*; the opioid neuropeptide GPCR OPRX/*OPRL1* and the olfactory GPCR OR1L4; the spermatogenesis-associated, calmodulin-binding protein SPT17/*SPATA17*; the ectonucleoside diphosphatase ENTP1/*ENTPD1*; the cystathionine beta-synthase CBS; the DNA methylation enzyme DNM3B/*DNMT3B*; the P-type ATPase AT12A/*ATP12A*; the putative P-glycoprotein-associated drug transporter EBP; the apoptosis suppressor XIAP; the protein tyrosine phosphatase PTN22/*PTPN22*; and the ephrin receptor tyrosine kinase EPHA8.

In passing, for target-based drug discovery purposes, it is notable that several specific members of extended gene families of potential drug discovery importance are revealed by DIGEX in these exploratory gene sets, for example, the PI3-kinase catalytic domain isoform P3C2B/*PIK3C2B* and the lysine demethylase KDM4D. PI3-kinases participate in the signaling pathways involved in cell proliferation and oncogenic cell survival, and the induction of P3C2B/*PIK3C2B* is therefore not surprising, since this protein has previously been identified as significantly correlated with cellular resistance to erlotinib [88]. However, Regorafenib also upregulates P3C2G/*PIK3C2G*, confirming this isoform, also, as a potential target in drug resistant GBM [89]. Likewise, although KDM5A has previously been identified in temozolomide resistant GBM cell lines [90], here we see Mardepodect upregulating KDM4D and KDM7A. The advent of small molecules specifically targeting individual lysine demethylase isoforms may open the way to more precise drug targeting within this extended family [91,92].

Many of the highly upregulated Exploratory targets seen in A172 cells are also present in T98G, including GTR3/*SLC2A3*; DUS1/*DUSP1*; the sterol biosynthesis enzymes HMCS1/*HMGCS1*; SCD; FDFT/*FDFT1*; DHCR7; MVD1/*MVD*; IDI1 and the multifunctional fatty acid biosynthesis enzyme FAS/*FASN*, as well as the additional steroid hormone biosynthesis enzymes 3BHS1/*HSD3B1* and DHB2/*HSD17B2* and ERG1/*SQLE*, the rate-determining enzyme in the steroidogenic pathway. Several highly upregulated Exploratory targets seen in A172 cells are also shared with U87MG: NR4A2; SGK1; KS6A2/*RPS6KA2*.

Top 200 Mardepodect-upregulated Exploratory targets seen only in T98G include the IGF-binding protein IBP4/*IGFBP4*; the membrane lipid remodeling phospholipase PA24A/*PLA2G4A*; the chromatin silencing histone H10/*H1F0*; the prostaglandin transporter SO2A1/*SLCO2A1*; the drug metabolizing methyltransferase NNMT; the histone demethylase KDM7A; the neurotrophin receptor signaling adapter BEX1; the transcription factor JUN; the hypoxia-inducible master transcription activator HIF1A; the serine/threonine protein kinases TNI3K/*TNNI3K* and NIM1/*NIM1K*; the MMP-9 activator MMP26; the histamine receptor GPCR HRH4; the tyrosine protein kinase FRK; and the GPCR specific serine/threonine kinase GRK5.

Together, these targets represent a prodigious amount of relatively unexplored drug discovery space. Systematic target validation studies are now required to establish experimentally how many of the exploratory targets within the Mardepodect-induced GBM cell phenotypes are valid as drug targets for GBM. We illustrate features of a possible chemical biology-driven target validation process below.

3.18. Downregulated Genes May Indicate Cell Cycle Control Imposed by Drug Treatment

The Pharos analysis of the genes that are coordinately downregulated by Mardepodect in the three GBM cell lines, is presented in Supplementary Table S15. As observed in the case of U87MG, above, these DIGEX profiles are dominated by reduced cell cycle and cell division gene expression.

Although a full analysis of the downregulated genes accompanying drug treatment is beyond the scope of this initial DIGEX study, it is clear from initial inspection that the downregulated gene sets contain many intriguing drug discovery targets, from well characterized enzymes such as ribonucleoside-diphosphate reductase RIR2/*RRM2*, to less well-known targets such as the serine protease F111B/*FAM111B*. The Venn analyses also show that most of the downregulated cell-cycle associated genes are differentially regulated between GBM cell types and the four drug treatments, suggesting a tight and precise downregulation of cell division, rather than random repression, possibly reflecting a more complex spatiotemporal control of cell division [93].

3.19. Summary of Drug-Induced Gene Expression (DIGEX) Analysis Results

An overall diagrammatic summary of the most highly upregulated drug-induced genes encoding potential drug targets, secretory proteins and cell surface antigens expressed in the three GBM cell lines is shown in Figure 6.

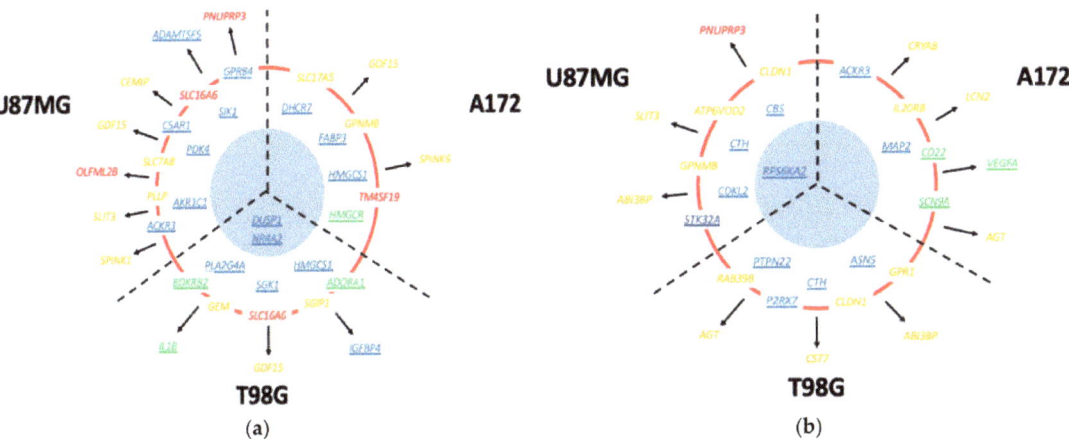

Figure 6. Summary of the most highly elevated drug induced genes encoding potential drug targets, secretory proteins and cell surface antigens expressed within the Top 25 gene set in the three GBM cell lines. (**a**) Mardepodect-treated cells; (**b**) Regorafenib-treated cells. Note the clear differences between the drug modulated phenotypes, both between GBM cell types and individual drug treatments. Targets underlined in green have existing FDA approved drugs; those underlined in blue have chemical leads but no approved drugs; those in yellow have only biological rationales, while those in red remain relatively unexplored.

3.20. Validating Individual Drug-Inducible Genes as Pharmacological Targets in GBM as Monotherapies and Drug Combinations

DIGEX profiling in conjunction with Pharos yields a rich vein of potential targets. With detailed bioinformatic analyses in hand, we moved to experimental validation of some of the targets themselves as potential GBM modulators.

To establish a screening sequence for potential combination therapies using Mardepodect as the initial drug, we identified a set of targets with cognate inhibitors to validate our triage strategy. These included:

- Two FDA approved inhibitors for HMGCoA reductase, Atorvastatin and Simvastatin. The gene encoding HMGCoA reductase (*HMGCR*) is in the Top 200 genes upregulated by Mardepodect in A172 and T98G cells but not U87MG. *HMGCR* is absent from the Regorafenib Top 200.
- Two exploratory inhibitors of the salt-inducible kinase SIK1, HG-9-91-01, and WH-4-023. The gene encoding SIK1 is present in the Top 200 genes upregulated by Mardepodect in all three GBM cells but absent from the Top 200 in Regorafenib-treated cells.
- Two inhibitors of the Janus Kinase JAK2, the FDA approved drug Ruxolitinib and the exploratory compound AZD1480. The gene encoding JAK2 is induced in U87MG by LY-294002 [20] but absent from the Top 200 upregulated genes in both Mardepodect and Regorafenib treated cells.
- Two inhibitors of the bradykinin B2 receptor, Icatibant and WIN 64338. The *BDKRB2* gene is in the Top 200 upregulated genes in Mardepodect treated T98G cells.

3.21. Combinations of the PDE10A Inhibitor Mardepodect and Regorafenib

Combination therapy is a major objective in GBM [9]. Although the screening sequence deployed here (DIGEX-Pharos-Pharmacology) was designed to uncover new drug discovery targets, it might also predict target combinations for validation. We therefore also determined whether any of the compounds we had identified individually to inhibit GBM cell proliferation were effective in combination.

As an initial experiment, we tested the two clinical compounds Mardepodect and Regorafenib in combination. Synergy between PI3K and cAMP signaling pathways has previously been suggested as potentially relevant in GBM [94]. We observed synergy in U87MG cells (with a maximum synergy score of 24), but modest antagonism between Mardepodect and Regorafenib in both T98G and A172 cells (with a maximum score of −21) (Figure 7).

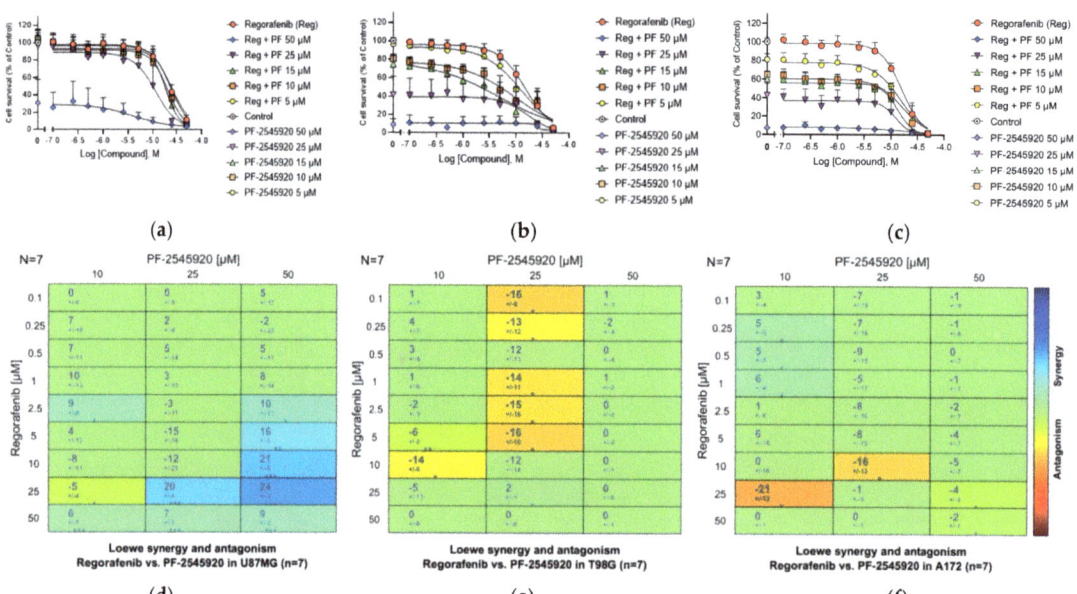

Figure 7. Anti-proliferative effect of combining Mardepodect and Regorafenib; (**a**) U87MG; (**b**) A172; (**c**) T98G cells. Data are presented as the mean ± standard error of the mean (SEM) (n = 7); (**d–f**), corresponding quantitative analyses of the same data using the Loewe method. Synergy is seen in U87MG cells, but antagonism in both T98G and A172 cells. Note: asterisks indicate the significance of synergy scores obtained following a one-sample t-test (* $p < 0.05$; ** $p < 0.001$; *** $p < 0.0001$).

3.22. HMGCoA Reductase

Our data indicated that HMGCoA reductase (HMDH/*HMGCR*) was upregulated in the Mardepodect-treated A172 cell line where it was the 33rd most upregulated gene. HMDH/*HMGCR* has recently been suggested as a therapeutic target in GBM [83] and upregulation of HMDH/*HMGCR* has previously been shown to positively regulate the growth and migration of the GBM cell lines U251 and U373 [95].

Both Atorvastatin and Simvastatin markedly inhibited cell proliferation (Figure 8a,b), with both U87MG and T98G cells showing synergy with Mardepodect (Figure 8c–h). A172 cells showed higher sensitivity to statin inhibition but showed antagonism upon combination of the statins with Mardepodect. Both Atorvastatin and Simvastatin are safe, widely prescribed FDA approved drugs, belonging to the lipophilic statin class which carries no borderline risk of causing glioma [96].

Additional genes associated with cholesterol biosynthesis—including *INSIG1*, *HMGCS1*, and *RNF145*—are also upregulated by Mardepodect in at least one of the three GBM cell lines studied here, warranting further examination of the pathway and its rate-limiting steps as adjunct therapeutic targets in GBM.

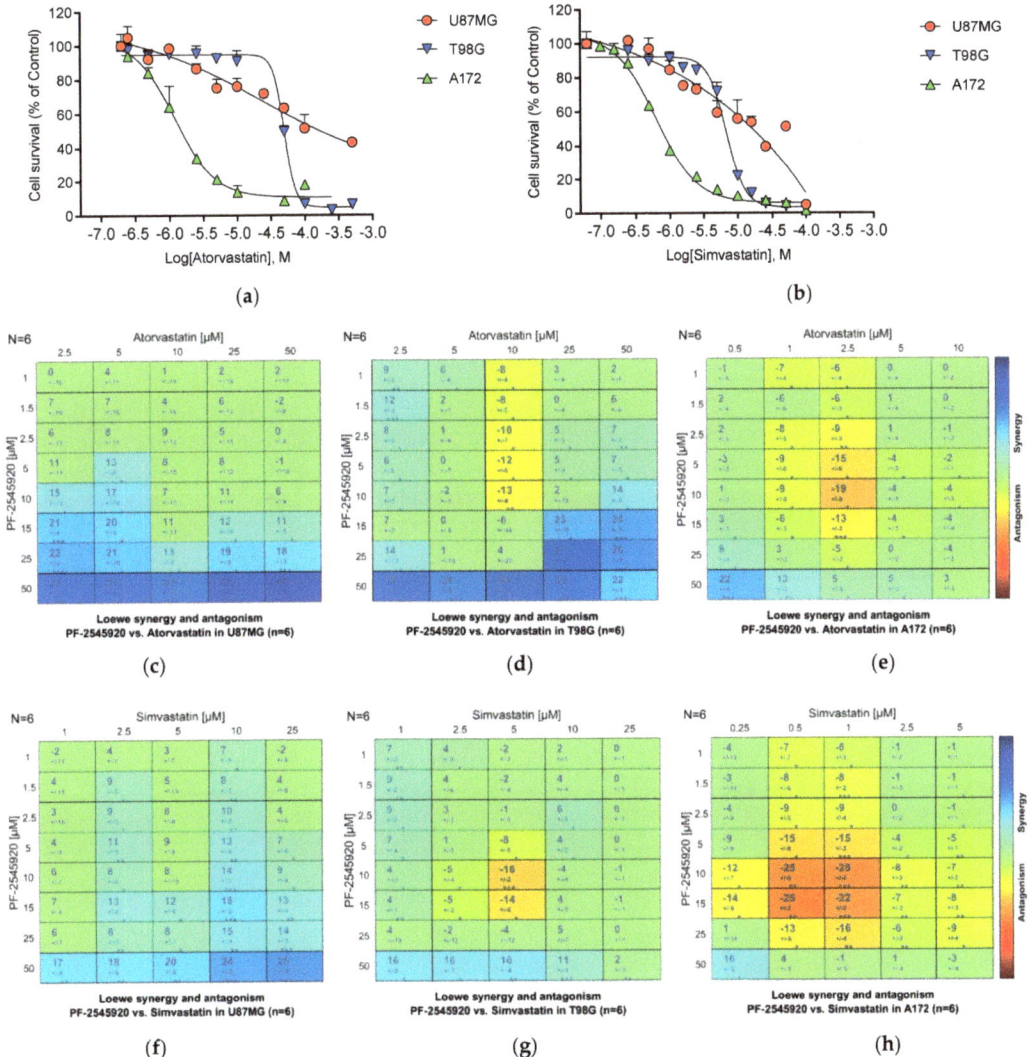

Figure 8. Anti-proliferative effects of HMGCoA reductase inhibitors on U87MG, A172 and T98G cells. (**a**) Atorvastatin; (**b**) Simvastatin. Data are presented as the mean ± standard error of the mean (SEM) (n = 3–6). Panels (**c**–**e**) show Loewe synergy plots for the combination of Atorvastatin and PF-2545920 in U87MG, T98G, and A172 glioblastoma cells, respectively. Synergy (in blue) was observed in U87MG and T98G cells at higher Mardepodect concentrations (with a maximal synergy score of 40), but signs of antagonism (in orange) were seen in A172 cells (synergy score of −25). Panels (**f**–**h**) show Loewe synergy plots for the combination of Simvastatin and PF-2545920 in U87MG, T98G, and A172 glioblastoma cells, respectively. Again, some synergy was observed in U87MG and T98G cells, with scores ranging from 16 to 25, with the combinations showing definite antagonism in A172 cells (with a score of −25). Note: asterisks indicate the significance of synergy scores obtained following a one-sample t-test (* $p < 0.05$; ** $p < 0.001$; *** $p < 0.0001$).

3.23. Salt-Inducible Kinase SIK1

Salt-inducible kinase isoform 1 (*SIK1*) is highly upregulated in all three GBM cells treated with Mardepodect (Table 3). Acting through their interaction with 14-3-3 proteins,

SIKs disrupt cAMP signaling, promoting inhibitory phosphorylation on CREB-regulated transcription coactivators [71,97].

We have previously shown that cAMP inhibits the growth of rat C6 glioma cells [20], and we know that the PDE10A inhibitor Mardepodect increases the levels of cAMP in the human GBM cell lines used here. Salt-inducible kinase (*SIK*) is also one of six genes associated with significantly shorter patient survival in GBM [98].

We used two commercially available compounds to investigate the effects of SIK inhibition on proliferation: HG-9-91-01, originally synthesized for studies of SIK involvement in inflammation [99], and WH-4-023, originally designed as a lymphocyte specific kinase (LCK) inhibitor but which has SIK inhibitory properties [100].

HG-9-91-01 is a pan-specific SIK inhibitor with an IC50 versus SIK1 of 0.92 nM, SIK2 of 6.6 nM, and SIK3 of 9.6 nM, with lower activity against the kinases NUAK2, SRC, LCK, YES, and BTK, and the FGFR and EphR families. WH-4-023 is also pan-specific towards the SIK family, with lower affinity on BTK, FGFR, JAK2, KDR, p38 alpha, SYK, TIE 2, and ZAP70.

Both inhibitors were anti-proliferative in all three GBM cell lines. The strong induction of *SIK1* upon Mardepodect treatment is consistent with GBM cells sensing elevated cAMP levels and raising *SIK1* mRNA levels to compensate for this. Considerably greater sensitivity to one of the SIK inhibitors, HG-9-91-01, was seen in A172 cells, but all three cell lines were inhibited by WH-4-023 to the same degree (Figure 9a,b).

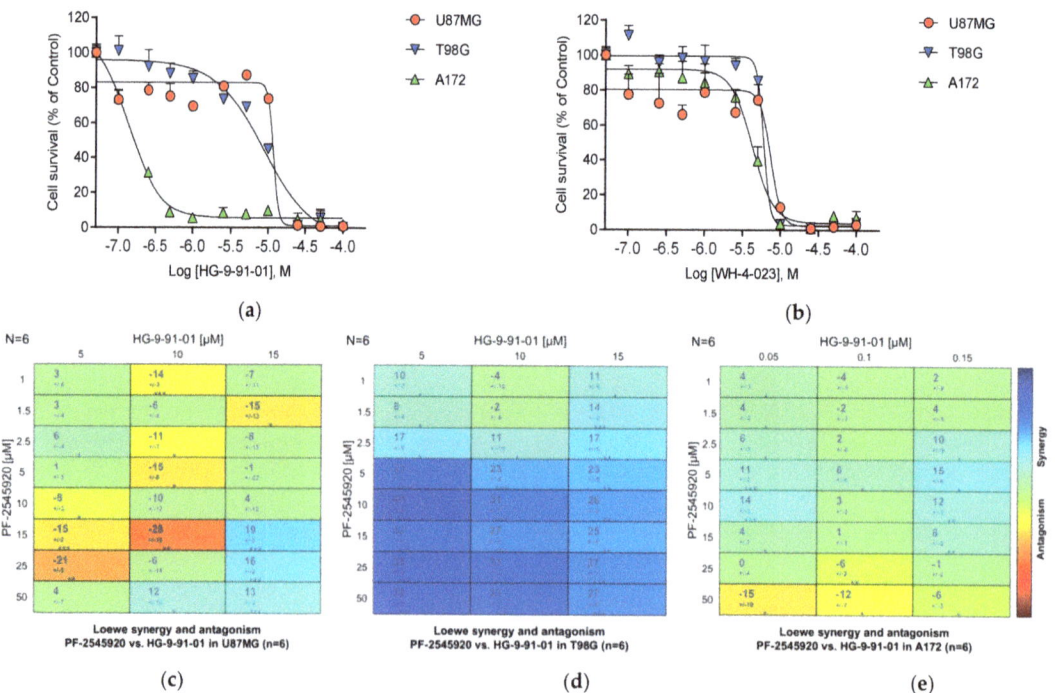

Figure 9. Anti-proliferative effects of SIK1 inhibitors on U87MG, A172 and T98G cells. (**a**) HG-9-91-01; (**b**) WH-4-023. Data are presented as the mean ± standard error of the mean (SEM) (n = 3–6). Panels (**c**–**e**) show Loewe synergy plots for the combination of HG-9-91-01 and PF-2545920 in U87MG, T98G, and A172 glioblastoma cells, respectively. T98G cells showed pronounced synergy. Note: Asterisks indicate the significance of synergy scores obtained following a one-sample t-test (* p < 0.05; ** p < 0.001; *** p < 0.0001).

Having seen marked inhibition of growth in the three cells by the two SIK inhibitors, we also tested Mardepodect in combination with the SIK inhibitor HG-9-91-01. Here, we observed strong synergy (with a synergy score rising to 40)—but only in T98G cells (Figure 9d). Both U87MG and A172 cells showed much lower synergy scores (Figure 9c,e).

The synergy between Mardepodect and HG-9-91-01 in T98G cells suggests an inducing drug (Mardepodect) synergizing with an inhibitor of an induced target (SIK1), with the two targets operating as a 'node' within the cAMP signaling pathway. Upregulation of induced targets within the cancer cell's survival programs has been suggested to promote drug resistance [101].

SIK1 is most upregulated by Mardepodect in U87MG cells, where it is the third most highly upregulated gene (Supplementary Table S15). One might imagine that U87MG cells would be more sensitive to SIK inhibition, but Mardepodect and HG-9-91-01 show only modest synergy in U87MG cells. In T98G cells, however, where strong synergy is seen, *SIK1* is only the 65th most upregulated gene, suggesting that in this case the degree of target upregulation alone does not predict combinatorial drug sensitivity.

A potentially important observation is that neither of the other two SIK subtypes, *SIK2* and *SIK3*, show pronounced induction upon Mardepodect treatment, implicating specific transcriptional selection of the *SIK1* subtype during drug response. Drug discovery focused on achieving SIK1 selectivity may therefore be a relevant objective in the design of effective GBM therapies. In this context, it is important to note that effective target validation by chemical biology is always dependent on the quality and selectivity of the chemical probes available [17,18].

As far as we know, no SIK inhibitors are in development as antiproliferative agents in GBM. However, topical SIK inhibitors are being developed as sunscreen agents in melanoma [102]. SIKs also mediate parathyroid hormone receptor activity in bone development and remodeling [103,104] and the inflammatory phenotype in activated myeloid cells [105,106]. SIK inhibitors, with their therapeutic potential for the treatment of inflammatory and autoimmune diseases, are thus a commercially attractive drug class which may possess the added advantage of being suitable for repurposing in GBM.

Our results confirm the general importance of the SIK pathway in GBM growth control. They also show that important growth mediators may be buried within DIGEX signatures, since *SIK1* is only the 41st most highly upregulated gene in Mardepodect-treated T98G cells and the 99th most highly upregulated gene in Mardepodect-treated A172 cells, despite being one of the most highly upregulated genes in Mardepodect-treated U87MG cells.

3.24. Janus Kinase JAK2

In previous studies, we observed upregulation of *JAK2* by LY-294002 in U87MG cells [20]. JAK2 plays a central role in phosphorylation of glioma-associated STAT3, a key component of the PI3K-signaling pathway [107]. The selective JAK2 inhibitors SAR317461 and AZD1480 have been reported to inhibit GBM proliferation via this pathway [108,109], and combining the approved EGFR inhibitors Erlotinib and Osimertinib with the JAK2 inhibitor AZD1480 induces irreversible apoptosis in GBM [110]. The JAK1/2 inhibitor, Ruxolitinib, is an approved drug for the treatment of polycythemia vera and myelofibrosis [111,112].

We examined the effects of both AZD1480 and Ruxolitinib on proliferation in the three GBM cell lines (Figure 10). Both compounds inhibit the growth of all three GBM cells. A172 cells showed greater sensitivity to AZD1480 than did U87MG, with T98G showing intermediate sensitivity, an order of potency previously observed by others for the JAK2 selective inhibitor SAR317461 [108].

We then tested the JAK2 inhibitor AZD1480 in combination with the prototypic PI3K inhibitor LY-294002 (Figure 10c–e). Here, strong synergy was seen in U87MG cells, with synergy scores rising to 54, with some synergy evident in T98G cells. No synergy was seen in A172 cells. Synergy was compound- and possibly subtype-specific, since the non-selective JAK1/2 inhibitor Ruxolitinib showed no synergy with LY-294002 in U87MG cells.

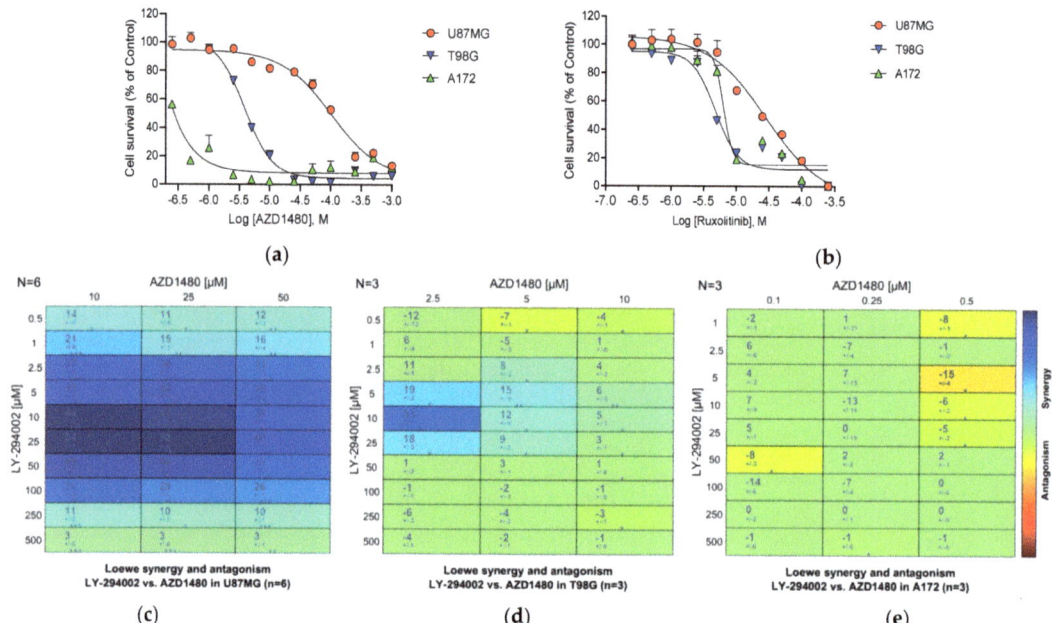

Figure 10. Anti-proliferative effects of JAK2 inhibitors on U87MG, A172 and T98G cells. (**a**) AZD1480; (**b**) Ruxolitinib. Data are presented as the mean ± standard error of the mean (SEM) (n = 3–6). Panels (**c**–**e**) show Loewe synergy plots for the combination of AZD1480 and LY-294002 in U87MG, T98G, and A172 glioblastoma cells, respectively. U87MG cells showed pronounced synergy for this combination, with synergy scores rising to >50. Note: Asterisks indicate the significance of synergy scores obtained following a one-sample t-test (* $p < 0.05$; ** $p < 0.001$; *** $p < 0.0001$).

Subtype selectivity in targeting kinases such as JAK2 and SIK1 in GBM will most likely be important in the clinic since we know that JAK and SIK subtypes play important roles in processes such as macrophage differentiation, dendritic cell function and innate immunity [104,105,113]. Balancing subtype selectivity may thus provide benefits in GBM immune recognition as well as GBM growth inhibition.

3.25. GPCRs

We noted prominent and specific upregulation of several genes encoding GPCRs in the DIGEX data (Supplementary Table S15), including *ADORA1*, which encodes the adenosine A1 receptor (highly upregulated in T98G cells by Mardepodect); *BDKRB2*, which encodes the bradykinin B2 receptor (highly upregulated in T98G cells by Mardepodect); *DRD2*, which encodes the dopamine D2 receptor (upregulated by Mardepodect in T98G cells); and *GPR84*, which encodes the orphan GPCR GPR84 (the most highly Mardepodect-upregulated gene in U87MG cells).

3.25.1. Bradykinin B2 Receptor (B_2R)

The gene encoding the B_2R, *BDKRB2*, was markedly upregulated in Mardepodect-treated T98G cells (Supplementary Table S15). B_2R is an EMT-related biomarker and predicts poor survival in glioma [114], while bradykinin itself enhances invasion of malignant glioma into the brain parenchyma [115]. Pharmacological studies in the human astrocytoma cell line D384 have shown the B_2R to be present and functionally linked to phospholipase C and inhibition of dopamine stimulated cyclic AMP accumulation [116].

Although the bradykinin receptor antagonist drug class represents an area of intense current drug discovery opportunity [117], only one bradykinin receptor ligand is currently used in clinical practice, the B_2R antagonist Icatibant/HOE-140 [118].

We tested Icatibant in GBM cells alongside the nonpeptide bradykinin B2 antagonist WIN 64338 [119]. Consistent with reports that the synthetic peptide Icatibant is metabolically vulnerable, Icatibant proved inactive as a growth inhibitor in our cellular models of GBM proliferation (Figure 11a). In contrast, the non-peptide B_2R antagonist WIN 64338 showed promising growth inhibitory activity against all three GBM cell lines (Figure 11b), confirming the potential involvement of B_2R signaling in GBM proliferation.

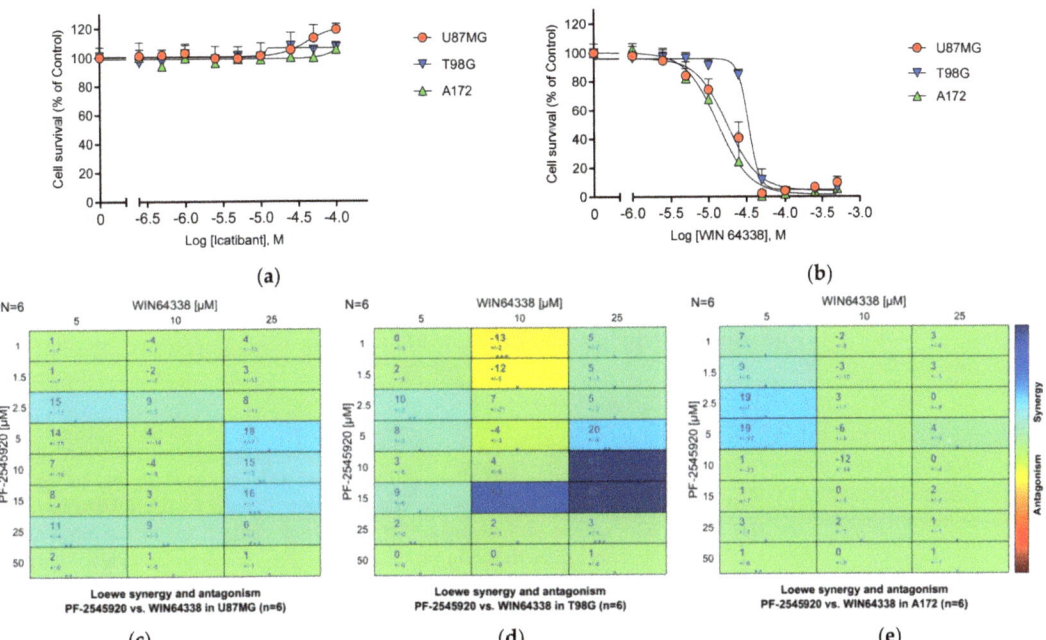

Figure 11. Anti-proliferative effects of bradykinin B2 antagonists on U87MG, A172 and T98G cells. (**a**) Icatibant; (**b**) WIN 64338. Data are presented as the mean ± standard error of the mean (SEM) (n = 6). Panels (**c**–**e**) show Loewe synergy plots for the combination of Mardepodect (PF-2545920) and WIN64338 in U87MG, T98G and A172 glioblastoma cells, respectively. T98G cells showed pronounced synergy, with synergy scores rising to 62. Note: Asterisks indicate the significance of synergy scores obtained following a one-sample t-test (* $p < 0.05$; ** $p < 0.001$; *** $p < 0.0001$).

Very interestingly, the T98G cell line, which showed marked upregulation of the *BDKRB2* gene after Mardepodect treatment, demonstrated pronounced synergy when Mardepodect was combined with WIN 64338 (Figure 11d). Neither U87MG or A172 cells showed comparable synergy (Figure 11c,e). Further examination of the comparative pharmacology of bradykinin signaling in these 3 GBM cell lines is merited.

3.25.2. Other GPCRs

GPCRs are the most common class of drug target [120] and are key targets in oncology [121]. We observed several upregulated genes encoding GPCRs in both Mardepodect- and Regorafenib-treated cells, including G Protein-coupled Receptor 37 (*GPR37*) and the dopamine D2 receptor *DRD2*, both of which, like B_2R, are Gi-coupled GPCRs [122,123]. GPR37 also acts as a cell survival factor [124], occurring as a complex with DRD2 at the cell surface where it exerts a neuroprotective effect [125,126].

Importantly, the DRD2 receptor is the target for the promising anticancer compound TIC10/ONC201 [127], currently in clinical trials for GBM [128]. Drug resistance to ONC201 has recently been observed [129], making pharmacological exploration of the signaling networks surrounding GPCRs such as GPR37, DRD2, AA1R/*ADORA1*, and BKRB2/*BDKRB2* of particular therapeutic relevance.

We have shown previously that increasing cAMP levels in glioma cells results in growth inhibition [29], suggesting that, in conjunction with the use of PDE inhibitors such as Mardepodect, raising intracellular cAMP levels in GBM cells by antagonizing Gi-linked GPCRs such as B_2R could be therapeutically relevant.

Another GPCR which merits future pharmacological follow-up in GBM is the orphan GPCR, GPR84. In Mardepodect-treated U87MG cells, *GPR84* was the most highly upregulated gene (Supplementary Table S15). GPR84 is a fatty-acid binding protein involved in fibrosis [130] and is also essential in the maintenance of cancer stem cells in acute myeloid leukemia [131]. A range of ligands is available for exploring its function [132].

3.26. Summary of the Compound Synergy Studies

These initial results show that synergy is often cell-type specific, especially evident in the LY-294002/AZD1480 combinations which showed strong synergy in U87MG cells. Cell-type specificity was also seen in Mardepodect/HG-9-91-01 combinations, with T98G cells on this occasion showing strongest synergy. In general, A172 cells exhibited lower levels of synergy than either U87MG or T98G cells, although they often showed higher compound sensitivities. Combinatorial testing of further inhibitors guided by the DIGEX data may enable additional synergies to be found.

4. Discussion

Previous work from our laboratory has used genome-wide drug-induced gene expression (DIGEX) as a method of defining the molecular phenotypes induced by growth inhibition in the GBM cell line U87MG [20]. In that study, we focused on two compounds, the prototypic PI3K inhibitor LY-294002, a pan-PI3K inhibitor with well-characterized multiple molecular modes of action [133,134], and Fucoxanthin, a marine algal natural product with anti-cancer growth inhibitory properties [135]. We were somewhat surprised to see the great variation in gene expression produced by these two growth inhibitors, having imagined that a single cell line such as U87MG, upon growth inhibition, would display a more restricted drug-induced phenotype.

To investigate these observations further, here we have used further growth inhibitors, including two clinical antiproliferative drugs, the PDE10A inhibitor Mardepodect and the multi-kinase inhibitor Regorafenib, profiling them in two additional GBM cell systems. Our results reinforce our earlier observations of the pleiotropic nature of the DIGEX response, uncovering a multitude of new drug response pathways, with relatively few genes expressed in common between treatments with these two further drugs and the two earlier compounds.

We were also expecting to see extensive crossover in DIGEX phenotypes between different cells treated with the same drugs, which we would then be able to interrogate for drug discovery further through a target-directed process such as MIPS (Mechanism-Informed Phenotypic Screening) [16]. In fact, the DIGEX process unveils highly divergent cell-specific gene signatures, revealing a distressingly complex combinatorial landscape from which future drug discovery campaigns for this challenging cancer will need to be prioritized.

Amongst these signatures, we can see the specific induction of several druggable targets that have been implicated previously in GBM growth (e.g., SGK1, NR4A2, discussed above). However, many targets represent completely new avenues for GBM drug discovery (e.g., LIPR3/*PNLIPRP3* and SIK1).

Amongst these emerging drug targets, we have confirmed two protein kinases, JAK2 and SIK1, as antiproliferative targets in their own right. When inhibited, both show synergy, on a cell-specific basis, with the primary drug used to generate the original DIGEX target landscapes. It is our hope that targeting the emerging properties of such drug-treated systems will reveal further actionable drug combinations.

While genome-wide transcriptomics provides a powerful platform for evaluating drug response in GBM, genetic technologies such as CRISPR and transposon mutagenesis are providing complementary information on the role of cancer drivers in tumor evolution [136,137]. Combining information from both sources promises to redefine the target landscape for drug discovery in GBM.

The DIGEX results also raise the possibility that the extreme drug resistance observed in GBM is at least partially due to the wide range of survival pathways that growth inhibition induces in GBM cells, indicating both the need for a broader range of effective drugs than we currently possess, and the informed use of our current armamentarium within personalized treatment schedules.

Our analyses based on gene annotations within the Pharos database, show that the current spectrum of clinically approved drugs available to address the GBM target space we define here, is relatively limited. Moreover, many of these drugs have been optimized and approved for indications in which CNS penetration has been minimized. There is a pressing need for rigorous validation of new molecular mechanisms as effective drug targets in GBM before embarking on costly programs of lead optimization. Combination therapy guided by emerging GBM biology will shorten these odds.

At a pharmacological level, our results are intriguing. Mardepodect, as a PDE inhibitor, would be expected to influence target cells through cyclic nucleotide signaling. However, scrutiny of the upregulated gene sets induced by this compound does not reveal a sustained effect on the expression of central cAMP or cGMP regulating processes, such as those operating through adenyl- or guanyl-cyclases. We do see upregulation of the genes encoding specific PDEs (*PDE4B*, *PDE4D*, and *PDE7B*) in Mardepodect-treated cells, but not *PDE10A* itself. The reason for this may be that the transcriptomics approach is measuring the emergence of a new steady-state within the drug-treated tumor cell population, involving more subtle regulation of localized cAMP- and cGMP-driven phosphorylation networks, as reported for PDE10A-regulated systems in the spiny neuron [138].

The three GBM cell types employed in this study are widely used as established GBM cell-based model systems [33]. Using this limited cell palette, well-defined drug response profiles emerge, with each cell line exhibiting characteristic DIGEX signatures. The fact that these GBM cell lines retain the capability of forming infiltrative tumors upon xenografting, yet respond so differently to drug challenges, may indicate a multi-dimensional phenotype containing features that are stably frozen in developmental time, yet capable of resurrection given the appropriate environment or selection pressure.

Designing experiments to capture the dynamic behavior of such pleiotropic systems is difficult and requires further studies across the drug dose–response and treatment timeframes to pinpoint key effectors—the current dataset is only a preliminary step on the way to understanding and exploiting the complex coordination of the GBM cell's drug response.

5. Conclusions

Glioblastoma (GBM) is a particularly challenging cancer, with few treatment options. Nevertheless, this dark landscape is gradually being illuminated by the application of powerful genomics technologies to define the molecular drivers underlying this complex cancer. Here, we have used transcriptomics, in the form of genome-wide drug-induced gene expression (DIGEX) analysis, to measure the changes in abundance of over 18,000 individual genes during drug treatment. We define these changes for three established GBM cell lines, identifying the key targets and pathways which these cells deploy to resist drug treatment. The good news is that we now have the genomic tools to interrogate and interpret these drug responses; the bad news is that the emerging landscape evoked in the cancer cell is both extremely complicated and highly pleiotropic.

Future therapy will rely heavily on diagnosing and targeting aggressive GBM cellular phenotypes, both before and after drug treatment, as part of personalized therapy programs. Using genome-wide information, we should be able to interrogate the therapeutic targets and signaling pathways emerging from this landscape, either individually, or at a phenotypic level, deploying integrated RNAi, CRISPR, chemical biology, and pharmacology platforms to identify and validate their relative importance to the proliferating GBM cell. Individual, personalized treatments will be essential if we are to address and overcome the pharmacological plasticity that GBM exhibits, and genome-wide DIGEX may represent a fast and comprehensive technology with which to validate and position future drugs and diagnostics for this challenging cancer.

One final thought. Although small molecule drug therapy has become central to the way we think of cancer treatment, alternative therapies—such as mRNA-directed vaccination and immunotherapy—are emerging as powerful treatment options. The GBM landscapes revealed by DIGEX and discussed here in the context of drug discovery, could well inform new diagnostics to support the development of multi-modal therapies, perhaps combining drug and vaccine treatment within personalized GBM therapy. A new age of phenotypic drug discovery?

Supplementary Materials: The following are available online at https://www.mdpi.com/article/10.3390/cancers13153780/s1, Supplementary Figure S1: PCA Analysis of transcriptomics data obtained for individual experiments: U87MG: control (blue), LY-294002 treated (red), Mardepodect treated (purple); A172: control (green), Mardepodect treated (aquamarine); T98G: control (orange), Mardepodect treated (sky blue). Data is tightly clustered within each treatment set ($n = 3$). Supplementary Figure S2: network analysis based on the 200 most elevated genes upon treatment with Mardepodect. (a) U87MG; (b) A172; (c) T98G cell line. Different clusters are represented in different colors. Lines represent the relations between various genes. Supplementary Figure S3: network analysis based on the 200 most lowered genes upon treatment with Mardepodect. (a) U87MG; (b) A172; (c) T98G cell line. Different clusters are represented in different colors. Lines represent the relations between various genes. Supplementary Figure S4: network analysis based on the 200 most elevated genes upon treatment with Regorafenib. (a) U87MG; (b) A172; (c) T98G cell line. Different clusters are represented in different colours. Lines represent the relations between various genes. Supplementary Figure S5: network analysis based on the 200 most lowered genes upon treatment with Regorafenib. (a) U87MG; (b) A172; (c) T98G cell line. Different clusters are represented in different colours. Lines represent the relations between various genes. Supplementary Table S1: compound specific genes amongst the top 200 genes with most elevated expression levels in U87MG treated with Mardepodect, Regorafenib, LY-294002 and Fucoxanthin, listed in order of decreasing fold change. Supplementary Table S2: four U87MG cell upregulated pathways with the lowest p-values, regulated by Mardepodect, Regorafenib, LY-294002 and Fucoxanthin, based on an analysis of the top 200 most elevated genes. Supplementary Table S3: pathway enrichment analysis based on top 200 genes with most elevated expression levels, upon treatment of U87MG cell lines. (a) with Mardepodect; (b) Regorafenib; (c) LY-294002; (d) Fucoxanthin. Supplementary Table S4: compound-specific genes amongst the top 200 genes with most reduced expression levels in U87MG treated with Mardepodect, Regorafenib, LY-294002 and Fucoxanthin; listed in order of increasing modulus of fold change. Supplementary Table S5: the four U87MG cell upregulated pathways with the lowest p-values, regulated by Mardepodect, Regorafenib, LY-294002 and Fucoxanthin, based on an analysis of the Top 200 most elevated genes. Supplementary Table S6: pathway enrichment analysis based on top 200 genes with most decreased expression levels, upon treatment of the U87MG cell line with (a) Mardepodect; (b) Regorafenib; (c) LY-294002; (d) Fucoxanthin. Supplementary Table S7: cell-specific genes amongst the top 200 genes with most elevated expression levels in U87MG, A172 and T98G cell lines, treated with Mardepodect, listed in order of decreasing fold change. Supplementary Table S8: cell-specific genes amongst the top 200 genes with most decreased expression levels in U87MG, A172 and T98G cell lines, treated with Mardepodect, listed in the order of increasing modulus of fold change. Supplementary Table S9: the four U87MG, A172 and T98G cell upregulated pathways with the lowest p-values, regulated by Mardepodect, based on an analysis of the Top 200 most elevated genes. Supplementary Table S10: pathway enrichment analysis based on the 200 genes with most elevated expression levels, upon treatment of cells with Mardepodect. (a) U87MG; (b) A172; (c) T98G. Supplementary Table S11: 4 U87MG, A172 and T98G cell downregulated pathways with the lowest p-values, regulated by Mardepodect, based on an analysis of the Top 200 genes with most lowered expression levels. Supplementary Table S12: pathway enrichment analysis based on top 200 genes with most lowered expression levels, upon treatment of cells with Mardepodect. (a) U87MG; (b) A172; (c) T98G. Supplementary Table S13: cell-specific genes amongst the top 200 genes with most elevated expression levels in U87MG, A172 and T98G cell lines, treated with Regorafenib, listed in the order of decreasing fold change. Supplementary Table S14: cell-specific genes amongst the top 200 genes with most decreased expression levels in U87MG, A172 and T98G cell lines, treated with Regorafenib, listed in the order of increasing modulus of fold change. Supplementary Table S15: the 200 genes with most elevated (a,c,e) or most lowered levels (b,d,f) of expression upon treatment, color coded according to the Pharos database classification*. (a,b) Mardepodect; (c,d) Regorafenib; (e,f) LY-294002 and Fucoxanthin.

Author Contributions: Conceptualization, D.S.B., V.S., L.-L.P., G.L. and L.K.; Methodology, L.-L.P., L.K., D.S.B. and G.L.; Software, L.-L.P. and V.S.; Validation, L.-L.P., L.K. and V.S.; Investigation, L.K. and L.-L.P.; Formal analysis, V.S., L.-L.P. and L.K.; Resources, D.S.B. and G.L.; Data curation, V.S. and L.-L.P.; Writing—original draft preparation, D.S.B.; Writing—review and editing, D.S.B. and V.S.; Visualization, V.S., L.K. and D.S.B.; Supervision, D.S.B. and G.L.; Project administration, D.S.B.; Funding acquisition, D.S.B. All authors have read and agreed to the published version of the manuscript.

Funding: This research was funded by the Brain Tumour Charity (UK) as part of the WINDOW Consortium, Grant number GN-000429, and the European Union Horizon 2020 Framework Programme for Research and Innovation (2014–2020), EC Grant Agreement Number 727892.

Institutional Review Board Statement: Not applicable.

Informed Consent Statement: Not applicable.

Data Availability Statement: All data used in this publication are reported within it.

Acknowledgments: The authors acknowledge the advice and encouragement of many colleagues, especially Paul England, Ed Zanders, Bart Westerman, and Fredrik Svensson. The publication is dedicated to Clare Bailey (1957–2011).

Conflicts of Interest: The authors declare no conflict of interest. The funders had no role in the design of the study; in the collection, analyses, or interpretation of data; in the writing of the manuscript, or in the decision to publish the results.

References

1. Sottoriva, A.; Spiteri, I.; Piccirillo, S.G.M.; Touloumis, A.; Collins, V.P.; Marioni, J.C.; Curtis, C.; Watts, C.; Tavare, S. Intratumor heterogeneity in human glioblastoma reflects cancer evolutionary dynamics. *Proc. Natl. Acad. Sci. USA* **2013**, *110*, 4009–4014. [CrossRef] [PubMed]
2. Carén, H.; Stricker, S.H.; Bulstrode, H.; Gagrica, S.; Johnstone, E.; Bartlett, T.E.; Feber, A.; Wilson, G.; Teschendorff, A.E.; Bertone, P.; et al. Glioblastoma stem cells respond to differentiation cues but fail to undergo commitment and terminal cell-cycle arrest. *Stem Cell Rep.* **2015**, *5*, 829–842. [CrossRef]
3. Engström, P.G.; Tommei, D.; Stricker, S.H.; Ender, C.; Pollard, S.M.; Bertone, P. Digital transcriptome profiling of normal and glioblastoma-derived neural stem cells identifies genes associated with patient survival. *Genome Med.* **2012**, *4*, 76. [CrossRef] [PubMed]
4. Wang, L.; Babikir, H.; Müller, S.; Yagnik, G.; Shamardani, K.; Catalan, F.; Kohanbash, G.; Alvarado, B.; Di Lullo, E.; Kriegstein, A.; et al. The phenotypes of proliferating glioblastoma cells reside on a single axis of variation. *Cancer Discov.* **2019**, *9*, 1708–1719. [CrossRef] [PubMed]
5. Neftel, C.; Laffy, J.; Filbin, M.G.; Hara, T.; Shore, M.E.; Rahme, G.J.; Richman, A.R.; Silverbush, D.; Shaw, M.L.; Hebert, C.M.; et al. An integrative model of cellular states, plasticity and genetics for glioblastoma. *Cell* **2019**, *178*, 835–849.e21. [CrossRef] [PubMed]
6. The ICGC/TCGA pan-cancer analysis of whole genomes consortium. Pan-cancer analysis of whole genomes. *Nature* **2020**, *578*, 82–93. [CrossRef]
7. Zanders, E.D.; Svensson, F.; Bailey, D.S. Therapy for glioblastoma: Is it working? *Drug Discov. Today* **2019**, *24*, 1193–1201. [CrossRef] [PubMed]
8. Saleem, H.; Abdul, K.U.; Küçükosmanoglu, A.; Houweling, M.; Cornelissen, F.M.G.; Heiland, D.H.; Hegi, M.E.; Kouwenhoven, M.C.M.; Bailey, D.; Würdinger, T.; et al. The ticking clock of EGFR therapy resistance in glioblastoma: Target independence or target compensation. *Drug Resist. Updates* **2019**, *43*, 29–37. [CrossRef]
9. Kast, R.E.; Boockvar, J.A.; Brüning, A.; Cappello, F.; Chang, W.-W.; Cvek, B.; Dou, Q.P.; Duenas-Gonzalez, A.; Efferth, T.; Focosi, D.; et al. A Conceptually New Treatment Approach for Relapsed Glioblastoma: Coordinated Undermining of Survival Paths with Nine Repurposed Drugs (CUSP9) by the International Initiative for Accelerated Improvement of Glioblastoma Care. *Oncotarget* **2013**, *4*, 502–530. [CrossRef]

10. Gromeier, M.; Brown, M.C.; Zhang, G.; Lin, X.; Chen, Y.; Wei, Z.; Beaubier, N.; Yan, H.; He, Y.; Desjardins, A.; et al. Very low mutation burden is a feature of inflamed recurrent glioblastomas responsive to cancer immunotherapy. *Nat. Commun.* **2021**, *12*, 352. [CrossRef] [PubMed]
11. Agliardi, G.; Liuzzi, A.R.; Hotblack, A.; De Feo, D.; Núñez, N.; Stowe, C.L.; Friebel, E.; Nannini, F.; Rindlisbacher, L.; Roberts, T.A.; et al. Intratumoral IL-12 delivery empowers CAR-t cell immunotherapy in a pre-clinical model of glioblastoma. *Nat. Commun.* **2021**, *12*, 444. [CrossRef]
12. Gupta, P.B.; Pastushenko, I.; Skibinski, A.; Blanpain, C.; Kuperwasser, C. Phenotypic plasticity: Driver of cancer initiation, progression and therapy resistance. *Cell Stem Cell* **2019**, *24*, 65–78. [CrossRef] [PubMed]
13. Liu, Y.; Yu, H.; Yoo, S.; Lee, E.; Laganà, A.; Parekh, S.; Schadt, E.E.; Wang, L.; Zhu, J. A network analysis of multiple myeloma related gene signatures. *Cancers* **2019**, *11*, 1452. [CrossRef]
14. Boumahdi, S.; Sauvage, D.F.J. The great escape: Tumour cell plasticity in resistance to targeted therapy. *Nat. Rev. Drug Discov.* **2020**, *19*, 39–56. [CrossRef]
15. Swinney, D.C.; Anthony, J. How were new medicines discovered? *Nat. Rev. Drug Discov.* **2011**, *10*, 507–519. [CrossRef] [PubMed]
16. Moffat, J.G.; Rudolph, J.; Bailey, D. Phenotypic screening in cancer drug discovery-past, present and future. *Nat. Rev. Drug Discov.* **2014**, *13*, 588–602. [CrossRef] [PubMed]
17. Blagg, J.; Workman, P. Choose and use your chemical probe wisely to explore cancer biology. *Cancer Cell* **2017**, *32*, 9–25. [CrossRef]
18. Jörg, M.; Madden, K.S. The right tools for the job: The central role for next generation chemical probes and chemistry-based target deconvolution methods in phenotypic drug discovery. *RSC Med. Chem.* **2021**, *12*, 646–665. [CrossRef]
19. Lyne, S.B.; Yamini, B. An alternative pipeline for glioblastoma therapeutics: A systematic review of drug repurposing in glioblastoma. *Cancers* **2021**, *13*, 1953. [CrossRef] [PubMed]
20. Pruteanu, L.-L.; Kopanitsa, L.; Módos, D.; Kletnieks, E.; Samarova, E.; Bender, A.; Gomez, L.D.; Bailey, D.S. Transcriptomics predicts compound synergy in drug and natural product treated glioblastoma cells. *PLoS ONE* **2020**, *15*, e0239551. [CrossRef] [PubMed]
21. Menniti, F.S.; Chappie, T.A.; Humphrey, J.M.; Schmidt, C.J. Phosphodiesterase 10A inhibitors: A novel approach to the treatment of the symptoms of schizophrenia. *Curr. Opin. Investig. Drugs* **2007**, *8*, 54–59. [PubMed]
22. Verhoest, P.R.; Chapin, D.S.; Corman, M.; Fonseca, K.; Harms, J.F.; Hou, X.; Marr, E.S.; Menniti, F.S.; Nelson, F.; O'Connor, R.; et al. Discovery of a novel class of phosphodiesterase 10a inhibitors and identification of clinical candidate 2-[4-(1-Methyl-4-Pyridin-4-Yl-1*H*-Pyrazol-3-Yl)-Phenoxymethyl]-Quinoline (PF-2545920) for the treatment of schizophrenia. *J. Med. Chem.* **2009**, *52*, 5188–5196. [CrossRef]
23. Walling, D.P.; Banerjee, A.; Dawra, V.; Boyer, S.; Schmidt, C.J.; de Martinis, N. Phosphodiesterase 10A inhibitor monotherapy is not an effective treatment of acute schizophrenia. *J. Clin. Psychopharmacol.* **2019**, *39*, 575–582. [CrossRef] [PubMed]
24. Rodrigues, F.B.; Wild, E.J. Clinical trials corner: September 2017. *J. Huntingt. Dis.* **2017**, *6*, 255–263. [CrossRef] [PubMed]
25. Grothey, A.; Blay, J.-Y.; Pavlakis, N.; Yoshino, T.; Bruix, J. Evolving role of regorafenib for the treatment of advanced cancers. *Cancer Treat. Rev.* **2020**, *86*, 101993. [CrossRef] [PubMed]
26. Wilhelm, S.M.; Dumas, J.; Adnane, L.; Lynch, M.; Carter, C.A.; Schütz, G.; Thierauch, K.-H.; Zopf, D. Regorafenib (BAY 73-4506): A new oral multikinase inhibitor of angiogenic, stromal and oncogenic receptor tyrosine kinases with potent preclinical antitumor activity. *Int. J. Cancer* **2011**, *129*, 245–255. [CrossRef]
27. Lombardi, G.; De Salvo, G.L.; Brandes, A.A.; Eoli, M.; Rudà, R.; Faedi, M.; Lolli, I.; Pace, A.; Daniele, B.; Pasqualetti, F.; et al. Regorafenib compared with lomustine in patients with relapsed glioblastoma (REGOMA): A multicentre, open-label, randomised, controlled, phase 2 trial. *Lancet Oncol.* **2019**, *20*, 110–119. [CrossRef]
28. Alexander, B.M.; Ba, S.; Berger, M.S.; Berry, D.A.; Cavenee, W.K.; Chang, S.M.; Cloughesy, T.F.; Jiang, T.; Khasraw, M.; Li, W.; et al. Adaptive global innovative learning environment for glioblastoma: GBM AGILE. *Clin. Cancer Res.* **2018**, *24*, 737–743. [CrossRef]
29. Safitri, D.; Harris, M.; Potter, H.; Yan Yeung, H.; Winfield, I.; Kopanitsa, L.; Svensson, F.; Rahman, T.; Harper, M.T.; Bailey, D.; et al. Elevated intracellular cAMP concentration mediates growth suppression in glioma cells. *Biochem. Pharmacol.* **2020**, *174*, 113823. [CrossRef]
30. Veroli, D.G.Y.; Fornari, C.; Wang, D.; Mollard, S.; Bramhall, J.L.; Richards, F.M.; Jodrell, D.I. Combenefit: An interactive platform for the analysis and visualization of drug combinations. *Bioinformatics* **2016**, *32*, 2866–2868. [CrossRef] [PubMed]
31. Irizarry, R.A. Exploration, normalization and summaries of high density oligonucleotide array probe level data. *Biostatistics* **2003**, *4*, 249–264. [CrossRef] [PubMed]
32. Nguyen, D.-T.; Mathias, S.; Bologa, C.; Brunak, S.; Fernandez, N.; Gaulton, A.; Hersey, A.; Holmes, J.; Jensen, L.J.; Karlsson, A.; et al. Pharos: Collating protein information to shed light on the druggable genome. *Nucleic Acids Res.* **2017**, *45*, D995–D1002. [CrossRef] [PubMed]
33. Svensson, F.; Westerman, B.; Würdinger, T.; Bailey, D. GBM drug bank—A new resource for glioblastoma drug discovery and informatics research. *Neuro Oncol.* **2018**, *20*, 1680–1681. [CrossRef] [PubMed]
34. Saelee, P.; Wongkham, S.; Puapairoj, A.; Khuntikeo, N.; Petmitr, S.; Chariyalertsak, S.; Sumethchotimaytha, W.; Karalak, A. Novel PNLIPRP3 and DOCK8 gene expression and prognostic implications of DNA loss on chromosome 10q25.3 in hepatocellular carcinoma. *Asian Pac. J. Cancer Prev.* **2009**, *10*, 501–506. [PubMed]

35. Junes-Gill, K.S.; Lawrence, C.E.; Wheeler, C.J.; Cordner, R.; Gill, T.G.; Mar, V.; Shiri, L.; Basile, L.A. Human hematopoietic signal peptide-containing secreted 1 (HHSS1) modulates genes and pathways in glioma: Implications for the regulation of tumorigenicity and angiogenesis. *BMC Cancer* **2014**, *14*, 920. [CrossRef] [PubMed]
36. The Human Protein Atlas: PNLIPRP3. Available online: https://www.proteinatlas.org/ENSG00000203837-PNLIPRP3 (accessed on 2 June 2021).
37. Liu, T.-T.; Liu, X.-T.; Chen, Q.-X.; Shi, Y. Lipase inhibitors for obesity: A review. *Biomed. Pharmacother.* **2020**, *128*, 110314. [CrossRef]
38. Whitelaw, J.A.; Lilla, S.; Paul, N.R.; Fort, L.; Zanivan, S.; Machesky, L.M. CYRI/Fam49 proteins represent a new class of rac1 interactors. *Commun. Integr. Biol.* **2019**, *12*, 112–118. [CrossRef]
39. Fort, L.; Batista, J.M.; Thomason, P.A.; Spence, H.J.; Whitelaw, J.A.; Tweedy, L.; Greaves, J.; Martin, K.J.; Anderson, K.I.; Brown, P.; et al. Fam49/CYRI interacts with rac1 and locally suppresses protrusions. *Nat. Cell Biol.* **2018**, *20*, 1159–1171. [CrossRef]
40. The Human Protein Atlas: FAM49A. Available online: https://www.proteinatlas.org/ENSG00000197872-FAM49A (accessed on 2 June 2021).
41. Kaplan, E.; Stone, R.; Hume, P.J.; Greene, N.P.; Koronakis, V. Structure of CYRI-B (FAM49B), a key regulator of cellular actin assembly. *Acta Crystallogr. Sect. D Struct. Biol.* **2020**, *76*, 1015–1024. [CrossRef] [PubMed]
42. Shnaper, S.; Desbaillets, I.; Brown, D.A.; Murat, A.; Migliavacca, E.; Schluep, M.; Ostermann, S.; Hamou, M.-F.; Stupp, R.; Breit, S.N.; et al. Elevated levels of MIC-1/GDF15 in the cerebrospinal fluid of patients are associated with glioblastoma and worse outcome. *Int. J. Cancer* **2009**, *125*, 2624–2630. [CrossRef]
43. Codó, P.; Weller, M.; Kaulich, K.; Schraivogel, D.; Silginer, M.; Reifenberger, G.; Meister, G.; Roth, P. Control of glioma cell migration and invasiveness by GDF-15. *Oncotarget* **2016**, *7*, 7732–7746. [CrossRef]
44. Roth, P.; Junker, M.; Tritschler, I.; Mittelbronn, M.; Dombrowski, Y.; Breit, S.N.; Tabatabai, G.; Wick, W.; Weller, M.; Wischhusen, J. GDF-15 contributes to proliferation and immune escape of malignant gliomas. *Clin. Cancer Res.* **2010**, *16*, 3851–3859. [CrossRef] [PubMed]
45. Wischhusen, J.; Melero, I.; Fridman, W.H. Growth/Differentiation Factor-15 (GDF-15): From biomarker to novel targetable immune checkpoint. *Front. Immunol.* **2020**, *11*, 951. [CrossRef] [PubMed]
46. Tang, Z.; Chen, H.; Zhong, D.; Wei, W.; Liu, L.; Duan, Q.; Han, B.; Li, G. TRIB3 facilitates glioblastoma progression via restraining autophagy. *Aging* **2020**, *12*, 25020–25034. [CrossRef] [PubMed]
47. Wang, S.; Wang, C.; Li, X.; Hu, Y.; Gou, R.; Guo, Q.; Nie, X.; Liu, J.; Zhu, L.; Lin, B. Down-Regulation of TRIB3 inhibits the progression of ovarian cancer via mek/erk signaling pathway. *Cancer Cell Int.* **2020**, *20*, 418. [CrossRef] [PubMed]
48. Lu, Y.; Li, L.; Chen, L.; Gao, Y.; Chen, X.; Cao, Y. TRIB3 confers glioma cell stemness via interacting with B-catenin. *Environ. Toxicol.* **2020**, *35*, 697–706. [CrossRef]
49. Li, Z.; Chen, Y.; An, T.; Liu, P.; Zhu, J.; Yang, H.; Zhang, W.; Dong, T.; Jiang, J.; Zhang, Y.; et al. Nuciferine inhibits the progression of glioblastoma by suppressing the SOX2-AKT/STAT3-Slug signaling pathway. *J. Exp. Clin. Cancer Res.* **2019**, *38*, 139. [CrossRef]
50. Sui, A.; Xu, Y.; Yang, J.; Pan, B.; Wu, J.; Guo, T.; Shen, Y.; Guo, X. The histone H3 Lys 27 demethylase KDM6B promotes migration and invasion of glioma cells partly by regulating the expression of SNAI1. *Neurochem. Int.* **2019**, *124*, 123–129. [CrossRef]
51. Min, D.-J.; Zhao, Y.; Monks, A.; Palmisano, A.; Hose, C.; Teicher, B.A.; Doroshow, J.H.; Simon, R.M. Identification of pharmacodynamic biomarkers and common molecular mechanisms of response to genotoxic agents in cancer cell lines. *Cancer Chemother. Pharm.* **2019**, *84*, 771–780. [CrossRef]
52. Tang, Q.; Ren, L.; Liu, J.; Li, W.; Zheng, X.; Wang, J.; Du, G. Withaferin A triggers G2/M arrest and intrinsic apoptosis in glioblastoma cells via ATF4-ATF3-CHOP axis. *Cell Prolif.* **2020**, *53*. [CrossRef]
53. Van Noorden, C.J.F.; Hira, V.V.V.; van Dijck, A.J.; Novak, M.; Breznik, B.; Molenaar, R.J. Energy metabolism in IDH1 wild-type and IDH1-Mutated glioblastoma stem cells: A novel target for therapy? *Cells* **2021**, *10*, 705. [CrossRef] [PubMed]
54. Perissi, V.; Aggarwal, A.; Glass, C.K.; Rose, D.W.; Rosenfeld, M.G. A corepressor/coactivator exchange complex required for transcriptional activation by nuclear receptors and other regulated transcription factors. *Cell* **2004**, *116*, 511–526. [CrossRef]
55. Hu, Y.; Ylivinkka, I.; Chen, P.; Li, L.; Hautaniemi, S.; Nyman, T.A.; Keski-Oja, J.; Hyytiäinen, M. Netrin-4 promotes glioblastoma cell proliferation through integrin B4 signaling. *Neoplasia* **2012**, *14*, 219–227. [CrossRef] [PubMed]
56. Tang, X.; Jang, S.-W.; Okada, M.; Chan, C.-B.; Feng, Y.; Liu, Y.; Luo, S.-W.; Hong, Y.; Rama, N.; Xiong, W.-C.; et al. Netrin-1 mediates neuronal survival through pike-l interaction with the dependence receptor UNC5B. *Nat. Cell Biol.* **2008**, *10*, 698–706. [CrossRef]
57. Pyrzynska, B.; Banach-Orlowska, M.; Teperek-Tkacz, M.; Miekus, K.; Drabik, G.; Majka, M.; Miaczynska, M. Multifunctional protein APPL2 contributes to survival of human glioma cells. *Mol. Oncol.* **2013**, *7*, 67–84. [CrossRef] [PubMed]
58. Shimizu, A.; Nakayama, H.; Wang, P.; König, C.; Akino, T.; Sandlund, J.; Coma, S.; Italiano, J.E.; Mammoto, A.; Bielenberg, D.R.; et al. Netrin-1 promotes glioblastoma cell invasiveness and angiogenesis by multiple pathways including activation of RhoA, Cathepsin B and CAMP-Response element-binding protein. *J. Biol. Chem.* **2013**, *288*, 2210–2222. [CrossRef]
59. Ylivinkka, I.; Hu, Y.; Chen, P.; Rantanen, V.; Hautaniemi, S.; Nyman, T.A.; Keski-Oja, J.; Hyytiäinen, M. Netrin-1 induced activation of notch signaling mediates glioblastoma cell invasion. *J. Cell Sci.* **2013**, *126*, 2459–2469. [CrossRef] [PubMed]
60. Emanuele, M.J.; Enrico, T.P.; Mouery, R.D.; Wasserman, D.; Nachum, S.; Tzur, A. Complex cartography: Regulation of E2F Transcription factors by Cyclin F and ubiquitin. *Trends Cell Biol.* **2020**, *30*, 640–652. [CrossRef]
61. Lee, S.; Park, Y.R.; Kim, S.; Park, E.; Kang, M.J.; So, I.; Chun, J.N.; Jeon, J. Geraniol suppresses prostate cancer growth through down-regulation of E2F8. *Cancer Med.* **2016**, *5*, 2899–2908. [CrossRef]

62. Teng, J.; Hejazi, S.; Hiddingh, L.; Carvalho, L.; de Gooijer, M.C.; Wakimoto, H.; Barazas, M.; Tannous, M.; Chi, A.S.; Noske, D.P.; et al. Recycling drug screen repurposes hydroxyurea as a sensitizer of glioblastomas to temozolomide targeting de novo DNA synthesis, irrespective of molecular subtype. *Neuro Oncol.* **2018**, *20*, 642–654. [CrossRef]
63. Mondal, P.; Sen, S.; Klein, B.J.; Tiwary, N.; Gadad, S.S.; Kutateladze, T.G.; Roy, S.; Das, C. TCF19 promotes cell proliferation through binding to the histone H3K4me3 mark. *Biochemistry* **2020**, *59*, 389–399. [CrossRef]
64. Hoffmann, S.; Pentakota, S.; Mund, A.; Haahr, P.; Coscia, F.; Gallo, M.; Mann, M.; Taylor, N.M.; Mailand, N. FAM111 protease activity undermines cellular fitness and is amplified by gain-of-function mutations in human disease. *EMBO Rep.* **2020**, *21*. [CrossRef] [PubMed]
65. Kawasaki, K.; Nojima, S.; Hijiki, K.; Tahara, S.; Ohshima, K.; Matsui, T.; Hori, Y.; Kurashige, M.; Umeda, D.; Kiyokawa, H.; et al. FAM111B enhances proliferation of *KRAS*-driven lung adenocarcinoma by degrading P16. *Cancer Sci.* **2020**, *111*, 2635–2646. [CrossRef] [PubMed]
66. Richter, J.D.; Bassell, G.J.; Klann, E. Dysregulation and restoration of translational homeostasis in fragile X syndrome. *Nat. Rev. Neurosci.* **2015**, *16*, 595–605. [CrossRef]
67. Tejero, R.; Huang, Y.; Katsyv, I.; Kluge, M.; Lin, J.Y.; Tome-Garcia, J.; Daviaud, N.; Wang, Y.; Zhang, B.; Tsankova, N.M.; et al. Gene signatures of quiescent glioblastoma cells reveal mesenchymal shift and interactions with niche microenvironment. *EBioMedicine* **2019**, *42*, 252–269. [CrossRef]
68. Emmerson, P.J.; Duffin, K.L.; Chintharlapalli, S.; Wu, X. GDF15 and growth control. *Front. Physiol.* **2018**, *9*, 1712. [CrossRef] [PubMed]
69. Cheng, K.; Shi, J.; Liu, Z.; Jia, Y.; Qin, Q.; Zhang, H.; Wan, S.; Niu, Z.; Lu, L.; Sun, J.; et al. A panel of five plasma proteins for the early diagnosis of hepatitis B virus-related hepatocellular carcinoma in individuals at risk. *EBioMedicine* **2020**, *52*, 102638. [CrossRef]
70. Dedobbeleer, M.; Willems, E.; Freeman, S.; Lombard, A.; Goffart, N.; Rogister, B. Phosphatases and solid tumors: Focus on glioblastoma initiation, progression and recurrences. *Biochem. J.* **2017**, *474*, 2903–2924. [CrossRef]
71. Sonntag, T.; Vaughan, J.M.; Montminy, M. 14-3-3 proteins mediate inhibitory effects of cAMP on Salt-inducible Kinases (SIK s). *FEBS J.* **2018**, *285*, 467–480. [CrossRef]
72. Ahmadi, M.; Amiri, S.; Pecic, S.; Machaj, F.; Rosik, J.; Łos, M.J.; Alizadeh, J.; Mahdian, R.; da Silva Rosa, S.C.; Schaafsma, D.; et al. Pleiotropic effects of statins: A focus on cancer. *Biochim. Biophys. Acta BBA Mol. Basis Dis.* **2020**, *1866*, 165968. [CrossRef]
73. Sunde, M.; McGrath, K.C.Y.; Young, L.; Matthews, J.M.; Chua, E.L.; Mackay, J.P.; Death, A.K. TC-1 is a novel tumorigenic and natively disordered protein associated with thyroid cancer. *Cancer Res.* **2004**, *64*, 2766–2773. [CrossRef]
74. Lei, J.; Li, W.; Yang, Y.; Lu, Q.; Zhang, N.; Bai, G.; Zhong, D.; Su, K.; Liu, B.; Li, X.; et al. TC-1 overexpression promotes cell proliferation in human non-small cell lung cancer that can be inhibited by PD173074. *PLoS ONE* **2014**, *9*, e100075. [CrossRef] [PubMed]
75. Cronin, R.; Brooke, G.N.; Prischi, F. The role of the P90 ribosomal S6 kinase family in prostate cancer progression and therapy resistance. *Oncogene* **2021**, *40*, 3775–3785. [CrossRef] [PubMed]
76. Sulzmaier, F.J.; Young-Robbins, S.; Jiang, P.; Geerts, D.; Prechtl, A.M.; Matter, M.L.; Kesari, S.; Ramos, J.W. RSK2 activity mediates glioblastoma invasiveness and is a potential target for new therapeutics. *Oncotarget* **2016**, *7*, 79869–79884. [CrossRef]
77. Mahajan-Thakur, S.; Bien-Möller, S.; Marx, S.; Schroeder, H.; Rauch, B. Sphingosine 1-Phosphate (S1P) signaling in glioblastoma multiforme-A systematic review. *Int. J. Mol. Sci.* **2017**, *18*, 2448. [CrossRef]
78. Loeffler, S.; Fayard, B.; Weis, J.; Weissenberger, J. Interleukin-6 induces transcriptional activation of Vascular Endothelial Growth Factor (VEGF) in astrocytes in vivo and regulates VEGF promoter activity in glioblastoma cells via direct interaction between STAT3 and Sp1. *Int. J. Cancer* **2005**, *115*, 202–213. [CrossRef] [PubMed]
79. Sferrazzo, G.; Di Rosa, M.; Barone, E.; Li Volti, G.; Musso, N.; Tibullo, D.; Barbagallo, I. Heme Oxygenase-1 in central nervous system malignancies. *J. Clin. Med.* **2020**, *9*, 1562. [CrossRef]
80. Shono, K.; Yamaguchi, I.; Mizobuchi, Y.; Kagusa, H.; Sumi, A.; Fujihara, T.; Nakajima, K.; Kitazato, K.T.; Matsuzaki, K.; Saya, H.; et al. Downregulation of the CCL2/CCR2 and CXCL10/CXCR3 axes contributes to antitumor effects in a mouse model of malignant glioma. *Sci. Rep.* **2020**, *10*, 15286. [CrossRef]
81. Groblewska, M.; Litman-Zawadzka, A.; Mroczko, B. The role of selected chemokines and their receptors in the development of gliomas. *Int. J. Mol. Sci.* **2020**, *21*, 3704. [CrossRef]
82. Ströbele, S.; Schneider, M.; Schneele, L.; Siegelin, M.D.; Nonnenmacher, L.; Zhou, S.; Karpel-Massle, G.; Westhoff, M.-A.; Halatsch, M.-E.; Debatin, K.-M. A potential role for the inhibition of PI3K signaling in glioblastoma therapy. *PLoS ONE* **2015**, *10*, e0131670. [CrossRef]
83. Ahmad, F.; Sun, Q.; Patel, D.; Stommel, J. Cholesterol metabolism: A potential therapeutic target in glioblastoma. *Cancers* **2019**, *11*, 146. [CrossRef]
84. Nakakuki, M.; Kawano, H.; Notsu, T.; Imada, K.; Mizuguchi, K.; Shimano, H. A novel processing system of sterol regulatory element-binding protein-1c regulated by polyunsaturated fatty acid. *J. Biochem.* **2014**, *155*, 301–313. [CrossRef] [PubMed]
85. Pharos: PNLIPRP3 (Pancreatic Lipase-Related Protein 3). Available online: https://pharos.nih.gov/targets/Q17RR3 (accessed on 2 June 2021).
86. Hattermann, K.; Held-Feindt, J.; Lucius, R.; Müerköster, S.S.; Penfold, M.E.T.; Schall, T.J.; Mentlein, R. The chemokine receptor CXCR7 is highly expressed in human glioma cells and mediates antiapoptotic effects. *Cancer Res.* **2010**, *70*, 3299–3308. [CrossRef]

87. Karki, K.; Li, X.; Jin, U.-H.; Mohankumar, K.; Zarei, M.; Michelhaugh, S.K.; Mittal, S.; Tjalkens, R.; Safe, S. Nuclear Receptor 4A2 (NR4A2) is a druggable target for glioblastomas. *J. Neuro Oncol.* **2020**, *146*, 25–39. [CrossRef] [PubMed]
88. Löw, S.; Vougioukas, V.I.; Hielscher, T.; Schmidt, U.; Unterberg, A.; Halatsch, M.E. Pathogenetic pathways leading to glioblastoma multiforme: Association between gene expressions and resistance to erlotinib. *Anticancer Res.* **2008**, *28*, 3729–3732. [PubMed]
89. Rahane, C.S.; Kutzner, A.; Heese, K. A cancer tissue-specific FAM72 expression profile defines a novel glioblastoma multiform (GBM) gene-mutation signature. *J. Neurooncol.* **2019**, *141*, 57–70. [CrossRef] [PubMed]
90. Banelli, B.; Carra, E.; Barbieri, F.; Würth, R.; Parodi, F.; Pattarozzi, A.; Carosio, R.; Forlani, A.; Allemanni, G.; Marubbi, D.; et al. The histone demethylase KDM5A is a key factor for the resistance to temozolomide in glioblastoma. *Cell Cycle* **2015**, *14*, 3418–3429. [CrossRef]
91. McAllister, T.E.; England, K.S.; Hopkinson, R.J.; Brennan, P.E.; Kawamura, A.; Schofield, C.J. Recent progress in histone demethylase inhibitors. *J. Med. Chem.* **2016**, *59*, 1308–1329. [CrossRef]
92. Banelli, B.; Daga, A.; Forlani, A.; Allemanni, G.; Marubbi, D.; Pistillo, M.P.; Profumo, A.; Romani, M. Small molecules targeting histone demethylase genes (KDMs) inhibit growth of temozolomide-resistant glioblastoma cells. *Oncotarget* **2017**, *8*, 34896–34910. [CrossRef]
93. Mahdessian, D.; Cesnik, A.J.; Gnann, C.; Danielsson, F.; Stenström, L.; Arif, M.; Zhang, C.; Le, T.; Johansson, F.; Shutten, R.; et al. Spatiotemporal dissection of the cell cycle with single-cell proteogenomics. *Nature* **2021**, *590*, 649–654. [CrossRef]
94. Fung, N.H.; Grima, C.A.; Widodo, S.S.; Kaye, A.H.; Whitehead, C.A.; Stylli, S.S.; Mantamadiotis, T. Understanding and exploiting cell signalling convergence nodes and pathway cross-talk in malignant brain cancer. *Cell. Signal.* **2019**, *57*, 2–9. [CrossRef]
95. Qiu, Z.; Yuan, W.; Chen, T.; Zhou, C.; Liu, C.; Huang, Y.; Han, D.; Huang, Q. HMGCR positively regulated the growth and migration of glioblastoma cells. *Gene* **2016**, *576*, 22–27. [CrossRef]
96. Cote, D.J.; Rosner, B.A.; Smith-Warner, S.A.; Egan, K.M.; Stampfer, M.J. Statin use, hyperlipidemia and risk of glioma. *Eur. J. Epidemiol.* **2019**, *34*, 997–1011. [CrossRef]
97. Taub, M. Salt inducible kinase signaling networks: Implications for acute kidney injury and therapeutic potential. *Int. J. Mol. Sci.* **2019**, *20*, 3219. [CrossRef]
98. Leone, P.E.; González, M.B.; Elosua, C.; Gómez-Moreta, J.A.; Lumbreras, E.; Robledo, C.; Santos-Briz, A.; Valero, J.M.; de la Guardia, R.D.; Gutiérrez, N.C.; et al. Integration of global spectral karyotyping, CGH arrays and expression arrays reveals important genes in the pathogenesis of glioblastoma multiforme. *Ann. Surg. Oncol.* **2012**, *19*, 2367–2379. [CrossRef] [PubMed]
99. Sundberg, T.B.; Liang, Y.; Wu, H.; Choi, H.G.; Kim, N.D.; Sim, T.; Johannessen, L.; Petrone, K.; Khor, B.; Graham, D.B.; et al. Development of chemical probes for investigation of salt-inducible kinase function in vivo. *ACS Chem. Biol.* **2016**, *11*, 2105–2111. [CrossRef]
100. Martin, M.W.; Newcomb, J.; Nunes, J.J.; McGowan, D.C.; Armistead, D.M.; Boucher, C.; Buchanan, J.L.; Buckner, W.; Chai, L.; Elbaum, D.; et al. Novel 2-Aminopyrimidine carbamates as potent and orally active inhibitors of Lck: Synthesis, SAR and in vivo antiinflammatory activity. *J. Med. Chem.* **2006**, *49*, 4981–4991. [CrossRef]
101. Tan, S.K.; Jermakowicz, A.; Mookhtiar, A.K.; Nemeroff, C.B.; Schürer, S.C.; Ayad, N.G. Drug repositioning in glioblastoma: A pathway perspective. *Front. Pharmacol.* **2018**, *9*, 218. [CrossRef] [PubMed]
102. Jeter, J.M.; Bowles, T.L.; Curiel-Lewandrowski, C.; Swetter, S.M.; Filipp, F.V.; Abdel-Malek, Z.A.; Geskin, L.J.; Brewer, J.D.; Arbiser, J.L.; Gershenwald, J.E.; et al. Chemoprevention agents for melanoma: A path forward into phase 3 clinical trials. *Cancer* **2019**, *125*, 18–44. [CrossRef] [PubMed]
103. Nishimori, S.; O'Meara, M.J.; Castro, C.D.; Noda, H.; Cetinbas, M.; da Silva Martins, J.; Ayturk, U.; Brooks, D.J.; Bruce, M.; Nagata, M.; et al. Salt-Inducible kinases dictate parathyroid hormone 1 receptor action in bone development and remodeling. *J. Clin. Investig.* **2019**, *129*, 5187–5203. [CrossRef]
104. Wein, M.N.; Foretz, M.; Fisher, D.E.; Xavier, R.J.; Kronenberg, H.M. Salt-Inducible kinases: Physiology, regulation by CAMP, and therapeutic potential. *Trends Endocrinol. Metab.* **2018**, *29*, 723–735. [CrossRef] [PubMed]
105. Clark, K.; MacKenzie, K.F.; Petkevicius, K.; Kristariyanto, Y.; Zhang, J.; Choi, H.G.; Peggie, M.; Plater, L.; Pedrioli, P.G.A.; McIver, E.; et al. Phosphorylation of CRTC3 by the salt-inducible kinases controls the interconversion of classically activated and regulatory macrophages. *Proc. Natl. Acad. Sci. USA* **2012**, *109*, 16986–16991. [CrossRef] [PubMed]
106. Sundberg, T.B.; Choi, H.G.; Song, J.-H.; Russell, C.N.; Hussain, M.M.; Graham, D.B.; Khor, B.; Gagnon, J.; O'Connell, D.J.; Narayan, K.; et al. Small-Molecule screening identifies inhibition of salt-inducible kinases as a therapeutic strategy to enhance immunoregulatory functions of dendritic cells. *Proc. Natl. Acad. Sci. USA* **2014**, *111*, 12468–12473. [CrossRef]
107. Brantley, E.C.; Benveniste, E.N. Signal transducer and activator of transcription-3: A molecular hub for signaling pathways in gliomas. *Mol. Cancer Res.* **2008**, *6*, 675–684. [CrossRef]
108. Mukthavaram, R.; Ouyang, X.; Saklecha, R.; Jiang, P.; Nomura, N.; Pingle, S.C.; Guo, F.; Makale, M.; Kesari, S. Effect of the JAK2/STAT3 inhibitor SAR317461 on human glioblastoma tumorspheres. *J. Transl. Med.* **2015**, *13*, 269. [CrossRef]
109. Ioannidis, S.; Lamb, M.L.; Wang, T.; Almeida, L.; Block, M.H.; Davies, A.M.; Peng, B.; Su, M.; Zhang, H.-J.; Hoffmann, E.; et al. Discovery of 5-Chloro-N^2-[(1 S)-1-(5-Fluoropyrimidin-2-Yl)Ethyl]-N^4-(5-Methyl-1 H-Pyrazol-3-Yl)Pyrimidine-2,4-Diamine (AZD1480) as a novel inhibitor of the Jak/Stat pathway. *J. Med. Chem.* **2011**, *54*, 262–276. [CrossRef] [PubMed]
110. Wong, R.A.; Luo, X.; Lu, M.; An, Z.; Haas-Kogan, D.A.; Phillips, J.J.; Shokat, K.M.; Weiss, W.A.; Fan, Q.W. Cooperative blockade of PKCα and JAK2 drives apoptosis in glioblastoma. *Cancer Res.* **2020**, *80*, 709–718. [CrossRef] [PubMed]

111. Quintás-Cardama, A.; Vaddi, K.; Liu, P.; Manshouri, T.; Li, J.; Scherle, P.A.; Caulder, E.; Wen, X.; Li, Y.; Waeltz, P.; et al. Preclinical characterization of the selective JAK1/2 inhibitor INCB018424: Therapeutic implications for the treatment of myeloproliferative neoplasms. *Blood* **2010**, *115*, 3109–3117. [CrossRef]
112. Roskoski, R. Janus Kinase (JAK) inhibitors in the treatment of inflammatory and neoplastic diseases. *Pharmacol. Res.* **2016**, *111*, 784–803. [CrossRef]
113. Darling, N.J.; Toth, R.; Arthur, J.S.C.; Clark, K. Inhibition of SIK2 and SIK3 during Differentiation enhances the anti-inflammatory phenotype of macrophages. *Biochem. J.* **2017**, *474*, 521–537. [CrossRef]
114. Yang, Y.; Wang, J.; Shi, F.; Shan, A.; Xu, S.; Lv, W. BDKRB2 is a novel EMT-related biomarker and predicts poor survival in glioma. *Aging* **2021**, *13*, 7499–7516. [CrossRef] [PubMed]
115. Seifert, S.; Sontheimer, H. Bradykinin enhances invasion of malignant glioma into the brain parenchyma by inducing cells to undergo amoeboid migration. *J. Physiol.* **2014**, *592*, 5109–5127. [CrossRef] [PubMed]
116. Balmforth, A.J.; Parkinson, F.E.; Altiok, N.; Fredholm, B.B. Identification of a B2-Bradykinin receptor linked to phospholipase c and inhibition of dopamine stimulated cyclic AMP accumulation in the human astrocytoma cell line D384. *Naunyn Schmiedeberg's Arch. Pharmacol.* **1992**, *346*. [CrossRef]
117. Lesage, A.; Gibson, C.; Marceau, F.; Ambrosi, H.-D.; Saupe, J.; Katzer, W.; Loenders, B.; Charest-Morin, X.; Knolle, J. In Vitro pharmacological profile of a new small molecule bradykinin B2 receptor antagonist. *Front. Pharmacol.* **2020**, *11*, 916. [CrossRef] [PubMed]
118. Hock, F.J.; Wirth, K.; Albus, U.; Linz, W.; Gerhards, H.J.; Wiemer, G.; Henke, S.; Breipohl, G.; König, W.; Knolle, J.; et al. Hoe 140 a new potent and long acting bradykinin-antagonist: In Vitro studies. *Br. J. Pharmacol.* **1991**, *102*, 769–773. [CrossRef] [PubMed]
119. Sawutz, D.G.; Salvino, J.M.; Dolle, R.E.; Casiano, F.; Ward, S.J.; Houck, W.T.; Faunce, D.M.; Douty, B.D.; Baizman, E.; Awad, M.M. The nonpeptide WIN 64338 is a bradykinin B2 receptor antagonist. *Proc. Natl. Acad. Sci. USA* **1994**, *91*, 4693–4697. [CrossRef]
120. Hauser, A.S.; Chavali, S.; Masuho, I.; Jahn, L.J.; Martemyanov, K.A.; Gloriam, D.E.; Babu, M.M. Pharmacogenomics of GPCR drug targets. *Cell* **2018**, *172*, 41–54.e19. [CrossRef]
121. Wu, V.; Yeerna, H.; Nohata, N.; Chiou, J.; Harismendy, O.; Raimondi, F.; Inoue, A.; Russell, R.B.; Tamayo, P.; Gutkind, J.S. Illuminating the Onco-GPCRome: Novel G protein–coupled receptor-driven oncocrine networks and targets for cancer immunotherapy. *J. Biol. Chem.* **2019**, *294*, 11062–11086. [CrossRef]
122. Meyer, R.C.; Giddens, M.M.; Schaefer, S.A.; Hall, R.A. GPR37 and GPR37L1 are receptors for the neuroprotective and glioprotective factors prosaptide and prosaposin. *Proc. Natl. Acad. Sci. USA* **2013**, *110*, 9529–9534. [CrossRef]
123. Yin, J.; Chen, K.-Y.M.; Clark, M.J.; Hijazi, M.; Kumari, P.; Bai, X.; Sunahara, R.K.; Barth, P.; Rosenbaum, D.M. Structure of a D2 dopamine receptor–G-protein complex in a lipid membrane. *Nature* **2020**, *584*, 125–129. [CrossRef]
124. Lundius, E.G.; Vukojević, V.; Hertz, E.; Stroth, N.; Cederlund, A.; Hiraiwa, M.; Terenius, L.; Svenningsson, P. GPR37 protein trafficking to the plasma membrane regulated by prosaposin and GM1 gangliosides promotes cell viability. *J. Biol. Chem.* **2014**, *289*, 4660–4673. [CrossRef]
125. Dunham, J.H.; Meyer, R.C.; Garcia, E.L.; Hall, R.A. GPR37 surface expression enhancement via N-terminal truncation or protein–protein interactions. *Biochemistry* **2009**, *48*, 10286–10297. [CrossRef] [PubMed]
126. Hertz, E.; Terenius, L.; Vukojević, V.; Svenningsson, P. GPR37 and GPR37L1 differently interact with dopamine 2 receptors in live cells. *Neuropharmacology* **2019**, *152*, 51–57. [CrossRef] [PubMed]
127. Allen, J.E.; Krigsfeld, G.; Mayes, P.A.; Patel, L.; Dicker, D.T.; Patel, A.S.; Dolloff, N.G.; Messaris, E.; Scata, K.A.; Wang, W.; et al. Dual inactivation of Akt and ERK by TIC10 signals Foxo3a nuclear translocation, trail gene induction and potent antitumor effects. *Sci. Transl. Med.* **2013**, *5*, 171ra17. [CrossRef]
128. Prabhu, V.V.; Morrow, S.; Rahman Kawakibi, A.; Zhou, L.; Ralff, M.; Ray, J.; Jhaveri, A.; Ferrarini, I.; Lee, Y.; Parker, C.; et al. ONC201 and imipridones: Anti-Cancer compounds with clinical efficacy. *Neoplasia* **2020**, *22*, 725–744. [CrossRef]
129. He, Y.; Li, J.; Koga, T.; Ma, J.; Dhawan, S.; Suzuki, Y.; Furnari, F.; Prabhu, V.V.; Allen, J.E.; Chen, C.C. Epidermal growth factor receptor as a molecular determinant of glioblastoma response to dopamine receptor D2 inhibitors. *Neuro Oncol.* **2021**, *23*, 400–411. [CrossRef] [PubMed]
130. Gagnon, L.; Leduc, M.; Thibodeau, J.-F.; Zhang, M.-Z.; Grouix, B.; Sarra-Bournet, F.; Gagnon, W.; Hince, K.; Tremblay, M.; Geerts, L.; et al. A newly discovered antifibrotic pathway regulated by two fatty acid receptors. *Am. J. Pathol.* **2018**, *188*, 1132–1148. [CrossRef] [PubMed]
131. Lynch, J.; Wang, J. G protein-coupled receptor signaling in stem cells and cancer. *Int. J. Mol. Sci.* **2016**, *17*, 707. [CrossRef]
132. Marsango, S.; Barki, N.; Jenkins, L.; Tobin, A.B.; Milligan, G. Therapeutic validation of an orphan g protein-coupled receptor: The case of GPR84. *Br. J. Pharm.* **2020**. [CrossRef]
133. Hayakawa, M.; Kaizawa, H.; Moritomo, H.; Koizumi, T.; Ohishi, T.; Okada, M.; Ohta, M.; Tsukamoto, S.; Parker, P.; Workman, P.; et al. Synthesis and biological evaluation of 4-morpholino-2-phenylquinazolines and related derivatives as novel PI3 kinase P110α inhibitors. *Bioorg. Med. Chem.* **2006**, *14*, 6847–6858. [CrossRef]
134. Gharbi, S.I.; Zvelebil, M.J.; Shuttleworth, S.J.; Hancox, T.; Saghir, N.; Timms, J.F.; Waterfield, M.D. Exploring the specificity of the PI3K family inhibitor LY294002. *Biochem. J.* **2007**, *404*, 15–21. [CrossRef] [PubMed]
135. Méresse, S.; Fodil, M.; Fleury, F.; Chénais, B. Fucoxanthin, a marine-derived carotenoid from brown seaweeds and microalgae: A promising bioactive compound for cancer therapy. *Int. J. Mol. Sci.* **2020**, *21*, 9273. [CrossRef] [PubMed]

136. Noorani, I.; Bradley, A.; de la Rosa, J. CRISPR and transposon in vivo screens for cancer drivers and therapeutic targets. *Genome Biol.* **2020**, *21*, 204. [CrossRef] [PubMed]
137. Noorani, I.; de la Rosa, J.; Choi, Y.H.; Strong, A.; Ponstingl, H.; Vijayabaskar, M.S.; Lee, J.; Lee, E.; Richard-Londt, A.; Friedrich, M.; et al. PiggyBac mutagenesis and exome sequencing identify genetic driver landscapes and potential therapeutic targets of EGFR-mutant gliomas. *Genome Biol.* **2020**, *21*, 181. [CrossRef]
138. Tejeda, G.S.; Whiteley, E.L.; Deeb, T.Z.; Bürli, R.W.; Moss, S.J.; Sheridan, E.; Brandon, N.J.; Baillie, G.S. Chorea-related mutations in PDE10A result in aberrant compartmentalization and functionality of the enzyme. *Proc. Natl. Acad. Sci. USA* **2020**, *117*, 677–688. [CrossRef] [PubMed]

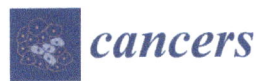

Editorial

Novel Treatment Strategies for Glioblastoma

Stanley S. Stylli [1,2]

[1] Department of Surgery, The University of Melbourne, The Royal Melbourne Hospital, Parkville, VIC 3050, Australia; sstylli@unimelb.edu.au or Stanley.stylli@mh.org.au
[2] Department of Neurosurgery, The Royal Melbourne Hospital, Parkville, VIC 3050, Australia

Received: 22 September 2020; Accepted: 6 October 2020; Published: 8 October 2020

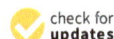

Abstract: Glioblastoma (GBM) is the most common primary central nervous system tumor in adults. It is a highly invasive disease, making it difficult to achieve a complete surgical resection, resulting in poor prognosis with a median survival of 12–15 months after diagnosis, and less than 5% of patients survive more than 5 years. Surgical, instrument technology, diagnostic and radio/chemotherapeutic strategies have slowly evolved over time, but this has not translated into significant increases in patient survival. The current standard of care for GBM patients involving surgery, radiotherapy, and concomitant chemotherapy temozolomide (known as the Stupp protocol), has only provided a modest increase of 2.5 months in median survival, since the landmark publication in 2005. There has been considerable effort in recent years to increase our knowledge of the molecular landscape of GBM through advances in technology such as next-generation sequencing, which has led to the stratification of the disease into several genetic subtypes. Current treatments are far from satisfactory, and studies investigating acquired/inherent resistance to current therapies, restricted drug delivery, inter/intra-tumoral heterogeneity, drug repurposing and a tumor immune-evasive environment have been the focus of intense research over recent years. While the clinical advancement of GBM therapeutics has seen limited progression compared to other cancers, developments in novel treatment strategies that are being investigated are displaying encouraging signs for combating this disease. This aim of this editorial is to provide a brief overview of a select number of these novel therapeutic approaches.

Keywords: glioblastoma; glioma; temozolomide; radiotherapy; immunotherapy; novel therapy; personalized treatment; drug repurposing

1. Introduction

It is more than 90 years since Percival Bailey and Harvey Cushing published the first classification of brain tumors [1] and devised the term 'glioblastoma multiforme', even though gliomas had been previously documented [2]. Gliomas are the most common malignant tumor in adults and they account for approximately 80% of all brain-related malignancies [3]. The twenty-second (22nd) statistical report (2012–2016; 408,133 records) published by CBTRUS (Central Brain Tumor Registry of the United States) is the largest population based primary brain tumor/central nervous system (CNS) tumor registry in the United States [3]. The average annual age-adjusted incidence rate of malignant brain/other CNS tumors was 7.08 per 100,000 and the most commonly occurring malignant brain/other CNS tumor was GBM (14.6% of all tumors; 48.3% of all malignant tumors; 25,510 malignant tumors expected in 2019). GBM also accounted for the majority of all gliomas (57.3%) with an incidence rate of 3.22 per 100,000. The five-year relative survival rate following diagnosis of a malignant brain/other CNS tumor was 35.8%, but this was significantly lower for GBM at 6.8%. The incidence also increases with age, with a median of 65 years. Surgical resection alone provided a survival benefit of approximately 3–6 months, which increased to 12.1 months with the inclusion of radiotherapy treatment and a further slight increase to 14.6 months was observed with the addition of concomitant and adjuvant temozolomide [4].

The World Health Organization (WHO), classifies brain tumors using a grading system, with grade I being the least aggressive and the best prognosis, to grade IV being the most malignant with the worst prognosis [5]. GBM can present as a de novo primary tumor (approximately 90% of GBM patients), without histological/clinical evidence of a lower grade lesion, or as a secondary GBM arising from lower grade gliomas, such as a diffuse astrocytoma or anaplastic astrocytoma. Primary and secondary GBMs are histopathologically indistinguishable; however, secondary GBM patients are generally younger, present with a more favorable prognosis, and differ in their molecular signature [6]. In 2010, The Cancer Genome Atlas (TCGA), presented a multidimensional analysis of 216 GBM tumor samples with the aim of characterizing the GBM genomic landscape. Several major genomic alterations were identified. Epidermal Growth Factor Receptor (EGFR) amplification/mutations, Phosphatase and tensin homolog (PTEN) deletion/mutations and CDKN2Ap16^{INK4a} were most frequently observed in primary GBM, whereas the genomic alterations common to secondary GBM included isocitrate dehydrogenase 1/2 (IDH1/2) or Tumor protein 53 (TP53) mutations [6,7]. IDH1 was also identified as the most reliable diagnostic molecular marker of secondary GBM, as the mutation occurred more frequently in secondary GBM patients which correlated with an improved overall survival [6].

Large scale genomic studies such as the TCGA led to the identification of four GBM clinical subtypes—mesenchymal, classical, proneural, and neural, characterized by abnormalities in EGFR, IDH1, neurofibromin 1 (NF1), and platelet-derived growth factor receptor A (PDGFRA). Mesenchymal GBMs display an overexpression of mesenchymal and astrocytic markers, in addition to an NF1 deletion, and are seen in older patients with a poor prognosis. The classical subtype is associated with EGFR amplification, is highly proliferative and observed in older patients, also with a poor prognosis. Aggressive, higher-grade tumors are associated with these two subtypes. Proneural and neural subtype GBMs are generally seen in younger patients, present with IDH1, PDGFRA, PIK3C, TP53 alterations (proneural), or genes involved in nervous system development (neural) and are less aggressive tumors. Subsequently, a new classification was proposed by Verhaak [8], ultimately leading to a 2016 update of the WHO Classification of CNS tumors based on the integration of molecular parameters into diagnostic procedures previously based only on histopathological features [9]. This molecular-based approach is critical in determining the potential response to current treatment protocols that may influence patient prognosis and the design and implementation of appropriately targeted therapies.

2. Therapeutic Strategies for Glioblastoma

2.1. Targeted Therapies

With the advancement of next-generation sequencing and the comprehensive molecular mapping of GBM, several potential targets have been identified and various strategies are being evaluated as treatments for GBM. IDH mutations, which exist in high numbers in secondary GBM, involve both a loss and gain of enzyme function [10]. There is an abnormal accumulation of 2-hydroxyglutarate (2-HG), which is a driver of tumorigenesis [11,12]. Several IDH inhibitors are currently being evaluated in clinical trials, including AG-120 (mIDH1 inhibitor), AG881 (non-specific IDH inhibitor), FT-21-2 (mIDH1 inhibitor), and IDH305 (an IDH1(R132H) inhibitor). EGFR inhibitors such as gefitinib, erlotinib, and afatinib have failed to show a survival benefit in GBM [13–15], even though they have been successful in other cancers. The activation of multiple receptor tyrosine kinase (RTK) pathways in GBM has also been proposed as a roadblock for single target-based strategies; therefore, efforts have been made to evaluate small molecule inhibitors with multiple targets such as Regorafenib. A phase II trial showed an increase in overall survival for recurrent GBM [16], while a current international phase I/II trial (GBM AGILE) is evaluating regorafenib with multiple treatment parameters for newly and recurrent GBM [17].

Depatuxizumab Mafodotin, also known as ABT-414, is an investigational anti-EGFR monoclonal antibody drug conjugate. ABT-414 targets the tumor cells by linking the anti-microtubule agent, monomethyl auristatin F, with an antibody directed against EGFR or mutant EGFRvIII. Participants within a phase I cohort who displayed EGFR amplification had a confirmed response, and this is currently being investigated in a phase II trial with ABT-414 and temozolomide in recurrent EGFR-amplified GBM. Monoclonal antibodies represent another class of targeted agents that have been used because of their high specificity and affinity to their targets. Bevacizumab, which binds to VEGF (vascular endothelial growth factor), inhibiting the growth of blood vessels, received accelerated FDA approval after encouraging phase I/II trials, but while phase III studies showed some extended progression-free survival, there was no observed overall survival benefit [18–20]. Cetuximab (EGFR monoclonal antibody), also failed to show survival benefits in phase II trials [21,22], identifying a potential weakness in the monoclonal antibody treatment strategy with incomplete tumor penetrance due to their size and restricted ability in crossing the blood brain barrier.

2.2. Chemotherapy

Since the landmark study in 2005 by Stupp [23], TMZ has been the first-line treatment following surgery and radiotherapy. This randomized clinical study demonstrated a significant survival benefit with the addition of TMZ to radiotherapy (27.2% versus 10.9% survival at 2 years). However, not all GBM patients respond to this treatment known as the Stupp protocol, while others may eventually display innate or acquired chemoresistance, ultimately resulting in tumor recurrence [24]. A positive prognostic indicator for TMZ-based chemotherapy for newly diagnosed GBM was correlated with MGMT gene methylation [25].

The DIRECTOR trial, investigating alternative schedules of TMZ treatment, found no difference in outcome between their treatment protocols, but they also observed that MGMT promoter methylation was a prognostic marker in the TMZ treatment of recurrent GBM patients [26]. DNA alkylating agents, known as nitrosoureas including lomustine (CCNU), carmustine (BCNU), and nimustine (ACNU) have been used in the treatment of GBM, but they are generally avoided due to the presence of systemic side effects including suppression of bone marrow and severe kidney/liver toxicities. However, improvement in the survival of recurrent and newly diagnosed GBM patients has been recently observed with the placement of carmustine wafers in the resection cavity, reducing systemic side effects [27]. Nevertheless, it is anticipated that the clinical efficacy of nitrosourea-based treatment protocols will be more prominent in GBM patients with tumors displaying MGMT promoter methylation [28,29].

Since the development of new therapeutics is associated with high costs and slow progress to successful implementation in the clinic, drug repurposing has emerged as an attractive strategy, due to lower costs and a shortened time for transition to the clinic for a new indication. For example, a study trialing Metformin, which is utilized in the management for diabetes mellitus type 2, demonstrated that the progression-free survival of patients with GBM and metformin-treated diabetes was significantly increased [30]. Furthermore, a combined analysis of 1731 patients in the AVAglio, CENTRIC, and CORE trials did not demonstrate a significant improvement in overall survival with metformin, but there was a significant hazard ratio observed for progression-free survival in these patients at baseline [31]. Nonsteroidal anti-inflammatory drugs such as celecoxib have been investigated due to encouraging results in pre-clinical laboratory-based studies [32,33]. The inclusion of celecoxib as an adjuvant to therapeutics such as temozolomide, while showing good tolerability, was inconclusive in terms of providing a significant survival benefit [34]. Currently, the DIRECT phase II/III multicenter trial is examining the efficacy of disulfiram (potent inhibitor of aldehyde dehydrogenase) in a randomized controlled study with GBM patients, due for primary completion at the end of 2021 [35].

Historically, a single-target, single-drug strategy has been the focus of drug discovery, laboratory-based studies, and clinical treatment. However, due to the genetic heterogeneity of GBM tumors, a multitarget approach with the repurposing of several drugs as a pharmacological treatment protocol has been considered and is underway. This was initially known as the CUSP9 trial, but it has undergone several modifications and is now known as CUSPv3 [36,37]. The genomic profiling of GBM tumors, coupled with the bioinformatic match-up of molecular abnormalities with drug libraries and the corresponding known drug targets in designing a personalized drug cocktail is being evaluated [38]. Numerous chemotherapeutic agents are under investigation, and it is beyond this editorial to discuss and list all the completed and ongoing trials. This information is available through the website www.clinicaltrials.gov.

2.3. Tumor Treating Fields (TTFields)

In 2011, a treatment technology known as tumor treating fields (TTFs), which utilizes intermediate frequency (200 KHz), low-intensity (1 V/cm) continuously delivered electric fields [39] to selectively target proliferating tumor cells by inhibiting mitosis was approved for the treatment of recurrent GBM by the FDA [40]. The first TTF device approved by the FDA, known as NovoTTF-100A (Optune®), manufactured by Novocure, is patient-operated, with the field generator being mounted on their shaved scalp. The results from the initial trials appear to be encouraging; when TTF was combined with TMZ chemotherapy, a significant increase in overall survival (20.9 months vs. 16 months) [41] compared to TMZ alone was observed, forming the foundation for further ongoing trials examining the efficacy of combining TTFields with chemotherapy in the treatment of GBM.

2.4. Laser Interstitial Therapy

Occasionally, GBM patients may not be candidates for surgical debulking of the tumor via an open craniotomy, and a relatively new technique known as 'Laser Interstitial Thermal Therapy' (LITT) is being trialed as a potential cytoreductive technique in destroying tumor cells via a localized elevated temperature [42–44]. It involves the insertion of an MRI-guided laser-tip probe into the tumor to deliver low-powered laser-induced thermotherapy. The initial studies have demonstrated that this therapy is safe [42], and an improved survival observed for patients with tumors where difficult surgical access may be achievable [45–48].

2.5. Radiotherapy

The current standard of care for GBM involves the combination of radiotherapy with chemotherapy [23]. Traditionally, whole brain radiation therapy was used. However due to the side effects of exposure of the normal brain to radiation, such as cognitive impairment, current practice utilizes focal radiotherapy treatment. The total radiotherapy dose of 60 Gy is normally delivered over 30 fractions of 2 Gy with adjuvant temozolomide [23], with the fractionated treatment allowing normal brain cells surrounding the tumor treatment area to recover between each treatment. Radiation dose escalation attempts have resulted in increased tissue damage and side effects, with no significant change in survival [49], hence there has been an effort in exploring other potential radiotherapy based strategies. Interstitial brachytherapy which requires the placement of radioactive isotopes (or seeds) into the surgical cavity is not an entirely new treatment, but due to continuing concerns such as radiation leakage into the surrounding brain, efforts into improving brachytherapy are underway, including the prolonged delivery of higher doses of radiation, use of alternative isotopes, and targeted delivery via the combination of isotopes with monoclonal antibodies. A treatment known as GammaTile, which involves inserting encapsulated radioactive cesium-131 seeds into the surgical cavity, was recently approved by the FDA for the treatment of GBM and has to date demonstrated feasibility and safety [50].

Proton Beam Therapy (PBT) has also been investigated as a therapeutic option for GBM, as the associated 'Bragg Peak Effect' reduces radiation exposure to the surrounding brain with the use of smaller treatment target volumes, providing for a lower risk of side effects such as neurocognitive decline. Dose escalation studies have been performed, with some observed toxicities [51,52], but it has also been shown to be a safe treatment option, resulting in a slight survival benefit for recurrent GBM [53]. Phase II trials are currently underway, evaluating the efficacy of PBT as a frontline treatment compared to standard dose radiotherapy with TMZ. The delivery of high dose radiation to the tumor can also be achieved via Gamma Knife Radiosurgery, which has been utilized for the treatment of recurrent GBM [54–56]. It has been observed that significant radiation-induced edema occurs in patients who receive high radiation doses; however, these adverse side effects were reduced, and patient survival prolonged when combined with bevacizumab [57,58].

2.6. Immunotherapies

Given the success that has been demonstrated with immunotherapeutic strategies in treating various cancers, there has been considerable effort into also translating this into a treatment for GBM patients. Traditionally, the brain is considered an immune-privileged organ due to the existence of the blood brain barrier (BBB) and the absence of a lymphatic drainage system. However, anti-tumor immune responses have been observed in brain tumors [59], which are proposed to be facilitated by the presence of a lymphatic system [60]. In general, immunotherapy has been more successful in treating tumors with a high mutational burden [61], but GBM has a low tumor mutational burden, while also displaying an immunosuppressive environment [62], and the added complication that chemotherapeutics can also promote an immunosuppressive effect [63]. Nevertheless, as immunotherapy involves harnessing the immune system to eradicate tumor cells, several different strategies have been explored with the goal to boost host immunity against GBM.

Immune checkpoint blockade has been utilized to achieve stimulation of the immune system with a significant effort focusing on blocking the binding of checkpoint receptors on immune cells such as Cytotoxic T-Lymphocyte Antigen 4 (CTLA-4) (early T-cell inhibition) and Programmed Cell Death protein 1 (PD-1) (late T-cell inhibition) to their corresponding ligands on tumor cells promoting a more effective T cell response against the tumor [64]. A number of checkpoint inhibitors that have been approved for use in several cancers have been trialed in the treatment of recurrent GBM, including nivolumab, pembrolizumab, durvalumab, atezolizumab [65]. The preliminary results have been less than inspiring; however, there are ongoing investigations into studying biomarkers that may identify which patients may respond to checkpoint blockade, the mutational load of the tumor as a predictor of response, administration of PD-1 antibodies prior to tumor resection to induce an early anti-tumor response, or analyze the effects of radiotherapy, which may be a synergistic facilitator of response to immunotherapy [66–69].

T-cell therapy involves the use of autologous T-cells, which are genetically engineered to express chimeric antigen receptor (CAR) constructs and have been FDA-approved for the treatment of hematologic malignancies. Several phase I trials have shown encouraging signs in terms of safety, feasibility and potential efficacy against relevant GBM surface antigens including IL13Ra2, HER2, EphA2 and EGFRVIII [70]. Even though the initial results have been promising, it is anticipated that, due to the high degree of heterogeneity exhibited by GBM tumors, T-cell therapy will be administered as a combination therapy, potentially with immune checkpoint blockade.

Vaccine-based strategies are also being investigated as a potential adoptive immunotherapy for GBM by stimulating an antigen-specific effector T cell response against tumor specific antigens (TSA) or tumor associated antigens (TAA). Several approaches have been utilized including cell-based protocols (patient-derived dendritic cell and autologous tumor cell vaccines) and non-cell based protocols (peptide and heat shock protein vaccines). Engineered peptide sequences that provide a targeted immunity against tumor associated antigens bound to major histocompatibility complexes form the basis of peptide vaccines. An example of two peptide vaccines are rindopepimut (EGFRvIII) [71–73] and SurVaxM (Survivin) [74,75]. While rindopepimut showed impressive responses in the early-phase studies [76], a survival benefit was not observed in the phase III evaluation [77]. However, a separate phase II study combining rindopepimut with temozolomide improved progression-free and overall survival for GBM patients [72], as well as the demonstration of encouraging results in a phase II study combining rindopepimut with bevacizumab in the treatment of recurrent GBM patients [78]. A phase II study evaluating SurVaxM has displayed improvements in progression-free and overall survival [74].

Heat shock proteins have also been utilized to deliver a variety of tumor antigens and are designed to create an anti-tumor inflammatory response. HSPPC-96 is one such vaccine, which has undergone a phase II, multicenter clinical trial for recurrent GBM [79]. Autologous tumor cell based vaccines use cytotoxic T lymphocytes that are induced with patient-derived tumor cells, which then subsequently elicit an immune response, once they are reintroduced back into the patient [80,81]. Dendritic cell vaccines rely on patient-derived dendritic cells that are exposed to purified tumor-specific antigens or tumor cell extracts derived from the tumor before being reintroduced to the patient, subsequently activating CD8+ and CD4+ T cells. A phase I trial with an autologous dendritic cell vaccine has demonstrated a correlation between the expression level of tumor-associated antigens on the glioma cells and prolonged overall/progression free patient survival [82]. Viral-based therapy that involves delivery of the gene of interest via viral vectors is also being investigated as a form of immunotherapy for treating GBM. Oncolytic viruses can selectively replicate in tumor cells, eliciting cytotoxic effects, ultimately providing an immunostimulatory effect. DNX-2401 is a replication-competent adenovirus that uses tumor-specific integrins to produce oncolytic effects [83,84], whereas PVSRIPO (attenuated polio-rhinovirus chimera) recognizes CD155 (poliovirus receptor), which is widely expressed in tumor cells [85,86].

3. Conclusions

The treatment of GBM continues to be a complex and difficult challenge. Previous attempts to find a cure have only resulted in a slight improvement in survival over the last 50 years, as the current 5-year survival rate remains low at <10% [25]. As there are limitations on the number of times the current therapeutic approach of surgery, radiotherapy, and chemotherapy can be utilized, the ideal novel therapeutic agent or treatment protocol, as part of a multimodal strategy, must function to eliminate any residual tumor. Ultimately, this may be achieved by the synergistic effects of combining a number of the current therapeutic strategies briefly outlined in this editorial, including a targeted therapy, immunotherapy, chemotherapy, or radiotherapy, as treatment resistance can potentially develop to a single therapy. The development of new and novel therapies has been aided by the considerable efforts to decipher the genomic landscape of GBM with the evolution of next generation sequencing, leading to modifications in tumor classification and the 'molecular' clinical management of some GBM patients.

Over time, the therapeutic options available will increase with additional targetable and actionable combinations of genomic mutations and alterations being uncovered, as only a small fraction to date have been demonstrated to have clinical implementation. Importantly, as tumor heterogeneity and patient-to-patient variability contributing to the growth of GBM and response to treatment is driven by the genomics of each tumor, a personalized treatment approach through the stratification of patients into molecular subgroups will be critical in their allocation to the most appropriate novel treatment strategy that will be available in the future management of GBM. The continued collaboration between researchers and clinicians, coupled with advancements in technology, both scientifically and clinically, provides for an optimistic future that new and effective treatments will be developed for GBM patients.

Funding: This research received no external funding.

Conflicts of Interest: The author declares no conflict of interest.

References

1. Bailey, P.C.H. *A Classification of the Tumors of the Glioma Group on a Histogenetic Basis with a Correlated Study of Prognosis*; Lippincott: Philadelphia, PA, USA, 1926. Available online: https://www.ncbi.nlm.nih.gov/pmc/articles/PMC1709238/?page=1 (accessed on 6 October 2020).
2. Bailey, P.; Cushing, H. Microchemical Color Reactions as an Aid to the Identification and Classification of Brain Tumors. *Proc. Natl. Acad. Sci. USA* **1925**, *11*, 82–84. [CrossRef] [PubMed]

3. Ostrom, Q.T.; Cioffi, G.; Gittleman, H.; Patil, N.; Waite, K.; Kruchko, C.; Barnholtz-Sloan, J.S. CBTRUS Statistical Report: Primary Brain and Other Central Nervous System Tumors Diagnosed in the United States in 2012–2016. *Neuro Oncol.* **2019**, *21*, v1–v100. [CrossRef] [PubMed]
4. Agnihotri, S.; Burrell, K.E.; Wolf, A.; Jalali, S.; Hawkins, C.; Rutka, J.T.; Zadeh, G. Glioblastoma, a brief review of history, molecular genetics, animal models and novel therapeutic strategies. *Arch. Immunol. Ther. Exp. (Warsz)* **2013**, *61*, 25–41. [CrossRef] [PubMed]
5. Louis, D.N.; Ohgaki, H.; Wiestler, O.D.; Cavenee, W.K.; Burger, P.C.; Jouvet, A.; Scheithauer, B.W.; Kleihues, P. The 2007 WHO classification of tumours of the central nervous system. *Acta Neuropathol.* **2007**, *114*, 97–109. [CrossRef] [PubMed]
6. Ohgaki, H.; Kleihues, P. The definition of primary and secondary glioblastoma. *Clin. Cancer Res.* **2013**, *19*, 764–772. [CrossRef]
7. Jiao, Y.; Killela, P.J.; Reitman, Z.J.; Rasheed, A.B.; Heaphy, C.M.; de Wilde, R.F.; Rodriguez, F.J.; Rosemberg, S.; Oba-Shinjo, S.M.; Nagahashi Marie, S.K.; et al. Frequent ATRX, CIC, FUBP1 and IDH1 mutations refine the classification of malignant gliomas. *Oncotarget* **2012**, *3*, 709–722. [CrossRef]
8. Verhaak, R.G.; Hoadley, K.A.; Purdom, E.; Wang, V.; Qi, Y.; Wilkerson, M.D.; Miller, C.R.; Ding, L.; Golub, T.; Mesirov, J.P.; et al. Integrated genomic analysis identifies clinically relevant subtypes of glioblastoma characterized by abnormalities in PDGFRA, IDH1, EGFR, and NF1. *Cancer Cell* **2010**, *17*, 98–110. [CrossRef]
9. Louis, D.N.; Perry, A.; Reifenberger, G.; von Deimling, A.; Figarella-Branger, D.; Cavenee, W.K.; Ohgaki, H.; Wiestler, O.D.; Kleihues, P.; Ellison, D.W. The 2016 World Health Organization Classification of Tumors of the Central Nervous System: A summary. *Acta Neuropathol.* **2016**, *131*, 803–820. [CrossRef]
10. Cohen, A.L.; Holmen, S.L.; Colman, H. IDH1 and IDH2 mutations in gliomas. *Curr. Neurol. Neurosci. Rep.* **2013**, *13*, 345. [CrossRef]
11. Killock, D. CNS cancer: Breaking boundaries—IDH mutations in glioma. *Nat. Rev. Clin. Oncol.* **2016**, *13*, 64. [CrossRef]
12. Kim, W.; Liau, L.M. IDH mutations in human glioma. *Neurosurg. Clin. N. Am.* **2012**, *23*, 471–480. [CrossRef] [PubMed]
13. Sepulveda-Sanchez, J.M.; Vaz, M.A.; Balana, C.; Gil-Gil, M.; Reynes, G.; Gallego, O.; Martinez-Garcia, M.; Vicente, E.; Quindos, M.; Luque, R.; et al. Phase II trial of dacomitinib, a pan-human EGFR tyrosine kinase inhibitor, in recurrent glioblastoma patients with EGFR amplification. *Neuro Oncol.* **2017**, *19*, 1522–1531. [CrossRef] [PubMed]
14. Kreisl, T.N.; Lassman, A.B.; Mischel, P.S.; Rosen, N.; Scher, H.I.; Teruya-Feldstein, J.; Shaffer, D.; Lis, E.; Abrey, L.E. A pilot study of everolimus and gefitinib in the treatment of recurrent glioblastoma (GBM). *J. Neurooncol.* **2009**, *92*, 99–105. [CrossRef]
15. Reardon, D.A.; Nabors, L.B.; Mason, W.P.; Perry, J.R.; Shapiro, W.; Kavan, P.; Mathieu, D.; Phuphanich, S.; Cseh, A.; Fu, Y.; et al. Phase I/randomized phase II study of afatinib, an irreversible ErbB family blocker, with or without protracted temozolomide in adults with recurrent glioblastoma. *Neuro Oncol.* **2015**, *17*, 430–439. [CrossRef] [PubMed]
16. Lombardi, G.; De Salvo, G.L.; Brandes, A.A.; Eoli, M.; Ruda, R.; Faedi, M.; Lolli, I.; Pace, A.; Daniele, B.; Pasqualetti, F.; et al. Regorafenib compared with lomustine in patients with relapsed glioblastoma (REGOMA): A multicentre, open-label, randomised, controlled, phase 2 trial. *Lancet Oncol.* **2019**, *20*, 110–119. [CrossRef]
17. Alexander, B.M.; Ba, S.; Berger, M.S.; Berry, D.A.; Cavenee, W.K.; Chang, S.M.; Cloughesy, T.F.; Jiang, T.; Khasraw, M.; Li, W.; et al. Adaptive Global Innovative Learning Environment for Glioblastoma: GBM AGILE. *Clin. Cancer Res.* **2018**, *24*, 737–743. [CrossRef]
18. Gilbert, M.R.; Sulman, E.P.; Mehta, M.P. Bevacizumab for newly diagnosed glioblastoma. *N. Engl. J. Med.* **2014**, *370*, 2048–2049. [CrossRef]
19. Hamza, M.A.; Mandel, J.J.; Conrad, C.A.; Gilbert, M.R.; Yung, W.K.; Puduvalli, V.K.; DeGroot, J.F. Survival outcome of early versus delayed bevacizumab treatment in patients with recurrent glioblastoma. *J. Neurooncol.* **2014**, *119*, 135–140. [CrossRef]
20. Gilbert, M.R.; Dignam, J.J.; Armstrong, T.S.; Wefel, J.S.; Blumenthal, D.T.; Vogelbaum, M.A.; Colman, H.; Chakravarti, A.; Pugh, S.; Won, M.; et al. A randomized trial of bevacizumab for newly diagnosed glioblastoma. *N. Engl. J. Med.* **2014**, *370*, 699–708. [CrossRef]

21. Neyns, B.; Sadones, J.; Joosens, E.; Bouttens, F.; Verbeke, L.; Baurain, J.F.; D'Hondt, L.; Strauven, T.; Chaskis, C.; In't Veld, P.; et al. Stratified phase II trial of cetuximab in patients with recurrent high–grade glioma. *Ann. Oncol.* **2009**, *20*, 1596–1603. [CrossRef]
22. Hasselbalch, B.; Lassen, U.; Hansen, S.; Holmberg, M.; Sorensen, M.; Kosteljanetz, M.; Broholm, H.; Stockhausen, M.T.; Poulsen, H.S. Cetuximab, bevacizumab, and irinotecan for patients with primary glioblastoma and progression after radiation therapy and temozolomide: A phase II trial. *Neuro Oncol.* **2010**, *12*, 508–516. [PubMed]
23. Stupp, R.; Mason, W.P.; van den Bent, M.J.; Weller, M.; Fisher, B.; Taphoorn, M.J.; Belanger, K.; Brandes, A.A.; Marosi, C.; Bogdahn, U.; et al. Radiotherapy plus concomitant and adjuvant temozolomide for glioblastoma. *N. Engl. J. Med.* **2005**, *352*, 987–996. [CrossRef] [PubMed]
24. Lee, S.Y. Temozolomide resistance in glioblastoma multiforme. *Genes Dis.* **2016**, *3*, 198–210. [CrossRef] [PubMed]
25. Stupp, R.; Hegi, M.E.; Mason, W.P.; van den Bent, M.J.; Taphoorn, M.J.; Janzer, R.C.; Ludwin, S.K.; Allgeier, A.; Fisher, B.; Belanger, K.; et al. Effects of radiotherapy with concomitant and adjuvant temozolomide versus radiotherapy alone on survival in glioblastoma in a randomised phase III study: 5–year analysis of the EORTC–NCIC trial. *Lancet Oncol.* **2009**, *10*, 459–466. [CrossRef]
26. Weller, M.; Tabatabai, G.; Kastner, B.; Felsberg, J.; Steinbach, J.P.; Wick, A.; Schnell, O.; Hau, P.; Herrlinger, U.; Sabel, M.C.; et al. MGMT Promoter Methylation Is a Strong Prognostic Biomarker for Benefit from Dose–Intensified Temozolomide Rechallenge in Progressive Glioblastoma: The DIRECTOR Trial. *Clin. Cancer Res.* **2015**, *21*, 2057–2064. [CrossRef]
27. Chowdhary, S.A.; Ryken, T.; Newton, H.B. Survival outcomes and safety of carmustine wafers in the treatment of high–grade gliomas: A meta–analysis. *J. Neurooncol.* **2015**, *122*, 367–382. [CrossRef]
28. Taal, W.; van der Rijt, C.C.; Dinjens, W.N.; Sillevis Smitt, P.A.; Wertenbroek, A.A.; Bromberg, J.E.; van Heuvel, I.; Kros, J.M.; van den Bent, M.J. Treatment of large low–grade oligodendroglial tumors with upfront procarbazine, lomustine, and vincristine chemotherapy with long follow–up: A retrospective cohort study with growth kinetics. *J. Neurooncol.* **2015**, *121*, 365–372. [CrossRef]
29. Taal, W.; Oosterkamp, H.M.; Walenkamp, A.M.; Dubbink, H.J.; Beerepoot, L.V.; Hanse, M.C.; Buter, J.; Honkoop, A.H.; Boerman, D.; de Vos, F.Y.; et al. Single–agent bevacizumab or lomustine versus a combination of bevacizumab plus lomustine in patients with recurrent glioblastoma (BELOB trial): A randomised controlled phase 2 trial. *Lancet Oncol.* **2014**, *15*, 943–953. [CrossRef]
30. Adeberg, S.; Bernhardt, D.; Ben Harrabi, S.; Bostel, T.; Mohr, A.; Koelsche, C.; Diehl, C.; Rieken, S.; Debus, J. Metformin influences progression in diabetic glioblastoma patients. *Strahlenther. Onkol.* **2015**, *191*, 928–935. [CrossRef]
31. Seliger, C.; Genbrugge, E.; Gorlia, T.; Chinot, O.; Stupp, R.; Nabors, B.; Weller, M.; Hau, P.; Group, E.B.T. Use of metformin and outcome of patients with newly diagnosed glioblastoma: Pooled analysis. *Int. J. Cancer* **2020**, *146*, 803–809. [CrossRef]
32. Sareddy, G.R.; Kesanakurti, D.; Kirti, P.B.; Babu, P.P. Nonsteroidal anti–inflammatory drugs diclofenac and celecoxib attenuates Wnt/beta–catenin/Tcf signaling pathway in human glioblastoma cells. *Neurochem. Res.* **2013**, *38*, 2313–2322. [CrossRef] [PubMed]
33. Chirasani, S.R.; Leukel, P.; Gottfried, E.; Hochrein, J.; Stadler, K.; Neumann, B.; Oefner, P.J.; Gronwald, W.; Bogdahn, U.; Hau, P.; et al. Diclofenac inhibits lactate formation and efficiently counteracts local immune suppression in a murine glioma model. *Int. J. Cancer* **2013**, *132*, 843–853. [CrossRef] [PubMed]
34. Stockhammer, F.; Misch, M.; Koch, A.; Czabanka, M.; Plotkin, M.; Blechschmidt, C.; Tuettenberg, J.; Vajkoczy, P. Continuous low–dose temozolomide and celecoxib in recurrent glioblastoma. *J. Neurooncol.* **2010**, *100*, 407–415. [CrossRef] [PubMed]
35. Jakola, A.S.; Werlenius, K.; Mudaisi, M.; Hylin, S.; Kinhult, S.; Bartek, J., Jr.; Salvesen, O.; Carlsen, S.M.; Strandeus, M.; Lindskog, M.; et al. Disulfiram repurposing combined with nutritional copper supplement as add–on to chemotherapy in recurrent glioblastoma (DIRECT): Study protocol for a randomized controlled trial. *F1000Res* **2018**, *7*, 1797. [CrossRef]
36. Kast, R.E.; Karpel–Massler, G.; Halatsch, M.E. CUSP9* treatment protocol for recurrent glioblastoma: Aprepitant, artesunate, auranofin, captopril, celecoxib, disulfiram, itraconazole, ritonavir, sertraline augmenting continuous low dose temozolomide. *Oncotarget* **2014**, *5*, 8052–8082. [CrossRef]

37. Skaga, E.; Skaga, I.O.; Grieg, Z.; Sandberg, C.J.; Langmoen, I.A.; Vik–Mo, E.O. The efficacy of a coordinated pharmacological blockade in glioblastoma stem cells with nine repurposed drugs using the CUSP9 strategy. *J. Cancer Res. Clin. Oncol.* **2019**, *145*, 1495–1507. [CrossRef]
38. Byron, S.A.; Tran, N.L.; Halperin, R.F.; Phillips, J.J.; Kuhn, J.G.; de Groot, J.F.; Colman, H.; Ligon, K.L.; Wen, P.Y.; Cloughesy, T.F.; et al. Prospective Feasibility Trial for Genomics–Informed Treatment in Recurrent and Progressive Glioblastoma. *Clin. Cancer Res.* **2018**, *24*, 295–305. [CrossRef]
39. Wenger, C.; Salvador, R.; Basser, P.J.; Miranda, P.C. The electric field distribution in the brain during TTFields therapy and its dependence on tissue dielectric properties and anatomy: A computational study. *Phys. Med. Biol.* **2015**, *60*, 7339–7357. [CrossRef]
40. Davies, A.M.; Weinberg, U.; Palti, Y. Tumor treating fields: A new frontier in cancer therapy. *Ann. N. Y. Acad. Sci.* **2013**, *1291*, 86–95. [CrossRef]
41. Stupp, R.; Taillibert, S.; Kanner, A.; Read, W.; Steinberg, D.; Lhermitte, B.; Toms, S.; Idbaih, A.; Ahluwalia, M.S.; Fink, K.; et al. Effect of Tumor–Treating Fields Plus Maintenance Temozolomide vs. Maintenance Temozolomide Alone on Survival in Patients With Glioblastoma: A Randomized Clinical Trial. *JAMA* **2017**, *318*, 2306–2316. [CrossRef]
42. Kamath, A.A.; Friedman, D.D.; Akbari, S.H.A.; Kim, A.H.; Tao, Y.; Luo, J.; Leuthardt, E.C. Glioblastoma Treated with Magnetic Resonance Imaging–Guided Laser Interstitial Thermal Therapy: Safety, Efficacy, and Outcomes. *Neurosurgery* **2019**, *84*, 836–843. [CrossRef] [PubMed]
43. Kim, A.H.; Tatter, S.; Rao, G.; Prabhu, S.; Chen, C.; Fecci, P.; Chiang, V.; Smith, K.; Williams, B.J.; Mohammadi, A.M.; et al. Laser Ablation of Abnormal Neurological Tissue Using Robotic NeuroBlate System (LAANTERN): 12–Month Outcomes and Quality of Life After Brain Tumor Ablation. *Neurosurgery* **2020**, *87*, E338–E346. [CrossRef] [PubMed]
44. Sloan, A.E.; Ahluwalia, M.S.; Valerio–Pascua, J.; Manjila, S.; Torchia, M.G.; Jones, S.E.; Sunshine, J.L.; Phillips, M.; Griswold, M.A.; Clampitt, M.; et al. Results of the NeuroBlate System first–in–humans Phase I clinical trial for recurrent glioblastoma: Clinical article. *J. Neurosurg.* **2013**, *118*, 1202–1219. [CrossRef] [PubMed]
45. Thomas, J.G.; Rao, G.; Kew, Y.; Prabhu, S.S. Laser interstitial thermal therapy for newly diagnosed and recurrent glioblastoma. *Neurosurg. Focus* **2016**, *41*, E12. [CrossRef]
46. Rahmathulla, G.; Recinos, P.F.; Kamian, K.; Mohammadi, A.M.; Ahluwalia, M.S.; Barnett, G.H. MRI–guided laser interstitial thermal therapy in neuro–oncology: A review of its current clinical applications. *Oncology* **2014**, *87*, 67–82. [CrossRef]
47. Mohammadi, A.M.; Hawasli, A.H.; Rodriguez, A.; Schroeder, J.L.; Laxton, A.W.; Elson, P.; Tatter, S.B.; Barnett, G.H.; Leuthardt, E.C. The role of laser interstitial thermal therapy in enhancing progression–free survival of difficult–to–access high–grade gliomas: A multicenter study. *Cancer Med.* **2014**, *3*, 971–979. [CrossRef]
48. Mohammadi, A.M.; Schroeder, J.L. Laser interstitial thermal therapy in treatment of brain tumors—The NeuroBlate System. *Expert Rev. Med. Devices* **2014**, *11*, 109–119. [CrossRef]
49. Barani, I.J.; Larson, D.A. Radiation therapy of glioblastoma. *Cancer Treat. Res.* **2015**, *163*, 49–73.
50. Gessler, D.J.; Ferreira, C.; Dusenbery, K.; Chen, C.C. GammaTile((R)): Surgically targeted radiation therapy for glioblastomas. *Future Oncol.* **2020**. [CrossRef]
51. Mizumoto, M.; Yamamoto, T.; Ishikawa, E.; Matsuda, M.; Takano, S.; Ishikawa, H.; Okumura, T.; Sakurai, H.; Matsumura, A.; Tsuboi, K. Proton beam therapy with concurrent chemotherapy for glioblastoma multiforme: Comparison of nimustine hydrochloride and temozolomide. *J. Neurooncol.* **2016**, *130*, 165–170. [CrossRef]
52. Mizumoto, M.; Yamamoto, T.; Takano, S.; Ishikawa, E.; Matsumura, A.; Ishikawa, H.; Okumura, T.; Sakurai, H.; Miyatake, S.; Tsuboi, K. Long–term survival after treatment of glioblastoma multiforme with hyperfractionated concomitant boost proton beam therapy. *Pract. Radiat Oncol.* **2015**, *5*, e9–16. [CrossRef] [PubMed]
53. Scartoni, D.; Amelio, D.; Palumbo, P.; Giacomelli, I.; Amichetti, M. Proton therapy re–irradiation preserves health–related quality of life in large recurrent glioblastoma. *J. Cancer Res. Clin. Oncol.* **2020**, *146*, 1615–1622. [CrossRef] [PubMed]
54. Larson, E.W.; Peterson, H.E.; Lamoreaux, W.T.; MacKay, A.R.; Fairbanks, R.K.; Call, J.A.; Carlson, J.D.; Ling, B.C.; Demakas, J.J.; Cooke, B.S.; et al. Clinical outcomes following salvage Gamma Knife radiosurgery for recurrent glioblastoma. *World J. Clin. Oncol.* **2014**, *5*, 142–148. [CrossRef] [PubMed]

55. Guseynova, K.; Liscak, R.; Simonova, G.; Novotny, J., Jr. Gamma knife radiosurgery for local recurrence of glioblastoma. *Neuro Endocrinol. Lett.* **2018**, *39*, 281–287. [PubMed]
56. Brehmer, S.; Grimm, M.A.; Forster, A.; Seiz-Rosenhagen, M.; Welzel, G.; Stieler, F.; Wenz, F.; Groden, C.; Mai, S.; Hanggi, D.; et al. Study Protocol: Early Stereotactic Gamma Knife Radiosurgery to Residual Tumor After Surgery of Newly Diagnosed Glioblastoma (Gamma–GBM). *Neurosurgery* **2019**, *84*, 1133–1137. [CrossRef]
57. Koga, T.; Saito, N. Efficacy and limitations of stereotactic radiosurgery in the treatment of glioblastoma. *Neurol. Med. Chir. (Tokyo)* **2012**, *52*, 548–552. [CrossRef]
58. Koga, T.; Maruyama, K.; Tanaka, M.; Ino, Y.; Saito, N.; Nakagawa, K.; Shibahara, J.; Todo, T. Extended field stereotactic radiosurgery for recurrent glioblastoma. *Cancer* **2012**, *118*, 4193–4200. [CrossRef]
59. D'Alessio, A.; Proietti, G.; Sica, G.; Scicchitano, B.M. Pathological and Molecular Features of Glioblastoma and Its Peritumoral Tissue. *Cancers (Basel)* **2019**, *11*, 469. [CrossRef]
60. Song, E.; Mao, T.; Dong, H.; Boisserand, L.S.B.; Antila, S.; Bosenberg, M.; Alitalo, K.; Thomas, J.L.; Iwasaki, A. VEGF–C–driven lymphatic drainage enables immunosurveillance of brain tumours. *Nature* **2020**, *577*, 689–694. [CrossRef]
61. Riviere, P.; Goodman, A.M.; Okamura, R.; Barkauskas, D.A.; Whitchurch, T.J.; Lee, S.; Khalid, N.; Collier, R.; Marebiona, M.; Frampton, G.M.; et al. High Tumor Mutational Burden Correlates with Longer Survival in Immunotherapy–Naive Patients with Diverse Cancers. *Mol. Cancer Ther.* **2020**. [CrossRef]
62. Liu, E.K.; Sulman, E.P.; Wen, P.Y.; Kurz, S.C. Novel Therapies for Glioblastoma. *Curr. Neurol. Neurosci. Rep.* **2020**, *20*, 19. [CrossRef] [PubMed]
63. Sengupta, S.; Marrinan, J.; Frishman, C.; Sampath, P. Impact of temozolomide on immune response during malignant glioma chemotherapy. *Clin. Dev. Immunol.* **2012**, *2012*, 831090. [CrossRef] [PubMed]
64. Maxwell, R.; Jackson, C.M.; Lim, M. Clinical Trials Investigating Immune Checkpoint Blockade in Glioblastoma. *Curr. Treat. Options Oncol.* **2017**, *18*, 51. [CrossRef] [PubMed]
65. Romani, M.; Pistillo, M.P.; Carosio, R.; Morabito, A.; Banelli, B. Immune Checkpoints and Innovative Therapies in Glioblastoma. *Front. Oncol.* **2018**, *8*, 464. [CrossRef]
66. Rajani, K.R.; Carlstrom, L.P.; Parney, I.F.; Johnson, A.J.; Warrington, A.E.; Burns, T.C. Harnessing Radiation Biology to Augment Immunotherapy for Glioblastoma. *Front. Oncol.* **2018**, *8*, 656. [CrossRef]
67. Le, D.T.; Durham, J.N.; Smith, K.N.; Wang, H.; Bartlett, B.R.; Aulakh, L.K.; Lu, S.; Kemberling, H.; Wilt, C.; Luber, B.S.; et al. Mismatch repair deficiency predicts response of solid tumors to PD–1 blockade. *Science* **2017**, *357*, 409–413. [CrossRef]
68. Bouffet, E.; Larouche, V.; Campbell, B.B.; Merico, D.; de Borja, R.; Aronson, M.; Durno, C.; Krueger, J.; Cabric, V.; Ramaswamy, V.; et al. Immune Checkpoint Inhibition for Hypermutant Glioblastoma Multiforme Resulting From Germline Biallelic Mismatch Repair Deficiency. *J. Clin. Oncol.* **2016**, *34*, 2206–2211. [CrossRef]
69. Cloughesy, T.F.; Mochizuki, A.Y.; Orpilla, J.R.; Hugo, W.; Lee, A.H.; Davidson, T.B.; Wang, A.C.; Ellingson, B.M.; Rytlewski, J.A.; Sanders, C.M.; et al. Neoadjuvant anti–PD–1 immunotherapy promotes a survival benefit with intratumoral and systemic immune responses in recurrent glioblastoma. *Nat. Med.* **2019**, *25*, 477–486. [CrossRef]
70. Bagley, S.J.; Desai, A.S.; Linette, G.P.; June, C.H.; O'Rourke, D.M. CAR T–cell therapy for glioblastoma: Recent clinical advances and future challenges. *Neuro Oncol.* **2018**, *20*, 1429–1438. [CrossRef]
71. Zussman, B.M.; Engh, J.A. Outcomes of the ACT III Study: Rindopepimut (CDX–110) Therapy for Glioblastoma. *Neurosurgery* **2015**, *76*, N17. [CrossRef]
72. Schuster, J.; Lai, R.K.; Recht, L.D.; Reardon, D.A.; Paleologos, N.A.; Groves, M.D.; Mrugala, M.M.; Jensen, R.; Baehring, J.M.; Sloan, A.; et al. A phase II, multicenter trial of rindopepimut (CDX–110) in newly diagnosed glioblastoma: The ACT III study. *Neuro Oncol.* **2015**, *17*, 854–861. [CrossRef] [PubMed]
73. Swartz, A.M.; Li, Q.J.; Sampson, J.H. Rindopepimut: A promising immunotherapeutic for the treatment of glioblastoma multiforme. *Immunotherapy* **2014**, *6*, 679–690. [CrossRef] [PubMed]
74. Fenstermaker, R.A.; Ciesielski, M.J.; Qiu, J.; Yang, N.; Frank, C.L.; Lee, K.P.; Mechtler, L.R.; Belal, A.; Ahluwalia, M.S.; Hutson, A.D. Clinical study of a survivin long peptide vaccine (SurVaxM) in patients with recurrent malignant glioma. *Cancer Immunol. Immunother.* **2016**, *65*, 1339–1352. [CrossRef] [PubMed]
75. Fenstermaker, R.A.; Ciesielski, M.J. Challenges in the development of a survivin vaccine (SurVaxM) for malignant glioma. *Expert Rev. Vaccines* **2014**, *13*, 377–385. [CrossRef]

76. Del Vecchio, C.A.; Wong, A.J. Rindopepimut, a 14–mer injectable peptide vaccine against EGFRvIII for the potential treatment of glioblastoma multiforme. *Curr. Opin. Mol. Ther.* **2010**, *12*, 741–754.
77. Weller, M.; Butowski, N.; Tran, D.D.; Recht, L.D.; Lim, M.; Hirte, H.; Ashby, L.; Mechtler, L.; Goldlust, S.A.; Iwamoto, F.; et al. Rindopepimut with temozolomide for patients with newly diagnosed, EGFRvIII–expressing glioblastoma (ACT IV): A randomised, double–blind, international phase 3 trial. *Lancet Oncol.* **2017**, *18*, 1373–1385. [CrossRef]
78. Reardon, D.A.; Desjardins, A.; Vredenburgh, J.J.; O'Rourke, D.M.; Tran, D.D.; Fink, K.L.; Nabors, L.B.; Li, G.; Bota, D.A.; Lukas, R.V.; et al. Rindopepimut with Bevacizumab for Patients with Relapsed EGFRvIII–Expressing Glioblastoma (ReACT): Results of a Double–Blind Randomized Phase II Trial. *Clin. Cancer Res.* **2020**, *26*, 1586–1594. [CrossRef]
79. Schuster, J.L.R.; Recht, L.D.; Reardon, D.A.; Paleologos, N.A.; Groves, M.D. Heat–shock protein peptide complex–96 vaccination for recurrent glioblastoma: A phase II, single–arm trial. *Neuro Oncol.* **2014**, *16*, 274–279.
80. Chamberlain, M.C. Is there a role for vaccine–based therapy in recurrent glioblastoma? *Neuro Oncol.* **2014**, *16*, 757. [CrossRef]
81. Reardon, D.A.; Wucherpfennig, K.W.; Freeman, G.; Wu, C.J.; Chiocca, E.A.; Wen, P.Y.; Curry, W.T., Jr.; Mitchell, D.A.; Fecci, P.E.; Sampson, J.H.; et al. An update on vaccine therapy and other immunotherapeutic approaches for glioblastoma. *Expert Rev. Vaccines* **2013**, *12*, 597–615. [CrossRef]
82. Phuphanich, S.; Wheeler, C.J.; Rudnick, J.D.; Mazer, M.; Wang, H.; Nuno, M.A.; Richardson, J.E.; Fan, X.; Ji, J.; Chu, R.M.; et al. Phase I trial of a multi–epitope–pulsed dendritic cell vaccine for patients with newly diagnosed glioblastoma. *Cancer Immunol. Immunother.* **2013**, *62*, 125–135. [CrossRef] [PubMed]
83. Lang, F.F.; Conrad, C.; Gomez–Manzano, C.; Yung, W.K.A.; Sawaya, R.; Weinberg, J.S.; Prabhu, S.S.; Rao, G.; Fuller, G.N.; Aldape, K.D.; et al. Phase I Study of DNX–2401 (Delta–24–RGD) Oncolytic Adenovirus: Replication and Immunotherapeutic Effects in Recurrent Malignant Glioma. *J. Clin. Oncol.* **2018**, *36*, 1419–1427. [CrossRef] [PubMed]
84. Philbrick, B.; Adamson, D.C. DNX–2401: An investigational drug for the treatment of recurrent glioblastoma. *Expert Opin. Investig. Drugs* **2019**, *28*, 1041–1049. [CrossRef] [PubMed]
85. Walton, R.W.; Brown, M.C.; Sacco, M.T.; Gromeier, M. Engineered Oncolytic Poliovirus PVSRIPO Subverts MDA5–Dependent Innate Immune Responses in Cancer Cells. *J. Virol.* **2018**, *92*. [CrossRef]
86. Desjardins, A.; Gromeier, M.; Herndon, J.E., 2nd; Beaubier, N.; Bolognesi, D.P.; Friedman, A.H.; Friedman, H.S.; McSherry, F.; Muscat, A.M.; Nair, S.; et al. Recurrent Glioblastoma Treated with Recombinant Poliovirus. *N. Engl. J. Med.* **2018**, *379*, 150–161. [CrossRef]

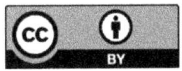

© 2020 by the author. Licensee MDPI, Basel, Switzerland. This article is an open access article distributed under the terms and conditions of the Creative Commons Attribution (CC BY) license (http://creativecommons.org/licenses/by/4.0/).

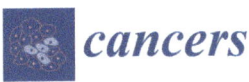

Article

KYP-2047, an Inhibitor of Prolyl-Oligopeptidase, Reduces GlioBlastoma Proliferation through Angiogenesis and Apoptosis Modulation

Sarah Adriana Scuderi [1], Giovanna Casili [1], Alessio Ardizzone [1], Stefano Forte [2], Lorenzo Colarossi [3], Serena Sava [3], Irene Paterniti [1], Emanuela Esposito [1,*], Salvatore Cuzzocrea [1] and Michela Campolo [1]

1. Department of Chemical, Biological, Pharmaceutical and Environmental Sciences, University of Messina, Viale Ferdinando Stagno D' Alcontres, 31-98166 Messina, ME, Italy; sarahadriana.scuderi@unime.it (S.A.S.); gcasili@unime.it (G.C.); aleardizzone@unime.it (A.A.); ipaterniti@unime.it (I.P.); salvator@unime.it (S.C.); michela.campolo@unime.it (M.C.)
2. IOM Ricerca Srl, Via Penninazzo 11, 95029 Viagrande, CT, Italy; stefano.forte@grupposamed.com
3. Istituto Oncologico del Mediterraneo, Via Penninazzo 7, 95029 Viagrande, CT, Italy; lorenzo.colarossi@grupposamed.com (L.C.); serena.sava@grupposamed.com (S.S.)
* Correspondence: eesposito@unime.it; Tel.: +39-090-6765208

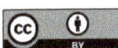

Simple Summary: Glioblastoma (GB) is the most aggressive brain tumor characterized by necrosis, excessive proliferation, and invasiveness. Despite relevant progress in conventional treatments, the survival rate for patients with GB remains low. The present study investigated the potential effect of KYP-2047, an inhibitor of the prolyl-oligopeptidase (POP or PREP), in an in vivo U87-xenograft model and in an in vitro study on human GB cells. This study demonstrated the abilities of KYP-2047 to counteract and reduce GB progression through angiogenesis and apoptosis modulation.

Abstract: Glioblastoma (GB) is the most aggressive tumor of the central nervous system (CNS), characterized by excessive proliferation, necrosis and invasiveness. The survival rate for patients with GB still remains low. Angiogenesis and apoptosis play a key role in the development of GB. Thus, the modulation of angiogenesis and apoptosis processes represent a possible strategy to counteract GB progression. This study aimed to investigate the potential effect of KYP-2047, an inhibitor of the prolyl-oligopeptidase (POP), known to modulate angiogenesis, in an in vivo U87-xenograft model and in an in vitro study on human GB cells. Our results showed that KYP-2047 at doses of 2.5 mg/kg and 5 mg/kg was able to reduce tumor burden in the xenograft-model. Moreover, KYP-2047 significantly reduced vascular endothelial-growth-factor (VEGF), angiopoietins (Ang) and endothelial-nitric-oxide synthase (eNOS) expression. In vitro study revealed that KYP-2047 at different concentrations reduced GB cells' viability. Additionally, KYP-2047 at the concentrations of 50 µM and 100 µM was able to increase the pro-apoptotic protein Bax, p53 and caspase-3 expression whereas Bcl-2 expression was reduced. Thus, KYP-2047 could represent a potential therapeutic treatment to counteract or reduce GB progression, thanks its abilities to modulate angiogenesis and apoptosis pathways.

Keywords: glioblastoma (GB); prolyl-oligopeptidase (POP); vascular endothelial growth factor (VEGF); transforming growth factor-β (TGF-β); angiopoietin (Ang); endothelial nitric oxide synthase (eNOS)

1. Introduction

Gliomas are the main neoplastic diseases affecting the central nervous system (CNS) [1]. Among gliomas, glioblastoma (GB) is the most common primary malignant tumor of CNS, with an incidence of about 3–4 cases per 100,000 people per year [2]. GB is classified by the World Health Organization (WHO) as grade IV astrocytoma, characterized by poorly differentiated neoplastic astrocytes with high mitotic activity, necrosis and vascular proliferation [2]. GB occurs more frequently in mature people aged between 45 and 75 years with a higher incidence in men than in women, associated with a poor quality of life [3]. GB is characterized by abnormal angiogenesis, apoptosis alteration and invasiveness [4]. Genome-wide expression studies in glioblastomas revealed that GB is associated with chromosomic alterations which can include deletions, amplifications or mutations which contribute to the development of GB [5]. In addition to genetic risk factors, other risk factors involved in the development of GB have been identified, such as exposure to ionizing radiation, ultraviolet rays, smoke, and pesticides [3,6]. The symptomatology of GB is varied, as it is related to the location and degree of infiltration of the tumor mass. Currently, standard treatment for GB includes surgical removal of the tumor, followed by the concomitant administration of chemotherapeutic agents such as temozolomide (TMZ) and radiotherapy [3]. However, the survival rate for patients with GB still remains low [7]; consequently, the identification of new therapeutic targets and new molecules able to reduce or arrest the progression of GB represents an important goal for cancer research. Many studies have focused on the role of angiogenesis and apoptosis in the development of GB [8,9]. It has been proposed that therapeutic resistance of GB is due to an up-regulation of anti-apoptotic proteins such as Bcl2 and a downregulation of pro-apoptotic proteins, leading to activation of oncogenes that promote tumor cell survival [9]. Moreover, also angiogenesis represents a key event for tumor growth and progression [10]; in fact, it has been demonstrated that several angiogenic factors such as vascular endothelial growth factor (VEGF) and angiopoietins (Ang) are up-regulated in GB that generate highly permeable and functionally immature blood vessels which contribute to tumor growth [8,10]. Recently, different studies have focused on the effect of KYP-2047 [11,12], a specific and potent inhibitor of the prolyl-oligopeptidase (POP or PREP), a serine protease involved in the angiogenesis process [11,12]. POP is present both in the brain and in peripheral tissues; it is involved in the hydrolysis of proline and in many other physiological functions [13]. KYP-2047 demonstrated the ability to modulate the angiogenesis process, but also cell cycle and differentiation [11–13]. Therefore, considering the key roles of angiogenesis and apoptosis in GB pathology, the aim of this study was to investigate the potential effect of KYP-2047 in an in vivo U87-xenograft model and in vitro model on human GB cells to counteract or reduce GB progression.

2. Materials and Methods

2.1. In Vivo Studies

2.1.1. Cell Line

The human GB cell line U-87 (U-87MG ATCC® HTB-14™ Homo sapiens brain Likely glioblastomas) was obtained from ATCC (American Type Culture Collection, Rockville, MD, USA). U-87 cells were cultured in 75 cm^2 flask with respectively Dulbecco's modified Eagle's medium (DMEM—Sigma-Aldrich® Catalog No. D5030; St. Louis, MO, USA) supplemented with antibiotics (penicillin 1000 units—streptomycin 0.1 mg/L, Sigma-Aldrich® Catalog No. P4333; St. Louis, MO, USA), L-glutamine (GlutaMAX™, ThermoFisher Scientific® Catalog No. 35050061; Waltham, MA, USA) and 10% (v/v) fetal bovine serum (FBS, Sigma-Aldrich® Catalog No. 12103C St. Louis, MO, USA) in a humidified atmosphere containing 5% CO_2 at 37 °C.

2.1.2. Animals

Wild-type nude male mice C57BL/6J were purchased from Jackson Laboratory (Bar Harbor, Hancock, ME, USA) and housed in microisolator cages under pathogen-free conditions on a 12 h light/12 h dark schedule for a week. Animals were fed a standard diet and water ad libitum. Animal experiments were in compliance with Italian regulations on protection of animals used for experimental and other scientific purposes (DM 116192) as well as European Union (EU) regulations (OJ of EC L 358/1 18 December 1986).

2.1.3. Experimental Design

The Xenograft tumor model was performed as previously described by Deng et al. [14]. The mice were inoculated subcutaneously with 3×10^6 human glioblastoma U-87 cells in 0.2 mL of phosphate buffered saline (PBS) and 0.1 mL matrigel (BD Bioscience, Bedford, MA, USA). Animals were treated with KYP-2047 at doses of 1 mg/kg, 2.5 mg/kg and 5 mg/kg every three days from day 7. KYP-2047 was dissolved in PBS with 0.001% of dimethyl sulfoxide (DMSO). After tumor cell inoculation, animals were monitored daily for morbidity and mortality [15]. At the thirty-fifth day, the animals were sacrificed and their tumors were excised and processed for analysis. Tumor volumes were measured non-invasively by using an electronic calliper. The tumor burden was calculated using the following formula: $0.5 \times$ length $\times$ width. The tumor size was measured every four days for 28 days. The tumor volume was calculated using an empirical formula, $V = 1/2 \times$ ((the shortest diameter) $2 \times$ (the longest diameter)). The experiments were performed three times to verify the data, using 25 animals for each experimental group.

Experimental groups:

The mice were randomly divided into four groups, as described below:

1. Control group (vehicle): weekly intravenous (IV) administration of saline.
2. Control group + KYP-2047 1 mg/kg: intraperitoneal (ip) administration of KYP-2047 1 mg/kg dissolved in PBS every three days from day 7.
3. Control group + KYP-2047 2.5 mg/kg: intraperitoneal (ip) administration of KYP-2047 2.5 mg/kg dissolved in PBS every three days from day 7.
4. Control group + KYP-2047 5 mg/kg: intraperitoneal (ip) administration of KYP-2047 5 mg/kg dissolved in PBS every three days from day 7.

Furthermore, the control group + KYP-2047 1 mg/kg was only subjected to histological evaluation, mean tumor burden and mean tumor weight, because it did not induce any beneficial effect; therefore, we decided to continue analyzing only KYP-2047 2.5 mg/kg and 5 mg/kg groups.

2.1.4. Histological Evaluation

Histological evaluation was performed as previously described by Esposito et al. [16]. Tumor samples were fixed with 10% neutral formalin, embedded in paraffin, and sectioned at 7 μm. Sections were deparaffinized with xylene and stained with hematoxylin and eosin. The slides were analyzed by a pathologist blinded to the treatment groups. All sections were analyzed using an Axiovision microscope (Zeiss, Milan, Italy).

2.1.5. Western Blot Analysis

Tumor samples from each mouse were suspended in extraction Buffer A (0.2 mM PMSF, 0.15 mM pepstatin A, 20 mM leupeptin, 1 mM sodium orthovanadate), homogenized at the highest setting for 2 min, and centrifuged at $12,000 \times g$ rpm for 4 min at 4 °C. Supernatants are the cytosolic fraction, whereas the pellets, containing enriched nuclei, were resuspended in Buffer B (1% Triton X-100, 150 mM NaCl, 10 mM TrisHCl pH 7.4, 1 mM EGTA, 1 mM EDTA, 0.2 mM PMSF, 20 mm leupeptin, 0.2 mM sodium orthovanadate) and centrifuged at $12,000 \times g$ rpm for 10 min at 4 °C; supernatants are the nuclear fraction. Protein concentration was estimated by the Bio-Rad protein assay using bovine serum albumin as standard. Then, tumor samples, in equal amounts of protein, were separated on 12% SDS-PAGE gel and transferred to nitrocellulose membrane as previously described [17]. The following primary antibodies were used: anti-vascular endothelial growth factor (VEGF) (1:500; Santa Cruz Biotechnology, Dallas, TX, USA; sc-7269); anti-endothelial nitric oxide synthase (eNOS) (1:500; Santa Cruz Biotechnology, Dallas, TX, USA; sc-376751); anti-angiopoietin 1 (Ang1) (1:500; Santa Cruz Biotechnology, Dallas, TX, USA; sc-517593); anti-angiopoietin 2 (Ang2) (1:500; Santa Cruz Biotechnology, Dallas, TX, USA; sc-74403); anti-Ki-67 (1:500; Santa Cruz Biotechnology, Dallas, TX, USA; sc-23900); anti-Bax (1:500; Santa Cruz Biotechnology, Dallas, TX, USA; sc-7480); anti-Bcl2 (1:500; Santa Cruz Biotechnology, Dallas, TX, USA; sc-7382). Antibody dilutions were made in PBS/5% w/v nonfat dried milk/0.1% Tween-20 (PMT) and membranes incubated overnight at 4 °C. Membranes were then incubated with secondary antibody (1:2000, Jackson ImmunoResearch, West Grove, PA, USA) for 1 h at room temperature. To ascertain that those blots were loaded with equal amounts of protein lysate, they were also incubated with β-actin antibody (for cytosolic fraction 1:500; Santa Cruz Biotechnology, Dallas, TX, USA; sc-8432) or lamin A/C (for nuclear fraction 1:500, Santa Cruz Biotechnology, Dallas, TX, USA; sc-376248). Signals were detected with an enhanced chemiluminescence (ECL) detection system reagent according to the manufacturer's instructions (Thermo Fisher, Waltham, MA, USA). The relative expression of the protein bands was quantified by densitometry with BIORAD ChemiDocTMXRS + software.

2.1.6. Immunohistochemical Localization of Vascular Endothelial-Growth-Factor (VEGF), Endothelial Nitric Oxide Synthase (eNOS), CD34, Ki-67, Bcl2 and Caspase-3

Immunohistochemical localization was performed as previously described by Esposito et al. [16]. Slides were incubated overnight using the following primary antibodies: VEGF (Santa Cruz Biotechnology, Dallas, TX, USA; 1:100 in PBS, v/v; sc-7269), eNOS (Santa Cruz Biotechnology, Dallas, TX, USA, 1:100 in PBS, v/v; sc-376751) anti-Bcl2 (1:100; Santa Cruz Biotechnology, Dallas, TX, USA; sc-7382); anti-caspase-3 (1:100, Santa Cruz Biotechnology, Dallas, TX, USA; sc-56053); anti-Ki-67 (1:100; Santa Cruz Biotechnology, Dallas, TX, USA; sc-23900); anti-CD34 (1:100; Santa Cruz Biotechnology, Dallas, TX, USA; sc-74499). At the end of the incubation with the primary antibodies, the sections were abundantly washed with PBS and incubated with a secondary antibody (Santa Cruz Biotechnology, Dallas, TX, USA) for 1 h at room temperature. The reaction was revealed by a chromogenic substrate (brown DAB), and counterstaining with NUCLEAR FAST-RED. The percentage of positive staining was measured using a computerized image analysis system (Leica QWin V3, Cambridge, UK). The images were acquired using an optical microscope (Zeiss, Axio Vision, Feldbach, Schweiz). For immunohistochemistry, the images were shown at a magnification of 20 × (50 μm of the bar scale).

2.1.7. Caspase-3 Activity Measurement

Caspase-3 activity in tumor lysate was measured using a colorimetric Assay Kit (cat#ab39401, Abcam, Cambridge, UK) as suggested by manufacturer's instruction.

2.1.8. RNA Isolation and Quantitative Real-Time Polymerase Chain Reaction (RT-qPCR)

Total RNA of tumor samples was isolated using TRIzol reagent (Invitrogen, Carlsbad, CA, USA) according to the manufacturer's instructions. RNA isolation was performed as previously described by Weinert et al. [18]. First-strand cDNA obtained from RNA samples was stored at −80 °C until use.

The mRNA expression levels of VEGF and eNOS in each sample, was measured using Power Up Sybr Master Mix (Applied Biosystems) and a QuantStudio Flex Real-Time Polymerase Chain Reaction (PCR) System (Applied Biosystems) [19]. The primer used for reverse transcriptase PCR were for VEGF: forward 5′-GAGCAGAAGTCCCATGAAGTGA-3′ and reverse 5′-CACAGGACGGCTTGAAGATGT-3′; eNOS: forward 5′-CCTGTGAGACCTT CTGTGTGG-3′ and reverse 5′-GGATCAGACCTGGCAGCAACT-3′. The mRNA expression levels were normalized to that of glyceraldehyde-3-phosphate dehydrogenase (GAPDH): forward: 5′-GGGCTGGCATTGCTCTCA-3′, reverse: 5′-TGCTGTAGCGTATTCATTG-3′. Each sample was analyzed in triplicate, and all tests were repeated at least three times.

2.1.9. Enzyme-Linked Immunosorbent Assay (ELISA) Kit

An enzyme-linked immunosorbent assay (ELISA) kit was performed to evaluate PREP expression in serum of each mice using Mouse PREP ELISA kit (cat#Q9QUR6 RayBiotech, Peachtree Corners, GA, USA) as suggested by manufacturer's instructions. The serum of each animal was collected and measured by ELISA kit once a week.

2.1.10. Immunofluorescence Assay

Immunofluorescence staining was performed as previously described by Campolo et al. [20]. Tumor samples were collected and processed for immunofluorescence staining. Tissue sections of 7 μm were incubated with the following primary antibody anti-CD34 at 37 °C overnight (1:100; Santa Cruz Biotechnology, Dallas, TX, USA; sc-74499). Then, tissue sections were washed with PBS and incubated with secondary antibody anti-mouse Alexa Fluor-488 antibody (1:1000 v/v, Molecular Probes, Altrincham, UK) for 1 h at 37 °C. For nuclear staining, 4′,6′-diamidino-2-phenylindole (DAPI; Hoechst, Frankfurt, Germany) (2 μg/mL) in PBS was added. Sections were observed and photographed at 40× magnification using a Leica DM2000 microscope.

2.2. In Vitro Studies

2.2.1. Cell Lines

U-87 MG (U-87 MG ATCC® HTB-14™ Homo sapiens brain likely glioblastomas), U-138MG (U-138 MG ATCC® HTB-16™ Homo sapiens brain glioblastoma IV grade), A-172 (A-172 ATCC® CRL-1620™ Homo sapiens brain glioblastoma) were obtained from ATCC (American Type Culture Collection, Rockville, MD, USA). The human GB cell lines were seeded in 75 cm² flask with respectively Dulbecco's modified Eagle's medium (DMEM—Sigma-Aldrich® Catalog No. D5030; St. Louis, MO, USA) supplemented with antibiotics (penicillin 1000 units—streptomycin 0.1 mg/L, Sigma-Aldrich® Catalog No. P4333; St. Louis, MO, USA), L-glutamine (GlutaMAX™, ThermoFisher Scientific® Catalog No. 35050061; Waltham, MA, USA) and 10% (v/v) FBS (Sigma-Aldrich® Catalog No. 12103C St. Louis, MO, USA) in a humidified atmosphere containing 5% CO_2 at 37 °C.

2.2.2. Cell Treatment

Human GB cells were plated on 96-well plates at a density of 4×10^4 cells/well to a final volume of 150 μL. After 24 h, GB cells were treated with KYP-2047 (Sigma-Aldrich®) for 24 h at increasing concentrations 0.01 μM, 0.1 μM, 0.5 μM, 1 μM, 10 μM, 30 μM, 50 μM and 100 μM dissolved in PBS.

Experimental Groups:

1. Control group (Ctr): human GB cell lines U-87, U-138 and A-172;
2. KYP-2047 0.01 μM group: GB cells treated with KYP-2047 0.01 μM;
3. KYP-2047 0.1 μM group: GB cells treated with KYP-2047 0.1 μM;
4. KYP-2047 0.5 μM group: GB cells treated with KYP-2047 0.5 μM;
5. KYP-2047 1 μM group: GB cells treated with KYP-2047 1 μM;
6. KYP-2047 10 μM group: GB cells treated with KYP-2047 10 μM;
7. KYP-2047 30 μM group: GB cells treated with KYP-2047 30 μM;
8. KYP-2047 50 μM group: GB cells treated with KYP-2047 50 μM;
9. KYP-2047 100 μM group: GB cells treated with KYP-2047 100 μM;

The experiments were repeated three times to verify the data.

For western blot analysis and immunofluorescence assay on U-87, A-172 and U-138 cells, we decided to continue to analyze only KYP-2047 at the concentrations of 50 μM and 100 μM because represented the most cytotoxic concentrations revealed by MTT assay.

2.2.3. Cell Viability Assay

Cell viability assay on U-87, U-138 and A-172 cells were performed using a mitochondria-dependent dye for live cells (tetrazolium dye; MTT) to formazan [20]. GB cells were pre-treated with increasing concentrations of KYP-2047 for 24 h. After 24 h, cells were incubated at 37 °C with MTT (0.2 mg/mL) for 1 h. The medium was removed, and the cells lysed with dimethyl sulfoxide (DMSO) (100 μL). The extent of reduction in MTT to formazan was quantified by measurement of optical density (OD) at 550 nm with a microplate rider.

2.2.4. Western Blot Analysis

Western blot analysis on U-87, A-172 and U-138 cell lysates was performed as previously described by Campolo et al. [20]. Human GB cells were washed with ice-cold PBS harvested and resuspended in Tris-HCl 20 mM pH 7.5, NaF 10 mM, 150 µL NaCl, 1% Nonidet P-40 and protease inhibitor cocktail (Roche). After 40 min, cell lysates were centrifuged at 16,000× g for 15 min at 4 °C. Protein concentration was estimated by the Bio-Rad protein assay using bovine serum albumin as standard. Samples were then heated at 95 °C for 5 min and equal amounts of protein separated on a 10–15% SDS-PAGE gel and transferred to a PVDF membrane (Immobilon-P). The membranes were incubated overnight at 4 °C with primary antibodies: anti-Bax (1:500; Santa Cruz Biotechnology, Dallas, TX, USA; sc-7480); anti-Bcl2 (1:500; Santa Cruz Biotechnology, Dallas, TX, USA; sc-7382); anti-p53 (1:500; Santa Cruz Biotechnology, Dallas, TX, USA; sc-126). To ascertain that blots were loaded with equal amounts of protein lysate, they were also incubated with the antibody β-actin for cytosolic fraction (1:500; Santa Cruz Biotechnology; Dallas, TX, USA. sc-8432) and lamin A/C for nuclear fraction (1:500; Santa Cruz Biotechnology; Dallas, TX, USA, sc-376248). Signals were detected with enhanced chemiluminescence (ECL) detection system reagent according to the manufacturer's instructions (Thermo Fisher, Waltham, MA, USA). The relative expression of the protein bands was quantified by densitometry with BIORAD ChemiDocTMXRS + software.

2.2.5. Immunofluorescence Assay for Transforming Growth Factor-β (TGF-β) and Caspase-3

Immunofluorescence assay was performed on U-87, A-172 and U-138 cells as previously described by Donaldson [21]. GB cells on glass cover slips were rinsed briefly in phosphate-buffered saline (PBS:0.15 M NaCl, 10 mM Na_2HPO_4, pH 7.4), permeabilized in 0.2% Triton X-100/PBS and blocked with 10% goat serum. The cells were stained overnight (O/N) at 4 °C with primary antibodies: anti-transforming growth factor-β (TGFβ, 1:50, Santa Cruz Biotechnology, Dallas, TX, USA; sc-130348) and anti-caspase-3 (1:50, Santa Cruz Biotechnology, Dallas, TX, USA; sc-56053). At the end of the incubation with the primary antibody, the sections were abundantly washed with PBS and incubated with a secondary antibody anti-mouse Alexa Fluor-488 antibody (1:1000 v/v Molecular Probes, UK) for 1 h at 37 °C. Sections were washed in PBS and for nuclear staining 4′,6′-diamidino-2-phenylindole (DAPI; Hoechst, Frankfurt; Germany) 2 µg/mL in PBS was added. Sections were observed and photographed at 40× magnification using a Leica DM2000 microscope (Leica, Axio Vision, Feldbach, Schweiz). All images were digitalized at a resolution of 8 bits into an array of 2560 × 1920 pixels. Optical sections of fluorescence specimens were obtained using a HeNe laser (543 nm), an ultraviolet (UV) laser (361–365 nm), and an argon laser (458 nm) at a 1 min, 2 s scanning speed with up to eight averages; 1.5 µm sections were obtained using a pinhole of 250. Contrast and brightness were established by examining the most brightly labeled pixels and applying settings that allowed clear visualization of structural details while keeping the highest pixel intensities close to 250.

2.3. Materials

KYP-2047 and all other chemicals were obtained by Sigma-Aldrich (Milan, Italy). All stock solutions were prepared in non-pyrogenic saline (0.9% NaCl, Baxter, Milan, Italy).

2.4. Statistical Analysis

All values are expressed as mean ± standard error of the mean (SEM) of "n" observations. Each analysis was performed three times with three samples replicates for each one. The results were analyzed by one-way analysis of variance (ANOVA) followed by a Bonferroni post hoc test for multiple comparisons. A p-value of less than 0.05 was considered significant.

3. Results

3.1. In Vivo Studies

3.1.1. Effect of KYP-2047 on Tumor Growth

The histological analysis of the control group (Figure 1A) showed a significant subcutaneous tumor mass, associated to an increase in necrosis and neutrophil infiltration; while the treatment with KYP-2047 at doses of 2.5 mg/kg and 5 mg/kg showed a reduction in tumor sections as well as neutrophil infiltration (Figure 1C,D), much more than KYP-2047 at the dose of 1 mg/kg (Figure 1B). Furthermore, we observed a marked reduction of mean tumor burden, tumor volume and tumor weight following KYP-2047 treatment at doses of 2.5 mg/kg and 5 mg/kg, much more than KYP-2047 1 mg/kg (Figure 1E–G). Moreover, to better understand if the expression levels of PREP changed during the course of treatment in the tumors, we decided to verify the expression of PREP during the treatment with KYP-2047 by ELISA kit. The results showed that KYP-2047 at doses of 2.5 mg/kg and 5 mg/kg was able to reduce significantly PREP levels particularly from day 14 (Figure 1H). During the course of treatment, no important change in animals' weight was seen (Figure 1I).

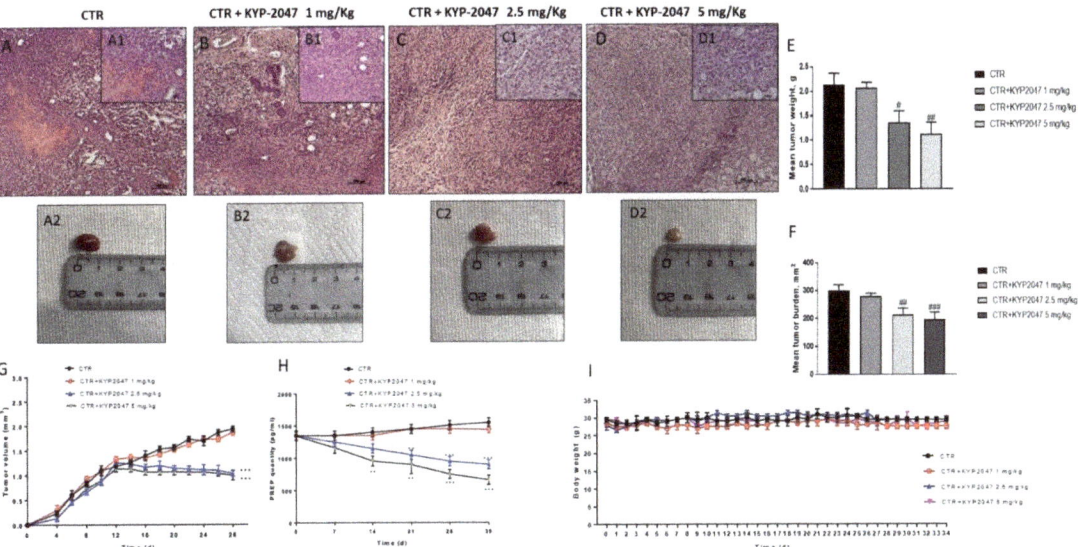

Figure 1. Effect of KYP-2047 on tumor growth. An elevated tumor mass was observed in the control group (**A**) while the treatment with KYP-2047 at doses of 2.5 mg/kg and 5 mg/kg significantly reduced tumor mass and neutrophil infiltration (**C,D**) more than KYP-2047 at dose of 1 mg/kg (**B**). Moreover, the panel (**E,F**) showed a reduction in tumor volume and tumor weight respectively following KYP-2047 treatment at doses of 2.5 mg/kg and 5 mg/kg without encountering important weight differences (Panel **I**). Additionally, the panel H showed a decrease of PREP expression following KYP-2047 treatment particularly from day 14. Data are representative of at least three independent experiments. Sections were observed and photographed at 10x magnification. (**E**) # $p < 0.05$ vs. CTR; ## $p < 0.01$ vs. CTR; (**F**) ## $p < 0.01$ vs. CTR; ### $p < 0.001$ vs. CTR. (**G**) *** $p < 0.001$ vs. CTR. (**H**) ** $p < 0.01$ vs. CTR; *** $p < 0.001$ vs. CTR.

3.1.2. Effect of KYP-2047 on Angiogenesis

Angiogenesis is an essential process for tumor growth [22]. GB is characterized by a deregulation of angiogenic growth factors as VEGF and eNOS expression, which play a key role in maintaining vascular homeostasis and vessel integrity [22–24]. Therefore, in this study we decided to investigate by immunohistochemical staining the levels of VEGF and eNOS. Our results demonstrated a significant increase of VEGF and eNOS levels in the control group (Figures 2A and 3A respectively); however, the treatment with KYP-2047 at doses of 2.5 mg/kg and 5 mg/kg significantly reduced their expression (Figure 2B,C, see immunohistochemistry score Figure 2D; Figure 3B,C, see immunohistochemistry score Figure 3D respectively) in a dose-dependent manner. These results were confirmed also by Western blot analysis and RT-qPCR, showing a significantly reduction of VEGF and eNOS expression in the groups treated with KYP-2047 at doses of 2.5 mg/kg and 5 mg/kg compared to control group (Figure 2M, see densitometric analysis Figure 2M1,N and Figure 3E, see densitometric analysis Figure 3E1,F).

Additionally, we evaluated the expression of CD34, a transmembrane glycoprotein involved in the process of newly-forming tumour vessels [25] by immunohistochemistry and immunofluorescence analysis. In this context, our results showed a significant reduction of CD34 expression in the groups treated with KYP-2047 at doses of 2.5 mg/kg and 5 mg/kg compared to control group (Figure 2E–G; see immunohistochemistry score Figure 2H) (Figure 2I–K; see CD34 ratio positive cells score Figure 2L).

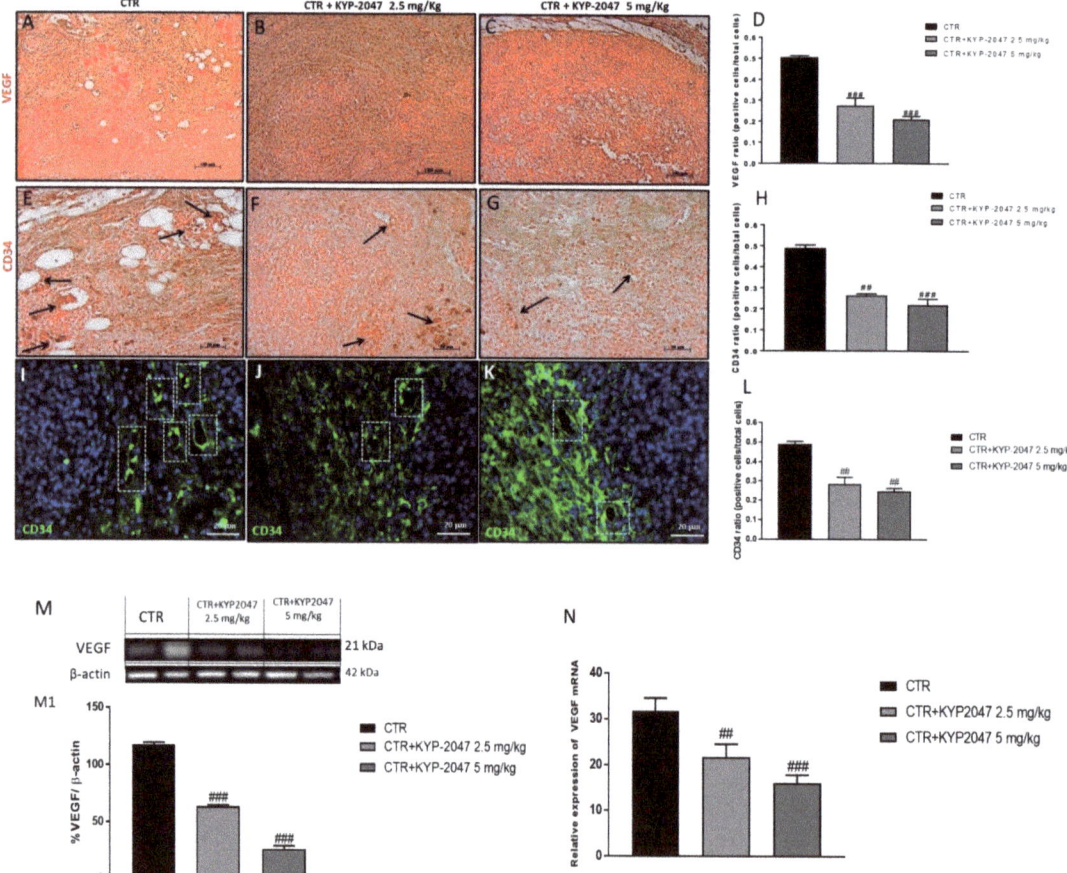

Figure 2. Effect of KYP-2047 on vascular endothelial-growth-factor (VEGF) and CD34 expression. Immunohistochemical staining showed a marked expression of VEGF and CD34 in the control group (A,E) whereas the treatment with KYP-2047 at doses of 2.5 mg/kg and 5 mg/kg significantly reduced their expression (B,C,F,G). Sections were observed and photographed at 10×, 20× and 40× magnification The data for VEGF were confirmed also by western blot analysis and quantitative real-time polymerase chain reaction (RT-qPCR), showing a decrease of VEGF expression following KYP-2047 treatment (M,N). Moreover, the data for CD34 were confirmed also by immunofluorescence assay (I,J,K). Data are representative of at least three independent experiments. (D) ### $p < 0.001$ vs. CTR; (H) ## $p < 0.01$ vs. CTR; ### $p < 0.001$ vs. CTR. (L) ## $p < 0.01$ vs. CTR; (M) ### $p < 0.001$ vs. CTR. (N) ## $p < 0.01$ vs. CTR; ### $p < 0.001$ vs. CTR.

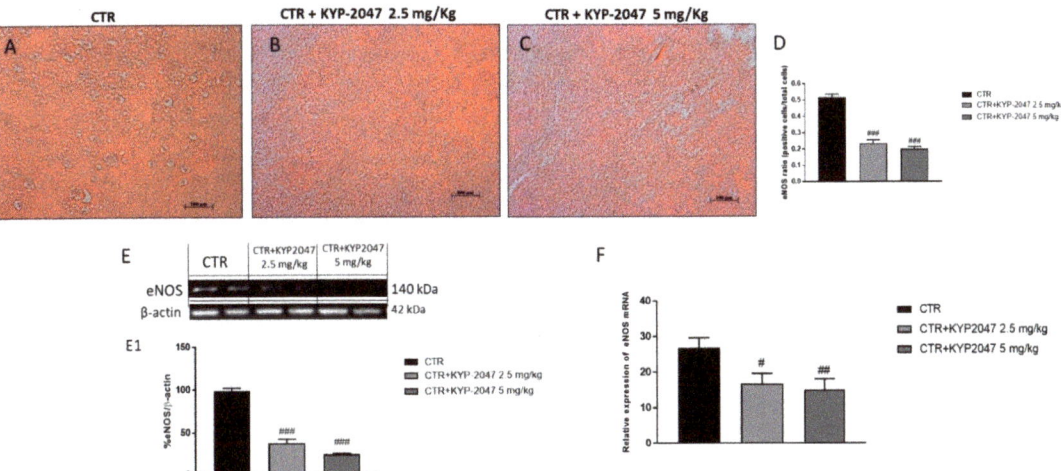

Figure 3. Effect of KYP-2047 on endothelial-nitric-oxide synthase (eNOS) expression. Immunohistochemical staining showed a marked expression of eNOS in the control group (**A**) whereas the treatment with KYP-2047 at doses of 2.5 mg/kg and 5 mg/kg significantly reduced its expression (**B,C**). Sections were observed and photographed at 10× magnification. The data were confirmed by Western blot analysis and RT-qPCR, showing a decrease of eNOS expression following KYP-2047 treatment (**E,F**). Data are representative of at least three independent experiments. (**D**) ### $p < 0.001$ vs. CTR; (**E**) ### $p < 0.001$ vs. CTR. (**F**) # $p < 0.05$ vs CTR; ## $p < 0.01$ vs. CTR.

Studies on angiogenesis have emphasized the importance of others angiogenic factors involved in tumor growth such as angiopoietins, in particular angiopoietin 1 (Ang1) and angiopoietin 2 (Ang2), currently proposed as biomarkers of GB [26,27]. Therefore, we detected Ang1 and Ang2 expression by Western blot analysis on tumor samples. Our results showed a significantly decrease of Ang1 and Ang2 levels following KYP-2047 treatment at doses of 2.5 mg/kg and 5 mg/kg compared to control group (Figure 4A, see densitometric analysis 4A1; Figure 4B, see densitometric analysis 4B1) in a dose-dependent manner.

Furthermore, we investigated the role of Ki-67, a nuclear protein associated with tumor proliferation and progression [28,29]. As shown in the Figure 4C, the blot revealed a marked expression of Ki-67 in the control group whereas the treatment with KYP-2047 at doses of 2.5 mg/kg and 5 mg/kg significantly reduced its expression (see densitometric analysis 4C1). Moreover, Ki-67 was evaluated also by immunohistochemistry assay confirming the results obtained as showed in the Figure 4D–F (see immunohistochemistry score 4G).

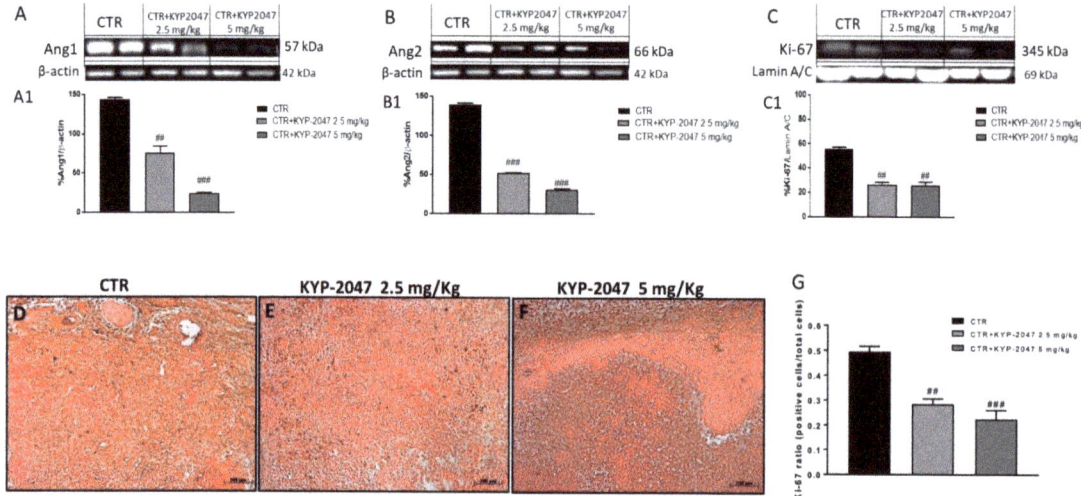

Figure 4. Effect of KYP-2047 on Ang1, Ang2 and Ki-67 expression. The blots revealed a significant increase of Ang1 and Ang2 expression in the control group while the treatment with KYP-2047 at doses of 2.5 mg/kg and 5 mg/kg significantly reduced their expression (**A**,**B**). Sections were observed and photographed at 10× magnification Moreover, the panel (**C**) revealed a significant increase of Ki-67 in the control group while the treatment with KYP-2047 at doses of 2.5 mg/kg and 5 mg/kg significantly decreased its expression. The data for Ki-67 was confirmed also by immunohistochemistry (**D**–**F**). Data are representative of at least three independent experiments. (**A**) ## $p < 0.01$ vs. CTR; ### $p < 0.001$ vs. CTR; (**B**) ### $p < 0.01$ vs. CTR; (**C**) ## $p < 0.01$ vs. CTR. (**G**) ## $p < 0.01$ vs. CTR; ### $p < 0.001$ vs. CTR.

3.1.3. Effect of KYP-2047 on Apoptosis Pathway

Considering the key role of apoptosis in GB progression [30], we evaluated the pro-apoptotic Bax, and anti-apoptotic Bcl2 protein by western blot analysis on tumor samples. The results showed that KYP-2047 was able to increase Bax expression and reduce Bcl2 expression (Figure 5A; see densitometric analysis 5A1; Figure 5B, see densitometric analysis 5B1). Moreover, the ability of KYP-2047 to modulate Bcl2 expression was confirmed by immunohistochemistry as shown in Figure 5C–E (see immunohistochemistry score Figure 5F). Furthermore, we detected caspase-3 levels by immunohistochemistry and by a colorimetric assay kit on tumor samples, showing that KYP2047 at doses of 2.5 and 5 mg/kg significantly increased caspase-3 activity compared to the control group (Figure 6A–C; see immunohistochemistry score Figure 6D,E

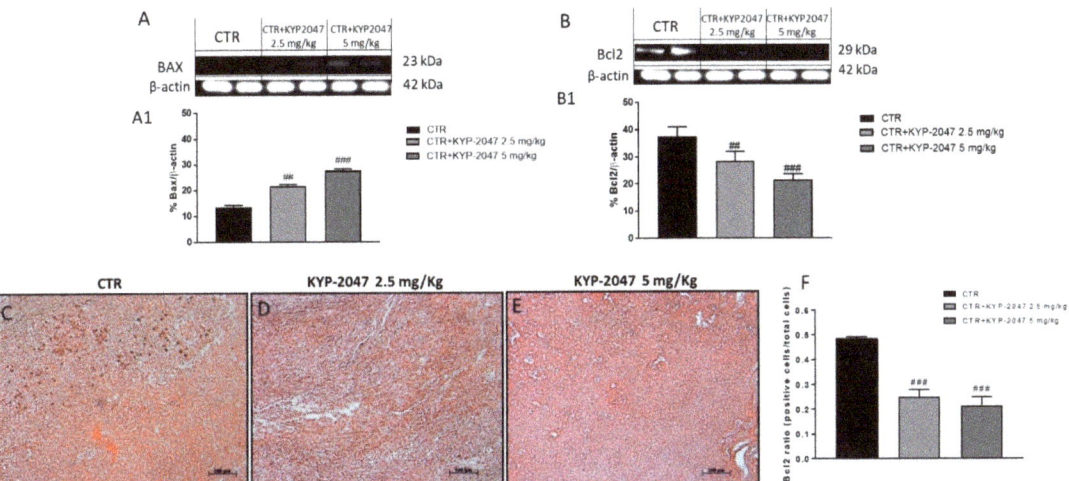

Figure 5. Effect of KYP-2047 on apoptosis pathway in the U87-xenograft model. The blots revealed an increase of pro-apoptotic Bax expression and a decrease of Bcl2 expression following KYP-2047 treatment compared to control group (**A**,**B**). Additionally, immunohistochemistry staining confirmed a decrease of Bcl2 expression after KYP-2047 treatment. (**C–F**). Sections were observed and photographed at 10× magnification. Data are representative of at least three independent experiments. (**A**) ## $p < 0.01$ vs. CTR; ### $p < 0.001$ vs. CTR; (**B**) ## $p < 0.01$ vs. CTR; ### $p < 0.001$ vs. CTR; (**F**) ### $p < 0.001$ vs. CTR.

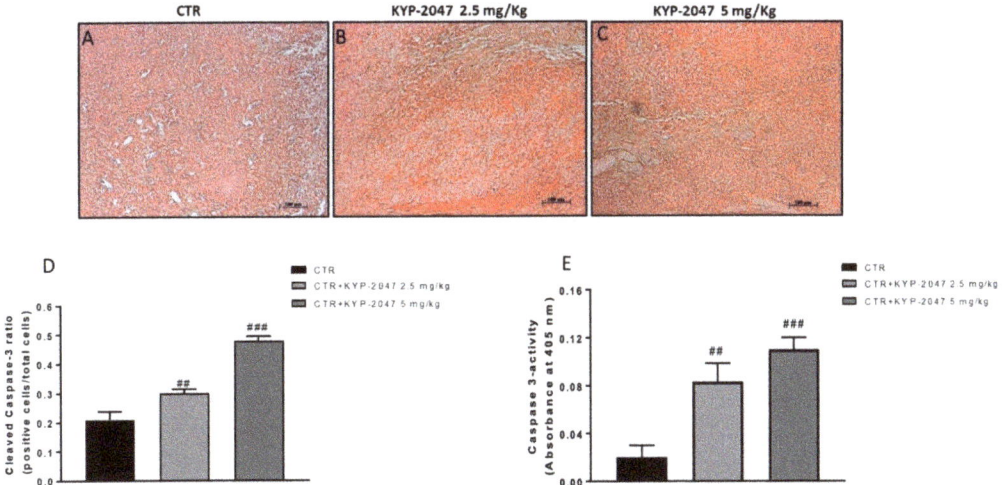

Figure 6. Effect of KYP-2047 on caspase-3 expression. Immunohistochemistry assay revealed an increase of cleaved-caspase-3 expression following KYP-2047 treatment at doses of 2.5 mg/kg and 5 mg/kg compared to control group (**A–C**). Sections were observed and photographed at 10× magnification. Additionally, the data for caspase-3 were confirmed also by a colorimetric assay kit as shown in the panel E. Data are representative of at least three independent experiments. (**D**) ## $p < 0.01$ vs. CTR; ### $p < 0.001$ vs. CTR; (**E**) ## $p < 0.01$ vs. CTR; ### $p < 0.001$ vs. CTR.

3.2. In Vitro Studies

3.2.1. Effect of KYP-2047 on Cell Viability

KYP-2047 cytotoxicity was evaluated incubating U-87, A-172 and U-138 cells with growing concentrations of KYP-2047 (0.01 µM, 0.1 µM, 0.5 µM, 1 µM, 10 µM, 30 µM, 50 µM and 100 µM) for 24 h. KYP-2047 treatment showed a significant decrease of cell viability in all three cell lines in a concentration dependent-manner as shown in the Figure 7A–C. Therefore, based on MTT results, we decided to continue testing for other analysis only KYP-2047 at concentrations of 50 µM and 100 µM on U-87, A172 and U138 cells because they represented the most cytotoxic concentrations.

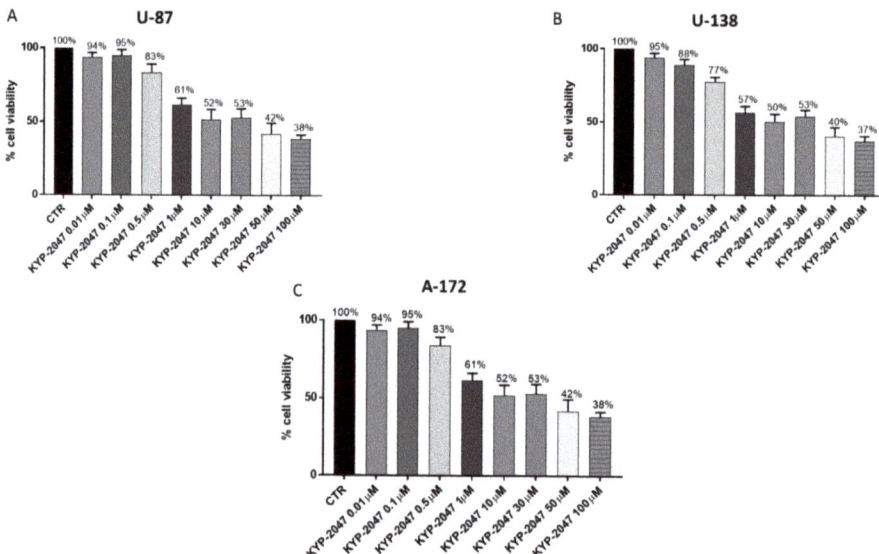

Figure 7. Effect of KYP-2047 on U-87, U-138 and A-172 cell viability. Cell viability was evaluated using MTT assay 24 h after KYP-2047 treatment at the concentrations of 0.01 µM, 0.1 µM, 0.5 µM, 1 µM, 10 µM, 30 µM, 50 µM and 100 µM. U-87, U-138 and A-172 cells showed a similar decrease of cell viability following KYP-2047 treatment in a concentration-dependent manner (**A–C**). Data are representative of at least three independent experiments.

3.2.2. Effect of KYP-2047 on Apoptosis Pathway

Apoptosis plays a key role in the development of cancer including GB [31]. Deregulation of apoptotic process is a relevant hallmark of a tumor [31], responsible not only for its progression but also for tumor resistance to therapies [32]. Therefore, we investigated the effect of KYP-2047 on the apoptosis pathway in U-87, A-172 and U-138 cell lysates evaluating the pro-apoptotic Bax, tumor suppressor p53 and anti-apoptotic Bcl2 protein by Western blot analysis (The original Western blot can be found in Figure S5). Our results revealed an increase of Bax and p53 levels following KYP-2047 treatment in U87 cell lysates performed for 24 h at the concentrations of 50 µM and 100 µM compared to control group (Figure 8A, see densitometric analysis 8A1; Figure 8B, see densitometric analysis 8B1, respectively); while Bcl2 expression was significantly reduced following KYP-2047 treatment compared to control group (Figure 8C; see densitometric analysis 8C1) in a concentration-dependent manner. The same results appear for A-172 and U-138 cell lysates, confirming an increase of pro-apoptotic Bax and p53 expression following KYP-2047 treatment compared to control group (Figure S1A, see densitometric analysis 1A1; Figure S1B, see densitometric analysis 1B1, respectively) (Figure S2A, see densitometric analysis 2A1; Figure S2B, see densitometric analysis 2B1, respectively) and a decrease of anti-apoptotic Bcl2 protein expression (Figure S1C; see densitometric analysis 1C) (Figure S2C; see densitometric analysis 2C1).

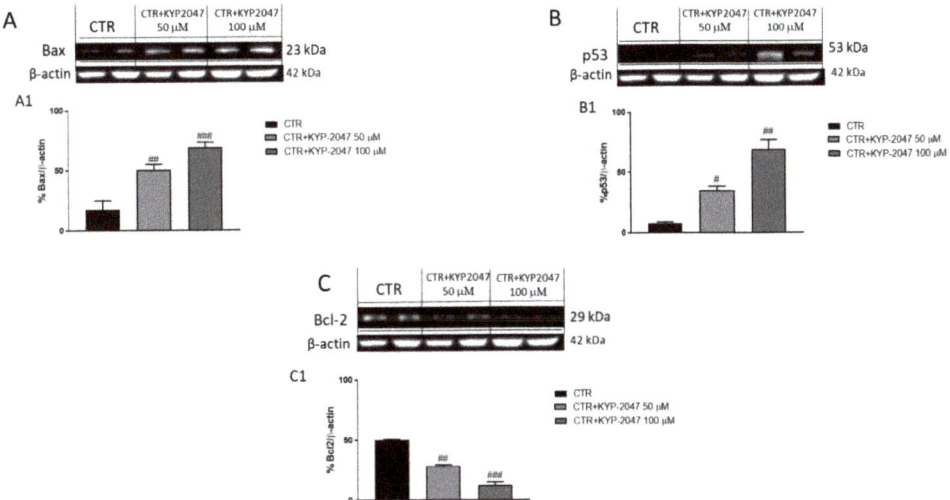

Figure 8. Effect of KYP-2047 on apoptosis pathway in U-87 cell lysates. The blots on U87 cell lysates revealed an increase of pro-apoptotic Bax and p53 expression following KYP-2047 treatment at the concentrations of 50 μM and 100 μM compared to control group (**A,B**). Moreover, KYP-2047 at the concentrations of 50 μM and 100 μM reduced significantly Bcl2 expression compared to control group (**C**). Data are representative of at least three independent experiments. (**A**) ## $p < 0.01$ vs. CTR; ### $p < 0.001$ vs. CTR; (**B**) # $p < 0.05$ vs. CTR; ## $p < 0.01$ vs. CTR; (**C**) ## $p < 0.01$ vs. CTR; ### $p < 0.001$ vs. CTR.

3.2.3. Effect of KYP-2047 on TGF-β and Caspase-3 Expression by Immunofluorescence Assay

Current studies have focused on the role of TGF-β in the tumor microenvironment suggesting that it plays a key role for GB progression [33,34]. Therefore, we investigated TGF-β expression by immunofluorescence assay on U-87, A-172 and U-138 cell lines. Our results confirmed a significant reduction of TGF-β expression after KYP-2047 treatment at the concentrations of 50 μM and 100 μM compared to the control group in U-87 cells (Figure 9A–C, see TGF-β ratio positive cells score Figure 9D), as well as in A-172 and U-138 cell lines (Figure S3A–C; see TGF-β ratio positive cells score 3D); (Figure S4A–C; see TGF-β ratio positive cells score 4D).

In addition to the regulation of the cell cycle and differentiation, TGF-β is able to induce apoptosis [35] promoting the activation of pro-apoptotic caspase-3, a member of the cysteine-aspartic acid protease family [36]. Thus, in this study we detected caspase-3 expression by immunofluorescence assay in all three GB cell lines. The results obtained showed an increase of caspase-3 expression following KYP-2047 treatment at the concentrations of 50 μM and 100 μM compared to the control group in U-87 cells (Figure 9E–G, see caspase-3 ratio positive cells score 9H) as well as in A-172 and U-138 cell lines in a concentration-dependent manner (Figure S3E–G; see caspase-3 ratio positive cells score 3H); (Figure S4E–G; see caspase-3 ratio positive cells score 4H).

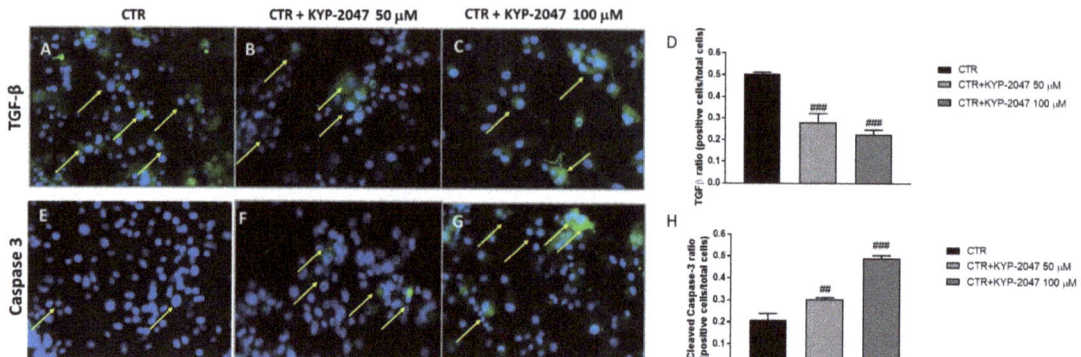

Figure 9. Effect of KYP-2047 on transforming growth factor-β (TGF-β) and caspase-3 expression in U-87 cells. Immunofluorescence assay performed on U-87 cells revealed a marked expression of TGF-β in the control group (**A**), while the treatment with KYP-2047 at the concentrations of 50 μM and 100 μM reduced significantly TGF-β expression (**B,C**). Additionally, immunofluorescence staining showed an increase of caspase-3 levels in the groups treated with KYP-2047 at the concentrations of 50 μM and 100 μM (**F,G**) compared to control group (**E**). Data are representative of at least three independent experiments. (**D**) ### $p < 0.001$ vs. CTR; (**H**) ## $p < 0.01$ vs. CTR; ### $p < 0.001$ vs. CTR.

4. Discussion

Glioblastoma (GB) is the most common and aggressive primary brain tumor in adults [37]. GB arise from glial cells but can also develop from astrocytic or neural stem/progenitor cells [38]. GB can be classified into primary and secondary subtypes, based on pre-existing lesion [38]. The primary GB subtype develops rapidly de novo in elderly patients without clinical or histologic evidence, whereas the secondary subtype develops from evolution of low-grade astrocytic tumours over the course of 4–5 years [38]. In the last decade, many studies have focused on the role of genetic mutations which contribute to GB initiation as TP53 and isocitrate dehydrogenase (IDH) mutations [37,39]. GB is characterized by a high degree of invasiveness, cell proliferation, angiogenesis and apoptosis alteration [2]. Despite scientific advances, the survival rate for patients with GB remains low and additional therapies are needed [12]. Previous studies have demonstrated that angiogenesis and apoptosis play a key role in GB pathology promoting cell survival and proliferation [10,31]. Therefore, the modulation of angiogenesis and apoptosis processes represent a valid strategy to counteract or reduce GB progression. KYP-2047 (4-phenylbutanoyl-L-prolyl-2(S)-cyanopyrrolidine) was developed as a highly specific and potent POP (or PREP) inhibitor, a serine protease involved in the angiogenesis process [40]. Recent studies revealed that KYP-2047 was able to modulate not only angiogenesis [11] but also cell cycle and differentiation [12,13]. Therefore, in this study we investigated the potential effect of KYP-2047 on angiogenesis and apoptosis pathways in an in vivo U87-xenograft model and in vitro study on the human GB cell line.

Firstly, we evaluated the ability of KYP-2047 to inhibit tumor growth in the xenograft model. Our results showed a high-grade necrosis and neutrophil infiltration in the control group, while KYP-2047 at higher doses significantly reduced subcutaneous tumor mass as well as neutrophil infiltration. Moreover, KYP-2047 significantly decreased mean tumor burden and tumor weight at higher doses, without encountering important weight differences.

Interestingly, treatment with KYP-2047 was able to reduce. PREP levels in serum of animals, particularly from day 14.

GB is one of the most highly angiogenic solid tumor [41]. Its tumor vasculature is both structurally and functionally abnormal, characterized by a dense network of vessels tortuous with increased diameter and thickened basement membranes [41]. Thus, angiogenesis is considered as a pathologic hallmark of GB, leading to VEGF activation, an angiogenic growth factor that promotes glioblastoma proliferation and CD34 activation, a transmembrane glycoprotein involved in the process of newly-forming tumour vessels [25,42]. Therefore, in this study we investigated VEGF and CD34 expression, showing that KYP-2047 at higher doses was able to reduce their expression significantly compared to the control group. Moreover, we investigated the role of eNOS, a relevant endothelial enzyme that modulates vascular homeostasis and vessel integrity [24]. In this context, our results showed that the control group was characterized by an increase of eNOS expression, whereas KYP-2047 significantly reduced eNOS expression.

The formation of new blood vessels is an essential process for GB growth [22]. In addition to VEGF, this process requires the involvement of other angiogenic factors as the angiopoietins, in particular angiopoietin 1 (Ang1) and angiopoietin 2 (Ang2) which have similar functions [26,43]. Previous studies revealed that Ang1 and Ang2 regulate vascular development and remodelling, promoting tumor growth [43,44]. Therefore, we decided to investigate the expression of Ang1 and Ang2 in GB; our results showed that the control group was characterized by an increase of Ang1 and Ang2 expression, while the treatment with KYP-2047 was able to significantly reduce their expression, inhibiting GB proliferation.

An increased vascularization provides to the tumor cells more oxygen and nutrients, promoting metastatic spread and cell proliferation [22]. In this context, Mastronardi et al. evaluated the correlation between angiogenesis and proliferation processes, through Ki-67 evaluation, a nuclear protein that regulates the cell cycle and differentiation [45]. Ki-67 is considered a relevant marker of tumor proliferation in GB [45,46]. Thus, we decided to evaluate Ki-67 expression, demonstrating that the control group was characterized by an increase of Ki-67 level, while KYP-2047 treatment was able to significantly reduce its expression.

Moreover, considering the key role of apoptosis in GB progression [3], we decided to investigate Bax, Bcl2 and caspase-3 expression in the U87-xenograft model, showing that KYP-2047 at doses of 2.5 mg/kg and 5 mg/kg was able to increase pro-apoptotic Bax and caspase-3 expression while Bcl2 expression was significantly reduced following KYP-2047 treatment.

To confirm the promising results obtained by an in vivo U87-xenograft model, we decided to conduct an in vitro model of GB on U-87, A-172 and U-138 cell lines. Firstly, we evaluated the cytotoxicity of KYP-2047 at different concentrations on U-87, A-172 and U-138 GB cells, demonstrating that KYP-2047 was able to significantly reduce cell viability in all three GB cell lines in a concentration-dependent manner.

Previous studies revealed that also apoptosis plays a key role in the development of GB [31,47]. It has been demonstrated that a down-regulation of apoptosis is associated with tumor survival [31,47]. Therefore, in this study we decided to evaluate the effect of KYP-2047 on the apoptosis pathway by evaluating protein levels of pro-apoptotic Bax, p53 and anti-apoptotic Bcl2 on U-87, A-172 and U-138 cell lysates. Our results revealed that KYP-2047 reduced Bcl2 expression, while Bax and p53 expression were significantly increased following KYP-2047 treatment in a concentration-dependent manner in all three GB cell lines, confirming apoptosis modulation.

Tumor proliferation is associated with an increase of TGF-β expression [48].

TGF-β regulates cell differentiation and apoptosis, promoting caspase-3 activation, a key regulator in apoptotic pathway [36]. Thus, we investigated the expression of TGF-β and caspase-3 in the in vitro model [49].

The results showed an increase of TGF-β expression in the control group while KYP-2047 treatment significantly reduced its expression in U-87, A-172 and U-138 cell lines. In addition, a marked increase of pro-apoptotic caspase-3 expression was revealed following KYP-2047 treatment, highlighting the ability of KYP-2047 to modulate apoptosis in all three GB cell lines.

Thus, the results obtained in an in vivo xenograft model and in an in vitro study on human GB cell lines revealed that KYP-2047 was able to reduce GB progression and growth by modulating angiogenesis and apoptosis pathways. Therefore, KYP-2047 could be considered as an alternative therapeutic strategy to counteract or reduce GB progression.

5. Conclusions

The data obtained revealed the ability of KYP-2047 to modulate angiogenesis and apoptosis pathways in an in vivo xenograft model and in an in vitro model of GB, reducing tumor progression. Therefore, on the basis of these results, KYP-2047 could represent an available strategy for the treatment of GB.

Supplementary Materials: The following are available online at https://www.mdpi.com/article/10.3390/cancers13143444/s1, Figure S1: Effect of KYP-2047 on apoptosis pathway in A-172 cell lysates., Figure S2: Effect of KYP-2047 on apoptosis pathway in U-138 cell lysates., Figure S3: Effect of KYP-2047 on TGF-β and Caspase3 expression in A-172 cells., Figure S4: Effect of KYP-2047 on TGF-β and Caspase3 expression in U-138 cells., Figure S5: Original western blot.

Author Contributions: S.A.S. prepared the manuscript; S.A.S., G.C., and A.A. performed experiments; S.F., L.C., and S.S. carried out formal analysis; I.P., E.E., and S.C. planned the experiments and critically revised the manuscript. M.C. supervised the research and revised the manuscript. All authors have read and agreed to the published version of the manuscript.

Funding: This research received no external funding.

Institutional Review Board Statement: This study was approved by the University of Messina Review Board for the care of animals, in compliance with Italian regulations on protection of animals (n° 368/2019-PR released on 14 May 2019). Animal care was in accordance with Italian regulations on the use of animals for the experiment (D.M.116192) as well as with the Council Regulation regulations (EEC) (O.J. of E.C. L 358/1 12/18/1986).

Informed Consent Statement: Not applicable.

Data Availability Statement: All data generated or analyzed during this study are included in this article.

Conflicts of Interest: The authors declare no conflict of interest.

References

1. DeAngelis, L.M. Brain tumors. *N. Engl. J. Med.* **2001**, *344*, 114–123. [CrossRef]
2. Hanif, F.; Muzaffar, K.; Perveen, K.; Malhi, S.M.; Simjee, S.U. Glioblastoma Multiforme: A Review of its Epidemiology and Pathogenesis through Clinical Presentation and Treatment. *Asian Pac. J. Cancer Prev.* **2017**, *18*, 3–9. [CrossRef]
3. Lieberman, F. Glioblastoma update: Molecular biology, diagnosis, treatment, response assessment, and translational clinical trials. *F1000Research* **2017**, *6*, 1892. [CrossRef]
4. Sattiraju, A.; Sai, K.K.S.; Mintz, A. Glioblastoma Stem Cells and Their Microenvironment. *Adv. Exp. Med. Biol.* **2017**, *1041*, 119–140. [CrossRef] [PubMed]
5. Lombardi, M.Y.; Assem, M. Glioblastoma Genomics: A Very Complicated Story. In *Glioblastoma*; De Vleeschouwer, S., Ed.; Codon Publications: Brisbane, Australia, 2017. [CrossRef]
6. Okada, M.; Miyake, K.; Tamiya, T. Glioblastoma Treatment in the Elderly. *Neurol. Med. Chir.* **2017**, *57*, 667–676. [CrossRef] [PubMed]
7. Cai, X.; Sughrue, M.E. Glioblastoma: New therapeutic strategies to address cellular and genomic complexity. *Oncotarget* **2018**, *9*, 9540–9554. [CrossRef]
8. Broekman, M.L.; Maas, S.L.N.; Abels, E.R.; Mempel, T.R.; Krichevsky, A.M.; Breakefield, X.O. Multidimensional communication in the microenvirons of glioblastoma. *Nat. Rev. Neurol.* **2018**, *14*, 482–495. [CrossRef] [PubMed]
9. Trejo-Solis, C.; Serrano-Garcia, N.; Escamilla-Ramirez, A.; Castillo-Rodriguez, R.A.; Jimenez-Farfan, D.; Palencia, G.; Calvillo, M.; Alvarez-Lemus, M.A.; Flores-Najera, A.; Cruz-Salgado, A.; et al. Autophagic and Apoptotic Pathways as Targets for Chemotherapy in Glioblastoma. *Int. J. Mol. Sci.* **2018**, *19*, 3773. [CrossRef] [PubMed]
10. Hundsberger, T.; Reardon, D.A.; Wen, P.Y. Angiogenesis inhibitors in tackling recurrent glioblastoma. *Expert Rev. Anticancer Ther.* **2017**, *17*, 507–515. [CrossRef] [PubMed]
11. Casili, G.; Lanza, M.; Scuderi, S.A.; Messina, S.; Paterniti, I.; Campolo, M.; Esposito, E. The Inhibition of Prolyl Oligopeptidase as New Target to Counteract Chronic Venous Insufficiency: Findings in a Mouse Model. *Biomedicines* **2020**, *8*, 604. [CrossRef]
12. Jalkanen, A.J.; Leikas, J.V.; Forsberg, M.M. KYP-2047 penetrates mouse brain and effectively inhibits mouse prolyl oligopeptidase. *Basic Clin. Pharmacol. Toxicol.* **2014**, *114*, 460–463. [CrossRef]

13. Myohanen, T.T.; Tenorio-Laranga, J.; Jokinen, B.; Vazquez-Sanchez, R.; Moreno-Baylach, M.J.; Garcia-Horsman, J.A.; Mannisto, P.T. Prolyl oligopeptidase induces angiogenesis both in vitro and in vivo in a novel regulatory manner. *Br. J. Pharmacol.* **2011**, *163*, 1666–1678. [CrossRef]
14. Deng, S.; Zhu, S.; Qiao, Y.; Liu, Y.J.; Chen, W.; Zhao, G.; Chen, J. Recent advances in the role of toll-like receptors and TLR agonists in immunotherapy for human glioma. *Protein Cell* **2014**, *5*, 899–911. [CrossRef] [PubMed]
15. Ovcharenko, D.; Chitjian, C.; Kashkin, A.; Fanelli, E.; Ovcharenko, V. Two dichloric compounds inhibit in vivo U87 xenograft tumor growth. *Cancer Biol. Ther.* **2019**, *20*, 1281–1289. [CrossRef]
16. Esposito, E.; Campolo, M.; Casili, G.; Lanza, M.; Franco, D.; Filippone, A.; Peritore, A.F.; Cuzzocrea, S. Protective Effects of Xyloglucan in Association with the Polysaccharide Gelose in an Experimental Model of Gastroenteritis and Urinary Tract Infections. *Int. J. Mol. Sci.* **2018**, *19*, 1844. [CrossRef]
17. Impellizzeri, D.; Bruschetta, G.; Di Paola, R.; Ahmad, A.; Campolo, M.; Cuzzocrea, S.; Esposito, E.; Navarra, M. The anti-inflammatory and antioxidant effects of bergamot juice extract (BJe) in an experimental model of inflammatory bowel disease. *Clin. Nutr.* **2015**, *34*, 1146–1154. [CrossRef]
18. Weinert, B.T.; Krishnadath, K.K.; Milano, F.; Pedersen, A.W.; Claesson, M.H.; Zocca, M.B. Real-time PCR analysis of genes encoding tumor antigens in esophageal tumors and a cancer vaccine. *Cancer Immun.* **2009**, *9*, 9. [PubMed]
19. Irrera, N.; D'Ascola, A.; Pallio, G.; Bitto, A.; Mannino, F.; Arcoraci, V.; Rottura, M.; Ieni, A.; Minutoli, L.; Metro, D.; et al. Beta-Caryophyllene Inhibits Cell Proliferation through a Direct Modulation of CB2 Receptors in Glioblastoma Cells. *Cancers* **2020**, *12*, 1038. [CrossRef]
20. Campolo, M.; Casili, G.; Lanza, M.; Filippone, A.; Paterniti, I.; Cuzzocrea, S.; Esposito, E. Multiple mechanisms of dimethyl fumarate in amyloid beta-induced neurotoxicity in human neuronal cells. *J. Cell. Mol. Med.* **2018**, *22*, 1081–1094. [CrossRef] [PubMed]
21. Donaldson, J.G. Immunofluorescence Staining. *Curr. Protoc. Cell Biol.* **2015**, *69*, 431–437. [CrossRef] [PubMed]
22. Ahir, B.K.; Engelhard, H.H.; Lakka, S.S. Tumor Development and Angiogenesis in Adult Brain Tumor: Glioblastoma. *Mol. Neurobiol.* **2020**, *57*, 2461–2478. [CrossRef] [PubMed]
23. Yang, X.; Li, X.; Luo, M.; Guo, Y.; Li, C.; Lv, D.; Cheng, Z.; Huang, L.; Shang, F.F.; Huang, B.; et al. Tubeimoside I promotes angiogenesis via activation of eNOS-VEGF signaling pathway. *J. Ethnopharmacol.* **2021**, *267*, 113642. [CrossRef]
24. Wood, K.C.; Cortese-Krott, M.M.; Kovacic, J.C.; Noguchi, A.; Liu, V.B.; Wang, X.; Raghavachari, N.; Boehm, M.; Kato, G.J.; Kelm, M.; et al. Circulating blood endothelial nitric oxide synthase contributes to the regulation of systemic blood pressure and nitrite homeostasis. *Arterioscler. Thromb. Vasc. Biol.* **2013**, *33*, 1861–1871. [CrossRef] [PubMed]
25. Chabowski, M.; Nowak, A.; Grzegrzolka, J.; Piotrowska, A.; Janczak, D.; Dziegiel, P. Comparison of Microvessel Density Using Nestin and CD34 in Colorectal Cancer. *Anticancer Res.* **2018**, *38*, 3889–3895. [CrossRef] [PubMed]
26. Sie, M.; Wagemakers, M.; Molema, G.; Mooij, J.J.; de Bont, E.S.; den Dunnen, W.F. The angiopoietin 1/angiopoietin 2 balance as a prognostic marker in primary glioblastoma multiforme. *J. Neurosurg.* **2009**, *110*, 147–155. [CrossRef]
27. Wang, P.F.; Li, H.L.; Qi, X.; Yao, K.; Han, S.; Liu, N.; Yang, Y.K.; Li, S.W.; Yan, C.X. Clinical significance of angiopoietin-like protein 3 expression in patients with glioblastoma. *Neoplasma* **2016**, *63*, 93–98. [CrossRef] [PubMed]
28. Rautiola, J.; Lampinen, A.; Mirtti, T.; Ristimaki, A.; Joensuu, H.; Bono, P.; Saharinen, P. Association of Angiopoietin-2 and Ki-67 Expression with Vascular Density and Sunitinib Response in Metastatic Renal Cell Carcinoma. *PLoS ONE* **2016**, *11*, e0153745. [CrossRef]
29. Zhang, J.; Cai, H.; Sun, L.; Zhan, P.; Chen, M.; Zhang, F.; Ran, Y.; Wan, J. LGR5, a novel functional glioma stem cell marker, promotes EMT by activating the Wnt/beta-catenin pathway and predicts poor survival of glioma patients. *J. Exp. Clin. Cancer Res.* **2018**, *37*, 225. [CrossRef]
30. Valdes-Rives, S.A.; Casique-Aguirre, D.; German-Castelan, L.; Velasco-Velazquez, M.A.; Gonzalez-Arenas, A. Apoptotic Signaling Pathways in Glioblastoma and Therapeutic Implications. *Biomed. Res. Int.* **2017**, *2017*, 7403747. [CrossRef]
31. Pistritto, G.; Trisciuoglio, D.; Ceci, C.; Garufi, A.; D'Orazi, G. Apoptosis as anticancer mechanism: Function and dysfunction of its modulators and targeted therapeutic strategies. *Aging* **2016**, *8*, 603–619. [CrossRef]
32. Kerr, J.F.; Wyllie, A.H.; Currie, A.R. Apoptosis: A basic biological phenomenon with wide-ranging implications in tissue kinetics. *Br. J. Cancer* **1972**, *26*, 239–257. [CrossRef]
33. Ahmad, F.; Ghosh, S.; Sinha, S.; Joshi, S.D.; Mehta, V.S.; Sen, E. TGF-beta-induced hCG-beta regulates redox homeostasis in glioma cells. *Mol. Cell. Biochem.* **2015**, *399*, 105–112. [CrossRef]
34. Margadant, C.; Sonnenberg, A. Integrin-TGF-beta crosstalk in fibrosis, cancer and wound healing. *EMBO Rep.* **2010**, *11*, 97–105. [CrossRef]
35. Siegel, P.M.; Massague, J. Cytostatic and apoptotic actions of TGF-beta in homeostasis and cancer. *Nat. Rev. Cancer* **2003**, *3*, 807–821. [CrossRef] [PubMed]
36. Zhang, S.; Ekman, M.; Thakur, N.; Bu, S.; Davoodpour, P.; Grimsby, S.; Tagami, S.; Heldin, C.H.; Landstrom, M. TGFbeta1-induced activation of ATM and p53 mediates apoptosis in a Smad7-dependent manner. *Cell Cycle* **2006**, *5*, 2787–2795. [CrossRef]
37. Wirsching, H.G.; Galanis, E.; Weller, M. Glioblastoma. *Handb. Clin. Neurol.* **2016**, *134*, 381–397. [CrossRef] [PubMed]
38. Soomro, S.H.; Ting, L.R.; Qing, Y.Y.; Ren, M. Molecular biology of glioblastoma: Classification and mutational locations. *J. Pak. Med. Assoc.* **2017**, *67*, 1410–1414.

39. SongTao, Q.; Lei, Y.; Si, G.; YanQing, D.; HuiXia, H.; XueLin, Z.; LanXiao, W.; Fei, Y. IDH mutations predict longer survival and response to temozolomide in secondary glioblastoma. *Cancer Sci.* **2012**, *103*, 269–273. [CrossRef]
40. Venalainen, J.I.; Garcia-Horsman, J.A.; Forsberg, M.M.; Jalkanen, A.; Wallen, E.A.; Jarho, E.M.; Christiaans, J.A.; Gynther, J.; Mannisto, P.T. Binding kinetics and duration of in vivo action of novel prolyl oligopeptidase inhibitors. *Biochem. Pharmacol.* **2006**, *71*, 683–692. [CrossRef] [PubMed]
41. Weathers, S.P.; de Groot, J. VEGF Manipulation in Glioblastoma. *Oncology* **2015**, *29*, 720–727. [PubMed]
42. Carmeliet, P. VEGF as a key mediator of angiogenesis in cancer. *Oncology* **2005**, *69* (Suppl. S3), 4–10. [CrossRef]
43. Tanaka, S.; Mori, M.; Sakamoto, Y.; Makuuchi, M.; Sugimachi, K.; Wands, J.R. Biologic significance of angiopoietin-2 expression in human hepatocellular carcinoma. *J. Clin. Investig.* **1999**, *103*, 341–345. [CrossRef]
44. Stoeltzing, O.; Ahmad, S.A.; Liu, W.; McCarty, M.F.; Parikh, A.A.; Fan, F.; Reinmuth, N.; Bucana, C.D.; Ellis, L.M. Angiopoietin-1 inhibits tumour growth and ascites formation in a murine model of peritoneal carcinomatosis. *Br. J. Cancer* **2002**, *87*, 1182–1187. [CrossRef] [PubMed]
45. Mastronardi, L.; Guiducci, A.; Puzzilli, F.; Ruggeri, A. Relationship between Ki-67 labeling index and survival in high-grade glioma patients treated after surgery with tamoxifen. *J. Neurosurg. Sci.* **1999**, *43*, 263–270. [PubMed]
46. Alkhaibary, A.; Alassiri, A.H.; AlSufiani, F.; Alharbi, M.A. Ki-67 labeling index in glioblastoma; does it really matter? *Hematol. Oncol. Stem. Cell Ther.* **2019**, *12*, 82–88. [CrossRef] [PubMed]
47. Wong, R.S. Apoptosis in cancer: From pathogenesis to treatment. *J. Exp. Clin. Cancer Res.* **2011**, *30*, 87. [CrossRef]
48. Katsuno, Y.; Lamouille, S.; Derynck, R. TGF-beta signaling and epithelial-mesenchymal transition in cancer progression. *Curr. Opin. Oncol.* **2013**, *25*, 76–84. [CrossRef]
49. Chio, C.C.; Chen, K.Y.; Chang, C.K.; Chuang, J.Y.; Liu, C.C.; Liu, S.H.; Chen, R.M. Improved effects of honokiol on temozolomide-induced autophagy and apoptosis of drug-sensitive and -tolerant glioma cells. *BMC Cancer* **2018**, *18*, 379. [CrossRef]

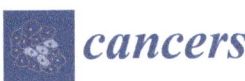

Review

FAM72, Glioblastoma Multiforme (GBM) and Beyond

Nguyen Thi Thanh Ho [1,†], Chinmay Satish Rahane [2,†], Subrata Pramanik [3], Pok-Son Kim [4], Arne Kutzner [5] and Klaus Heese [1,*]

1. Graduate School of Biomedical Science and Engineering, Hanyang University, 222 Wangsimni-ro, Seongdong-gu, Seoul 133-791, Korea; nguyenho1408@hanyang.ac.kr
2. Maharashtra Institute of Medical Education and Research, Talegaon Dabhade, Maharashtra 410507, India; chinsanity@gmail.com
3. Institute of Biotechnology, RWTH Aachen University, Worringerweg 3, 52074 Aachen, Germany; s.pramanik@biotec.rwth-aachen.de
4. Department of Mathematics, Kookmin University, 77 Jeongneung-ro, Seongbuk-gu, Seoul 136-702, Korea; pskim@kookmin.ac.kr
5. Department of Information Systems, College of Computer Science, Hanyang University, 222 Wangsimni-ro, Seongdong-gu, Seoul 133-791, Korea; kutzner@hanyang.ac.kr
* Correspondence: klaus@hanyang.ac.kr
† Contributed equally to the study.

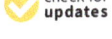

Citation: Ho, N.T.T.; Rahane, C.S.; Pramanik, S.; Kim, P.-S.; Kutzner, A.; Heese, K. FAM72, Glioblastoma Multiforme (GBM) and Beyond. *Cancers* **2021**, *13*, 1025. https://doi.org/10.3390/cancers13051025

Academic Editors: Stanley Stylli and Giulio Cabrini

Received: 25 January 2021
Accepted: 22 February 2021
Published: 1 March 2021

Publisher's Note: MDPI stays neutral with regard to jurisdictional claims in published maps and institutional affiliations.

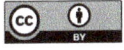

Copyright: © 2021 by the authors. Licensee MDPI, Basel, Switzerland. This article is an open access article distributed under the terms and conditions of the Creative Commons Attribution (CC BY) license (https://creativecommons.org/licenses/by/4.0/).

Simple Summary: Glioblastoma multiforme (GBM) is a serious and aggressive cancer disease that has not allowed scientists to rest for decades. In this review, we consider the new gene pair |-SRGAP2–FAM72-| and discuss its role in the cell cycle and the possibility of defining new therapeutic approaches for the treatment of GBM and other cancers via this gene pair |-SRGAP2–FAM72-|.

Abstract: Neural stem cells (NSCs) offer great potential for regenerative medicine due to their excellent ability to differentiate into various specialized cell types of the brain. In the central nervous system (CNS), NSC renewal and differentiation are under strict control by the regulation of the pivotal SLIT-ROBO Rho GTPase activating protein 2 (SRGAP2)—Family with sequence similarity 72 (FAM72) master gene (i.e., |-SRGAP2–FAM72-|) via a divergent gene transcription activation mechanism. If the gene transcription control unit (i.e., the intergenic region of the two sub-gene units, SRGAP2 and FAM72) gets out of control, NSCs may transform into cancer stem cells and generate brain tumor cells responsible for brain cancer such as glioblastoma multiforme (GBM). Here, we discuss the surveillance of this |-SRGAP2–FAM72-| master gene and its role in GBM, and also in light of FAM72 for diagnosing various types of cancers outside of the CNS.

Keywords: brain cancer; cell cycle; differentiation; glioblastoma; proliferation; RAS; SRGAP2; stem cell; TP53

1. Introduction

The human brain is a unique organ that can perform higher cognitive functions and is therefore different from all other species. Its uniqueness is reflected in the expression of four paralog gene pairs |-SRGAP2–FAM72-| (A–D) [1,2]. FAM72 is active in proliferating neural stem cells (NSCs) found in the brain hippocampus [1–5]. There are four specific FAM72 (A–D) paralogs associated with four respective SRGAP2 paralogs on human chromosome 1 (chr 1), but only one such gene pair co-exists as the |-SRGAP2–FAM72-| master gene in all other notochord containing vertebrates (Figure 1a) [1,2,6,7].

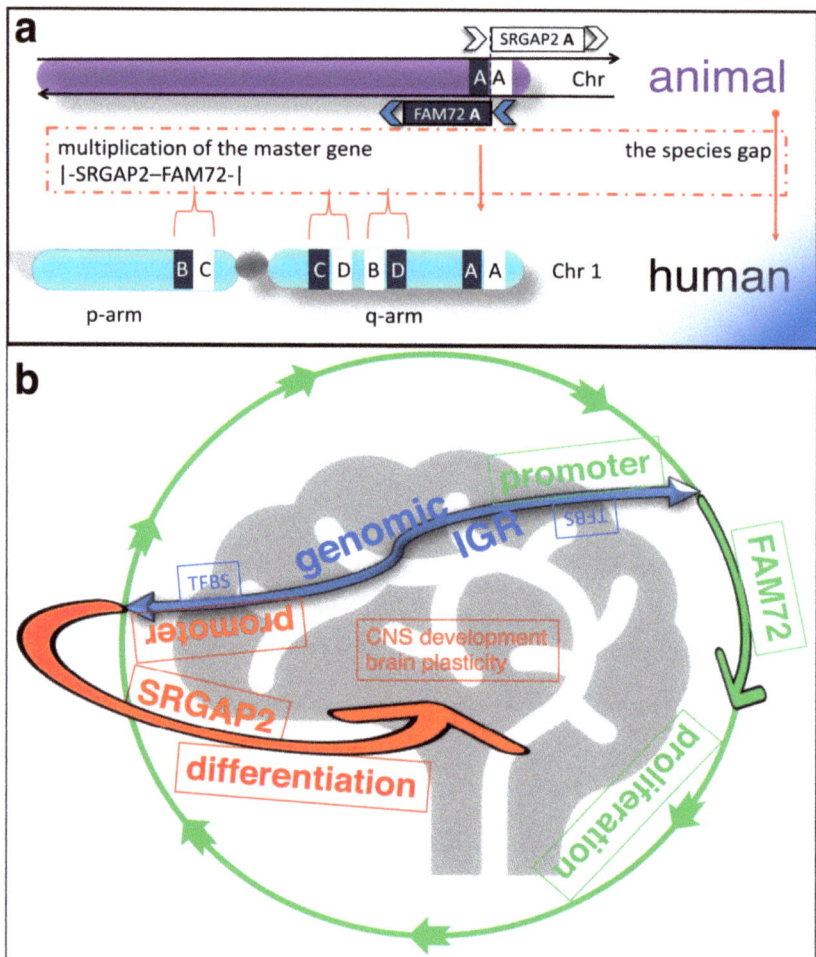

Figure 1. Overview scheme of the |-SRGAP2–FAM72-| master gene expression across the phylogenetic tree. (**a**) While humans express four master genes on chr 1, all other notochord containing vertebrates carry only one such master gene; other species do not show any such master gene, and thus far, no species have been found that show two or three such master genes. FAM72 shows four exons (149 amino acids (aa)), SRGAP2 is composed of 22 exons (1071 aa), and both sub-genes are separated by a 4-kbp intergenic region (IGR). The four paralogous gene pairs A–D are located on opposite strands from one another [1,2,5]. (**b**) Simplified divergent gene transcription paradigm scheme of the novel pivotal |-SRGAP2–FAM72-| master gene in the brain. The |-SRGAP2–FAM72-| master gene resides within a nucleosome-depleted region with the IGR (blue), containing potential transcription factor (TF)-binding sites (BS) (TFBS) between the SRGAP2 (red) and FAM72 (green) genes indicated. Reverse-oriented SRGAP2 (red) and FAM72 (green) genes are expressed from opposite DNA strands [1,8]. The dual IGR promotor controls the two reverse-oriented reciprocal functional-dependent genes FAM72 and SRGAP2, respectively, located on opposite DNA strands. If FAM72 gene is activated by TFs, then the transcription of the SRGAP2 gene is activated until it is actively terminated early and vice versa for neuronal differentiation; accordingly, if FAM72 is in the 'on' modus, SRGAP2 is switched off and vice versa [8–11]. Through this mechanism, FAM72 maintains renewal and proliferation of a critical mass of NSCs during brain development while SRGAP2 promotes escape of the cell cycle fostering neuronal differentiation and brain plasticity [5,8]. This structure represents a novel paradigm for controlling the transcription of divergent genes in regulating NSC gene expression and may allow for novel therapeutic approaches to restore or improve higher cognitive functions and cure cancers (Figure 2).

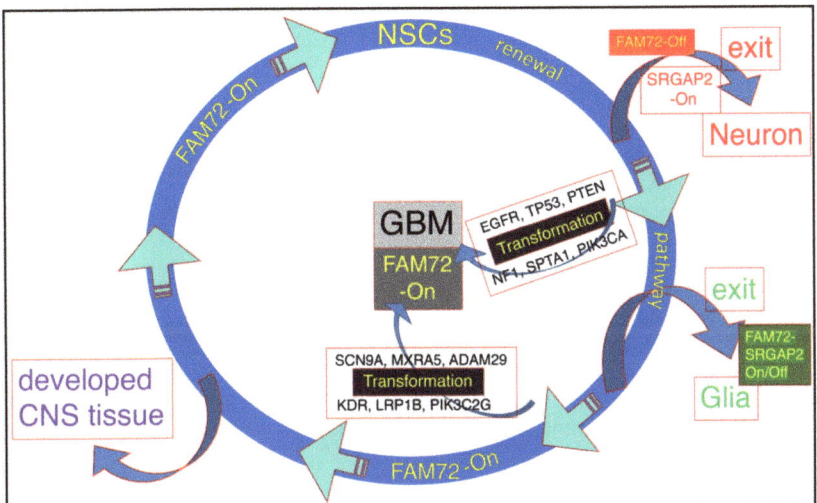

Figure 2. Overview of the |-SRGAP2–FAM72-| master gene expression in GBM [12]. As long as FAM72 remains in the on modus, NSCs keep proliferating. For neuronal differentiation and brain plasticity, FAM72 needs to be switched off to allow SRGAP2 activation and brain development. The activity of the |-SRGAP2–FAM72-| master gene expression during glia cell differentiation is less clear. Since glia cells have the capacity to proliferate, FAM72 might be switched on or off [13–15]. Eventually, mutations in GBM-specific driver genes: epidermal growth factor receptor (EGFR), tumor protein p53 (TP53), phosphatase and tensin homolog (PTEN), neurofibromin 1 (NF1), spectrin alpha, erythrocytic 1 (SPTA1) and phosphatidylinositol-4,5-bisphosphate 3-kinase catalytic subunit alpha (PIK3CA) or sodium voltage-gated channel alpha subunit 9 (SCN9A), matrix remodeling associated 5 (MXRA5), a disintegrin and metalloprotease domain 29 (ADAM29), kinase insert domain receptor (KDR), phosphatidylinositol-4-phosphate 3-kinase catalytic subunit type 2 gamma (PIK3C2G), and low-density lipoprotein receptor related protein 1B (LRP1B) induce NSC transformation into cancer stem cells (CSCs) while FAM72 is still in the on modus [12].

2. Physiological Function of the |-SRGAP2–FAM72-| Master Gene

Endogenous FAM72 expression has been shown in the hippocampal dentate gyrus [3], where the |-SRGAP2–FAM72-| master-gene regulates NSC renewal, neurogenesis and brain plasticity [4,5]. Here, the |-SRGAP2–FAM72-| master-gene is under a divergent gene expression control (Figure 1b) [5,8]. Thus, FAM72 expression is switched on to promote NSC renewal and proliferation and is switched off (concomitantly SRGAP2 is switched on) to foster differentiation, neuritogenesis, synaptic plasticity, and brain development (Figure 1b) [4,5,8,16–21]. However, this divergent expression paradigm is currently restricted to neural tissue [5,8] and apoptosis is induced if it gets out of control (i.e., neuronal expression of FAM72 forces reentry into the cell cycle) [3].

3. Pathophysiological Function of the |-SRGAP2–FAM72-| Master Gene—FAM72 Expression in Various Types of Cancer

Early studies revealed that FAM72 was overexpressed outside the nervous system in various types of cancer with the protein kinase C signaling pathway activated in neuroblastoma and breast adenocarcinoma (e.g., MCF-7 and MDA-MB-231 cells) [3] and uracil DNA glycosylase-2 as a binding partner in malignant colon cancers [22]. FAM72B was identified as a member of a 7-gene signature in prostate cancer [23], and it was also upregulated in multiple non-neuronal tissues as well [12]. FAM72B, C, and D were also among the highly upregulated genes in B-cell lymphoma [24]. Recently, FAM72D has been identified as a specific proliferation marker in multiple myelomas [25]. Moreover, we reported increased mean expression of FAM72 paralogs across human tumors compared to control tissues, except in cases of skin cutaneous melanoma, kidney chromophobes, and pheochromocytomas. This indicates that neuronal FAM72 paralogs are being expressed in non-neuronal proliferating tumor tissue cells [12].

3.1. The |-SRGAP2–FAM72-| Master Gene in Brain Cancer

Previously, we correlated FAM72 (A–D) mRNA expression z-scores and highly mutated protooncogenes as well as unique mutated genes in deceased GBM patients. mRNA expression and mutation data for GBM was retrieved from cBioportal. Normalized mRNA expression z-score data were computed for all GBM samples and the data for FAM72 (A–D) paralogs were grouped in bins with a size of 0.7 z-score units and correlated with genes showing high numbers of tissue-specific gene mutations. Linear regression was determined first between the FAM72 (A–D) paralogs and then between all available genes in the GBM study, then visualized using online Python-based Bokeh software. A complex brain-specific gene-mutation signature: EGFR, TP53, PTEN, NF1, SPTA1, PIK3CA or SCN9A, MXRA5, ADAM29, KDR, PIK3C2G, and LRP1B was identified that correlated with high FAM72 expression and may lead to cell cycle activation, cell transformation, and cell proliferation. This led to the identification of several pivotal driver genes responsible for the transformation of NSCs into CSCs and GBM (Figure 2) [12].

On the other hand, the partner gene SRGAP2 showed no change in expression in GBM. SRGAP2 is reported to be a tumor suppressor [26], and its expression is usually induced when FAM72 expression is blocked. NSCs stop proliferating during neural differentiation and neuronal synaptogenesis [4,5,8,16–21], but may lead to apoptosis in non-neuronal tissue or proliferating cancerous cells [3,5]. Genomic rearrangements causing loss of physiological functions of SRGAP2 may enhance cell motility and metastasis [26].

3.2. The |-SRGAP2–FAM72-| Master Gene in Other Cancerous Tissues

Our recent large-scale tissue analysis demonstrated that the Ki-67 gene (MKI67) and FAM72 paralogs are co-expressed in proliferating cells in NSCs and also outside neuronal tissue (i.e., in cancer cells across various tissues) (Figure 3, Supplementary Materials Figure S1). FAM72 does not appear to be a protooncogene and the reciprocal expression dependency of SRGAP2 and FAM72 seems to be limited to the nervous system. Outside the nervous system, FAM72 expression appears to be induced by a different cancer-causing oncogene [12,27,28].

3.3. FAM72 in Adrenocortical Carcinoma

Our understanding of the molecular mechanism driving ACC has advanced. Alterations in the components of the WNT1/β-catenin, EGFR, and TP53 pathways are prominent markers in ACC [29–32]. CTNNB1 and TP53 mutations are mutually exclusive in aggressive adrenal cancers [36]. Activating mutations in CTNNB1 have been observed in approximately 25% of adrenocortical cancers [37]. TP53 mutations have been observed in more than 50% of child patients, but only in 4% of adult patients of ACC [38,39].

Recently, we identified a complex novel ACC-specific gene signature: CRIPAK, DGKZ, GARS1, LRIG1, ZFPM1, and ZNF517, which was significantly, specifically, and most repeatedly mutated in ACC and correlated with high FAM72 expression (Figure 3) [28]. This gene set is involved in tumor suppression and cellular proliferation and thus could be useful for the prognosis and development of therapeutic approaches for the treatment of ACC.

Experimental evidence indicates that EGFR signaling is an anchor body through which proliferative pathways can be initiated and most of the proto-oncogenes in ACC act downstream of EGFR. Moreover, in ACC, LRIG1 mutations would cause a continuous expression of the EGFR signaling cascade, thereby causing cellular proliferation. Inhibition of EGFR via tumor suppressor LRIG1 is thus a key step in regulating (either partially or fully) the consequent signaling cascades. Mutations in GARS1 also serve to increase proliferation via a cascade that is, however, independent of the phosphoinositide-3-kinase (PI3K)/mitogen-activated protein kinase 1 (MAPK1)/WNT1 signaling pathways. Mutations in our novel gene set thus appear to be more influential in ACC tumorigenesis than those described in earlier studies and could serve as a powerful therapeutic target [28,29].

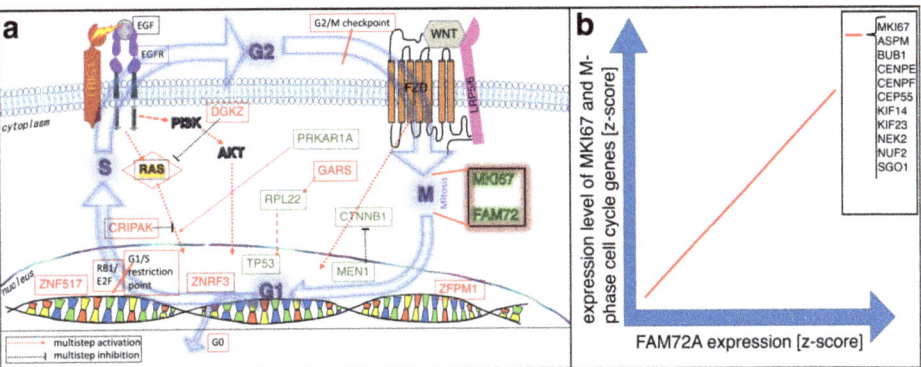

Figure 3. Experimental evidence-based schematic illustration of FAM72 and MKI67 co-activation in adrenocortical carcinoma (ACC). (**a**) Mutations in ACC-specific driver proto-onco- or tumor-suppressor-genes (red and green color) push the cell through the cell cycle and mediate MKI67 as well as FAM72 expression during the M-phase. Red-colored proto-oncogenes (or tumor-suppressor genes) are from Rahane et al. [28], while green-colored proto-oncogenes (or tumor-suppressor genes) are from Zheng et al. [29]; additional ACC-specific cell cycle information are from Assié et al. [30], Lippert et al. [31], and Pereira et al. [32]. Tumor suppressor LRIG1 interferes with EGFR signaling and might be a druggable protein of primary interest [33–35]. (**b**) Schematic illustration of mRNA expression correlation between FAM72A on the one hand and M-phase cell cycle genes, including MKI67, on the other hand. FAM72A expression correlates with the expression of cell cycle phase-specific genes across various human cancer tissue. Genes specifically associated with the late G2- to M-phase of the cell cycle, including ASPM, BUB1, CENPE, CENPF, CEP55, KIF14, KIF23, NEK2, NUF2, and SGO1 (ASPM, BUB1, CEP55, KIF14, KIF23, and NEK2 are involved either with spindle formation or with regulation; CENPE, CENPF, NUF2, and SGO1 are involved in the centromere-kinetochore complex) [12,28]. ASPM, Assembly factor for spindle microtubules; BUB1, Budding uninhibited by benzimidazoles 1 mitotic checkpoint serine/threonine kinase; CENPE, Centromere protein E; CENPF, Centromere protein F; CEP55, Centrosomal protein 55; CRIPAK, Cysteine-rich p21-activated protein kinase 1 inhibitor; CTNNB1, Catenin beta 1; DGKZ, Diacylglycerol kinase zeta; FZD, Frizzleds; GARS1, Glycyl-tRNA synthetase 1; KIF14/23, Kinesin family member 14/23; LRIG1, Leucine rich repeats and immunoglobulin-like domains 1; NEK2, Never in mitosis gene a-related kinase 2; NUF2, NUF2 component of NDC80 kinetochore complex; RPL22, Ribosomal protein L22; PRKAR1A, Protein kinase cAMP-dependent type I regulatory subunit alpha; RAS, Rat sarcoma; SGO1, Shugoshin 1; WNT1, Wingless and Int-1 family member 1; ZFPM1, Zinc finger protein, friend of GATA family member 1; ZNF517, Zinc finger protein 517; ZNRF3, Zinc and ring finger 3.

4. FAM72 and Its Role in the Cell Cycle

4.1. FAM72 in the M-Phase of the Cell Cycle

FAM72 (A–D) is highly expressed when promoting NSC and cancer cell proliferation and are present in the G2/M phase of the cell cycle [2,5,12,28]. It has been shown that knock-down of FAM72A in NSCs blocks cell proliferation and causes cell differentiation [4]. In line with this, FAM72B knockdown experiments showed that cell proliferation was reduced in human fibroblasts [40], suggesting that FAM72B also has a common role in promoting cell proliferation, similar to the other FAM72 members. Cell cycle specific expression analysis revealed that FAM72 (A–D) activity occurred particularly during the G2/M-phase, but not during the G1/S-phase (Figure 3b) [12,28].

NSC or cancer cell fate is determined based on specific E2 factor transcription factor E2Fx TFs (x = 1, 2, 3, 4 and 6, i.e., E2F1, E2F2, E2F3, E2F4, E2F6 such as E2F6 in a complex with transcription factor dimerization partner 1 [TFDP1]) bound to the promoter within the IGR of the |-SRGAP2–FAM72-| master gene. We found that FAM72 expression correlates with the expression of a baculoviral inhibitor of apoptosis protein (IAP) repeat (BIR)-containing 5 (BIRC5, also known as survivin), Forkhead box M1 (FOXM1), LIN9, LIN54 (partially), and retinoblastoma binding protein 4 (RBBP4) (Lin53, partially) and also with pivotal E2Fx TFs in various cancer tissues including brain glioma. Other genes showed either weak (TFDP1 and TFDP2) or no correlation (oligodendrocyte marker OLIG2, tumor suppressor family with sequence similarity 107 member A [FAM107A]), paired box protein Pax-6 (PAX6), and ten eleven translocation protein 2 (tet methylcytosine dioxygenases 2, TET2), and LIN37) (Figure 4, Supplementary Materials Figures S2–S16).

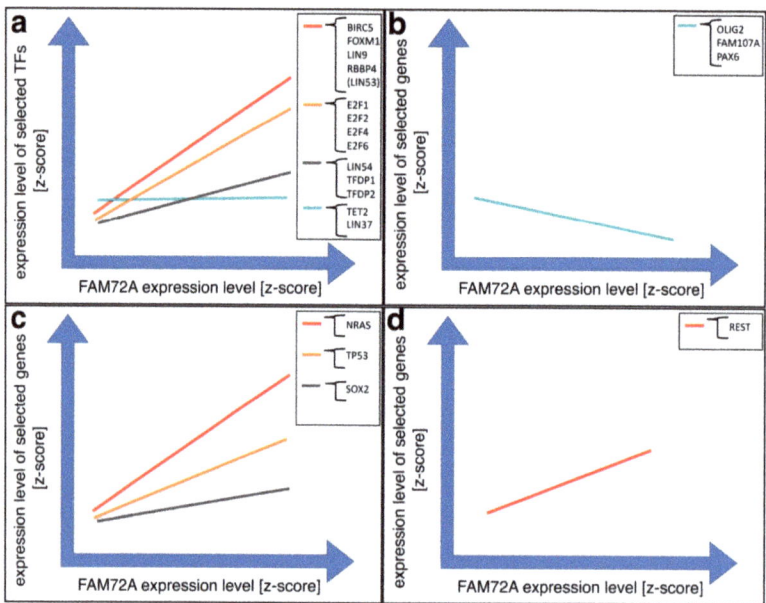

Figure 4. Schematic illustration of mRNA expression correlation of FAM72A compared with several other GBM-relevant genes, including E2Fx TFs. (**a**) FAM72A expression correlates with the expression of selected genes and TFs (Supplementary Materials Figures S2–S17). (**b**) FAM72A expression does not correlate with the expression of OLIG2, FAM107A nor with PAX6 (Supplementary Materials Figures S7, S12, and S13). (**c**) FAM72A expression correlates with neuroblastoma rat sarcoma proto-oncogene (NRAS), TP53, and weakly with sex determining region Y (SRY) box transcription factor 2 (SOX2) in glioma (Supplementary Materials Figures S18–S20). (**d**) FAM72A expression correlates with RE1 silencing transcription factor (REST) in glioma (Supplementary Materials Figure S21).

4.2. FAM72 in the G0 Stage of the Cell Cycle

Some studies showed that retinoblastoma transcriptional corepressor 1 (RB1) may cause the cell to go into the G0 phase with different cell fates: Quiescent G0 with reversible return option to reenter the cell cycle for proliferation, post-mitotic G0 with irreversible cell differentiation, or cell senescence G0, eventually leading to apoptosis [41,42]. Our data suggest that the |-SRGAP2–FAM72-| master gene induces the RB1 pathway (eventually via TP53 acetylation) to push cells into the G0 stage concomitantly with SRGAP2 expression, supporting neural survival and stabilizing a neuronal phenotype at stage G0 [8].

As we reported recently, the dual IGR promoter has an important role in regulating divergent gene transcription of both directions of the |-SRGAP2–FAM72-| master gene [8]. In the context of rat PC12 cells (a well-known neuronal cell model to study neurogenesis [8,43–48]), Fam72a expression (in proliferating PC12 cells stimulated by the mitogen Egf) or Srgap2 expression (in differentiating PC12 cells stimulated by nerve growth factor (Ngf)) was enhanced upon growth factor (Ngf or Egf)-mediated stimulation. Strikingly, under serum-withdrawal-induced stress and bi-directional IGR control, Egf-stimulated PC12 cells were kept alive for a long period of time with Fam72a expression, while Ngf-stimulated PC12 cells remained in a G0 stage co-expressing Srgap2 and Fam72a without proliferation [5,8].

4.3. Governance of FAM72 Expression: The IGR and Its TFBSs

A comparative genome analysis of the IGR (located between the SRGAP2 and FAM72 genes within the I-SRGAP2–FAM72-I master gene on the one hand and the gene promoters of several G2/M-phase-specific cell cycle genes on the other hand) revealed potential common regulatory elements (i.e., common TFBSs), driving the expression of those cell cycle genes and FAM72 to promote and maintain cell proliferation (Figures 3b, 4 and 5a,b). We found that many genes with increased expression during the late G2/M-phase of the cell cycle including all human FAM72 paralogs shared the same TFBS motifs for GATA binding protein 2 (GATA2) [12], E2F4, E2F6, and TFDP1 (Figures 4 and 5a,b). This indicates that their expression is co-regulated in concert with the FAM72 paralogs and implies a common temporal and spatial function, particularly fostering cell proliferation, eventually associated with the RAS signaling pathway [49–53].

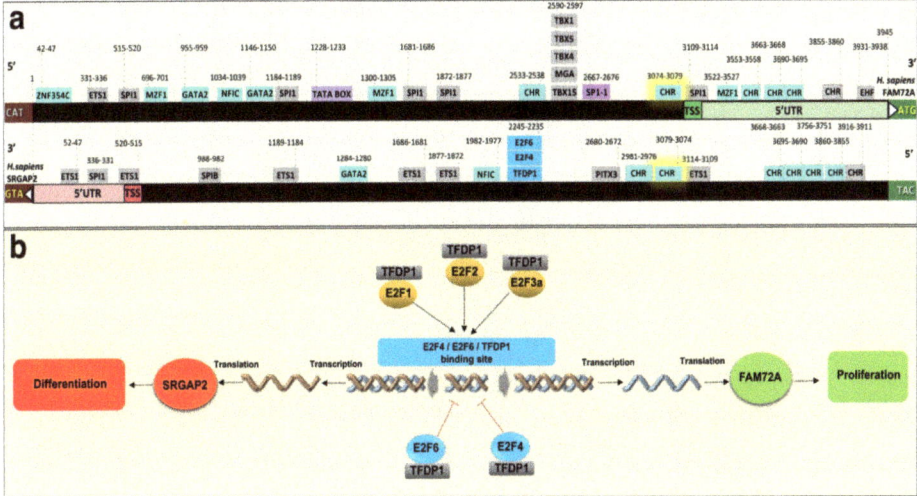

Figure 5. Integrated diagram for putative TFBSs in the intergenic region IGR between the transcription start sites (TSS) of FAM72A and SRGAP2, using the Ensembl and JASPAR databases, and the effect on the cell cycle. (**a**) Putative TFBSs on the IGR between SRGAP2 and FAM72A coding sequences in *Homo sapiens*. Multiple TFBSs are present for binding of the TFs GATA2, SPI1, MZF1, EGR1, SP1, and E2Fx (x = 1, 2, 3, 4 and 6). The open reading frames (ORFs) for FAM72A and SRGAP2 are indicated on the right and left sides, respectively. TFs that are common between FAM72 (A–D) and selected M-phase cell cycle genes are in pale blue. Investigation of the potential TFBSs on the IGR shows that FAM72A is a cell cycle gene particularly active in mitosis and under control of the DREAM and MMB-FOXM1 complexes acting on the CHR BS to regulate I-SRGAP2–FAM72A-I. The DREAM complex is composed of TFDP1, RBL2, or RBL1, the repressor E2F TF E2F4 or E2F5 and the MuvB core complex (containing LIN9, LIN37, LIN52, RBBP4 (LIN53), LIN54). The MMB–FOXM1 complex is composed of the MuvB complex (dissociated from the DREAM complex), MYBL2, and FOXM1. Notably, the CHR site (pale blue) located next to the TSS of the FAM72A gene has the highest potential to be targeted for driving FAM72A gene expression. (**b**) The crucial E2F4/E2F6/TFDP1 BS in cell fate decision. The consensus E2F4/E2F6/TFDP1 BS within the IGR could become occupied by an E2Fx family member depending on cell demand during specific cell phase stages and may be crucial for cell fate decision to activate either FAM72A (for cell proliferation and renewal) or SRGAP2 (for neural differentiation). Chr, chromosome; CHR, Cell cycle gene homology region; E2F1/2/3/4/6, E2 factor TF 1/2/3/4/6; EGR1, early growth response 1; EHF, ETS homologous factor; ETS1, E26 transformation specific proto-oncogene 1; GATA2, GATA binding protein 2; MGA, MAX dimerization protein; MZF1, Myeloid zinc finger 1; NFIC, Nuclear factor I C; SP1-1, Specificity protein 1 TFBS 1; SPI1, Spleen focus forming virus proviral integration oncogene 1; TBX15/TBX1/TBX4, T-box TFBS 15/1/4; TFDP1, TF dimerization partner 1; ZNF345C, Zinc finger protein 345C.

Additional comparative genome analysis between the FAM72 and MKI67 gene promoters also revealed common potential TFBSs for the TFs GATA2, E26 transformation specific proto-oncogene 1 (ETS1), myeloid zinc finger 1 (MZF1), and nuclear factor I C (NFIC), zinc finger protein 345C (ZNF354C) (Figures 3b and 5a) [12].

To further understand the mechanism of IGR-controlled |-SRGAP2–FAM72-| master gene expression, we performed bioinformatic analysis of TFBSs on the IGR (Figure 5a) [54]. The predicted TFBSs appear to partly explain our questions raised based on their ability to control the cell cycle and transcription regulation of this |-SRGAP2–FAM72-| master gene pair via its IGR. Specifically, we discovered E2F4, E2F6, and TFDP1 TFBSs present on the IGRs of the |-SRGAP2–FAM72A-|, |-SRGAP2C–FAM72B-|, |-SRGAP2D–FAM72C-|, and |-SRGAP2B–FAM72D-| gene pairs (Figure 5a,b). This indicates the participation of a heterodimeric E2Fx/TFDP1 complex, which may contribute to the divergent gene transcription control of FAM72A and SRGAP2, respectively (Figure 5a,b). The E2Fx family is known to consist of TF members, which all play important roles in the cell cycle control. The E2F4/E2F6/TFDP1 predicted sites on the IGR are assumed as binding sites for E2Fx family members with both gene activation or repression abilities [55–57]. Interchangeable roles of E2Fx family members were revealed by a comprehensive ChIP analysis of E2F1 (e.g., E2F1-3a activators), E2F4 (e.g., E2F4-5 canonical repressors), and E2F6 (e.g., E2F6-8 atypical repressors) in normal and tumor cells [55], while loss of one E2F member could cause a function compensation by the other E2Fs to ensure cell cycle operation [58,59]. Specifically, E2F6 encodes a member of a family of TFs that plays a crucial role in the control of the cell cycle, of which the protein lacks the transactivation and tumor suppressor protein association domains found in other E2Fx family members, and it contains a modular suppression domain that functions in the inhibition of transcription. It interacts in a complex with chromatin modifying factors. Moreover, TFDP1 encodes a member of a family of TFs that heterodimerize with E2Fx proteins to enhance their DNA-binding activity and promote transcription from E2Fx target genes. The encoded protein functions as part of this complex to control the transcriptional activity of numerous genes involved in cell cycle progression from G1 to the S phase.

In the CNS, E2Fx TFs such as E2F1, E2F2, E2F3, and E2F4, along with the pocket proteins (PPs including RB1, RB-like pocket proteins RBL1 (p107) and RBL2 (p130)), regulate NSC self-renewal via pivotal genes including SOX2, PAX6, fibroblast growth factor 2 (FGF2), distal-less homeobox 1 and 2 (DLX1, DLX2), neogenin 1 (NEO1), and neuropilin 1 (NRP1) as well as the Notch and sonic hedgehog (SHH) pathways [60–70]. Interestingly, E2F4 establishes a proper cell fate both in conjunction with or without RB1 [71,72].

Detailed spatiotemporal expression analysis of E2Fx TFs unraveled specific E2Fx activators (E2F3A) and canonical (E2F4) and atypical (E2F8) E2Fx TF repressors during the cell cycle [73]. An orchestrated accumulation of different E2Fx TF combinations control gene expression in proliferating (E2F3A-8-4) and differentiating (E2F3A-4) cells. The sequential nuclear accumulation and disappearance of E2F3A, E2F8, and E2F4 form an E2F module used to drive waves of activation and repression that support cell-cycle-dependent oscillations in gene expression necessary for cell proliferation and cell divisions. Another E2Fx TF module composed of E2F3A and E2F4 is used to extinguish cell-cycle-dependent gene expression in cells programmed to exit the cell cycle and differentiate. With an activity in the G2 phase and a TFBS within the IGR, E2F4 seems to be among the pivotal TFs controlling the |-SRGAP2–FAM72-| master gene (Figure 5).

Since E2F4 may have both functions of gene activation and repression, we assume that E2F4 could be the key that could repress FAM72A and support SRGAP2 expression during differentiation. This is consistent with the finding that E2F4 permanently accumulates in the nucleus of differentiating and differentiated cells [73].

With these important discoveries about the |-SRGAP2–FAM72-| master gene and its regulatory role regarding cell fate decision [5,8], we looked for partners to cooperate with these two genes. Among the possible candidates, E2Fx TFs and their regulatory partners, the PPs RB1, RBL1 and RBL2, are widespread and dynamic epigenetic stem cell regulators [69]. The E2Fx consensus TFBS on the IGR shows an ability to interact with various E2Fx TFs, which in turn, can bind to the IGR and govern FAM72 as well as SRGAP2 expression (Figure 5). The RB1 and E2Fx TFs make complexes called RB-E2Fx, which cooperate with a protein complex called DREAM (dimerization partner (DP), RB-like, E2F and multi-vulval class B (MuvB)), repressing G1/S cell cycle genes to move the cell cycle forward to the G2/M phase [74–76]. The conserved human DREAM complex thus has been described as an important master regulator of cell cycle genes with a decisive role in coordinating cell cycle progression [75–81].

The DREAM complex comprises TFDP1, RBL1, or RBL2, the repressor E2Fx TFs E2F4 or E2F5 and the MuvB core complex (containing LIN9, LIN37, LIN52, RBBP4 (also known as LIN53), LIN54).

LIN9, a component of the DREAM core complex, encodes a tumor suppressor protein that inhibits DNA synthesis and oncogenic transformation through association with the RB1 protein. It also interacts with a complex of other cell cycle regulators to repress cell cycle-dependent gene expression in non-dividing cells [82].

RBBP4 is a chromatin remodeling factor that encodes a ubiquitously expressed nuclear protein that belongs to a highly conserved subfamily of WD-repeat proteins [83,84]. It is involved in histone (de-) acetylation and chromatin assembly and remodeling. RBBP4 is also part of co-repressor complexes, which are integral components of transcriptional silencing. It is found among several cellular proteins that bind directly to RB1 to regulate cell proliferation and also seems to be involved in transcriptional repression of E2Fx-responsive genes [85,86].

As an integral subunit of the DREAM complex, LIN54 is a pivotal regulator of cell cycle genes, which binds to the cell division control 2 (CDC2) promoter for cell cycle progression [87].

Previously, we described FAM72 (A–D) expression specifically during the G2/M phase [12,28]. Other scientists have verified that the DREAM and MMB-FOXM1 complexes can bind genomic cell cycle gene homology region (CHR) motifs, suggesting that DREAM and MMB-FOXM1 are crucially involved in regulating FAM72 (A–D) expression during the G2/M phase (Figures 5 and 6) [12,75,76,88]. Indeed, the DREAM complex was verified to bind to the FAM72 promoter, most probably via the CHR BS on the IGR. Notably, the CHR element is conserved on the IGR across all FAM72 (A–D) (Figure 5a) [75,76]. Genome-wide association studies and experimental validation have verified FAM72D as a G2/M cell cycle gene modulated by the DREAM and MMB-FOXM1 complexes [75,76]. These complexes bind and regulate FAM72D through a CHR BS on the IGR.

The DREAM complex interacts with the CHR element and E2Fx TFBSs to inhibit G1/S cell cycle gene expression until MuvB dissociates away to associate with MMB-FOXM1 to push the cell cycle into the G2/M phase [75,76]. During quiescence and early G1 phase of the cell cycle, the DREAM–MuvB complex represses cell cycle-promoting gene expression. When the stages end, it becomes deactivated, while the MuvB complex dissociates away to associate with v-myb avian myeloblastosis viral oncogene homolog-like 2 (MYBL2) and FOXM1, forming the MMB–FOXM1 complex. This new complex promotes late cell cycle gene expression and is required to pass through the G2/M phases [80]. FOXM1 gets phosphorylated during the M phase and regulates the expression of several cell cycle genes such as cyclin B1 (CCNB1) and cyclin D1 (CCND1). It is a crucial TF also found in fostering GBM development and progression by regulating key factors involved in cell proliferation, epithelial to mesenchymal transition (EMT), invasion, angiogenesis, and upregulating WNT1/β-catenin signaling [89].

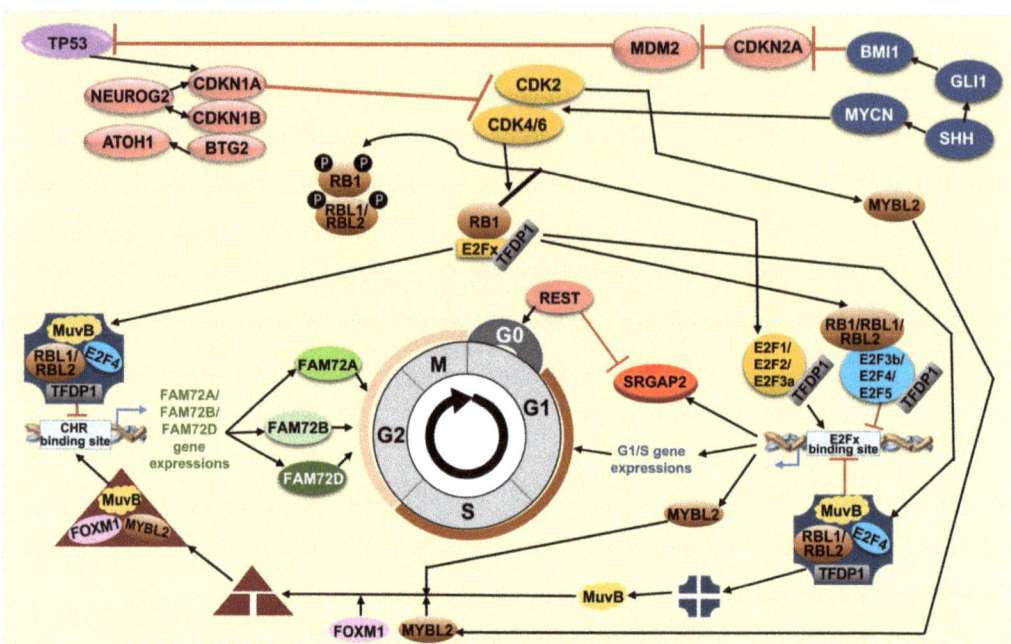

Figure 6. FAM72 paralog-specific cell cycle signaling mediated by various TFs. DREAM (blue rectangle) is composed of TFDP1, RBL1 or RBL2, the E2Fx TFs E2F4, or E2F5 and the MuvB core complex (consists of LIN9, LIN37, LIN52, RBBP4 (LIN53), LIN54). During quiescence/G0 and early G1 phases of the cell cycle, DREAM represses cell cycle gene expression. When these G0/G1 stages end, DREAM gets inactivated so that the MuvB complex dissociates away to form a new complex with the MYBL2 and FOXM1 called the MMB-FOXM1 complex (red triangle, MuvB, MYBL2 and FOXM1). This new complex promotes late cell cycle gene expression and is required to pass through the G2/M phases [80]. At the end of the M-phase, REST inhibits neuronal gene expression (such as SRGAP2) to allow re-entry into a new cycle, thus maintaining NSC renewal and FAM72 expression. Once it receives a neurogenic signal, REST is degraded, FAM72 expression is blocked, and SGRAP2 expression is initiated for neuronal differentiation. ATOH1, Atonal basic helix-loop-helix (bHLH) TF 1; BMI1, B cell-specific Moloney murine leukemia virus integration site 1; BTG2, B-cell translocation gene 2;CDK2/4/6, Cyclin dependent kinase 2/4/6; CDKN1A/1B/2A, Cyclin dependent kinase inhibitor 1A/1B/2A; FOXM1, Forkhead box M1; GLI1, Glioma-associated oncogene family zinc finger 1; MDM2, Murine double minute 2; MuvB, Multi-vulval class B complex; MYBL2, v-myb avian myeloblastosis viral oncogene homolog-like 2; MYCN, v-myc avian myelocytomatosis viral oncogene neuroblastoma derived; NEUROG2, Neurogenin 2; REST, Transcriptional repressor RE1 silencing transcription factor; SHH, Sonic hedgehog signaling molecule.

The cell cycle promoting regulation indeed comes from the interaction between the FOXM1 protein—a part of the MMB-FOXM1 complex—and the FAM72A [75,76,78,81], FAM72B [40,75,76,78,81], and FAM72D [25,75,76,78,81] promotors, confirming that all FAM72 (A–D) paralogs are regulated by this pathway during the G2/M phase in proliferating cells (i.e., NSCs and cancer cells). Since the FAM72 function may contribute to the mitotic spindle or the kinetochore-centromere complex formations and activities, loss of MMB-FOXM1 or FAM72 (A–D) function may cause spindle assembly chaos and mitotic catastrophe (Figure 6) [12,25].

Taken together, FAM72A, FAM72B, and FAM72D might be regulated by the DREAM complex as well as the RB-E2F3b/4/5 complex to be suppressed for a while by interacting with the putative E2F4/E2F6/TFDP1 TFBS, until the E2F1/2/3a/activators promote essential G1/S gene expressions and thereby foster cell cycle progression into G2/M phases and FAM72 activation via the MMB–FOXM1 complex. Thus, cell cycle progression and control depend on targeting the genomic E2F4/E2F6/TFDP1 TFBS (for G1/S phase) and the CHR motif (for G2/M phase) on the IGR with pivotal regulators involved such as DREAM, the RB family members-E2Fx-, and the MMB-FOXM1 complexes.

4.4. FAM72 Expression and the RE1 Silencing Transcription Factor

REST was initially identified as a transcriptional repressor that represses neuronal genes in non-neuronal tissues [90,91]. However, depending on the cellular context, this gene can act as either an oncogene or a tumor suppressor, and its specific role in glioma remains controversial [92,93]. The encoded protein is a member of the Kruppel-type zinc finger transcription factor family. It represses transcription by binding a DNA sequence element called the neuron-restrictive silencer element [94,95]. The protein is also found in undifferentiated neuronal progenitor cells and it is thought that this repressor may act as a master negative regulator of neurogenesis [96–98]. Alternatively-spliced transcript variants have been described [99]. Expression correlation analyses showed a weak correlation of FAM72A with REST in glioma (Figure 4d).

4.5. FAM72 Expression and Long Non-Coding RNAs

Additionally, it has been hypothesized that IGR regulation of the |-SRGAP2–FAM72-| master gene is susceptible to long non-coding RNAs (lncRNAs) [1,5,8]. Long non-coding RNAs (LncRNAs) are of particular interest due to the wide variety of roles they play in gene regulation. LncRNAs have been reported to regulate transcription (via epigenetic mechanisms [100,101]) as well as pluripotency and cellular reprogramming [102] and have been implicated in a variety of diseases, notably cancers of the breast [103], colon [104], stomach [105], lymph [24], and the CNS [106].

Recent reports about the oncogenic role of lncRNA revealed interactions between a lncRNA and the centrosomal protein CEP112 as well as the breast cancer type 1 susceptibility protein BRCA1, which resulted in mitotic abnormalities and malignancies [107]. The particular lncRNA, called genomic instability inducing RNA (Ginir), functions normally during embryonic development and is enriched in the brain. The expression of Ginir, along with its partner genomic instability inducing RNA antisense (Giniras), was regulated in a spatio-temporal manner and overexpression of Ginir led to tumorigenesis [107]. This ties in with the role of lncRNA in FAM72 expression. Since FAM72 is also expressed predominantly in NSCs, it is likely that the transcription of the |-SRGAP2–FAM72-| master gene is regulated by a similar pair of lncRNAs on the IGR. FAM72 co-expresses with centrosomal proteins in cancer tissues [12], and it is possible that dysfunction of the lncRNA on the IGR would lead to loss of control over FAM72 expression, thereby leading to cellular proliferation.

4.6. Anti-Apoptotic Features of |-SRGAP2–FAM72-| via TP53

Our previous study showed an early anti-apoptotic rescue program activated via the IGR-based expression of the |-Srgap2–Fam72a-| master gene under serum-free stress conditions in rat PC12 cells. Tp53 was thought to influence Fam72 activities in this stress response to rescue cells from apoptosis by driving them into the G0 phase, a possible new anti-apoptotic functional ability of Fam72a [8]. This anti-apoptotic activity of Fam72a was recently consolidated with its highly correlated expression with BIRC5 (Figure 4, Supplementary Materials Figure S2) [108], a member of the family of IAPs that prevent apoptotic cell death [109]. IAP family members usually contain multiple BIR domains, but BIRC5 encodes a protein with only a single BIR domain. The encoded protein also lacks a C-terminus RING finger domain. Along with FAM72A, the FOXM1 protein was also found to be similarly co-regulated with BIRC5 [108]. BIRC5 expression is high in most tumors; however, its usefulness as a prognostic marker is still a controversial issue [110,111].

Although TP53-mediated impact on FAM72 might be indirect, we found a TATA box and a SP1-1 TFBS on the IGR, which could be bound by TP53 with high affinity, thereby eventually affecting FAM72 directly or indirectly by blocking those positions for other TFs (Figure 5) [112–114].

On the other hand, TP53 could also bind SP1-1 TFBS on the IGR for transcription regulation by competing with the SP1 protein. To enter G0, downregulation of cell division cycle 25C (CDC25C), another key molecule for cell cycle progression through the G2/M phase [115–117], is mediated by TP53 via two independent mechanisms. One of these involves direct binding to the CDC25C promoter [114].

In another scenario, FAM72 expression was regulated by both DREAM and MMB–FOXM1 complexes under the control of TP53, particularly in cancer cells [75,76]. Through inhibition of cyclin-dependent kinase (CDK) activity by the CDK inhibitor 1A (encoded by CDKN1A), FAM72A and FAM72D were downregulated by TP53 in response to DNA damage via interfering with the DREAM and MMB-FOXM1 complex binding via the CHR BS motifs on the IGR. This prevents the FAM72A and FAM72D expressions, respectively, thus confirming FAM72A and FAM72D as G2/M-phase-promoting cell cycle genes (Figures 5 and 7) [75].

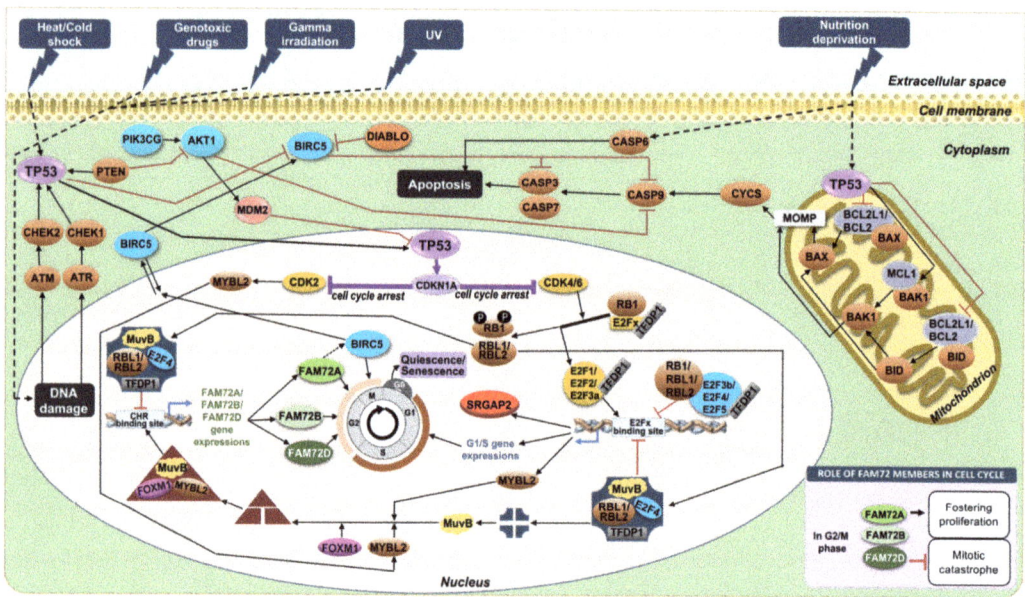

Figure 7. The influence of TP53 on FAM72 paralogs directly regulates the cell cycle in cancer. Upon a stressful DNA-damaging signal (e.g., gamma irradiation), TP53 gets activated to mediate cell arrest in G0 to give the cell quiescence for cell repair or, if impossible, to induce the alternative pathway for apoptosis. TP53-mediated cell cycle arrest is conveyed by CDKN1A (p21) causing inhibition of the cell-cycle promoting the CDK4/6-E2Fx pathway; consequently, the G1/S phase genes remain blocked. The TP53-CDKN1A-CDK4/6 pathway also causes activation of DREAM, which in turn blocks FAM72 expression via the CHR element within the IGR of the |-SRGAP2–FAM72-| master gene.

Notably, investigation of TP53 interaction network showed that FAM72A, FAM72B, and FAM72D expressions positively and negatively correlated with TP53 expression in multiple types of cancer under unknown pathways. All FAM72 and TP53 are expressed increasingly in kidney renal papillary-cell carcinoma, but are only highly expressed in FAM72B and TP53 in pancreatic adeno-carcinoma, pheochromocytoma, and paraganglioma. In contrast, the TP53 expression went down, while the three FAM72 were upregulated in lung adeno-carcinoma and prostate adeno-carcinoma [118]. The correlations indicate that all members of the FAM72 family have important roles in tumorigenesis and crossing regulation with the tumor suppressor TP53.

Taken together, FAM72A, FAM72B, and FAM72D can be regulated by the DREAM complex by interacting with the putative E2Fx BS from cell cycle G0/G1/S phases, which are controlled by the RB-E2Fx complex—a specific E2Fx TF complex for cell cycle gene expressions. This pathway was also regulated through inhibition of CDKN1A coordinated by TP53 (Figures 5 and 7). In summary, all FAM72 (A–D) paralogs and TP53 appear to have strictly correlated expression patterns with a possible crucial functional impact on each other. On the topic of interfering with FAM72 expression in the context of tumor cell proliferation, the tumor suppressor TP53-FAM72 linked pathway could be important as an option to inhibit cancer cell proliferation.

The TP53-CDKN1A pathway also takes away the MYBL2 phosphorylation by CDK2, resulting in the activation of MMB-FOXM1, which in turn, could act on the CHR element on the IGR of |-SRGAP2–FAM72-| master gene for FAM72 activation [119,120]. If the DNA damage is too strong (e.g., causing a mutation in a cancer driver proto-oncogene or even in TP53 itself), G2/M phase genes and FAM72 expression remains at high level fostering cancer cell proliferation [12,75,76,78,81]. AKT1, AK strain transforming serine/threonine kinase 1; ATM, Ataxia-telangiectasia mutated serine/threonine kinase; ATR, Ataxia telangiectasia and Rad3-related serine/threonine kinase; BAK1, BCL2 antagonist/killer 1; BAX, BCL2 associated X; BCL2, B cell lymphoma 2; BCL2L1, BCL2 like 1; BID, Bcl-2 homology 3 interacting domain death agonist; CASP3/6/7/9, Caspase 3/6/7/9; CHEK1/2, Checkpoint kinase 1/2; CYCS, Cytochrome c, somatic; DIABLO, Direct inhibitor of apoptosis binding protein with low pI; MCL1, Myeloid cell leukemia 1; MOMP, Mitochondrial outer membrane permeabilization; PIK3CG, Phosphatidylinositol-4,5-bisphosphate 3-kinase catalytic subunit gamma.

5. Methylation of FAM72 in Cancerous Tissues

DNA methylation is a well-studied epigenetic modification and involves the covalent attachment of a methyl group to the 5-carbon residue of cytosine [121]. These attachments usually occur on genomic regions with a high density of CpG nucleotides, called CpG islands, but methylation has also been reported in non-CpG regions [122]. Modifications in DNA methylation have been reported from various disorders including multiple sclerosis, diabetes, multiple human cancers as well as neurological disorders [123–127]. Both hyper- and hypomethylation at the CpG islands have been associated with cancers, and there has been a lot of work to understand the mechanisms regulating this behavior [128–130].

We verified the hypomethylation of FAM72A in GBM, which revealed that expression of FAM72A in GBM could depend on its methylation status [12]. Investigation of the methylation status of FAM72A in non-neuronal tissues revealed that increased expression of FAM72A in lung and uterine cancer tissues appeared to be rather independent of its methylation status (Figure 8a). However, methylation-expression analysis of breast and liver cancer tissues showed an increase in mRNA expression corresponding to a decrease in promoter methylation. The methylation status of the FAM72 promoter thus appears to be important—to a certain extent—in some tissues, namely GBM, breast, and liver cancers, whereas other factors come into play in other non-neuronal tissues. The increased FAM72 expression in non-neuronal tissues is driven by somatic mutations in oncogenes, which would then trigger the signaling cascade for promoting cellular proliferation and fostering tumorigenesis and metastasis [12]. Another factor responsible for increased FAM72 expression could be binding of TFs, which regulate other proliferative genes. We described GATA2 as one of the candidates that could regulate both FAM72 as well as prophase/metaphase cell cycle genes [12].

Comparing the corresponding methylation-expression statuses in SRGAP2 revealed that there is no clear difference in its methylation status, which correlates to no or minor changes in its expression status across the same cancer tissues. Indeed, SRGAP2 itself shows no changes in its comparatively higher expression (with FAM72A) with slight differences in promoter methylation of SRGAP2 in breast, liver, lung, and uterine cancers (Figure 8). However, a decrease of methylation (demethylation) on the SRGAP2 gene body in GBM with no changes in its gene expression indicates that this genomic methylation does not affect SRGAP2 gene expression itself, but may rather have an impact on the other coupled gene FAM72A (Figure 8). This also fits with SRGAP2's established role in neuronal differentiation, synaptic maturation as well as neuronal migration [5,8,16,17,26,131]. Usually, SRGAP2 is mobilized to foster neuronal differentiation and synaptic plasticity [4,5,8,16–21]. However, in non-neuronal cells, SRGAP2 expression is needed for rearranging the cytoskeleton required for cell-specific locomotion and motility and, if genomic rearranging occurs within the genomic SRGAP2 body, its tumor suppressor function is abolished, and metastasis is induced [26,132–134]. Overall, however, it appears that in cancer tissues including GBM [135], the methylation status does not have a major impact on the |-SRGAP2–FAM72-| master gene.

In the brain, the hypothalamus, cerebral cortex, and hippocampus have been reported to be rich sources of oxidized 5-methylcytosine (5mC), thus converting it to 5-hydroxymethylcytosine (5hmC) [139] on enhancers [140]. Demethylation (5hmC) is significantly increased when NSCs and neural progenitor cells (NPGs) differentiate into neurons [141]. This is in contrast to the hypomethylation observed during oncogenesis in FAM72 or the lack of methylation changes observed in SRGAP2, thus confirming that the proliferative and neurogenic mechanisms occur via completely different mechanisms under normal and pathophysiological conditions in the |-SRGAP2–FAM72-| master gene. 5mC-loss/5hmC-gain loci are enriched in active enhancers and motifs for key binding factors involved with neurogenic genes during neurogenesis, as is expected for neurogenic SRGAP2 expression during neuronal differentiation under physiological conditions [142]. The TET1-3 proteins are connected with neural fate decisions [141–144]. TET2 is a key protein involved in the development and cancer regulating gene expression via oxidization of 5mCs, thereby promoting locus-specific reversal of DNA methylation [145,146]. Thus, TET2 mutations are associated with multiple neurodegenerative diseases [147] and variations of the TET2 gene in either non-coding or coding regions might cause alterations of the homeostasis of key aging-related processes [147].

This indicates that TET2 and the 5mC/5hmC mechanism may contribute to |-SRGAP2–FAM72-| master gene activity during neurogenesis (e.g., the 5hmC-gain of neurogenic SRGAP2 during neural differentiation) (Figure 9). Partially differentiated NSCs going into NPGs might be able to concurrently express FAM72 and SRGAP2, thus not resulting in complete loss of 5mC and still gaining some 5hmC. The full 5hmC-gain needed is met only once neurogenic commitment is accomplished, when SRGAP2 is sufficiently expressed and FAM72A expression is completely blocked (e.g., in post-mitotic differentiated neurons).

Moreover, multiple myeloma [25] and breast cancers [25] showed that FAM72 expression may be dependent on its methylation status. Demethylation (5mC → 5hmC) of FAM72D occurs mainly in intronic enhancers (but outside the IGR area) and could activate FAM72D to maintain mitotic fidelity. This probably also works for the other FAM72 member expressions such as FAM72A, FAM72B, and FAM72C (due to high homology (99%) in amino acid sequences) [25]. As for GBM, Kan et al. could not identify epigenetically affected FAM72, though our data showed a change in the methylation status (Figure 8) [12,135].

This observation is also in line with our results obtained in PC12 cells [8]. The hypothesis here is whether GATA2 TFBS (present three times on the IGR of the human |-SRGAP2–FAM72-| master gene, Figure 5) can act as a binding target for this pioneering TF since GATA2 may not directly mediate DNA methylation, but may have an impact on DNA packaging controlled by histone methylation and acetylation [142,148]. GATA TFs can either activate gene expression by synergy with another co-activator (which recruits a histone methyltransferase and/or a histone acetyl transferase) or repress gene expression by cooperating with a co-repressor to recruit a histone demethylase and/or a histone deacetylase [148]. Thus, the GATA2 TFBSs on the IGR may play important roles in the governance of the |-SRGAP2–FAM72-| master gene expression and require further investigation.

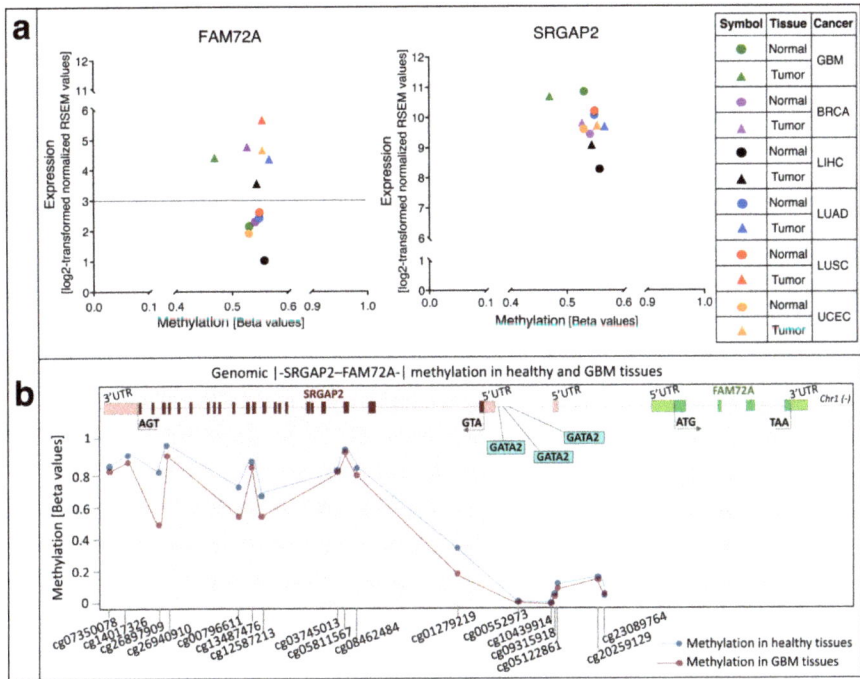

Figure 8. (**a**) Comparison between methylation status and expression levels of FAM72A and SRGAP2 across normal and tumor tissues in GBM, breast, lung, uterine, and liver cancers. Mean methylation beta values were plotted against mean RNA-sequencing by expectation-maximization (RSEM) expression values (log2-transformed normalized RSEM values). Circles indicate normal tissues and triangles indicate cancer tissues. Green symbols indicate GBM data, purple symbols indicate breast invasive carcinoma data, black symbols indicate liver hepatocellular carcinoma data, blue symbols indicate lung adenocarcinoma data, red symbols indicate lung squamous cell carcinoma data, and orange symbols indicate uterine corpus endometrial carcinoma data. In the case of FAM72A, the differences in methylation status between normal and cancer tissues vary among GBM, breast, and liver cancer, where less methylation leads to a two-fold difference in FAM72A expression in cancer tissues. Methylation status between normal and cancer tissues is similar in lung and uterine cancer tissues. In the case of lung tissues, the cancer samples show higher FAM72A expression and a higher methylation status as well, indicating that the FAM72A promoter methylation alone may not be responsible for its increased expression but other factors such as mutations in cancer driver-oncogenes may promote increased FAM72 expression and foster cancer cell proliferation [12,28]. For SRGAP2, the differences in methylation status between normal and cancer tissues is not significant, except eventually for GBM. However, there are no significant changes in SRGAP2 expression in most tissues. Hence, the change of methylation levels within the genomic SRGAP2 area in GBM does not affect SRGAP2 expression. Mean beta values as well as mean mRNA expression values were retrieved from the Wanderer database [136]. BRCA, breast cancer (breast invasive carcinoma); GBM, glioblastoma multiforme; LIHC, liver hepatocellular carcinoma; LUAD, lung adenocarcinoma; LUSC, lung squamous cell carcinoma; UCEC, uterine corpus endometrial carcinoma. (**b**) Investigation of the specific methylation probes on the genomic |-SRGAP2–FAM72A-| master gene in both normal and GBM tissues. Demethylation is described as a decrease in the methylation score of all probes bound to cancer tissue genomes compared to normal tissue genomes. Unfortunately, most probes are focused on the genomic SRGAP2 gene body and IGR area, while no probes could be identified to bind to the genomic FAM72 gene body area. As above, almost no change of SRGAP2 expression level was observed throughout many cancer types including GBM. In contrast, the discovered demethylations may have an impact on regulating the other part of the |-SRGAP2–FAM72-| master gene (i.e., modulating FAM72A expression). The probe information was retrieved from the HumanMethylation450 v1.2 manifest file on the Illumina database (https://support.illumina.com/downloads/infinium_humanmethylation450_product_files.html) (accessed date: 20 December 2020) and aligned the source sequences to genome reference consortium human build 38 patch release 13 (GRCh38.p13) using the BLAST-like alignment tool (BLAT) function from the Integrative Genomics Viewer (IGV) [137,138].

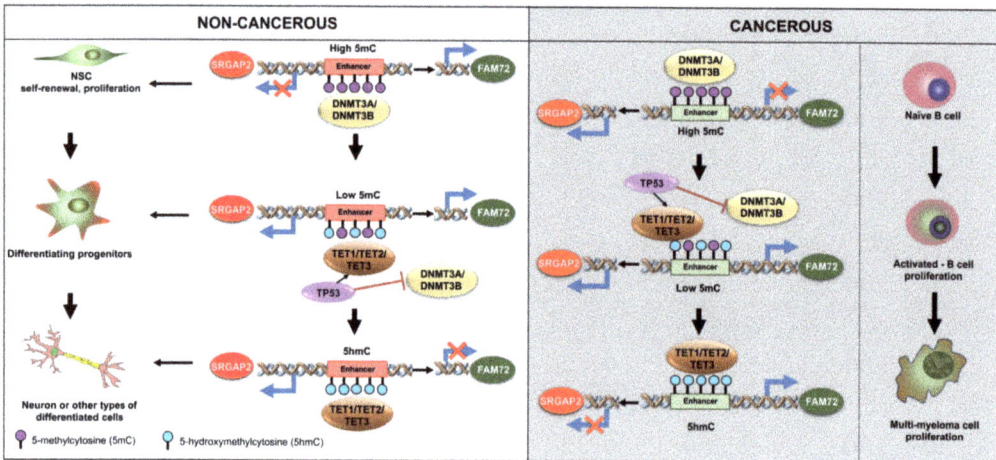

Figure 9. Effects of methylation and demethylation on the expression of the master gene |-SRGAP2–FAM72-|. The epigenetic modifications during neurogenesis can control FAM72 expression for cell fate decision. Dysregulation causes CSC formation and tumorigenesis. In proliferating (non-cancerous) NSCs, demethylation or hypomethylation (such as 5-hydroxymethylcytosine (5hmC) or the loss of the methyl group in the 5-methylcytosine nucleotide (5mC)), were demonstrated to activate neurogenic genes such as SRGAP2 to mediate neural differentiation [142]. As a consequence, FAM72 is deactivated. In cancer, demethylation is crucial for FAM72 activation during CSC proliferation. In the case of glioma genesis, FAM72 is silenced in glia progenitor cells until activated TP53 replaces the methylation factors DNA methyltransferase 3 alpha/beta (DNMT3A/DNMT3B) for demethylation factors TET1/TET2/TET3 so that FAM72 is activated for proliferation and forming GBM cells, which is in line with the genomic hypomethylation of the FAM72 promoter region in our previous study (Figure 8) [12,149,150]. FAM72 expression is activated outside the CNS only under cancerous conditions by mutated protooncogenes and genomic FAM72 demethylation by TET family members to support the proliferation of cancerous cells including multiple myeloma [25,151].

6. FAM72 and FAM107A in GBM

FAM107A (also known as downregulated in renal cell carcinoma 1 [DRR1]) is a novel unique protein family that exhibits functional similarity with heat shock proteins (HSPs) during the cellular stress response with diverse functions in cancer and the nervous system [152]. Recent evidence indicates that FAM107A is involved in GBM invasion and progression, possibly through the induction of EMT activation by phosphorylation of AKT1 [153]. Accordingly, antibody (against glioblastoma stem cells surface markers glycoprotein cluster of differentiation 44 (CD44) and ephrin receptor A2 (EPHA2)-antisense oligodeoxynucleotides (ASOs) strategy against FAM107A) were established for the treatment of GBM [154].

In agreement with FAM107A as a tumor suppressor gene [152,155,156], FAM72A shows a negative expression correlation in GBM (Figure 4b).

7. FAM72 and Its Role as a Potential Biomarker in Clinical Cancer Diagnostics

Liquid biopsies carrying circulating tumor-derived material, also called the "tumor circulome," consist of circulating tumor DNA (ctDNA), circulating tumor RNA (ctRNA), circulating tumor proteins (ctPs), tumor-derived extracellular vesicles (EVs), tumor-educated platelets (TEPs), and circulating tumor cells (CTCs), among others, which have promising diagnostic potential at each stage of cancer [157]. Liquid biopsies have a great potential to overcome existing limitations of tissue biopsies, particularly in light of sampling and analysis of such liquid biological sources, typically blood, for cancer diagnosis, screening, and prognosis. The 'tumor circulome' can be directly or indirectly used as a source of cancer biomarkers in liquid biopsies, particularly ctDNA, ctRNA, and ctPs. FAM72, at the ctDNA, ctRNA, and ctP level, could possibly serve as biomarkers for clinical diagnostics of cancer as its expression is usually limited to proliferating NSCs.

8. FAM72 and Its Role in Cancer Therapy: Therapeutic Options against Tumorigenic FAM72

Targeting FAM72 could thus be a viable treatment method for several cancer types outside the CNS because knockout of neural-specific FAM72 gene function in non-neuronal tissue may cause spindle assembly defects outside the CNS, followed by cell differentiation, senescence, or death by mitotic catastrophe in all non-neuronal proliferating cancer cells. FAM72 is an attractive target for therapy as it is a proliferative marker expressed during the late G2/M-phase of the cell cycle as well as its low expression in normal non-neuronal tissues [3,12,158], and multiple potential approaches are possible.

8.1. Therapeutic Options against Tumorigenic FAM72: RNA Interference (RNAi)

RNAi has emerged as a very effective tool for in vivo selective silencing of gene transcription, and substantial progress has been made in analyzing the therapeutic potential of various RNAi products. There are certain advantages of using RNAi for cancer therapy including the ability to target any gene including FAM72A [4], low dosages, and extended inhibition after a single dose [159]. Recently conducted clinical trials against solid tumors are promising, with the RNAi being delivered via nanoparticles [159,160]. Short hairpin-loop RNAs (shRNAs) have been demonstrated to knockdown FAM72A activity, leading to differentiation in NSCs [4]. This proves the efficacy of the approach in developing therapy against FAM72. Another approach would be to target both small interfering RNAs (siRNAs) as well as telomerase reverse transcriptase and/or MKI67 [161]. Briefly, the authors constructed adenovirus containing siRNAs targeting both MKI67 as well as the telomerase reverse transcriptase. Gene silencing for multiple oncogenes using more than one siRNA have been demonstrated before [162], and the experiment by Fang et al. [161] inhibited renal cancer cells in vitro. An oncolytic vector containing siRNAs targeted toward FAM72A as well as telomerase reverse transcriptases could prove effective without affecting normal cells, especially in non-neuronal tissues.

Another approach would be the application of ASOs. ASOs are synthetically generated nucleotide sequences, about 12–25 bases long, which can be tailored according to the target sequence of interest. Intracellular binding of the ASO to its target mRNA results in RNAse cleavage, thereby leading to a lack of mRNA translation and protein formation. Currently, there are approximately 90 ongoing clinical cancer trials evaluating treatment with ASOs, with a majority being in phase I [163,164]. Animal models have proved the efficacy in inhibiting tumor formation using MKI67 ASOs, however, issues remain with optimizing dosage and nuclease degradation susceptibility [165,166]. There have been some successes using ASO cancer trials. OT-101, a phosphorothioate ASO designed for the targeted inhibition of human transforming growth factor beta 2 (TGFβ2) mRNA, has proceeded to the phase I/II clinical trial and demonstrated encouraging results [167]. AZD9150, a STAT3-inhibiting ASO, has demonstrated tumor suppressive activity in lung and lymphoma models as well as in a phase1b trial of pretreated lymphoma patients [168,169]. Another group reported that AZD9150 increases drug sensitivity and decreases tumorigenicity in neuroblastomas [170]. Recruitment for AZD9150 trials in colorectal, pancreatic, and lung cancer is ongoing (NCT02983578) [171].

Although RNAi-based drug therapeutic trials have been ongoing for some time, it was only in 2018 that the Food and Drug Administration (FDA) approved the first RNAi-based drug ONPATTRO, which is used to treat transthyretin amyloidosis. Due to a better understanding of the clinical development process required for RNAi therapeutics, more candidates are presently in development and trials, especially for cancer [172]. Selection and design of a delivery vector for RNA duplexes targeted toward FAM72 would be critical. Benayoun et al. have already demonstrated RNA silencing for FAM72, utilizing shRNA lentiviral constructs [4]. Alternatively, gRNA delivery via any of the methods above-mentioned could be performed to knockout FAM72.

8.2. Therapeutic Options against Tumorigenic FAM72: CRISPR-Cas9

An alternative mechanism to knockout FAM72 in cancer tissues would be to use the clustered regularly interspersed short palindromic repeats (CRISPR)-CRISPR-associated protein (Cas) 9 gene editing tool. Briefly, CRISPR and Cas target foreign viral DNA as part of the adaptive immune system in bacteria [173]. A combination of trans-activating RNA (tracrRNA) and CRISPR targeting RNA (crRNA), together known as small guide RNA (sgRNA or sg FAM72-RNA), guide Cas proteins to the targeted foreign viral (or tumorigenic FAM72) DNA, which is then degraded [174]. The sg FAM72-RNA in combination with the Cas9 protein from Streptococcus pyogenes form the popular CRISPR-Cas9 gene editing tool [175–177]. A nuclease deficient Cas9 (dCas9) system combined with a transcriptional repressor protein such as the Kruppel-associated box (KRAB) [178,179] that target the transcription start site for FAM72 would be ideal to knockdown FAM72 in vivo at the site of the tumor [179–183]. Since FAM72 is overexpressed in non-neuronal cancer tissues, such a system would only affect the cancer tissues, leading to greater specificity. The delivery mechanism could be via lipid nanoparticles, similar to siRNA (Figure 10) [184].

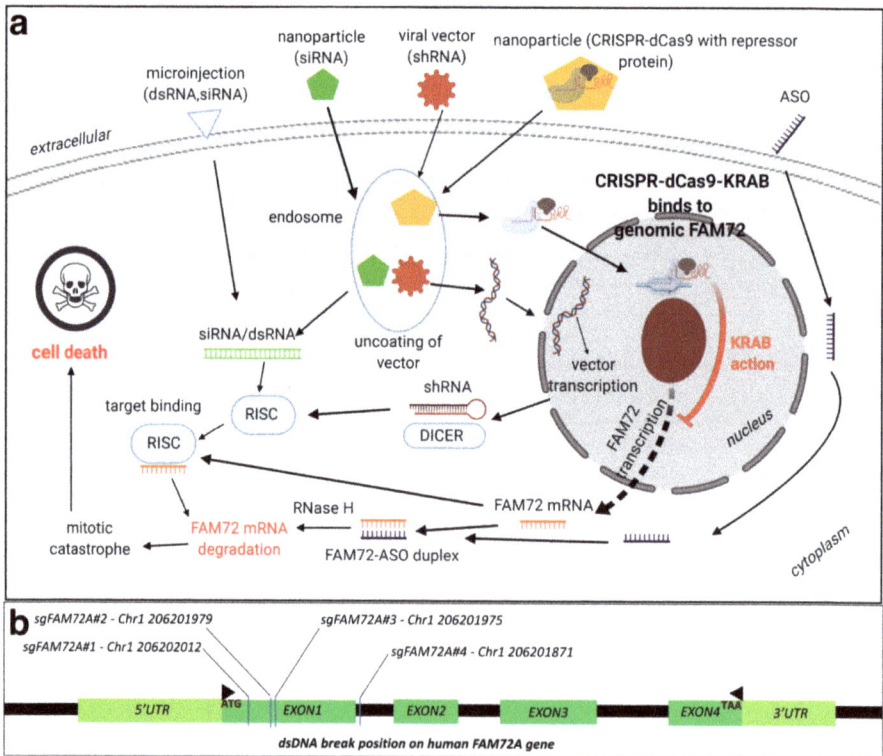

Figure 10. (**a**) Mechanisms of FAM72 knockdown using RNAi and CRISPR for the possible treatment of various types of cancer. Exogenous double-stranded RNA (dsRNA) or siRNA can be delivered via microinjection or lipid nanoparticles. The dsRNA or siRNA is released from the endosome after which it binds to the RNA-induced silencing complex (RISC). This complex then binds to the FAM72 mRNA, leading to the degradation of the whole complex. If shRNA is delivered via plasmid or viral vectors, the RNA is processed in the nucleus and exported into the cytoplasm. The Dicer enzyme processes shRNA into siRNA and then binds it to the RISC, followed by loading onto the target mRNA, and the resulting complex is degraded as before. Alternatively, the CRISPR-dCas9 with a transcriptional repressor protein is delivered via lipid nanoparticles. After entering the endosome, the CRISPR-dCas9 complex is released and it enters the nucleus. The Cas9 nuclease is directed to the target DNA by its bound sgRNA. Following binding of the dCas9 complex with the FAM72 target DNA, the repressor will attach to the transcriptional start site of FAM72, thereby resulting in a knockdown of transcription

and thus, prevention of spindle formation causing mitotic catastrophe followed by cell death. ASOs delivered into the cell binding directly to the mRNA transcript, resulting in RNAse degradation. Cas, CRISPR-associated proteins; CRISPR, clustered regularly interspersed short palindromic repeats; dCas9, nuclease deficient Cas9; dsDNA/RNA, double stranded DNA/RNA; KRAB, Kruppel-associated box; sgRNA, single guide RNA; shRNA, short hairpin loop RNA; siRNA, small interfering RNA. (**b**) Double-strand break positions of CRISPR/Cas9 application on the human FAM72A gene. The sgFAM72A#1, sgFAM72A#2, sgFAM72A#3, sgFAM72A#4 have been used to target and break within exon 1 of FAM72A to interrupt FAM72A gene transcription. sgFAM72A, single guide FAM72A: target DNA positions to be recognized and cleaved by the CRISPR/Cas9 system for FAM72A gene expression knockout.

8.3. Therapeutic Options against Tumorigenic FAM72: Chemotherapy

FAM72 and its paralogs could also be targeted via chemotherapy options using targeted drugs. We conducted an *in silico* binding study to predict potential ligand binding sites on FAM72A [185]. We found potential Zn^{2+} and Fe^{3+} binding sites along with possible binding for the organic compound RSM: (2s)-2-(acetylamino)-N-methyl-4-[(R)-methylsulfinyl] butanamide) [185].

Structure-based drug design (SBDD) is rapidly growing with the development of new technologies (e.g., high-throughput screening, molecular docking, pharmacophore mapping, quantitative structure-activity/property/toxicity relationship (QSAR/QSPR/QSTR), and virtual screening) to interpret, guide, and advance experimental biomedical research to achieve success in anti-cancer drug discovery [186–190]. SBDD methods analyze three-dimensional (3D) structures of macromolecule, typically of proteins or RNA, to identify key sites and interactions, which are important for their specific biological functions [187]. Understanding key sites and interactions can be used to design potential drug candidates that can interfere with essential interactions of the target protein and thus interrupt signaling pathways for survival and progression of cancer cells [187,191]. This requires knowledge of the 3D structure of the drug candidate and how its shape and charge cause it to interact with its biological target, ultimately revealing a therapeutic effect [187,192].

As discussed above in this review, increasing evidence indicates that FAM72 is a potential therapeutic target for the treatment of cancers [1,3,8,158], especially GBM [12] and ACC [28]. In essence, 3D protein structures and understanding ligand–protein interactions of FAM72 represent the key and even obligatory steps in FAM72-targated drug design for the development of a useful treatment for GBM and ACC. There is an urgent need to advance the FAM72-targeted drug design process, and we employed a comprehensive in silico 3D protein determination strategy to determine the 3D protein structure of FAM72A and further identify potential ligand–protein interactions of FAM72A (Figure 11) [185]. An integrated approach combining homology modeling and de novo modeling was applied to obtain a reliable 3D protein structure of FAM72A [185]. In the homology modeling, a homologous template search was performed in various databases (e.g., National Center for Biotechnology Information-Protein Data Bank (NCBI-PDB), Phyre2, 3D-JIGSAW, Swiss Model, and RaptorX) [185]. Additionally, 3D FAM72A protein structure models were also obtained from Phyre2, 3DJIGSAW, Swiss Model, and RaptorX tools. Furthermore, an optimized prediction with the Modeller program [193–195] using templates, 1YQ3_D, 4OGC_A, 4OGE_A, 3GA3_A, 3MCA_B, 1I8D_B, 4M0M_A, 2FJA_A, and 3UK7_A (obtained from NCBI-PDB, Phyre2, 3D-JIGSAW, Swiss Model, and RaptorX) revealed that the monomeric 3D FAM72A protein structure, based on the 3GA3_A template, was the most reliable model in terms of stereochemical parameter evaluations (i.e., G-factor, Ramachandran plot analysis, and additional comparative iterative threading assembly refinement (I-TASSER) analysis) [185]. To this end, protein-ligand binding site prediction based on BioLiP protein function database screening (based on COACH, TM-SITE, S-SITE, COFACTOR, and ConCavity methods) [196,197] revealed that FAM72A is a Zn^{2+}- or Fe^{3+}-containing protein, which could potentially interact with the organic molecule RSM (Figure 11) [185]. Taken together, these data suggest a theoretical view of the 3D structure model of FAM72A and its ligand-binding sites [185]. In our view, these structural and protein–ligand interaction data provide a basis of FAM72A protein ligand-binding sites, which require further investigation using well-defined in vitro and in vivo experiments to confirm the therapeutic activity of the suggested compound as potential leads for drug discovery screenings for the treatment of FAM72A-driven cancers (e.g., GBM and ACC) [185].

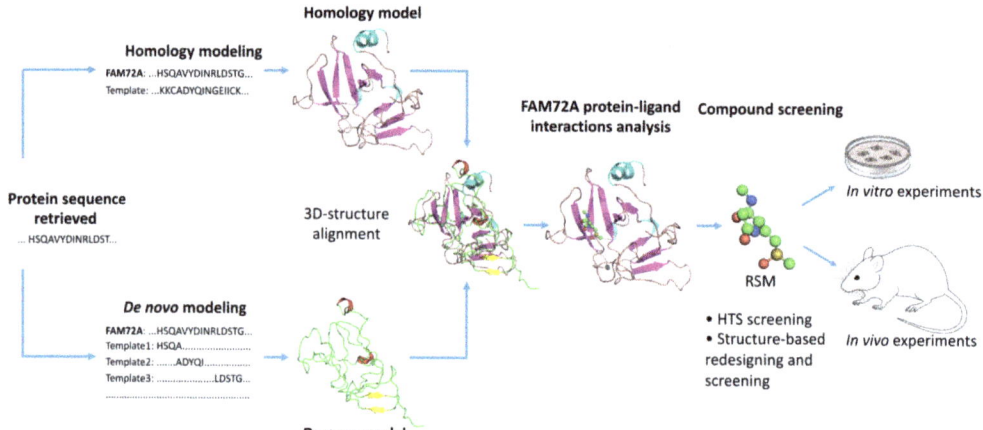

Figure 11. Structure based anti-cancer drug screening for the treatment of FAM72A-mediated cancers. Based on an in silico 3D protein structure model of FAM72A and its ligand-binding sites, the potential hit molecule RSM has been proposed for possible further therapeutic activity evaluations via in vitro and in vivo experiments.

9. Conclusions

The |-SRGAP2–FAM72-| master gene appears to be a pivotal genomic unit involved in brain development and synaptic plasticity. However, in light of the tissue-specific governance of this master gene, it remains to be seen what differentiates and regulates the expression of the |-FAM72–SRGAP2-| master gene across neuronal and non-neuronal tissues. This knowledge might be crucial for the specific biomedical interference with tumorigenic cell proliferation targeting FAM72.

Supplementary Materials: The following are available online at https://www.mdpi.com/2072-6694/13/5/1025/s1, Supplementary Figures S1–S21: Correlation of Fam72A mRNA expression with mRNA expression of MKI67, BIRC5 (survivin), E2F1, E2F2, E2F4, E2F6, FAM107A, FOXM1, LIN9, LIN37, LIN54, OLIG2, PAX6, RBBP4, TET2, TFDP1, TFDP2, TP53, SOX2, NRAS, and REST, respectively, across various TCGA human cancer tissues.

Funding: This study was supported by the Basic Science Research Program through the National Research Foundation of Korea (NRF), which was funded by the Ministry of Education (2019R1F1A1056445). This work was partly supported by an Institute of Information & Communications Technology Planning & Evaluation (IITP) grant funded by the Korean government (MSIT) (No. 2020-0-01373, Artificial Intelligence Graduate School Program (Hanyang University)) and the research fund of Hanyang University (HY- 202000000700017, 202000000790014).

Acknowledgments: We would like to thank Hanyang University for providing a scholarship to N.T.T.H.

Conflicts of Interest: The authors have no conflict of interests to declare.

References

1. Kutzner, A.; Pramanik, S.; Kim, P.S.; Heese, K. All-or-(N)One—An epistemological characterization of the human tumorigenic neuronal paralogous FAM72 gene loci. *Genomics* **2015**, *106*, 278–285. [CrossRef]
2. Ho, N.T.; Kim, P.S.; Kutzner, A.; Heese, K. Cognitive Functions: Human vs. Animal—4:1 Advantage |-FAM72-SRGAP2-|. *J. Mol. Neurosci.* **2017**, *61*, 603–606. [CrossRef]
3. Nehar, S.; Mishra, M.; Heese, K. Identification and characterisation of the novel amyloid-beta peptide-induced protein p17. *FEBS Lett.* **2009**, *583*, 3247–3253. [CrossRef]

4. Benayoun, B.A.; Pollina, E.A.; Ucar, D.; Mahmoudi, S.; Karra, K.; Wong, E.D.; Devarajan, K.; Daugherty, A.C.; Kundaje, A.B.; Mancini, E.; et al. H3K4me3 breadth is linked to cell identity and transcriptional consistency. *Cell* **2014**, *158*, 673–688. [CrossRef]
5. Ho, N.T.T.; Kutzner, A.; Heese, K. Brain plasticity, cognitive functions and neural stem cells: A pivotal role for the brain-specific neural master gene |-SRGAP2-FAM72-|. *Biol. Chem.* **2017**, *399*, 55–61. [CrossRef]
6. Dennis, M.Y.; Nuttle, X.; Sudmant, P.H.; Antonacci, F.; Graves, T.A.; Nefedov, M.; Rosenfeld, J.A.; Sajjadian, S.; Malig, M.; Kotkiewicz, H.; et al. Evolution of human-specific neural SRGAP2 genes by incomplete segmental duplication. *Cell* **2012**, *149*, 912–922. [CrossRef]
7. Geschwind, D.H.; Konopka, G. Neuroscience: Genes and human brain evolution. *Nature* **2012**, *486*, 481–482. [CrossRef]
8. Ho, N.T.T.; Kutzner, A.; Heese, K. A Novel Divergent Gene Transcription Paradigm-the Decisive, Brain-Specific, Neural |-Srgap2-Fam72a-| Master Gene Paradigm. *Mol. Neurobiol.* **2019**, *56*, 5891–5899. [CrossRef]
9. Chen, Y.; Pai, A.A.; Herudek, J.; Lubas, M.; Meola, N.; Jarvelin, A.I.; Andersson, R.; Pelechano, V.; Steinmetz, L.M.; Jensen, T.H.; et al. Principles for RNA metabolism and alternative transcription initiation within closely spaced promoters. *Nat. Genet.* **2016**, *48*, 984–994. [CrossRef]
10. Lacadie, S.A.; Ibrahim, M.M.; Gokhale, S.A.; Ohler, U. Divergent transcription and epigenetic directionality of human promoters. *FEBS J.* **2016**, *283*, 4214–4222. [CrossRef]
11. Ibrahim, M.M.; Karabacak, A.; Glahs, A.; Kolundzic, E.; Hirsekorn, A.; Carda, A.; Tursun, B.; Zinzen, R.P.; Lacadie, S.A.; Ohler, U. Determinants of promoter and enhancer transcription directionality in metazoans. *Nat. Commun.* **2018**, *9*, 4472. [CrossRef]
12. Rahane, C.S.; Kutzner, A.; Heese, K. A cancer tissue-specific FAM72 expression profile defines a novel glioblastoma multiform (GBM) gene-mutation signature. *J. Neurooncol.* **2019**, *141*, 57–70. [CrossRef]
13. Schneider, J.; Karpf, J.; Beckervordersandforth, R. Role of Astrocytes in the Neurogenic Niches. In *Methods in Molecular Biology*; Springer: Berlin, Germany, 2019; Volume 1938, pp. 19–33. [CrossRef]
14. Cassé, F.; Richetin, K.; Toni, N. Astrocytes' Contribution to Adult Neurogenesis in Physiology and Alzheimer's Disease. *Front. Cell. Neurosci.* **2018**, *12*, 432. [CrossRef]
15. Brandao, M.; Simon, T.; Critchley, G.; Giamas, G. Astrocytes, the rising stars of the glioblastoma microenvironment. *Glia* **2019**, *67*, 779–790. [CrossRef]
16. Charrier, C.; Joshi, K.; Coutinho-Budd, J.; Kim, J.E.; Lambert, N.; de Marchena, J.; Jin, W.L.; Vanderhaeghen, P.; Ghosh, A.; Sassa, T.; et al. Inhibition of SRGAP2 function by its human-specific paralogs induces neoteny during spine maturation. *Cell* **2012**, *149*, 923–935. [CrossRef]
17. Fossati, M.; Pizzarelli, R.; Schmidt, E.R.; Kupferman, J.V.; Stroebel, D.; Polleux, F.; Charrier, C. SRGAP2 and Its Human-Specific Paralog Co-Regulate the Development of Excitatory and Inhibitory Synapses. *Neuron* **2016**, *91*, 356–369. [CrossRef]
18. Geschwind, D.H.; Rakic, P. Cortical evolution: Judge the brain by its cover. *Neuron* **2013**, *80*, 633–647. [CrossRef]
19. Rincic, M.; Rados, M.; Krsnik, Z.; Gotovac, K.; Borovecki, F.; Liehr, T.; Brecevic, L. Complex intrachromosomal rearrangement in 1q leading to 1q32.2 microdeletion: A potential role of SRGAP2 in the gyrification of cerebral cortex. *Mol. Cytogenet.* **2016**, *9*, 19. [CrossRef]
20. Subramanian, J.; Nedivi, E. Filling the (SR)GAP in Excitatory/Inhibitory Balance. *Neuron* **2016**, *91*, 205–207. [CrossRef]
21. Jiao, Q.; Wang, L.; Zhang, S.; Wang, Y.; Yan, H.; Ma, W.; Jin, W.; Lu, H.; Liu, Y. Dynamic expression of srGAP2 in cell nuclei and cytoplasm during the differentiation of rat neural stem cells in vitro. *Mol. Med. Rep.* **2016**, *14*, 4599–4605. [CrossRef]
22. Guo, C.; Zhang, X.; Fink, S.P.; Platzer, P.; Wilson, K.; Willson, J.K.; Wang, Z.; Markowitz, S.D. Ugene, a newly identified protein that is commonly overexpressed in cancer and binds uracil DNA glycosylase. *Cancer Res.* **2008**, *68*, 6118–6126. [CrossRef]
23. Rajan, P.; Stockley, J.; Sudbery, I.M.; Fleming, J.T.; Hedley, A.; Kalna, G.; Sims, D.; Ponting, C.P.; Heger, A.; Robson, C.N.; et al. Identification of a candidate prognostic gene signature by transcriptome analysis of matched pre- and post-treatment prostatic biopsies from patients with advanced prostate cancer. *BMC Cancer* **2014**, *14*, 977. [CrossRef]
24. Zhu, D.; Fang, C.; Li, X.; Geng, Y.; Li, R.; Wu, C.; Jiang, J.; Wu, C. Predictive analysis of long non-coding RNA expression profiles in diffuse large B-cell lymphoma. *Oncotarget* **2017**, *8*, 23228–23236. [CrossRef]
25. Chatonnet, F.; Pignarre, A.; Serandour, A.A.; Caron, G.; Avner, S.; Robert, N.; Kassambara, A.; Laurent, A.; Bizot, M.; Agirre, X.; et al. The hydroxymethylome of multiple myeloma identifies FAM72D as a 1q21 marker linked to proliferation. *Haematologica* **2020**, *105*, 774–783. [CrossRef]
26. Marko, T.A.; Shamsan, G.A.; Edwards, E.N.; Hazelton, P.E.; Rathe, S.K.; Cornax, I.; Overn, P.R.; Varshney, J.; Diessner, B.J.; Moriarity, B.S.; et al. Slit-Robo GTPase-Activating Protein 2 as a metastasis suppressor in osteosarcoma. *Sci. Rep.* **2016**, *6*, 39059. [CrossRef]
27. Whitfield, M.L.; George, L.K.; Grant, G.D.; Perou, C.M. Common markers of proliferation. *Nat. Rev. Cancer* **2006**, *6*, 99–106. [CrossRef]
28. Rahane, C.S.; Kutzner, A.; Heese, K. Establishing a human adrenocortical carcinoma (ACC)-specific gene mutation signature. *Cancer Genet.* **2019**, *230*, 1–12. [CrossRef]
29. Zheng, S.; Cherniack, A.D.; Dewal, N.; Moffitt, R.A.; Danilova, L.; Murray, B.A.; Lerario, A.M.; Else, T.; Knijnenburg, T.A.; Ciriello, G.; et al. Comprehensive Pan-Genomic Characterization of Adrenocortical Carcinoma. *Cancer Cell* **2016**, *29*, 723–736. [CrossRef]
30. Assie, G.; Letouze, E.; Fassnacht, M.; Jouinot, A.; Luscap, W.; Barreau, O.; Omeiri, H.; Rodriguez, S.; Perlemoine, K.; Rene-Corail, F.; et al. Integrated genomic characterization of adrenocortical carcinoma. *Nat. Genet.* **2014**, *46*, 607–612. [CrossRef]

31. Lippert, J.; Appenzeller, S.; Liang, R.; Sbiera, S.; Kircher, S.; Altieri, B.; Nanda, I.; Weigand, I.; Gehrig, A.; Steinhauer, S.; et al. Targeted Molecular Analysis in Adrenocortical Carcinomas: A Strategy Toward Improved Personalized Prognostication. *J. Clin. Endocrinol. Metab.* **2018**, *103*, 4511–4523. [CrossRef]
32. Pereira, S.S.; Monteiro, M.P.; Bourdeau, I.; Lacroix, A.; Pignatelli, D. Mechanisms of endocrinology: Cell cycle regulation in adrenocortical carcinoma. *Eur. J. Endocrinol.* **2018**, *179*, R95–R110. [CrossRef]
33. Zhang, Q.; Shi, W.; Wang, Q.; Zhu, Y.; Zhai, C.; Wang, J.; Yan, X.; Chai, L.; Li, M. Clinicopathological and prognostic significance of leucine-rich repeats and immunoglobulin-like domains protein 1 (LRIG1) in malignant tumors: A meta-analysis. *J. Cancer* **2018**, *9*, 2895–2909. [CrossRef]
34. Torigoe, H.; Yamamoto, H.; Sakaguchi, M.; Youyi, C.; Namba, K.; Sato, H.; Shien, K.; Soh, J.; Suzawa, K.; Tomida, S.; et al. Tumor-suppressive effect of LRIG1, a negative regulator of ErbB, in non-small cell lung cancer harboring mutant EGFR. *Carcinogenesis* **2018**, *39*, 719–727. [CrossRef]
35. Mao, F.; Wang, B.; Xiao, Q.; Cheng, F.; Lei, T.; Guo, D. LRIG proteins in glioma: Functional roles, molecular mechanisms, and potential clinical implications. *J. Neurol. Sci.* **2017**, *383*, 56–60. [CrossRef]
36. Ragazzon, B.; Libe, R.; Gaujoux, S.; Assie, G.; Fratticci, A.; Launay, P.; Clauser, E.; Bertagna, X.; Tissier, F.; de Reynies, A.; et al. Transcriptome analysis reveals that p53 and {beta}-catenin alterations occur in a group of aggressive adrenocortical cancers. *Cancer Res.* **2010**, *70*, 8276–8281. [CrossRef]
37. Tissier, F.; Cavard, C.; Groussin, L.; Perlemoine, K.; Fumey, G.; Hagnere, A.M.; Rene-Corail, F.; Jullian, C.; Gicquel, C.; Bertagna, X.; et al. Mutations of beta-catenin in adrenocortical tumors: Activation of the Wnt signaling pathway is a frequent event in both benign and malignant adrenocortical tumors. *Cancer Res.* **2005**, *65*, 7622–7627. [CrossRef]
38. Herrmann, L.J.; Heinze, B.; Fassnacht, M.; Willenberg, H.S.; Quinkler, M.; Reisch, N.; Zink, M.; Allolio, B.; Hahner, S. TP53 germline mutations in adult patients with adrenocortical carcinoma. *J. Clin. Endocrinol. Metab.* **2012**, *97*, E476–E485. [CrossRef]
39. Raymond, V.M.; Else, T.; Everett, J.N.; Long, J.M.; Gruber, S.B.; Hammer, G.D. Prevalence of germline TP53 mutations in a prospective series of unselected patients with adrenocortical carcinoma. *J. Clin. Endocrinol. Metab.* **2013**, *98*, E119–E125. [CrossRef]
40. Giotti, B.; Chen, S.H.; Barnett, M.W.; Regan, T.; Ly, T.; Wiemann, S.; Hume, D.A.; Freeman, T.C. Assembly of a parts list of the human mitotic cell cycle machinery. *J. Mol. Cell. Biol.* **2019**, *11*, 703–718. [CrossRef]
41. Ajioka, I. Coordination of proliferation and neuronal differentiation by the retinoblastoma protein family. *Dev. Growth Differ.* **2014**, *56*, 324–334. [CrossRef]
42. Hardwick, L.J.; Ali, F.R.; Azzarelli, R.; Philpott, A. Cell cycle regulation of proliferation versus differentiation in the central nervous system. *Cell Tissue Res.* **2015**, *359*, 187–200. [CrossRef]
43. Vaudry, D.; Stork, P.J.; Lazarovici, P.; Eiden, L.E. Signaling pathways for PC12 cell differentiation: Making the right connections. *Science* **2002**, *296*, 1648–1649. [CrossRef]
44. Greene, L.A.; Tischler, A.S. Establishment of a noradrenergic clonal line of rat adrenal pheochromocytoma cells which respond to nerve growth factor. *Proc. Natl. Acad. Sci. USA* **1976**, *73*, 2424–2428.
45. Jensch, A.; Thomaseth, C.; Radde, N.E. Sampling-based Bayesian approaches reveal the importance of quasi-bistable behavior in cellular decision processes on the example of the MAPK signaling pathway in PC-12 cell lines. *BMC Syst. Biol.* **2017**, *11*, 11. [CrossRef]
46. Offermann, B.; Knauer, S.; Singh, A.; Fernandez-Cachon, M.L.; Klose, M.; Kowar, S.; Busch, H.; Boerries, M. Boolean Modeling Reveals the Necessity of Transcriptional Regulation for Bistability in PC12 Cell Differentiation. *Front. Genet.* **2016**, *7*, 44. [CrossRef]
47. Santos, S.D.; Verveer, P.J.; Bastiaens, P.I. Growth factor-induced MAPK network topology shapes Erk response determining PC-12 cell fate. *Nat. Cell Biol.* **2007**, *9*, 324–330. [CrossRef]
48. Moriguchi, T.; Gotoh, Y.; Nishida, E. Activation of two isoforms of mitogen-activated protein kinase kinase in response to epidermal growth factor and nerve growth factor. *Eur. J. Biochem.* **1995**, *234*, 32–38.
49. Tipping, A.J.; Pina, C.; Castor, A.; Hong, D.; Rodrigues, N.P.; Lazzari, L.; May, G.E.; Jacobsen, S.E.; Enver, T. High GATA-2 expression inhibits human hematopoietic stem and progenitor cell function by effects on cell cycle. *Blood* **2009**, *113*, 2661–2672. [CrossRef]
50. Kumar, M.S.; Hancock, D.C.; Molina-Arcas, M.; Steckel, M.; East, P.; Diefenbacher, M.; Armenteros-Monterroso, E.; Lassailly, F.; Matthews, N.; Nye, E.; et al. The GATA2 transcriptional network is requisite for RAS oncogene-driven non-small cell lung cancer. *Cell* **2012**, *149*, 642–655. [CrossRef]
51. Vicente, C.; Vazquez, I.; Conchillo, A.; Garcia-Sanchez, M.A.; Marcotegui, N.; Fuster, O.; Gonzalez, M.; Calasanz, M.J.; Lahortiga, I.; Odero, M.D. Overexpression of GATA2 predicts an adverse prognosis for patients with acute myeloid leukemia and it is associated with distinct molecular abnormalities. *Leukemia* **2012**, *26*, 550–554. [CrossRef]
52. Vicente, C.; Conchillo, A.; Garcia-Sanchez, M.A.; Odero, M.D. The role of the GATA2 transcription factor in normal and malignant hematopoiesis. *Crit. Rev. Oncol. Hematol.* **2012**, *82*, 1–17. [CrossRef]
53. Zheng, R.; Blobel, G.A. GATA Transcription Factors and Cancer. *Genes Cancer* **2010**, *1*, 1178–1188. [CrossRef]
54. Fornes, O.; Castro-Mondragon, J.A.; Khan, A.; van der Lee, R.; Zhang, X.; Richmond, P.A.; Modi, B.P.; Correard, S.; Gheorghe, M.; Baranasic, D.; et al. JASPAR 2020: Update of the open-access database of transcription factor binding profiles. *Nucl. Acids Res.* **2020**, *48*, D87–D92. [CrossRef]

55. Xu, X.; Bieda, M.; Jin, V.X.; Rabinovich, A.; Oberley, M.J.; Green, R.; Farnham, P.J. A comprehensive ChIP-chip analysis of E2F1, E2F4, and E2F6 in normal and tumor cells reveals interchangeable roles of E2F family members. *Genome Res.* **2007**, *17*, 1550–1561. [CrossRef]
56. Zheng, N.; Fraenkel, E.; Pabo, C.O.; Pavletich, N.P. Structural basis of DNA recognition by the heterodimeric cell cycle transcription factor E2F-DP. *Genes Dev.* **1999**, *13*, 666–674. [CrossRef]
57. Wells, J.; Boyd, K.E.; Fry, C.J.; Bartley, S.M.; Farnham, P.J. Target gene specificity of E2F and pocket protein family members in living cells. *Mol. Cell. Biol.* **2000**, *20*, 5797–5807. [CrossRef]
58. To, B.; Andrechek, E.R. Transcription factor compensation during mammary gland development in E2F knockout mice. *PLoS ONE* **2018**, *13*, e0194937. [CrossRef]
59. Kong, L.J.; Chang, J.T.; Bild, A.H.; Nevins, J.R. Compensation and specificity of function within the E2F family. *Oncogene* **2007**, *26*, 321–327. [CrossRef]
60. Vanderluit, J.L.; Ferguson, K.L.; Nikoletopoulou, V.; Parker, M.; Ruzhynsky, V.; Alexson, T.; McNamara, S.M.; Park, D.S.; Rudnicki, M.; Slack, R.S. p107 regulates neural precursor cells in the mammalian brain. *J. Cell. Biol.* **2004**, *166*, 853–863. [CrossRef]
61. Vanderluit, J.L.; Wylie, C.A.; McClellan, K.A.; Ghanem, N.; Fortin, A.; Callaghan, S.; MacLaurin, J.G.; Park, D.S.; Slack, R.S. The Retinoblastoma family member p107 regulates the rate of progenitor commitment to a neuronal fate. *J. Cell. Biol.* **2007**, *178*, 129–139. [CrossRef]
62. Ruzhynsky, V.A.; McClellan, K.A.; Vanderluit, J.L.; Jeong, Y.; Furimsky, M.; Park, D.S.; Epstein, D.J.; Wallace, V.A.; Slack, R.S. Cell cycle regulator E2F4 is essential for the development of the ventral telencephalon. *J. Neurosci.* **2007**, *27*, 5926–5935. [CrossRef]
63. McClellan, K.A.; Ruzhynsky, V.A.; Douda, D.N.; Vanderluit, J.L.; Ferguson, K.L.; Chen, D.; Bremner, R.; Park, D.S.; Leone, G.; Slack, R.S. Unique requirement for Rb/E2F3 in neuronal migration: Evidence for cell cycle-independent functions. *Mol. Cell. Biol.* **2007**, *27*, 4825–4843. [CrossRef]
64. McClellan, K.A.; Vanderluit, J.L.; Julian, L.M.; Andrusiak, M.G.; Dugal-Tessier, D.; Park, D.S.; Slack, R.S. The p107/E2F pathway regulates fibroblast growth factor 2 responsiveness in neural precursor cells. *Mol. Cell. Biol.* **2009**, *29*, 4701–4713. [CrossRef]
65. Jiang, S.X.; Sheldrick, M.; Desbois, A.; Slinn, J.; Hou, S.T. Neuropilin-1 is a direct target of the transcription factor E2F1 during cerebral ischemia-induced neuronal death in vivo. *Mol. Cell. Biol.* **2007**, *27*, 1696–1705. [CrossRef]
66. Andrusiak, M.G.; McClellan, K.A.; Dugal-Tessier, D.; Julian, L.M.; Rodrigues, S.P.; Park, D.S.; Kennedy, T.E.; Slack, R.S. Rb/E2F regulates expression of neogenin during neuronal migration. *Mol. Cell. Biol.* **2011**, *31*, 238–247. [CrossRef]
67. Ghanem, N.; Andrusiak, M.G.; Svoboda, D.; Al Lafi, S.M.; Julian, L.M.; McClellan, K.A.; De Repentigny, Y.; Kothary, R.; Ekker, M.; Blais, A.; et al. The Rb/E2F pathway modulates neurogenesis through direct regulation of the Dlx1/Dlx2 bigene cluster. *J. Neurosci.* **2012**, *32*, 8219–8230. [CrossRef]
68. Julian, L.M.; Vandenbosch, R.; Pakenham, C.A.; Andrusiak, M.G.; Nguyen, A.P.; McClellan, K.A.; Svoboda, D.S.; Lagace, D.C.; Park, D.S.; Leone, G.; et al. Opposing regulation of Sox2 by cell-cycle effectors E2f3a and E2f3b in neural stem cells. *Cell Stem Cell* **2013**, *12*, 440–452. [CrossRef]
69. Julian, L.M.; Blais, A. Transcriptional control of stem cell fate by E2Fs and pocket proteins. *Front. Genet.* **2015**, *6*, 161. [CrossRef]
70. Julian, L.M.; Liu, Y.; Pakenham, C.A.; Dugal-Tessier, D.; Ruzhynsky, V.; Bae, S.; Tsai, S.Y.; Leone, G.; Slack, R.S.; Blais, A. Tissue-specific targeting of cell fate regulatory genes by E2f factors. *Cell Death Differ.* **2016**, *23*, 565–575. [CrossRef]
71. Hsu, J.; Sage, J. Novel functions for the transcription factor E2F4 in development and disease. *Cell Cycle* **2016**, *15*, 3183–3190. [CrossRef]
72. Hsu, J.; Arand, J.; Chaikovsky, A.; Mooney, N.A.; Demeter, J.; Brison, C.M.; Oliverio, R.; Vogel, H.; Rubin, S.M.; Jackson, P.K.; et al. E2F4 regulates transcriptional activation in mouse embryonic stem cells independently of the RB family. *Nat. Commun.* **2019**, *10*, 2939. [CrossRef]
73. Cuitino, M.C.; Pecot, T.; Sun, D.; Kladney, R.; Okano-Uchida, T.; Shinde, N.; Saeed, R.; Perez-Castro, A.J.; Webb, A.; Liu, T.; et al. Two Distinct E2F Transcriptional Modules Drive Cell Cycles and Differentiation. *Cell Rep.* **2019**, *27*, 3547–3560. [CrossRef]
74. Bertoli, C.; Skotheim, J.M.; de Bruin, R.A. Control of cell cycle transcription during G1 and S phases. *Nat. Rev. Mol. Cell. Biol.* **2013**, *14*, 518–528. [CrossRef]
75. Fischer, M.; Grossmann, P.; Padi, M.; DeCaprio, J.A. Integration of TP53, DREAM, MMB-FOXM1 and RB-E2F target gene analyses identifies cell cycle gene regulatory networks. *Nucl. Acids Res.* **2016**, *44*, 6070–6086. [CrossRef]
76. Uxa, S.; Bernhart, S.H.; Mages, C.F.S.; Fischer, M.; Kohler, R.; Hoffmann, S.; Stadler, P.F.; Engeland, K.; Muller, G.A. DREAM and RB cooperate to induce gene repression and cell-cycle arrest in response to p53 activation. *Nucl. Acids Res.* **2019**, *47*, 9087–9103. [CrossRef]
77. Schade, A.E.; Oser, M.G.; Nicholson, H.E.; DeCaprio, J.A. Cyclin D-CDK4 relieves cooperative repression of proliferation and cell cycle gene expression by DREAM and RB. *Oncogene* **2019**, *38*, 4962–4976. [CrossRef]
78. Schade, A.E.; Fischer, M.; DeCaprio, J.A. RB, p130 and p107 differentially repress G1/S and G2/M genes after p53 activation. *Nucl. Acids Res.* **2019**, *47*, 11197–11208. [CrossRef]
79. Sadasivam, S.; DeCaprio, J.A. The DREAM complex: Master coordinator of cell cycle-dependent gene expression. *Nat. Rev. Cancer* **2013**, *13*, 585–595. [CrossRef]
80. Sadasivam, S.; Duan, S.; DeCaprio, J.A. The MuvB complex sequentially recruits B-Myb and FoxM1 to promote mitotic gene expression. *Genes Dev.* **2012**, *26*, 474–489. [CrossRef]

81. Fischer, M.; Muller, G.A. Cell cycle transcription control: DREAM/MuvB and RB-E2F complexes. *Crit. Rev. Biochem. Mol. Biol.* **2017**, *52*, 638–662. [CrossRef]
82. Litovchick, L.; Sadasivam, S.; Florens, L.; Zhu, X.; Swanson, S.K.; Velmurugan, S.; Chen, R.; Washburn, M.P.; Liu, X.S.; DeCaprio, J.A. Evolutionarily conserved multisubunit RBL2/p130 and E2F4 protein complex represses human cell cycle-dependent genes in quiescence. *Mol. Cell* **2007**, *26*, 539–551. [CrossRef]
83. Zhang, W.; Tyl, M.; Ward, R.; Sobott, F.; Maman, J.; Murthy, A.S.; Watson, A.A.; Fedorov, O.; Bowman, A.; Owen-Hughes, T.; et al. Structural plasticity of histones H3-H4 facilitates their allosteric exchange between RbAp48 and ASF1. *Nat. Struct. Mol. Biol.* **2013**, *20*, 29–35. [CrossRef]
84. Murzina, N.V.; Pei, X.Y.; Zhang, W.; Sparkes, M.; Vicente-Garcia, J.; Pratap, J.V.; McLaughlin, S.H.; Ben-Shahar, T.R.; Verreault, A.; Luisi, B.F.; et al. Structural basis for the recognition of histone H4 by the histone-chaperone RbAp46. *Structure* **2008**, *16*, 1077–1085. [CrossRef]
85. Qian, Y.W.; Wang, Y.C.; Hollingsworth, R.E., Jr.; Jones, D.; Ling, N.; Lee, E.Y. A retinoblastoma-binding protein related to a negative regulator of Ras in yeast. *Nature* **1993**, *364*, 648–652. [CrossRef]
86. Kitamura, H.; Ozono, E.; Iwanaga, R.; Bradford, A.P.; Okuno, J.; Shimizu, E.; Kurayoshi, K.; Kugawa, K.; Toh, H.; Ohtani, K. Identification of novel target genes specifically activated by deregulated E2F in human normal fibroblasts. *Genes Cells* **2015**, *20*, 739–757. [CrossRef]
87. Schmit, F.; Cremer, S.; Gaubatz, S. LIN54 is an essential core subunit of the DREAM/LINC complex that binds to the cdc2 promoter in a sequence-specific manner. *FEBS J.* **2009**, *276*, 5703–5716. [CrossRef]
88. Engeland, K. Cell cycle arrest through indirect transcriptional repression by p53: I have a DREAM. *Cell Death Differ.* **2018**, *25*, 114–132. [CrossRef]
89. Wang, Z.; Zhang, S.; Siu, T.L.; Huang, S. Glioblastoma multiforme formation and EMT: Role of FoxM1 transcription factor. *Curr. Pharm. Des.* **2015**, *21*, 1268–1271. [CrossRef]
90. Coulson, J.M. Transcriptional regulation: Cancer, neurons and the REST. *Curr. Biol.* **2005**, *15*, R665–R668. [CrossRef]
91. Lunyak, V.V.; Rosenfeld, M.G. No rest for REST: REST/NRSF regulation of neurogenesis. *Cell* **2005**, *121*, 499–501. [CrossRef]
92. Negrini, S.; Prada, I.; D'Alessandro, R.; Meldolesi, J. REST: An oncogene or a tumor suppressor? *Trends Cell. Biol.* **2013**, *23*, 289–295. [CrossRef]
93. Li, C.; Wang, Z.; Tang, X.; Zeng, L.; Fan, X.; Li, Z. Molecular mechanisms and potential prognostic effects of REST and REST4 in glioma (Review). *Mol. Med. Rep.* **2017**, *16*, 3707–3712. [CrossRef]
94. Zhao, Y.; Zhu, M.; Yu, Y.; Qiu, L.; Zhang, Y.; He, L.; Zhang, J. Brain REST/NRSF Is Not Only a Silent Repressor but Also an Active Protector. *Mol. Neurobiol.* **2017**, *54*, 541–550. [CrossRef]
95. Ren, X.; Kerppola, T.K. REST interacts with Cbx proteins and regulates polycomb repressive complex 1 occupancy at RE1 elements. *Mol. Cell. Biol.* **2011**, *31*, 2100–2110. [CrossRef]
96. Niklison-Chirou, M.V.; Agostini, M.; Amelio, I.; Melino, G. Regulation of Adult Neurogenesis in Mammalian Brain. *Int. J. Mol. Sci.* **2020**, *21*, 4869. [CrossRef]
97. Mozzi, A.; Guerini, F.R.; Forni, D.; Costa, A.S.; Nemni, R.; Baglio, F.; Cabinio, M.; Riva, S.; Pontremoli, C.; Clerici, M.; et al. REST, a master regulator of neurogenesis, evolved under strong positive selection in humans and in non human primates. *Sci. Rep.* **2017**, *7*, 9530. [CrossRef]
98. Urban, N.; Blomfield, I.M.; Guillemot, F. Quiescence of Adult Mammalian Neural Stem Cells: A Highly Regulated Rest. *Neuron* **2019**, *104*, 834–848. [CrossRef]
99. Chen, G.L.; Miller, G.M. Alternative REST Splicing Underappreciated. *eNeuro* **2018**, *5*. [CrossRef]
100. Shafik, A.; Schumann, U.; Evers, M.; Sibbritt, T.; Preiss, T. The emerging epitranscriptomics of long noncoding RNAs. *Biochim. Biophys. Acta* **2016**, *1859*, 59–70. [CrossRef]
101. Bonasio, R.; Shiekhattar, R. Regulation of transcription by long noncoding RNAs. *Annu. Rev. Genet.* **2014**, *48*, 433–455. [CrossRef]
102. Yan, P.; Luo, S.; Lu, J.Y.; Shen, X. Cis- and trans-acting lncRNAs in pluripotency and reprogramming. *Curr. Opin. Genet. Dev.* **2017**, *46*, 170–178. [CrossRef]
103. Hansji, H.; Leung, E.Y.; Baguley, B.C.; Finlay, G.J.; Askarian-Amiri, M.E. Keeping abreast with long non-coding RNAs in mammary gland development and breast cancer. *Front. Genet.* **2014**, *5*, 379. [CrossRef]
104. Han, D.; Wang, M.; Ma, N.; Xu, Y.; Jiang, Y.; Gao, X. Long noncoding RNAs: Novel players in colorectal cancer. *Cancer Lett.* **2015**, *361*, 13–21. [CrossRef]
105. Wang, J.; Sun, J.; Wang, J.; Song, Y.; Gao, P.; Shi, J.; Chen, P.; Wang, Z. Long noncoding RNAs in gastric cancer: Functions and clinical applications. *Onco Targets Ther.* **2016**, *9*, 681–697. [CrossRef]
106. Pastori, C.; Wahlestedt, C. Involvement of long noncoding RNAs in diseases affecting the central nervous system. *RNA Biol.* **2012**, *9*, 860–870. [CrossRef]
107. Panda, S.; Setia, M.; Kaur, N.; Shepal, V.; Arora, V.; Singh, D.K.; Mondal, A.; Teli, A.; Tathode, M.; Gajula, R.; et al. Noncoding RNA Ginir functions as an oncogene by associating with centrosomal proteins. *PLoS Biol.* **2018**, *16*, e2004204. [CrossRef]
108. Zhang, L.; Wei, Y.; Yan, X.; Li, N.; Song, H.; Yang, L.; Wu, Y.; Xi, Y.F.; Weng, H.W.; Li, J.H.; et al. Survivin is a prognostic marker and therapeutic target for extranodal, nasal-type natural killer/T cell lymphoma. *Ann. Transl. Med.* **2019**, *7*, 316. [CrossRef]
109. Altieri, D.C. Survivin—The inconvenient IAP. *Semin. Cell Dev. Biol.* **2015**, *39*, 91–96. [CrossRef]

110. Preusser, M.; Gelpi, E.; Matej, R.; Marosi, C.; Dieckmann, K.; Rossler, K.; Budka, H.; Hainfellner, J.A. No prognostic impact of survivin expression in glioblastoma. *Acta Neuropathol.* **2005**, *109*, 534–538. [CrossRef]
111. Tong, X.; Yang, P.; Wang, K.; Liu, Y.; Liu, X.; Shan, X.; Huang, R.; Zhang, K.; Wang, J. Survivin is a prognostic indicator in glioblastoma and may be a target of microRNA-218. *Oncol. Lett* **2019**, *18*, 359–367. [CrossRef]
112. Farmer, G.; Friedlander, P.; Colgan, J.; Manley, J.L.; Prives, C. Transcriptional repression by p53 involves molecular interactions distinct from those with the TATA box binding protein. *Nucl. Acids Res.* **1996**, *24*, 4281–4288. [CrossRef]
113. Truant, R.; Xiao, H.; Ingles, C.J.; Greenblatt, J. Direct interaction between the transcriptional activation domain of human p53 and the TATA box-binding protein. *J. Biol. Chem.* **1993**, *268*, 2284–2287.
114. St Clair, S.; Giono, L.; Varmeh-Ziaie, S.; Resnick-Silverman, L.; Liu, W.J.; Padi, A.; Dastidar, J.; DaCosta, A.; Mattia, M.; Manfredi, J.J. DNA damage-induced downregulation of Cdc25C is mediated by p53 via two independent mechanisms: One involves direct binding to the cdc25C promoter. *Mol. Cell* **2004**, *16*, 725–736. [CrossRef]
115. Giono, L.E.; Resnick-Silverman, L.; Carvajal, L.A.; St Clair, S.; Manfredi, J.J. Mdm2 promotes Cdc25C protein degradation and delays cell cycle progression through the G2/M phase. *Oncogene* **2017**, *36*, 6762–6773. [CrossRef]
116. Liu, K.; Lu, R.; Zhao, Q.; Du, J.; Li, Y.; Zheng, M.; Zhang, S. Association and clinicopathologic significance of p38MAPK-ERK-JNK-CDC25C with polyploid giant cancer cell formation. *Med. Oncol.* **2019**, *37*, 6. [CrossRef]
117. Liu, K.; Zheng, M.; Lu, R.; Du, J.; Zhao, Q.; Li, Z.; Li, Y.; Zhang, S. The role of CDC25C in cell cycle regulation and clinical cancer therapy: A systematic review. *Cancer Cell Int.* **2020**, *20*, 213. [CrossRef]
118. Wang, X.; Sun, Q. TP53 mutations, expression and interaction networks in human cancers. *Oncotarget* **2017**, *8*, 624–643. [CrossRef]
119. Musa, J.; Aynaud, M.M.; Mirabeau, O.; Delattre, O.; Grunewald, T.G. MYBL2 (B-Myb): A central regulator of cell proliferation, cell survival and differentiation involved in tumorigenesis. *Cell Death Dis.* **2017**, *8*, e2895. [CrossRef]
120. Bayley, R.; Ward, C.; Garcia, P. MYBL2 amplification in breast cancer: Molecular mechanisms and therapeutic potential. *Biochim. Biophys. Acta Rev. Cancer* **2020**, *1874*, 188407. [CrossRef]
121. Sant, K.E.; Nahar, M.S.; Dolinoy, D.C. DNA methylation screening and analysis. *Methods Mol. Biol* **2012**, *889*, 385–406. [CrossRef]
122. Lister, R.; Pelizzola, M.; Dowen, R.H.; Hawkins, R.D.; Hon, G.; Tonti-Filippini, J.; Nery, J.R.; Lee, L.; Ye, Z.; Ngo, Q.M.; et al. Human DNA methylomes at base resolution show widespread epigenomic differences. *Nature* **2009**, *462*, 315–322. [CrossRef]
123. Bibikova, M.; Barnes, B.; Tsan, C.; Ho, V.; Klotzle, B.; Le, J.M.; Delano, D.; Zhang, L.; Schroth, G.P.; Gunderson, K.L.; et al. High density DNA methylation array with single CpG site resolution. *Genomics* **2011**, *98*, 288–295. [CrossRef]
124. Guo, J.U.; Su, Y.; Shin, J.H.; Shin, J.; Li, H.; Xie, B.; Zhong, C.; Hu, S.; Le, T.; Fan, G.; et al. Distribution, recognition and regulation of non-CpG methylation in the adult mammalian brain. *Nat. Neurosci.* **2014**, *17*, 215–222. [CrossRef]
125. Zhang, T.Y.; Meaney, M.J. Epigenetics and the environmental regulation of the genome and its function. *Annu. Rev. Psychol.* **2010**, *61*, 439–466. [CrossRef]
126. Feng, J.; Fan, G. The role of DNA methylation in the central nervous system and neuropsychiatric disorders. *Int. Rev. Neurobiol.* **2009**, *89*, 67–84. [CrossRef]
127. Rauscher, G.H.; Kresovich, J.K.; Poulin, M.; Yan, L.; Macias, V.; Mahmoud, A.M.; Al-Alem, U.; Kajdacsy-Balla, A.; Wiley, E.L.; Tonetti, D.; et al. Exploring DNA methylation changes in promoter, intragenic, and intergenic regions as early and late events in breast cancer formation. *BMC Cancer* **2015**, *15*, 816. [CrossRef]
128. Ehrlich, M. DNA methylation in cancer: Too much, but also too little. *Oncogene* **2002**, *21*, 5400–5413. [CrossRef]
129. Esteller, M. CpG island hypermethylation and tumor suppressor genes: A booming present, a brighter future. *Oncogene* **2002**, *21*, 5427–5440. [CrossRef]
130. Kulis, M.; Esteller, M. DNA methylation and cancer. *Adv. Genet.* **2010**, *70*, 27–56. [CrossRef]
131. Guez-Haddad, J.; Sporny, M.; Sasson, Y.; Gevorkyan-Airapetov, L.; Lahav-Mankovski, N.; Margulies, D.; Radzimanowski, J.; Opatowsky, Y. The Neuronal Migration Factor srGAP2 Achieves Specificity in Ligand Binding through a Two-Component Molecular Mechanism. *Structure* **2015**, *23*, 1989–2000. [CrossRef]
132. Fritz, R.D.; Menshykau, D.; Martin, K.; Reimann, A.; Pontelli, V.; Pertz, O. SrGAP2-Dependent Integration of Membrane Geometry and Slit-Robo-Repulsive Cues Regulates Fibroblast Contact Inhibition of Locomotion. *Dev. Cell* **2015**, *35*, 78–92. [CrossRef]
133. Ren, C.; Yuan, Q.; Braun, M.; Zhang, X.; Petri, B.; Zhang, J.; Kim, D.; Guez-Haddad, J.; Xue, W.; Pan, W.; et al. Leukocyte Cytoskeleton Polarization Is Initiated by Plasma Membrane Curvature from Cell Attachment. *Dev. Cell* **2019**, *49*, 206–219.e7. [CrossRef]
134. Mason, F.M.; Heimsath, E.G.; Higgs, H.N.; Soderling, S.H. Bi-modal regulation of a formin by srGAP2. *J. Biol. Chem.* **2011**, *286*, 6577–6586. [CrossRef]
135. Kan, S.; Chai, S.; Chen, W.; Yu, B. DNA methylation profiling identifies potentially significant epigenetically-regulated genes in glioblastoma multiforme. *Oncol. Lett.* **2019**, *18*, 1679–1688. [CrossRef]
136. Diez-Villanueva, A.; Mallona, I.; Peinado, M.A. Wanderer, an interactive viewer to explore DNA methylation and gene expression data in human cancer. *Epigenet. Chromatin* **2015**, *8*, 22. [CrossRef]
137. Robinson, J.T.; Thorvaldsdottir, H.; Winckler, W.; Guttman, M.; Lander, E.S.; Getz, G.; Mesirov, J.P. Integrative genomics viewer. *Nat. Biotechnol.* **2011**, *29*, 24–26. [CrossRef]
138. Thorvaldsdottir, H.; Robinson, J.T.; Mesirov, J.P. Integrative Genomics Viewer (IGV): High-performance genomics data visualization and exploration. *Brief. Bioinform.* **2013**, *14*, 178–192. [CrossRef]

139. Munzel, M.; Globisch, D.; Bruckl, T.; Wagner, M.; Welzmiller, V.; Michalakis, S.; Muller, M.; Biel, M.; Carell, T. Quantification of the sixth DNA base hydroxymethylcytosine in the brain. *Angew. Chem. Int. Ed. Engl.* **2010**, *49*, 5375–5377. [CrossRef]
140. Yu, M.; Hon, G.C.; Szulwach, K.E.; Song, C.X.; Zhang, L.; Kim, A.; Li, X.; Dai, Q.; Shen, Y.; Park, B.; et al. Base-resolution analysis of 5-hydroxymethylcytosine in the mammalian genome. *Cell* **2012**, *149*, 1368–1380. [CrossRef]
141. Stricker, S.H.; Gotz, M. DNA-Methylation: Master or Slave of Neural Fate Decisions? *Front. Neurosci.* **2018**, *12*, 5. [CrossRef]
142. Noack, F.; Pataskar, A.; Schneider, M.; Buchholz, F.; Tiwari, V.K.; Calegari, F. Assessment and site-specific manipulation of DNA (hydroxy-)methylation during mouse corticogenesis. *Life Sci. Alliance* **2019**, *2*. [CrossRef]
143. Santiago, M.; Antunes, C.; Guedes, M.; Sousa, N.; Marques, C.J. TET enzymes and DNA hydroxymethylation in neural development and function—How critical are they? *Genomics* **2014**, *104*, 334–340. [CrossRef]
144. Dabrowski, M.J.; Wojtas, B. Global DNA Methylation Patterns in Human Gliomas and Their Interplay with Other Epigenetic Modifications. *Int. J. Mol. Sci.* **2019**, *20*, 3478. [CrossRef]
145. Rasmussen, K.D.; Helin, K. Role of TET enzymes in DNA methylation, development, and cancer. *Genes Dev.* **2016**, *30*, 733–750. [CrossRef]
146. Wang, L.; Ozark, P.A.; Smith, E.R.; Zhao, Z.; Marshall, S.A.; Rendleman, E.J.; Piunti, A.; Ryan, C.; Whelan, A.L.; Helmin, K.A.; et al. TET2 coactivates gene expression through demethylation of enhancers. *Sci. Adv.* **2018**, *4*, eaau6986. [CrossRef]
147. Cochran, J.N.; Geier, E.G.; Bonham, L.W.; Newberry, J.S.; Amaral, M.D.; Thompson, M.L.; Lasseigne, B.N.; Karydas, A.M.; Roberson, E.D.; Cooper, G.M.; et al. Non-coding and Loss-of-Function Coding Variants in TET2 are Associated with Multiple Neurodegenerative Diseases. *Am. J. Hum. Genet.* **2020**, *106*, 632–645. [CrossRef]
148. Tremblay, M.; Sanchez-Ferras, O.; Bouchard, M. GATA transcription factors in development and disease. *Development* **2018**, *145*. [CrossRef]
149. Lin, R.K.; Wang, Y.C. Dysregulated transcriptional and post-translational control of DNA methyltransferases in cancer. *Cell Biosci.* **2014**, *4*, 46. [CrossRef]
150. Tovy, A.; Spiro, A.; McCarthy, R.; Shipony, Z.; Aylon, Y.; Allton, K.; Ainbinder, E.; Furth, N.; Tanay, A.; Barton, M.; et al. p53 is essential for DNA methylation homeostasis in naive embryonic stem cells, and its loss promotes clonal heterogeneity. *Genes Dev.* **2017**, *31*, 959–972. [CrossRef]
151. Tsherniak, A.; Vazquez, F.; Montgomery, P.G.; Weir, B.A.; Kryukov, G.; Cowley, G.S.; Gill, S.; Harrington, W.F.; Pantel, S.; Krill-Burger, J.M.; et al. Defining a Cancer Dependency Map. *Cell* **2017**, *170*, 564–576. [CrossRef]
152. Nakajima, H.; Koizumi, K. Family with sequence similarity 107: A family of stress responsive small proteins with diverse functions in cancer and the nervous system (Review). *Biomed. Rep.* **2014**, *2*, 321–325. [CrossRef]
153. Ma, Y.S.; Wu, Z.J.; Bai, R.Z.; Dong, H.; Xie, B.X.; Wu, X.H.; Hang, X.S.; Liu, A.N.; Jiang, X.H.; Wang, G.R.; et al. DRR1 promotes glioblastoma cell invasion and epithelial-mesenchymal transition via regulating AKT activation. *Cancer Lett.* **2018**, *423*, 86–94. [CrossRef]
154. Arnold, A.E.; Malek-Adamian, E.; Le, P.U.; Meng, A.; Martinez-Montero, S.; Petrecca, K.; Damha, M.J.; Shoichet, M.S. Antibody-Antisense Oligonucleotide Conjugate Downregulates a Key Gene in Glioblastoma Stem Cells. *Mol. Ther. Nucl. Acids* **2018**, *11*, 518–527. [CrossRef]
155. Yamato, T.; Orikasa, K.; Fukushige, S.; Orikasa, S.; Horii, A. Isolation and characterization of the novel gene, TU3A, in a commonly deleted region on 3p14.3->p14.2 in renal cell carcinoma. *Cytogenet. Cell Genet.* **1999**, *87*, 291–295. [CrossRef]
156. Wang, L.; Darling, J.; Zhang, J.S.; Liu, W.; Qian, J.; Bostwick, D.; Hartmann, L.; Jenkins, R.; Bardenhauer, W.; Schutte, J.; et al. Loss of expression of the DRR 1 gene at chromosomal segment 3p21.1 in renal cell carcinoma. *Genes Chromosomes Cancer* **2000**, *27*, 1–10. [CrossRef]
157. De Rubis, G.; Rajeev Krishnan, S.; Bebawy, M. Liquid Biopsies in Cancer Diagnosis, Monitoring, and Prognosis. *Trends Pharmacol. Sci.* **2019**, *40*, 172–186. [CrossRef]
158. Heese, K. The protein p17 signaling pathways in cancer. *Tumour Biol.* **2013**, *34*, 4081–4087. [CrossRef]
159. Zuckerman, J.E.; Davis, M.E. Clinical experiences with systemically administered siRNA-based therapeutics in cancer. *Nat. Rev. Drug Discov.* **2015**, *14*, 843–856. [CrossRef]
160. Wittrup, A.; Lieberman, J. Knocking down disease: A progress report on siRNA therapeutics. *Nat. Rev. Genet.* **2015**, *16*, 543–552. [CrossRef]
161. Fang, L.; Cheng, Q.; Li, W.; Liu, J.; Li, L.; Xu, K.; Zheng, J. Antitumor activities of an oncolytic adenovirus equipped with a double siRNA targeting Ki67 and hTERT in renal cancer cells. *Virus Res.* **2014**, *181*, 61–71. [CrossRef]
162. Zhang, J.; Ding, M.; Xu, K.; Mao, L.; Zheng, J. shRNA-armed conditionally replicative adenoviruses: A promising approach for cancer therapy. *Oncotarget* **2016**, *7*, 29824–29834. [CrossRef]
163. Bennett, C.F.; Swayze, E.E. RNA targeting therapeutics: Molecular mechanisms of antisense oligonucleotides as a therapeutic platform. *Annu. Rev. Pharmacol. Toxicol.* **2010**, *50*, 259–293. [CrossRef]
164. Castanotto, D.; Stein, C.A. Antisense oligonucleotides in cancer. *Curr. Opin. Oncol.* **2014**, *26*, 584–589. [CrossRef]
165. Yang, C.; Zhang, J.; Ding, M.; Xu, K.; Li, L.; Mao, L.; Zheng, J. Ki67 targeted strategies for cancer therapy. *Clin. Transl. Oncol.* **2018**, *20*, 570–575. [CrossRef]
166. Kausch, I.; Lingnau, A.; Endl, E.; Sellmann, K.; Deinert, I.; Ratliff, T.L.; Jocham, D.; Sczakiel, G.; Gerdes, J.; Bohle, A. Antisense treatment against Ki-67 mRNA inhibits proliferation and tumor growth in vitro and in vivo. *Int. J. Cancer* **2003**, *105*, 710–716. [CrossRef]

167. D'Cruz, O.J.; Qazi, S.; Hwang, L.; Ng, K.; Trieu, V. Impact of targeting transforming growth factor beta-2 with antisense OT-101 on the cytokine and chemokine profile in patients with advanced pancreatic cancer. *Onco Targets Ther.* **2018**, *11*, 2779–2796. [CrossRef]
168. Hong, D.; Kurzrock, R.; Kim, Y.; Woessner, R.; Younes, A.; Nemunaitis, J.; Fowler, N.; Zhou, T.; Schmidt, J.; Jo, M.; et al. AZD9150, a next-generation antisense oligonucleotide inhibitor of STAT3 with early evidence of clinical activity in lymphoma and lung cancer. *Sci. Transl. Med.* **2015**, *7*, 314ra185. [CrossRef]
169. Reilley, M.J.; McCoon, P.; Cook, C.; Lyne, P.; Kurzrock, R.; Kim, Y.; Woessner, R.; Younes, A.; Nemunaitis, J.; Fowler, N.; et al. STAT3 antisense oligonucleotide AZD9150 in a subset of patients with heavily pretreated lymphoma: Results of a phase 1b trial. *J. Immunother. Cancer* **2018**, *6*, 119. [CrossRef]
170. Odate, S.; Veschi, V.; Yan, S.; Lam, N.; Woessner, R.; Thiele, C.J. Inhibition of STAT3 with the Generation 2.5 Antisense Oligonucleotide, AZD9150, Decreases Neuroblastoma Tumorigenicity and Increases Chemosensitivity. *Clin. Cancer Res.* **2017**, *23*, 1771–1784. [CrossRef]
171. Takakura, K.; Kawamura, A.; Torisu, Y.; Koido, S.; Yahagi, N.; Saruta, M. The Clinical Potential of Oligonucleotide Therapeutics against Pancreatic Cancer. *Int. J. Mol. Sci.* **2019**, *20*, 3331. [CrossRef]
172. Setten, R.L.; Rossi, J.J.; Han, S.P. The current state and future directions of RNAi-based therapeutics. *Nat. Rev. Drug Discov.* **2019**, *18*, 421–446. [CrossRef]
173. Barrangou, R.; Fremaux, C.; Deveau, H.; Richards, M.; Boyaval, P.; Moineau, S.; Romero, D.A.; Horvath, P. CRISPR provides acquired resistance against viruses in prokaryotes. *Science* **2007**, *315*, 1709–1712. [CrossRef]
174. Jinek, M.; Chylinski, K.; Fonfara, I.; Hauer, M.; Doudna, J.A.; Charpentier, E. A programmable dual-RNA-guided DNA endonuclease in adaptive bacterial immunity. *Science* **2012**, *337*, 816–821. [CrossRef]
175. Mali, P.; Yang, L.; Esvelt, K.M.; Aach, J.; Guell, M.; DiCarlo, J.E.; Norville, J.E.; Church, G.M. RNA-guided human genome engineering via Cas9. *Science* **2013**, *339*, 823–826. [CrossRef]
176. Cong, L.; Ran, F.A.; Cox, D.; Lin, S.; Barretto, R.; Habib, N.; Hsu, P.D.; Wu, X.; Jiang, W.; Marraffini, L.A.; et al. Multiplex genome engineering using CRISPR/Cas systems. *Science* **2013**, *339*, 819–823. [CrossRef]
177. Gasiunas, G.; Barrangou, R.; Horvath, P.; Siksnys, V. Cas9-crRNA ribonucleoprotein complex mediates specific DNA cleavage for adaptive immunity in bacteria. *Proc. Natl. Acad. Sci. USA* **2012**, *109*, E2579–E2586. [CrossRef]
178. Wang, X.; Ma, S.; Liu, Y.; Lu, W.; Sun, L.; Zhao, P.; Xia, Q. Transcriptional repression of endogenous genes in BmE cells using CRISPRi system. *Insect Biochem. Mol. Biol.* **2019**, *111*, 103172. [CrossRef]
179. MacLeod, R.S.; Cawley, K.M.; Gubrij, I.; Nookaew, I.; Onal, M.; O'Brien, C.A. Effective CRISPR interference of an endogenous gene via a single transgene in mice. *Sci. Rep.* **2019**, *9*, 17312. [CrossRef]
180. Kampmann, M. CRISPRi and CRISPRa Screens in Mammalian Cells for Precision Biology and Medicine. *ACS Chem. Biol.* **2018**, *13*, 406–416. [CrossRef]
181. Qi, L.S.; Larson, M.H.; Gilbert, L.A.; Doudna, J.A.; Weissman, J.S.; Arkin, A.P.; Lim, W.A. Repurposing CRISPR as an RNA-guided platform for sequence-specific control of gene expression. *Cell* **2013**, *152*, 1173–1183. [CrossRef]
182. Dominguez, A.A.; Lim, W.A.; Qi, L.S. Beyond editing: Repurposing CRISPR-Cas9 for precision genome regulation and interrogation. *Nat. Rev. Mol. Cell. Biol.* **2016**, *17*, 5–15. [CrossRef]
183. Gilbert, L.A.; Larson, M.H.; Morsut, L.; Liu, Z.; Brar, G.A.; Torres, S.E.; Stern-Ginossar, N.; Brandman, O.; Whitehead, E.H.; Doudna, J.A.; et al. CRISPR-mediated modular RNA-guided regulation of transcription in eukaryotes. *Cell* **2013**, *154*, 442–451. [CrossRef]
184. Finn, J.D.; Smith, A.R.; Patel, M.C.; Shaw, L.; Youniss, M.R.; van Heteren, J.; Dirstine, T.; Ciullo, C.; Lescarbeau, R.; Seitzer, J.; et al. A Single Administration of CRISPR/Cas9 Lipid Nanoparticles Achieves Robust and Persistent In Vivo Genome Editing. *Cell Rep.* **2018**, *22*, 2227–2235. [CrossRef]
185. Pramanik, S.; Kutzner, A.; Heese, K. Lead discovery and in silico 3D structure modeling of tumorigenic FAM72A (p17). *Tumour Biol.* **2015**, *36*, 239–249. [CrossRef]
186. Kalyaanamoorthy, S.; Chen, Y.P. Structure-based drug design to augment hit discovery. *Drug Discov. Today* **2011**, *16*, 831–839. [CrossRef]
187. Yu, W.; MacKerell, A.D., Jr. Computer-Aided Drug Design Methods. In *Methods in Molecular Biology*; Springer: Berlin, Germany, 2017; Volume 1520, pp. 85–106. [CrossRef]
188. Schneider, G.; Fechner, U. Computer-based de novo design of drug-like molecules. *Nat. Rev. Drug Discov.* **2005**, *4*, 649–663. [CrossRef]
189. Pramanik, S.; Roy, K. Predictive modeling of chemical toxicity towards Pseudokirchneriella subcapitata using regression and classification based approaches. *Ecotoxicol. Environ. Saf.* **2014**, *101*, 184–190. [CrossRef]
190. Pramanik, S.; Roy, K. Exploring QSTR modeling and toxicophore mapping for identification of important molecular features contributing to the chemical toxicity in Escherichia coli. *Toxicol. In Vitro* **2014**, *28*, 265–272. [CrossRef]
191. van Montfort, R.L.; Workman, P. Structure-based design of molecular cancer therapeutics. *Trends Biotechnol.* **2009**, *27*, 315–328. [CrossRef]
192. Acharya, C.; Coop, A.; Polli, J.E.; Mackerell, A.D., Jr. Recent advances in ligand-based drug design: Relevance and utility of the conformationally sampled pharmacophore approach. *Curr. Comput. Aided Drug Des.* **2011**, *7*, 10–22. [CrossRef]
193. Fiser, A.; Sali, A. Modeller: Generation and refinement of homology-based protein structure models. *Methods Enzymol.* **2003**, *374*, 461–491. [CrossRef]

194. Marti-Renom, M.A.; Stuart, A.C.; Fiser, A.; Sanchez, R.; Melo, F.; Sali, A. Comparative protein structure modeling of genes and genomes. *Annu. Rev. Biophys. Biomol. Struct.* **2000**, *29*, 291–325. [CrossRef]
195. Webb, B.; Sali, A. Comparative Protein Structure Modeling Using MODELLER. *Curr. Protoc. Bioinform.* **2016**, *54*, 5.6.1–5.6.37. [CrossRef]
196. Yang, J.; Roy, A.; Zhang, Y. BioLiP: A semi-manually curated database for biologically relevant ligand-protein interactions. *Nucl. Acids Res.* **2013**, *41*, D1096–D1103. [CrossRef]
197. Yang, J.; Roy, A.; Zhang, Y. Protein-ligand binding site recognition using complementary binding-specific substructure comparison and sequence profile alignment. *Bioinformatics* **2013**, *29*, 2588–2595. [CrossRef]

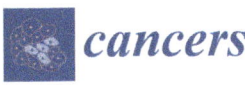

Review

Glioblastoma: Emerging Treatments and Novel Trial Designs

Vincenzo Di Nunno [1,*], Enrico Franceschi [1], Alicia Tosoni [1], Lidia Gatto [1], Raffaele Lodi [2], Stefania Bartolini [1] and Alba Ariela Brandes [1]

1. Department of Oncology, AUSL Bologna, Via Altura 3, 40139 Bologna, Italy;
   e.franceschi@ausl.bologna.it (E.F.); a.tosoni@ausl.bologna.it (A.T.); lidia.gatto@ausl.bologna.it (L.G.); stefania.bartolini@ausl.bologna.it (S.B.); alba.brandes@ausl.bologna.it (A.A.B.)
2. Istituto delle Scienze Neurologiche di Bologna, Istituto di Ricovero e Cura a Carattere Scientifico (IRCCS), 10139 Bologna, Italy; raffaele.lodi@isnb.it
* Correspondence: vincenzo.dinunno@ausl.bologna.it; Tel.: +39-0516225697

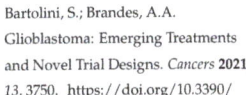

Citation: Di Nunno, V.; Franceschi, E.; Tosoni, A.; Gatto, L.; Lodi, R.; Bartolini, S.; Brandes, A.A. Glioblastoma: Emerging Treatments and Novel Trial Designs. *Cancers* **2021**, *13*, 3750. https://doi.org/10.3390/cancers13153750

Academic Editor: Stanley Stylli

Received: 25 June 2021
Accepted: 21 July 2021
Published: 26 July 2021

Publisher's Note: MDPI stays neutral with regard to jurisdictional claims in published maps and institutional affiliations.

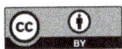

Copyright: © 2021 by the authors. Licensee MDPI, Basel, Switzerland. This article is an open access article distributed under the terms and conditions of the Creative Commons Attribution (CC BY) license (https://creativecommons.org/licenses/by/4.0/).

Simple Summary: Nowadays, very few systemic agents have shown clinical activity in patients with glioblastoma, making the research of novel therapeutic approaches a critical issue. Fortunately, the availability of novel compounds is increasing thanks to better biological knowledge of the disease. In this review we want to investigate more promising ongoing clinical trials in both primary and recurrent GBM. Furthermore, a great interest of the present work is focused on novel trial design strategies.

Abstract: Management of glioblastoma is a clinical challenge since very few systemic treatments have shown clinical efficacy in recurrent disease. Thanks to an increased knowledge of the biological and molecular mechanisms related to disease progression and growth, promising novel treatment strategies are emerging. The expanding availability of innovative compounds requires the design of a new generation of clinical trials, testing experimental compounds in a short time and tailoring the sample cohort based on molecular and clinical behaviors. In this review, we focused our attention on the assessment of promising novel treatment approaches, discussing novel trial design and possible future fields of development in this setting.

Keywords: glioblastoma; newly diagnosed glioblastoma; recurrent glioblastoma; GBM; new trial design

1. Introduction

Glioblastoma (GBM) is the most common primary brain tumor, with an estimated incidence of 3.22/100,000 persons in the United States and a five-year overall survival of only 6.8% [1,2]. Nowadays, GBM can be diagnosed as a diffuse astrocytic glioma without IDH and H3R gene mutations, with microvascular proliferation, necrosis, and/or peculiar molecular features such as TERT mutation, EGFR amplification, and/or gain of chromosome 7 combined with the loss of chromosome 10 [3–6]. According to the EANO guidelines for the diagnosis and treatment of diffuse gliomas of adulthood, isocitrate dehydrogenase (IDH)-mutated glioblastoma should be better defined as a grade 4 IDH-mutant astrocytoma [6].

Current management of patients with GBM employs maximal safe resection surgery followed by radiation and chemotherapy [2,7–10].

Recurrent GBM can be managed by different approaches [11–13], including loco-regional treatment and systemic treatments [2,14–19].

The prognosis of patients with GBM remains poor, with an estimated overall survival (OS) of 12–18 months from primary diagnosis and a life expectancy of 5–10 months after the diagnosis of recurrent GBM [20–22].

Since treatments provided are not curative, guidelines strongly recommend the patient's inclusion in clinical trials [2,23].

In the last decade, several novel discoveries about the molecular, genomic, and biological background of the disease have been determined. Nonetheless, none of these improvements translated into a significant progress in terms of therapeutic options. Indeed, several drugs and approaches showing promising results in early studies failed to confirm a clinical improvement on large randomized trials. Furthermore, the enrollment on clinical trials is limited, with only 10% of GBM patients being enrolled in a clinical study [24,25].

The purpose of the present paper is to investigate possible reasons related to the lack of therapeutic improvements on GBM, focusing on possible improvements in terms of trial planning and design. We also reviewed more promising experimental systemic treatments for patients in early phase of development, as well as in patients with newly diagnosed and recurrent GBM.

2. Therapeutic Targets on GBM

Several biological obstacles make the development novel effective drugs difficult [26,27]. These are represented by (1) the blood–brain and blood– tumor - brain barrier which makes the passage of therapeutic compounds difficult, (2) the extreme heterogeneity of the disease, and finally (3) the capacity to develop molecular mechanisms able to promote treatment resistance to antitumoral treatment. All these elements reduce the development of novel target agents. Nonetheless, the increasing knowledge of the molecular mechanisms related to disease development and progression has allowed the identification of several attractive targets for the systemic management of GBM (Table 1) [26,27]. The majority of these targets are represented by tyrosine kinase (TK) receptors.

Table 1. Clinical trials cited in the text. MGMT: methylation of the O(6)-methylguanine-DNA methyltransferase, TMZ: temozolomide.

Trial Name	Phase	Experimental Compounds	Setting
NCT02386826	I	Capmatinib and bevacizumab	Newly diagnosed and recurrent GBM
NCT04077866	I/II	B7-HR CAR-T	Glioblastoma cells expressing B7-H3
NCT04741984 DEMAND	I	Pp65CMV antigen monocytes	Newly diagnosed MGMT unmethylated GBM
NCT04047706	I	BMS-986205 + Nivolumab	Newly diagnosed GBM
NCT03294486 ONCOVIRAC	I/II	Combination of TG002 and 5-flucytosine	Recurrent GBM
NCT03714334	I	DNX-2440	Recurrent GBM
NCT02062827	I	M032-HSV1	Newly diagnosed GBM or recurrent GBM.
NCT03663725 StrateGlio	III	Intensified TMZ protocol	Newly diagnosed GBM
NCT03899857 PERGOLA	II	Pembrolizumab	Newly diagnosed GBM
NCT04396860	II/III	Ipilimumab + nivolumab	Newly diagnosed GBM-MGMT unmethylated
NCT03776071	III	Enzastaurin	Newly diagnosed GBM
NCT04704154	II	Regorafenib + nivolumab	Recurrent GBM
NCT04277221	III	Autologous Dendritic Cell/Tumor antigen	Recurrent GBM

The amplification of the epidermal growth factor receptor can be found in about 50% of GBMs [28], and several agents targeting this pathway have been investigated in GBMs (a discussion of treatments proposed for EGFR inhibition is included in Section 4. Recurrent GBM). Other than EGFR, some other TK receptors have gained particular interest.

Altered tumor vascularization is one of the hallmarks of the disease and there are at least two TK receptors whose inhibition could be associated with angiogenesis regression and tumor responses. These are the vascular endothelial growth factor receptor (VEGFR) and the platelet-delivered growth factor receptor (PDGFR) [16,29]. Several small TK inhibitors (TKIs) targeting one or both of these two receptors have been tested without significant benefit [16]. Imatinib, pazopanib, cediranib, sunitinib, sorafenib, nintedanib, tivozanib, dovitinib, crenolanib, and cabozantinib are all oral TKIs that failed to show a significant clinical benefit on patients with GBM [16]. The mesenchymal–epithelial transition (MET) receptor is another pathway that could be activated in GBM cells [30]. Although the multi-target and MET inhibitor cabozantinib showed only a modest effect on GBM [31] (weighted by a high adverse events rate), the oral MET inhibitor capmatinib is under investigation for patients with GBM, in combination with bevacizumab (NCT02386826).

The epidermal growth factor receptor 2 (HER2) amplification is a driver molecule that is well-targeted by several target compounds in breast cancer. This receptor can be amplified also in GBM cells [32]. However, to date, no agents targeting HER2 have shown clinical efficacy on patients with GBM. Indeed, the oral inhibitors lapatinib and neratinib failed to show a significant impact on patients with GBM and in patients with brain metastases from solid tumors [33,34]. The novel oral TKI tucatinib has been shown to pass through the blood–brain barrier, reaching therapeutic concentrations in the brain [35]. Although this could be an effective treatment on patients with HER2-altered GBM, no trials are investigating this agent.

The management of several solid tumors has been revolutionized by the advent of immune-checkpoint inhibitors. Briefly, these agents can restore an inhibited immune response against tumors and are effective also on brain metastases from solid malignancies [36]. Their role will be further discussed in the next paragraph. Nonetheless, some other immunological approaches are assuming particular interest in the hematological and solid tumor treatment field [37]. Chimeric antigen receptor T cells (CAR-Ts) and chimeric antigen receptor macrophage (CAR-Ms) are surely two of the most enthusiastic approaches, involving the genomic recombination of T cells or macrophages which are oriented against tumor cells. Although there is little data regarding the safety and efficacy of this approach on GBM, several early phase studies are assessing this strategy on patients with GBM (NCT04077866, NCT04741984). Nonetheless, it is still unclear which could be the optimal cell manufacture and administration process. Of interest, some data are suggesting that CAR-Ms could be key strategies for GBM management, mainly thanks to the better penetration of the macrophage into the tumor-associated microenvironment (NCT04741984) [38].

Indoleamine 2,3-dioxygenase (IDO) 1 and 2 are catabolic enzymes involved in the degradation of tryptophan. IDO is supposed to promote a negative regulation of immune response, and it has the potential to inhibit both innate and adaptive responses against the tumor [39]. Although these agents have been already tested on GBM, the combinations of IDO inhibitors such as indoximod, epacadostat, BMS-986205, [40,41] and immune checkpoint, chemotherapy, and/or radiation treatment is under assessment in several different trials (NCT04047706).

Oncolytic viruses are reprogrammed viruses able to specifically target tumor cells, replicating and killing them [42–45]. Previous studies suggested a potential effective role of these agents against GBM in preclinical models and within early clinical studies [42–45]. Thus, several trials are testing these agents on GBM patients (NCT03294486, NCT03714334, NCT02062827).

3. Newly Diagnosed GBM

Since 2005, the post-surgical standard treatment of GBM is surgical resection followed by temozolomide (TMZ), concomitant with and adjuvant to radiotherapy (60 Gy over six weeks), leading to a median survival time of 14.6 months [9]. The benefit from TMZ is greater in patients who present MGMT promoter methylation, which epigenetically silences the gene [7].

Different improvements of the current protocol have been tested in recent years.

Two trials demonstrating an improvement in overall survival with standard treatment have not been fully incorporated in the actual therapeutic scenario for different reasons. Tumor-treating fields (TTFields) is an antimitotic treatment modality, which acts by delivering a low-intensity (200 kHZ) electric field within the brain, alternating electric fields to the tumor. Through this action, TTFields interferes with GBM cell division and organelle assembly. The efficacy of incorporating TTFields in the standard first line treatment has been explored in the EF-14 trial [46]. In this randomized trial, 695 GBM patients, after completed concomitant radio chemotherapy, were randomized to TTFields plus maintenance TMZ or TMZ alone. The addition of TTFields lead to a significant increase in PFS (6.7 vs. 4.0 months, HR, 0.63; 95% CI, 0.52–0.76; $p < 0.001$) and OS (20.0 vs. 16.0 months HR, 0.63; 95% CI, 0.53–0.76; $p < 0.001$) over standard treatment, without significant difference in adverse events. Despite the FDA approving TTFields for newly diagnosed GBM in 2015, the use in clinical practice remains limited (3–12% of patients with newly diagnosed GBM) due to patients declining to wear the device, combined with difficulty in understanding the mechanism of action, doubts about the favorable outcome of existing studies, and the high costs of the treatment (to date, this treatment strategy is mainly adopted by USA, Israel, and Switzerland).

The CeTeG/NOA-09 German trial has randomized 141 MGMT-methylated GBM patients to standard TMZ concomitant with and adjuvant to radiotherapy, or to six cycles of a lomustine and TMZ combination in addition to radiotherapy [47]. Median OS was 31.4 months in the TMZ group, compared to 48.1 months in the lomustine–TMZ group (hazard ratio (HR) 0.60; 95% CI, 0.35–1.03; $p = 0.0492$). There was no difference in terms of progression-free survival (PFS), while adverse events of grade 3 or higher were observed in 51% and 59% of patients in the TMZ group and lomustine–TMZ group, respectively. However, the study presents some significant limitations. First, the small cohort of patients limits the validity of the results and presents the possibility of biases. Furthermore, the low number of randomized patients is in contrast with the high number of MGMT-methylated screened patients, with an accrual rate of only 60%. Another interesting issue was the improvement in OS which was not associated to a PFS benefit. This was not observed in previous newly diagnosed GBM phase III trials [9,46], and was not explained by differences in subsequent treatments at recurrence/progression.

Moreover, no survival benefit has been demonstrated with TMZ dose-dense regimens [48] or with extension of maintenance treatment up to 12 cycles [49]. To further explore this setting, the ANOCEF group proposes a randomized trial (NCT03663725) comparing standard treatment versus an intensified arm consisting of one TMZ cycle started between day 2 and 15 after surgery, followed by TMZ concomitant to radiotherapy, followed by maintenance TMZ until progression, intolerance, the patient's or the physician's decision.

Given the potential role of hypoxia in the biology of GBM, the addition of antiangiogenic therapy with bevacizumab has been investigated in two large phase III randomized trials in the first line setting [50,51]. Despite prolonging PFS in both trials, the addition of bevacizumab failed to demonstrate an overall survival improvement. Moreover, bevacizumab was associated with an increase in adverse events.

The introduction of immune checkpoint inhibitors (ICIs) has recently revolutionized the therapeutic scenario in a number of different cancer types. ICIs act as inhibitors of immune-checkpoints, restoring an inhibited immune-response against the tumor. Two phase III clinical trials investigated nivolumab (a programmed death receptor-1 (PD-1) inhibitor) in combination with radiation therapy in patients with unmethylated MGMT GBM (CheckMate-498; NCT02617589), and in association with radiation therapy plus concomitant and adjuvant temozolomide in patients with methylated MGMT glioblastoma CheckMate-548; NCT02667587). Unfortunately, none of these trials showed significant improvement in terms of OS and PFS for patients receiving nivolumab.

Another immunotherapy first line phase II trial, PERGOLA (NCT03899857) is evaluating the addition of pembrolizumab to standard treatment in newly diagnosed GBM patients.

The ICIs combination with ipilimumab and nivolumab has been initially studied in exploratory phase I cohorts. In these patients there was a significant rate of high-grade adverse events, with a discontinuation rate due to toxicity accounting for 20.30 [52]; thus, this combination strategy has not being further assessed in the subsequent phase III trials. The ICI ipilimumab and nivolumab combination is now being retested in a phase II/III study in newly diagnosed MGMT unmethylated GBM patients, comparing the usual treatment with radiation therapy and TMZ to radiation therapy in combination with ipilimumab and nivolumab (NCT04396860).

The role of active immunotherapy via vaccine injection is being explored in the ongoing study of dendritic cell (DC) immunotherapy against cancer stem cells. In this study, newly diagnosed GBM patients are vaccinated during standard treatment with ex vivo generated DCs transfected with mRNA from autologous tumor stem cells, survivin, and hTERT.

Enzastaurin (enz) inhibits protein kinase C-beta, angiogenesis, and has a direct cytotoxic activity against glioma cells [53]. Previous phase II studies carried out in recurrent high-grade glioma and in newly diagnosed MGMT unmethylated GBM patients did not show any significant single-agent activity [54,55]. However, the recent discovery of a novel biomarker, de novo genomic marker 1 (DGM1), a germline polymorphism on chromosome 8, highly correlated with response to enz in both lymphoma and GBM [56], has prompted the clinical development of this drug. In particular, GBM patients with DGM1+ assessment receiving enz had a median OS of 18 months versus 12.8 months in DGM1− patients (HR 0.68; 95% CI, 0.25–1.81; $p = 0.12$). Given these data, a randomized double-blind, placebo-controlled phase III study of enz added to temozolomide during and following radiotherapy in newly diagnosed GBM with or without DGM1 has been recently launched in the US (NCT03776071).

The phase III trial EORTC 1709 evaluating the addition of marizomib, a novel brain-penetrant pan-proteasome inhibitor, to standard TMZ/RT→TMZ in newly diagnosed GBM has been prematurely closed by IDMC, after evidence of more frequent grade 3/4 treatment-emergent adverse events compared to the standard therapy group (42.6% vs. 20.5%), including ataxia, hallucinations, and headache. The study did not show a significant impact on OS or PFS over standard treatment in [57].

Adaptive platform trials allow the testing of several experimental drugs at the same time, developing a more efficient and cost-effective mechanism for accelerating treatment approval for patients. In the neuro-oncology field, the GBM AGILE study (NCT03970447) is evaluating several experimental compounds on patients with newly diagnosed and recurrent GBM, tailoring each experimental arm according to the molecular assessment of the disease. AGILE opened for patient enrollment in 2019, and site activation is ongoing in the US, whereas expansion to Canada, Europe, and China are under progress. The trial is evaluating a new treatment arm using regorafenib, paxalisib, and VAL-083 in maintenance period in newly diagnosed GBM after concomitant treatment [58].

Despite available treatments, GBM inevitably recurs, demonstrating a poor overall prognosis with a two-year survival rate of less than 20%. Nevertheless, it should be highlighted that a small proportion of patients achieve a long survival of over three years, but the molecular prognostic and predictive background dividing long-term (LTS) from short-term survivors (STS) is still poorly understood. Nonetheless, some studies investigated the clinical and molecular behaviors of LTS. Overall, LTS were younger at diagnosis, female, and presented MGMT methylation. The sphingomyelin metabolism was also increased in these patients [59–61]. With the aim to understand biological background of LTS, EORTC is conducting the EORTC 1419 Eternity trial (NCT03770468). This prospective and retrospective multicentric clinical epidemiological study will evaluate the molecular genetics, and host-derived and clinical determinants of GBM patients with an overall survival of more than five years.

4. Recurrent GBM

Effective treatment options are limited, and new therapeutic strategies are desperately needed. As of yet, nitrosoureas are still considered the standard of care for recurrent GBM. Several tyrosine kinase inhibitors (TKIs) and monoclonal antibodies (mAbs) targets have been investigated in the last few years with limited results [14,15,17,18,62–65], while many others are in clinical development in recent clinical trials.

About 50% of all GBM patients present an amplification of the epidermal growth factor receptor (*EGFR*) gene which represents a driver mutation in GBM. Most frequent EGRF mutations are represented by EGFRA289D, EGFRA289T, and EGFRA289V [28]. Nonetheless, agents targeting this receptor failed to show a significant survival impact on patients with GBM [66–68].

Recently, depatuxizumab mafodotin (depatux−m, ABT414), an antibody-drug conjugate that consists of an antibody directed against EGFR and EGFRvIII, conjugated to a toxin (monomethyl auristatin F), was evaluated in the INTELLANCE-2/EORTC_1410 randomized phase II study [69]. Patients receiving depatux-m and TMZ had a trend towards improved survival (primary analysis: HR 0.71; 95% CI, 0.50–1.02; $p = 0.06$; second follow up analysis: HR 0.66; 95% CI, 0.48–0.93; $p = 0.024$), corresponding to a median OS difference of 9.6 months (deatux-m + TMZ) versus 8.2 months (TMZ). The presence of EGFR single-nucleotide variations (SNVs) was shown to predict an improved outcome in the depatux−m + TMZ arm. These SNVs result in a receptor that is hypersensitive to low-affinity EGFR ligands, which can explain the increased activity of depatux−m and TMZ [70].

Antiangiogenic approaches have been investigated since 2007, with bevacizumab being the most studied agent [14,19,71–78]. Despite promising results in terms of progression-free survival across multiple studies, these results did not translate into an overall survival benefit in the randomized phase III EORTC 26101 trial that compared bevacizumab and lomustine with lomustine alone (9.1 vs. 8.6 months, hazard ratio for death, 0.95; 95% CI, 0.74–1.21; $p = 0.65$)

More recently, regorafenib, an oral multi-kinase inhibitor targeting VEGFR-1, -2, -3, TIE 2, PDGFR, FGFR, KIT, RAF-1, RET, and BRAF has been investigated in the randomized phase II trial REGOMA, which has been approved for the management of recurrent glioblastoma by the EMA (European Medicines Agency) [17]; this trial showed a median OS of 7.4 months in the regorafenib arm vs. 5.6 in the lomustine arm. Thus, this agent has been included in other ongoing trials (i.e., the AGILE study) or in combination with other agents (i.e., Nivolumab, NCT04704154). Alteration of the cyclin-dependent kinase 4–6 (CDK4–6) pathway is a common event in GBM. A phase II trial evaluated the role of palbociclib in recurrent GBM patients with RB1 proficiency. Despite adequate penetration in tumor tissue, palbociclib showed limited activity with a median PFS of 5 weeks and a median survival of 15.4 weeks [79]. Similarly, in another phase II trial in patients with recurrent GBM and with evidence of CDKN2A/B loss and intact RB, abemaciclib showed a six-month PFS of 9.37% (95% CI, 2.4–22.7%), a median PFS was 55 days (95% CI, 49–56 days), and a median OS of 384 days (95% CI, 228–488).

Larotrectinib is a selective TRK inhibitor that showed an impressive response rate and also durable disease control in GBM patients. The study [80], presented at the 2019 ASCO meeting, evaluated 18 cases with primary brain tumors, including six (32%) patients with GBM. A disease control rate was achieved in 100% of patients (in 14 evaluable patients), with a disease control rate ≥ 16 and 24 weeks in 79% and 71% of patients, respectively; the median PFS was 11 months (95% CI, 2.8–Not Reached). At the recent 2021 ASCO meeting, data regarding larotrectinib suggested that better results were obtained in pediatric patients with brain tumors, while no partial responses were seen in adult glioma patients.

Agents targeting BRAF inhibit the downstream altered MAPK pathway, which is often altered in solid tumors and is also an important driver of cell proliferation in glioma patients. V600E is the most frequent mutation in the BRAF gene described in gliomas, occurring in about 5% of adults [81]. Vemurafenib and dabrafenib, selective oral tyrosine kinase inhibitors of the oncogenic BRAF V600 kinase, have been tested in BRAF mutant melanoma patients. The role of vemurafenib in BRAF V600-mutant gliomas has been investigated in the VE-BASKET trial [82], which evaluated 24 patients (six GBM, five anaplastic astrocytoma, one high grade glioma not otherwise specified, and twelve with other histologies). For high-grade glioma patients, the response rate was 9%, the median PFS was 5.3 months, and the median survival was 11.9 months. Combined inhibition of BRAF and MEK in gliomas was also investigated in the ROAR basket trial [83]; in the group of high-grade gliomas response rate was 27%, and the disease control rate was 57%.

Immunotherapies have also been investigated in recurrent GBM. The Check-Mate-143 trial evaluating nivolumab (a PD-1 inhibitor) versus bevacizumab in recurrent GBM was negative in the general population [18]. Nonetheless, the response duration was longer in the nivolumab (11.1 months) arm as compared to the bevacizumab arm (5.3 months). The corticosteroid use did not impact survival in the bevacizumab arm, while reduced doses were associated with an improved clinical outcome in the nivolumab treatment arm (HR, 0.59; 95% CI, 0.36–0.95). Moreover, a trend toward a longer survival was observed in MGMT-methylated patients without any baseline corticosteroids receiving nivolumab over bevacizumab (17.0 vs. 10.1 months; HR, 0.58; 95% CI, 0.30–1.11).

Pembrolizumab was also evaluated as a "neoadjuvant" treatment for recurrent GBM in an Ivy Foundation Early Phase Clinical Trials Consortium randomized study. Cloughesy and Colleagues evaluated the survival and immune response obtained when using pembrolizumab before and/or after surgery in 35 recurrent GBM patients [84]. Patients in the "neoadjuvant" arm with continued adjuvant therapy following surgery reported a significant increase in survival compared to patients treated with pembrolizumab only after surgery, with a median survival of 13.7 months in the "neoadjuvant/adjuvant" arm vs. 7.5 months in the "adjuvant"-only arm (HR: 0.39; 95% CI, 0.17–0.94; $p = 0.04$). Interestingly, treatment with pembrolizumab before surgery was associated with upregulation of T cell- and interferon-γ-related gene expression, but downregulation of cell cycle-related gene expression within the tumor.

Another immunotherapy approach consists of vaccination against EGFRvIII, a GBM-specific EGFR driver mutation [85]. Rindopepimut in combination with bevacizumab, or a control injection of keyhole limpet hemocyanin in combination with bevacizumab, were investigated in a randomized phase II trial in recurrent EGFRvIII-positive GBM patients. The primary endpoint was PFS at six months, which was 28% for rindopepimut and 16% for the control ($p = 0.12$); the analysis of survival, a secondary endpoint, showed a statistically significant advantage in the rindopepimut–bevacizumab arm (HR 0.53; 95% CI, 0.32–0.88; $p = 0.01$). Additionally, in a randomized phase III study investigating rindopepimut in patients with newly diagnosed GBM, this agent did not improve OS compared to the standard of care [86].

Another immunotherapy approach consists of active immunization (i.e., dendritic cells or peptide vaccines). Dendritic cells (DCs) are antigen-presenting cells able to induce adaptive immunity. Due to promising results from a phase III trial in a newly diagnosed setting [87] with an autologous tumor lysate-pulsed dendritic cell vaccine (DCVax®-L), similar approaches are now under investigation in phase III trials in the recurrent setting GBM (NCT04277221).

5. Problematic Issues on Interventional Trials: The Glioblastoma Paradox

The lack of therapeutic improvements in the last years appears even more disappointing considering the increasing scientific understanding of the disease and the large availability of novel potential active compounds to test.

This paradox makes GBM a unique disease in which the availability of key molecular and biological insight does not translate into the development of new drugs.

The presence of the blood–brain barrier, the heterogeneous and complex biology of the disease, and the lack of sufficient investment are possible explanations of this failure.

Nonetheless, some concerns emerge about the modality by which these novel compounds are tested therefore the clinical trial landscape (Table 2).

Table 2. Challenges and innovations of trial design planning for patients with glioblastoma.

Challenges of Clinical Trials Design on GBM	Innovation Proposed
A small number of patients benefit from inclusion in clinical trials	The inclusion of patients should be encouraged through the development of inter-center networks and improvement of organizational phases. Investments in trial planning and facilities for patients enrolled in clinical trials can increase the number of patients in clinical trials [88–90].
Reduced reliability from phase II study	Inclusion of comparator arm in this setting and also randomization in phase II studies [91].
A large number of patients are required for randomization in an early setting	Bayesian models with flexible and adaptive trial designs offer to test more compounds at the same time (comparing them to a shared comparator arm) with a reduced number of patients [92].
A long time from the trial start to the final result	(1) Bayesian adaptive randomized (AR) studies [93–95] (2) Use of different endpoints such as a composed PFS-OS endpoint or ORR through assessment of learning algorithms [96].
A large number of novel compounds in pre-clinical phases	Phase 0 trials [97].
Molecular heterogeneity of the disease	Umbrella trial in which treatment arm allocation is driven by the molecular composition of the disease [98].

In 2018, Vanderbeek A.M. et al. published the results of a survey of clinical trials reported on clinicaltrials.gov, including GBM patients in the United States from 2005 to 2016 [25]. Interestingly, they reported over 400 clinical trials of which the majority were represented by phase I/II and phase II studies (60%) [25].

Of note, the authors found a very high rate of uncompleted and terminated trials with one to ten studies concluded due to lack of accrual, funding, or futility (no clinical advantage emerging at early assessment) [25]. Moreover, there was a median time to study completion of three to four years in phase II studies. These data appear even more surprising considering that only 5 of 249 phase I/II and phase II trials were randomized. Phase III trials were a minority, representing only 7% of all clinical trials assessed. Twelve of sixteen phase III trials were supported by a previous phase II study, and the overall population enrolled in these trials represented 26% of the total population assessed on clinical trials between 2005 and 2016 [25].

The authors concluded that only one to ten (8–11%) patients entered into clinical trials, which is a very frustrating result considering the rate of terminated trials due to lack of accrual [25].

Another well-known problematic issue related to interventional trials on GBM is the weakness of surrogate efficacy endpoints [50,51,95,99,100]. Indeed, progression-free survival (PFS) and overall response rate (ORR) is successfully adopted in clinical trials assessing novel compounds on solid malignancies as they provide a reliable prediction of other outcomes of interest, such as clinical improvement and overall survival (OS). The use of surrogate endpoints of OS could be important as they can reduce the time of the study. Nonetheless, the relationship between OS and surrogate such as PFS and ORR is extremely uncertain on GBM as survival benefit cannot reflect the improvement of PFS or ORR [50,51,95,99,100], especially in the case of antiangiogenic treatments. The post-progressive survival is a composite outcome, which has been assessed in a large series of over a thousand patients with GBM, and represents an interesting surrogate endpoint [101].

The research of reliable surrogates of OS acquires great importance in the assessment of novel agents in GBM.

The availability of novel potentially active drugs is increasing as biological and genomic assessment of the disease becomes even more clear. Furthermore, it has been demonstrated that GBM is not a unique disease as its molecular behaviors can drastically modify the clinical presentation, progression, and response to treatment. The larger the availability of novel compounds, the higher the need for interventional trials. This can be complicated considering the low incidence of the disease.

To date, only a few patients benefit from interventional clinical trials. The rate of terminated study due to lack of accrual is relatively high even if patients are strongly required, considering the increasing availability of novel agents. Additionally, the time to study completion is long, requiring years due to the absence of reliable surrogate endpoints of overall survival. Finally, the distribution of patients could be unbalanced, since the majority of them are enrolled in phase III trials with a relatively small number of patients enrolled in early phase I and II studies. This can lead to an unpowered early efficacy study, exposed to the risk of unclear information. The result is the early termination of potentially active compounds and a further unsuccessful test (on phase III) of unactive drugs.

Excluding financial and biological problems related to the development of new effective compounds, these issues may represent a strong limitation to the clinical progress of GBM management.

Improving Interventional Clinical Trials Design on GBM

The primary field of improvement is represented by organizational improvement and the need for investment in the research of active compounds, trial planning, and patients on trial tutelage [88–90].

Patients with GBM should be referred to reference centers and the development of inter-center networks providing early information about active trials should be encouraged. Similarly, the participation of patients in clinical trials could be encouraged through facilities allowing patient mobility, permanence in the experimental center during the trial course and follow up, and job and economic safeguarding of patients and caregivers. These elements could reduce the number of early terminated trials, as well as increase the number of patients who could benefit from a clinical trial (Table 2).

From the organizational point of view, there are several fields of improvement of clinical trials in GBM [88–90].

The introduction of a comparator arm in phase II study has provided a more accurate estimation of the efficacy of the novel compound under investigation [91], however, again, the transition from a positive randomized phase II [14,15,17,18,64,68,73,86,102–105] trial with a limited number of patients to a large phase III trial was negative [77]. Nonetheless, early randomized studies require more time for their completion and a higher number of patients as compared to single-arm phase II studies. To avoid these limitations, the incorporation of Bayesian statistics in trial design is a winning strategy [92]. Classical trials test a hypothesis among a distinct population, in a study with a pre-planned sample size dimension which conditions the power of the study.

The hypothesis of the Bayesian model is not fixed, but its probability (for example to be true or false) is constantly modified during the study due to the increasing amount of data acquired. For example, the Bayesian adaptive randomized (AR) study can use the data accumulating in the course of the same trial to modify the treatment allocation according to the potentially more efficient interventional arms [92].

In 2012, Trippa L. et al. acquired data from different phase II trials assessing four different compounds. In their simulation, authors allocated these same patients into a Bayesian AR study, assessing the same interventional arms [92]. Results of this simulation were surprising, as the same findings of the previous phase II studies were confirmed without loss in statistical power and with a significantly lower number of patients required [92].

Nowadays, Bayesian AR is commonly adopted in clinical trial design and represents a significant improvement in terms of quality of the research due to the possibility of testing more treatments with a shared comparator arm, at the same time reducing the number of patients required.

Another commonly adopted strategy to overcome the need for a comparator arm, and thus the randomization, is the adoption of a historical cohort based on previous findings in clinical trials [91]. This strategy exposes the risk of several biases for different reasons. First, outcomes such as the survival of patients with GBM are not static values, as there is a trend showing increases in time even if there is no modification of treatment standards [91,106]. In addition, it has been well demonstrated that the inter-trial variability reflects a variable distribution of the outcome of interest, which significantly increases the risk of underestimating or overestimating the benchmarks [91]. This final result poses a very high risk of achieving false positive or negative observations in phase II trials, leading to a subsequent assessment of inactive compounds or the early termination of the study of an active drug [91].

Even if OS remains the best available clinical endpoint, the research of a novel surrogate endpoint is still a clinical need.

The PFS improvement failed to show an improvement in OS across different clinical trials [50,51,95,99,100]. Nonetheless, PFS expressed as the rate of patients progressing at a specified interval of time is commonly adopted in GBM clinical trials [50,51,95,99,100]. Again, Bayesian AR trials can offer a possible solution to this problem [96]. Thanks to the flexibility of the Bayesian AR trial, the incoming data provided in the course of the clinical trial can allow early determination of whether concordance between OS and PFS exists, therefore allowing, in case of concordance, decision-making results based on the assessment of PFS alone [96].

There are several problems related to response assessment in patients with GBM [107–110]. Indeed, response assessment must involve other data in addition to dimensional and imaging criteria. The type of treatment provided and the molecular background of the disease are mandatory elements to estimate response to treatment. Integration of molecular and clinical data with imaging improves ORR estimation; nonetheless, functional imaging provided by magnetic resonance imaging (MRI) and positron emission tomography (PET) is increasing as to allow a more reliable distinction of progression/response to treatment [107–113]. Criteria of response assessment have been modified and reflects the type of treatment provided [107,108].

Novel technologies are currently employing the use of artificial intelligence algorithms which can, based on the data provided and learned, assess the disease [114,115], and improve the use of this endpoint.

Innovative trials on GBM are represented by AGILE, INSIGhT, and N2M2 trials [93,94,98].

The Adaptive Global Innovative Learning Environment (GBM AGILE) is a novel, multi-arm, platform trial which is composed of two different statistical designs [93]. The first phase is a Bayesian AR stage in which several compounds are tested with a common control. Through this phase, the aim is to isolate the active compounds and determine the population in which this is expected to be more effective, preventing and reducing the number of patients receiving ineffective treatments. Regarding this last point, results of the experimental arm investigating the CC-115 compound within the INSIGhT trial have been recently reported [116]. Thanks to the adaptive study design of the INSIGhT trial, a reduced number of patients received the experimental treatment which showed significant toxicity and lack of clinical efficacy [116]. Once that a promising active compound has been established, it proceeds to the second phase which involves classical fixed randomization to confirm the result of the Bayesian step [93]. Other advantages of this platform are represented by the inclusion of novel compounds at any time during the study. In addition, biomarkers can be assessed during each phase of the study allowing a fast discovery and validation of prognostic/predictive biological markers [93].

In addition, the INSIGhT trials employed a Bayesian AR in the first step [94]. Different from AGILE, in the INSIGhT trial, only patients with newly diagnosed unmethylated GBM without the isocitrate dehydrogenase (IDH) R132H gene mutation have been included. A key inclusion criterion is also represented by complete genomic data for biomarker groupings [94]. This trial is currently testing three different compounds simultaneously and comparing them to the standard represented by radiation and adjuvant temozolomide [94]. Preliminary results of the abemaciclib treatment arm have been recently reported showing no OS advantage for patients receiving the CDK inhibitor [117].

The paradigm of the precision medicine era is the administration of drugs tailored based on the biological background of tumor disease. AGILE and INSIGhT offer the possibility to test more drugs rapidly, isolating the population where the novel agent is more effective.

The NCT Neuro Master Match (N2M2) offers a different solution, as the goal of this trial is to primarily identify the target population, then provide the drug which can result in a clinical improvement based on the biological background of the disease [98]. This is an umbrella trial for patients with unmethylated IDH wild-type GBM [98]. The design of the study is composed of two parts; the discovery phase provides a molecular and neuropathological assessment of the disease to detect predefined biomarkers for targeted treatments, while the treatment phase employs a stratification of the population based on the results obtained in the discovery phase. The Bayesian model is employed to provide continuous monitoring of toxicity in phase I, while the efficacy endpoint is represented by six-month progression-free survival [98].

Despite umbrella and molecular tailored designs being extremely attractive, it should be noted that GBM is a heterogeneous disease and that the isolation of potentially predictive biomarkers may not reflect a sensitivity to defined novel compounds.

One proposed type of trial that specifically aims to target agents is represented by "phase 0" studies [97] (Figure 1).

Due to the protection offered by the blood–brain barrier (BBB) and the blood-tumor–brain barrier, several drugs failed to show a clinical effect on GBM. Phase 0 studies can rapidly assess pharmacological effects of the compounds on a patient's tumors, also discovering if and how much the compounds pass the BBB and penetrate the tumor tissue. Briefly, the study design requires that patients assume the study drug one to two weeks before preplanned surgery. After surgery, there is an in vivo assessment of tumor tissue, cerebrospinal fluid, and/or blood. Vogelbaum M.A. et al. recently reviewed all phase 0 and phase 0-like studies carried out between 1993 and 2018, establishing that phase 0 study in neuro-oncology should include patients in which tumor resection is planned, and involve clinical doses of the investigational agent, a tissue sample from each part of the tumor (including enhancing and non-enhancing portions of the tumor), and the assessment of specific drug-related target effects [97].

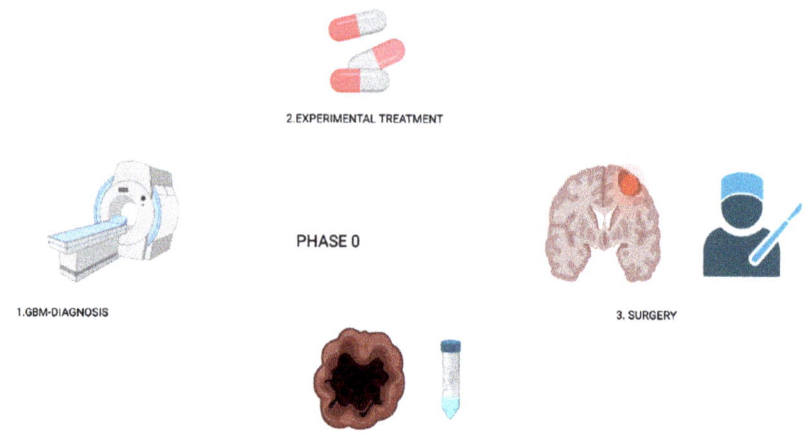

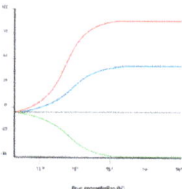

Figure 1. Phase 0 study overall design.

6. Conclusions

Glioblastoma represents a clinical challenge for oncologists and researchers. The increasing knowledge of molecular mechanisms related to disease onset and progression has allowed the development of several novel compounds which should be assessed among clinical trials. The need to test more and more compounds at the same time led to the development of a next generation of trials adopting a Bayesian design. In addition, phase 0 trials can detect early and perform an in vivo assessment of drugs able to penetrate the tumor tissue, stopping further development of drugs unable to cross the blood–brain barrier. All these elements will surely contribute to the development of effective treatments against the disease, as well as to allow patients access to experimental compounds.

Author Contributions: Conceptualization, V.D.N., E.F., A.T., and A.A.B.; writing original draft preparation, V.D.N., E.F., A.T., A.A.B., L.G., and S.B.; editing, R.L. and A.A.B.; supervision, R.L. and A.A.B. All authors have read and agreed to the published version of the manuscript.

Funding: This research received no external funding.

Conflicts of Interest: The authors declare no conflict of interest.

References

1. Ostrom, Q.T.; Cioffi, G.; Gittleman, H.; Patil, N.; Waite, K.; Kruchko, C.; Barnholtz-Sloan, J.S. CBTRUS Statistical Report: Primary Brain and Other Central Nervous System Tumors Diagnosed in the United States in 2012–2016. *Neuro Oncol.* **2019**, *21*, v1–v100. [CrossRef] [PubMed]
2. Wen, P.Y.; Weller, M.; Lee, E.Q.; Alexander, B.M.; Barnholtz-Sloan, J.S.; Barthel, F.P.; Batchelor, T.T.; Bindra, R.S.; Chang, S.M.; Chiocca, E.A.; et al. Glioblastoma in adults: A Society for Neuro-Oncology (SNO) and European Society of Neuro-Oncology (EANO) consensus review on current management and future directions. *Neuro Oncol.* **2020**, *22*, 1073–1113. [CrossRef] [PubMed]

3. Brat, D.J.; Aldape, K.; Colman, H.; Figrarella-Branger, D.; Fuller, G.N.; Giannini, C.; Holland, E.C.; Jenkins, R.B.; Kleinschmidt-DeMasters, B.; Komori, T.; et al. cIMPACT-NOW update 5: Recommended grading criteria and terminologies for IDH-mutant astrocytomas. *Acta Neuropathol.* **2020**, *139*, 603–608. [CrossRef] [PubMed]
4. Brat, D.J.; Aldape, K.; Colman, H.; Holland, E.C.; Louis, D.N.; Jenkins, R.B.; Kleinschmidt-DeMasters, B.K.; Perry, A.; Reifenberger, G.; Stupp, R.; et al. cIMPACT-NOW update 3: Recommended diagnostic criteria for "Diffuse astrocytic glioma, IDH-wildtype, with molecular features of glioblastoma, WHO grade IV". *Acta Neuropathol.* **2018**, *136*, 805–810. [CrossRef]
5. Louis, D.N.; Wesseling, P.; Aldape, K.; Brat, D.J.; Capper, D.; Cree, I.A.; Eberhart, C.; Figarella-Branger, D.; Fouladi, M.; Fuller, G.N.; et al. cIMPACT-NOW update 6: New entity and diagnostic principle recommendations of the cIMPACT-Utrecht meeting on future CNS tumor classification and grading. *Brain Pathol.* **2020**, *30*, 844–856. [CrossRef]
6. Weller, M.; van den Bent, M.; Preusser, M.; Le Rhun, E.; Tonn, J.C.; Minniti, G.; Bendszus, M.; Balana, C.; Chinot, O.; Dirven, L.; et al. EANO guidelines on the diagnosis and treatment of diffuse gliomas of adulthood. *Nat. Rev. Clin. Oncol.* **2021**, *18*, 170–186. [CrossRef]
7. Hegi, M.E.; Diserens, A.C.; Gorlia, T.; Hamou, M.F.; de Tribolet, N.; Weller, M.; Kros, J.M.; Hainfellner, J.A.; Mason, W.; Mariani, L.; et al. MGMT gene silencing and benefit from temozolomide in glioblastoma. *N. Engl. J. Med.* **2005**, *352*, 997–1003. [CrossRef] [PubMed]
8. Perry, J.R.; Laperriere, N.; O'Callaghan, C.J.; Brandes, A.A.; Menten, J.; Phillips, C.; Fay, M.; Nishikawa, R.; Cairncross, J.G.; Roa, W.; et al. Short-Course Radiation plus Temozolomide in Elderly Patients with Glioblastoma. *N. Engl. J. Med.* **2017**, *376*, 1027–1037. [CrossRef] [PubMed]
9. Stupp, R.; Mason, W.P.; van den Bent, M.J.; Weller, M.; Fisher, B.; Taphoorn, M.J.; Belanger, K.; Brandes, A.A.; Marosi, C.; Bogdahn, U.; et al. Radiotherapy plus concomitant and adjuvant temozolomide for glioblastoma. *N. Engl. J. Med.* **2005**, *352*, 987–996. [CrossRef]
10. Tosoni, A.; Franceschi, E.; Ermani, M.; Bertorelle, R.; Bonaldi, L.; Blatt, V.; Brandes, A.A. Temozolomide three weeks on and one week off as first line therapy for patients with recurrent or progressive low grade gliomas. *J. Neurooncol.* **2008**, *89*, 179–185. [CrossRef] [PubMed]
11. Le Rhun, E.; Preusser, M.; Roth, P.; Reardon, D.A.; van den Bent, M.; Wen, P.; Reifenberger, G.; Weller, M. Molecular targeted therapy of glioblastoma. *Cancer Treat. Rev.* **2019**, *80*, 101896. [CrossRef]
12. Lombardi, G.; Idbaih, A.; Le Rhun, E.; Preusser, M.; Zagonel, V.; French, P. A New Landscape for Systemic Pharmacotherapy of Recurrent Glioblastoma? *Cancers* **2020**, *12*, 3775. [CrossRef] [PubMed]
13. Weller, M.; Le Rhun, E. How did lomustine become standard of care in recurrent glioblastoma? *Cancer Treat. Rev.* **2020**, *87*, 102029. [CrossRef]
14. Brandes, A.A.; Finocchiaro, G.; Zagonel, V.; Reni, M.; Caserta, C.; Fabi, A.; Clavarezza, M.; Maiello, E.; Eoli, M.; Lombardi, G.; et al. AVAREG: A phase II, randomized, noncomparative study of fotemustine or bevacizumab for patients with recurrent glioblastoma. *Neuro Oncol.* **2016**, *18*, 1304–1312. [CrossRef]
15. Brandes, A.A.; Tosoni, A.; Franceschi, E.; Blatt, V.; Santoro, A.; Faedi, M.; Amistà, P.; Gardiman, M.; Labianca, R.; Bianchini, C.; et al. Fotemustine as second-line treatment for recurrent or progressive glioblastoma after concomitant and/or adjuvant temozolomide: A phase II trial of Gruppo Italiano Cooperativo di Neuro-Oncologia (GICNO). *Cancer Chemother. Pharmacol.* **2009**, *64*, 769–775. [CrossRef]
16. Di Nunno, V.; Franceschi, E.; Tosoni, A.; Di Battista, M.; Gatto, L.; Lamperini, C.; Minichillo, S.; Mura, A.; Bartolini, S.; Brandes, A.A. Treatment of recurrent glioblastoma: State-of-the-art and future perspectives. *Expert Rev. Anticancer Ther.* **2020**, *20*, 785–795. [CrossRef] [PubMed]
17. Lombardi, G.; De Salvo, G.L.; Brandes, A.A.; Eoli, M.; Rudà, R.; Faedi, M.; Lolli, I.; Pace, A.; Daniele, B.; Pasqualetti, F.; et al. Regorafenib compared with lomustine in patients with relapsed glioblastoma (REGOMA): A multicentre, open-label, randomised, controlled, phase 2 trial. *Lancet Oncol.* **2019**, *20*, 110–119. [CrossRef]
18. Reardon, D.A.; Brandes, A.A.; Omuro, A.; Mulholland, P.; Lim, M.; Wick, A.; Baehring, J.; Ahluwalia, M.S.; Roth, P.; Bähr, O.; et al. Effect of Nivolumab vs Bevacizumab in Patients with Recurrent Glioblastoma: The CheckMate 143 Phase 3 Randomized Clinical Trial. *JAMA Oncol.* **2020**, *6*, 1003–1010. [CrossRef]
19. Wick, W.; Gorlia, T.; Bendszus, M.; Taphoorn, M.; Sahm, F.; Harting, I.; Brandes, A.A.; Taal, W.; Domont, J.; Idbaih, A.; et al. Lomustine and Bevacizumab in Progressive Glioblastoma. *N. Engl. J. Med.* **2017**, *377*, 1954–1963. [CrossRef] [PubMed]
20. Lamborn, K.R.; Yung, W.K.; Chang, S.M.; Wen, P.Y.; Cloughesy, T.F.; DeAngelis, L.M.; Robins, H.I.; Lieberman, F.S.; Fine, H.A.; Fink, K.L.; et al. Progression-free survival: An important end point in evaluating therapy for recurrent high-grade gliomas. *Neuro Oncol.* **2008**, *10*, 162–170. [CrossRef]
21. Stupp, R.; Hegi, M.E.; Mason, W.P.; van den Bent, M.J.; Taphoorn, M.J.; Janzer, R.C.; Ludwin, S.K.; Allgeier, A.; Fisher, B.; Belanger, K.; et al. Effects of radiotherapy with concomitant and adjuvant temozolomide versus radiotherapy alone on survival in glioblastoma in a randomised phase III study: 5-year analysis of the EORTC-NCIC trial. *Lancet Oncol.* **2009**, *10*, 459–466. [CrossRef]
22. Wu, W.; Lamborn, K.R.; Buckner, J.C.; Novotny, P.J.; Chang, S.M.; O'Fallon, J.R.; Jaeckle, K.A.; Prados, M.D. Joint NCCTG and NABTC prognostic factors analysis for high-grade recurrent glioma. *Neuro Oncol.* **2010**, *12*, 164–172. [CrossRef]

23. Nabors, L.B.; Portnow, J.; Ahluwalia, M.; Baehring, J.; Brem, H.; Brem, S.; Butowski, N.; Campian, J.L.; Clark, S.W.; Fabiano, A.J.; et al. Central Nervous System Cancers, Version 3.2020, NCCN Clinical Practice Guidelines in Oncology. *J. Natl. Compr. Canc Netw.* **2020**, *18*, 1537–1570. [CrossRef]
24. Cihoric, N.; Tsikkinis, A.; Minniti, G.; Lagerwaard, F.J.; Herrlinger, U.; Mathier, E.; Soldatovic, I.; Jeremic, B.; Ghadjar, P.; Elicin, O.; et al. Current status and perspectives of interventional clinical trials for glioblastoma—Analysis of ClinicalTrials.gov. *Radiat. Oncol.* **2017**, *12*, 1. [CrossRef] [PubMed]
25. Vanderbeek, A.M.; Rahman, R.; Fell, G.; Ventz, S.; Chen, T.; Redd, R.; Parmigiani, G.; Cloughesy, T.F.; Wen, P.Y.; Trippa, L.; et al. The clinical trials landscape for glioblastoma: Is it adequate to develop new treatments? *Neuro Oncol.* **2018**, *20*, 1034–1043. [CrossRef] [PubMed]
26. Muir, M.; Gopakumar, S.; Traylor, J.; Lee, S.; Rao, G. Glioblastoma multiforme: Novel therapeutic targets. *Expert Opin. Ther. Targets* **2020**, *24*, 605–614. [CrossRef]
27. Wang, Z.; Peet, N.P.; Zhang, P.; Jiang, Y.; Rong, L. Current development of glioblastoma therapeutic agents. *Mol. Cancer Ther.* **2021**. [CrossRef] [PubMed]
28. Binder, Z.A.; Thorne, A.H.; Bakas, S.; Wileyto, E.P.; Bilello, M.; Akbari, H.; Rathore, S.; Ha, S.M.; Zhang, L.; Ferguson, C.J. Epidermal growth factor receptor extracellular domain mutations in glioblastoma present opportunities for clinical imaging and therapeutic development. *Cancer Cell* **2018**, *34*, 163–177.e167. [CrossRef]
29. Franceschi, E.; De Biase, D.; Di Nunno, V.; Pession, A.; Tosoni, A.; Gatto, L.; Tallini, G.; Visani, M.; Lodi, R.; Bartolini, S. The clinical and prognostic role of ALK in glioblastoma. *Pathol. Res. Pract.* **2021**, *221*, 153447. [CrossRef]
30. Cheng, F.; Guo, D. MET in glioma: Signaling pathways and targeted therapies. *J. Exp. Clin. Cancer Res.* **2019**, *38*, 1–13. [CrossRef] [PubMed]
31. Wen, P.Y.; Drappatz, J.; De Groot, J.; Prados, M.D.; Reardon, D.A.; Schiff, D.; Chamberlain, M.; Mikkelsen, T.; Desjardins, A.; Holland, J. Phase II study of cabozantinib in patients with progressive glioblastoma: Subset analysis of patients naive to antiangiogenic therapy. *Neuro Oncol.* **2018**, *20*, 249–258. [CrossRef] [PubMed]
32. Wang, Z.; Sun, D.; Chen, Y.-J.; Xie, X.; Shi, Y.; Tabar, V.; Brennan, C.W.; Bale, T.A.; Jayewickreme, C.D.; Laks, D.R. Cell lineage-based stratification for glioblastoma. *Cancer Cell* **2020**, *38*, 366–379.e368. [CrossRef]
33. Yu, A.; Faiq, N.; Green, S.; Lai, A.; Green, R.; Hu, J.; Cloughesy, T.F.; Mellinghoff, I.; Nghiemphu, P.L. Report of safety of pulse dosing of lapatinib with temozolomide and radiation therapy for newly-diagnosed glioblastoma in a pilot phase II study. *J. Neuro Oncol.* **2017**, *134*, 357–362. [CrossRef] [PubMed]
34. Freedman, R.A.; Gelman, R.S.; Wefel, J.S.; Melisko, M.E.; Hess, K.R.; Connolly, R.M.; Van Poznak, C.H.; Niravath, P.A.; Puhalla, S.L.; Ibrahim, N. Translational breast cancer research consortium (TBCRC) 022: A phase II trial of neratinib for patients with human epidermal growth factor receptor 2–positive breast cancer and brain metastases. *J. Clin. Oncol.* **2016**, *34*, 945. [CrossRef] [PubMed]
35. Garcia-Alvarez, A.; Papakonstantinou, A.; Oliveira, M. Brain Metastases in HER2-Positive Breast Cancer: Current and Novel Treatment Strategies. *Cancers* **2021**, *13*, 2927. [CrossRef]
36. Nunno, V.D.; Nuvola, M.; Mosca, M.; Maggio, I.; Gatto, L.; Tosoni, A.; Lodi, R.; Franceschi, E.; Brandes, A.A. Clinical efficacy of immune checkpoint inhibitors in patients with brain metastases. *Immunotherapy* **2021**, *13*, 419–432. [CrossRef] [PubMed]
37. Marei, H.E.; Althani, A.; Afifi, N.; Hasan, A.; Caceci, T.; Pozzoli, G.; Cenciarelli, C. Current progress in chimeric antigen receptor T cell therapy for glioblastoma multiforme. *Cancer Med.* **2021**. [CrossRef] [PubMed]
38. Gatto, L.; Nunno, V.D.; Franceschi, E.; Brandes, A.A. Chimeric antigen receptor macrophage for glioblastoma immunotherapy: The way forward. *Future Med.* **2021**. [CrossRef]
39. Uyttenhove, C.; Pilotte, L.; Théate, I.; Stroobant, V.; Colau, D.; Parmentier, N.; Boon, T.; Van den Eynde, B.J. Evidence for a tumoral immune resistance mechanism based on tryptophan degradation by indoleamine 2, 3-dioxygenase. *Nat. Med.* **2003**, *9*, 1269–1274. [CrossRef]
40. Zhai, L.; Ladomersky, E.; Lauing, K.L.; Wu, M.; Genet, M.; Gritsina, G.; Győrffy, B.; Brastianos, P.K.; Binder, D.C.; Sosman, J.A. Infiltrating T cells increase IDO1 expression in glioblastoma and contribute to decreased patient survival. *Clin. Cancer Res.* **2017**, *23*, 6650–6660. [CrossRef]
41. Le Naour, J.; Galluzzi, L.; Zitvogel, L.; Kroemer, G.; Vacchelli, E. Trial watch: IDO inhibitors in cancer therapy. *Oncoimmunology* **2020**, *9*, 1777625. [CrossRef] [PubMed]
42. Zhang, Q.; Liu, F. Advances and potential pitfalls of oncolytic viruses expressing immunomodulatory transgene therapy for malignant gliomas. *Cell Death Dis.* **2020**, *11*, 1–11. [CrossRef]
43. Tyler, M.; Ulasov, I.; Sonabend, A.; Nandi, S.; Han, Y.; Marler, S.; Roth, J.; Lesniak, M. Neural stem cells target intracranial glioma to deliver an oncolytic adenovirus in vivo. *Gene Ther.* **2009**, *16*, 262–278. [CrossRef] [PubMed]
44. Philbrick, B.; Adamson, D.C. DNX-2401: An investigational drug for the treatment of recurrent glioblastoma. *Expert Opin. Investig. Drugs* **2019**, *28*, 1041–1049. [CrossRef]
45. Patel, D.M.; Foreman, P.M.; Nabors, L.B.; Riley, K.O.; Gillespie, G.Y.; Markert, J.M. Design of a phase I clinical trial to evaluate M032, a genetically engineered HSV-1 expressing IL-12, in patients with recurrent/progressive glioblastoma multiforme, anaplastic astrocytoma, or gliosarcoma. *Hum. Gene Ther. Clin. Dev.* **2016**, *27*, 69–78. [CrossRef]

46. Stupp, R.; Taillibert, S.; Kanner, A.; Read, W.; Steinberg, D.; Lhermitte, B.; Toms, S.; Idbaih, A.; Ahluwalia, M.S.; Fink, K.; et al. Effect of Tumor-Treating Fields Plus Maintenance Temozolomide vs Maintenance Temozolomide Alone on Survival in Patients With Glioblastoma: A Randomized Clinical Trial. *JAMA* **2017**, *318*, 2306–2316. [CrossRef]
47. Herrlinger, U.; Tzaridis, T.; Mack, F.; Steinbach, J.P.; Schlegel, U.; Sabel, M.; Hau, P.; Kortmann, R.D.; Krex, D.; Grauer, O.; et al. Lomustine-temozolomide combination therapy versus standard temozolomide therapy in patients with newly diagnosed glioblastoma with methylated MGMT promoter (CeTeG/NOA-09): A randomised, open-label, phase 3 trial. *Lancet* **2019**, *393*, 678–688. [CrossRef]
48. Gilbert, M.R.; Wang, M.; Aldape, K.D.; Stupp, R.; Hegi, M.E.; Jaeckle, K.A.; Armstrong, T.S.; Wefel, J.S.; Won, M.; Blumenthal, D.T.; et al. Dose-dense temozolomide for newly diagnosed glioblastoma: A randomized phase III clinical trial. *J. Clin. Oncol.* **2013**, *31*, 4085–4091. [CrossRef]
49. Blumenthal, D.T.; Gorlia, T.; Gilbert, M.R.; Kim, M.M.; Burt Nabors, L.; Mason, W.P.; Hegi, M.E.; Zhang, P.; Golfinopoulos, V.; Perry, J.R.; et al. Is more better? The impact of extended adjuvant temozolomide in newly diagnosed glioblastoma: A secondary analysis of EORTC and NRG Oncology/RTOG. *Neuro Oncol.* **2017**, *19*, 1119–1126. [CrossRef]
50. Chinot, O.L.; Wick, W.; Mason, W.; Henriksson, R.; Saran, F.; Nishikawa, R.; Carpentier, A.F.; Hoang-Xuan, K.; Kavan, P.; Cernea, D.; et al. Bevacizumab plus radiotherapy-temozolomide for newly diagnosed glioblastoma. *N. Engl. J. Med.* **2014**, *370*, 709–722. [CrossRef]
51. Gilbert, M.R.; Dignam, J.J.; Armstrong, T.S.; Wefel, J.S.; Blumenthal, D.T.; Vogelbaum, M.A.; Colman, H.; Chakravarti, A.; Pugh, S.; Won, M.; et al. A randomized trial of bevacizumab for newly diagnosed glioblastoma. *N. Engl. J. Med.* **2014**, *370*, 699–708. [CrossRef] [PubMed]
52. Omuro, A.; Vlahovic, G.; Lim, M.; Sahebjam, S.; Baehring, J.; Cloughesy, T.; Voloschin, A.; Ramkissoon, S.H.; Ligon, K.L.; Latek, R.; et al. Nivolumab with or without ipilimumab in patients with recurrent glioblastoma: Results from exploratory phase I cohorts of CheckMate 143. *Neuro Oncol.* **2018**, *20*, 674–686. [CrossRef] [PubMed]
53. Graff, J.R.; McNulty, A.M.; Hanna, K.R.; Konicek, B.W.; Lynch, R.L.; Bailey, S.N.; Banks, C.; Capen, A.; Goode, R.; Lewis, J.E.; et al. The protein kinase Cbeta-selective inhibitor, Enzastaurin (LY317615.HCl), suppresses signaling through the AKT pathway, induces apoptosis, and suppresses growth of human colon cancer and glioblastoma xenografts. *Cancer Res.* **2005**, *65*, 7462–7469. [CrossRef] [PubMed]
54. Kreisl, T.N.; Kotliarova, S.; Butman, J.A.; Albert, P.S.; Kim, L.; Musib, L.; Thornton, D.; Fine, H.A. A phase I/II trial of enzastaurin in patients with recurrent high-grade gliomas. *Neuro Oncol.* **2010**, *12*, 181–189. [CrossRef]
55. Wick, W.; Steinbach, J.P.; Platten, M.; Hartmann, C.; Wenz, F.; von Deimling, A.; Shei, P.; Moreau-Donnet, V.; Stoffregen, C.; Combs, S.E. Enzastaurin before and concomitant with radiation therapy, followed by enzastaurin maintenance therapy, in patients with newly diagnosed glioblastoma without MGMT promoter hypermethylation. *Neuro Oncol.* **2013**, *15*, 1405–1412. [CrossRef]
56. Butowski, N.; Chang, S.M.; Lamborn, K.R.; Polley, M.Y.; Pieper, R.; Costello, J.F.; Vandenberg, S.; Parvataneni, R.; Nicole, A.; Sneed, P.K.; et al. Phase II and pharmacogenomics study of enzastaurin plus temozolomide during and following radiation therapy in patients with newly diagnosed glioblastoma multiforme and gliosarcoma. *Neuro Oncol.* **2011**, *13*, 1331–1338. [CrossRef]
57. Roth, P.; Reijneveld, J.C.; Gorlia, T.; Dhermain, F.; Vos, F.Y.F.L.D.; Vanlancker, M.; O'Callaghan, C.J.; Rhun, E.L.; Bent, M.J.V.D.; Mason, W.P.; et al. EORTC 1709/CCTG CE.8: A phase III trial of marizomib in combination with standard temozolomide-based radiochemotherapy versus standard temozolomide-based radiochemotherapy alone in patients with newly diagnosed glioblastoma. *J. Clin. Oncol.* **2019**, *37*, TPS2072. [CrossRef]
58. Buxton, M.B.; Alexander, B.M.; Berry, D.A.; Cavenee, W.K.; Colman, H.; Groot, J.F.D.; Ellingson, B.M.; Gordon, G.B.; Khasraw, M.; Lassman, A.B.; et al. GBM AGILE: A global, phase II/III adaptive platform trial to evaluate multiple regimens in newly diagnosed and recurrent glioblastoma. *J. Clin. Oncol.* **2020**, *38*, TPS2579. [CrossRef]
59. Burgenske, D.M.; Yang, J.; Decker, P.A.; Kollmeyer, T.M.; Kosel, M.L.; Mladek, A.C.; Caron, A.A.; Vaubel, R.A.; Gupta, S.K.; Kitange, G.J. Molecular profiling of long-term IDH-wildtype glioblastoma survivors. *Neuro Oncol.* **2019**, *21*, 1458–1469. [CrossRef]
60. Richardson, T.E.; Kumar, A.; Xing, C.; Hatanpaa, K.J.; Walker, J.M. Overcoming the Odds: Toward a Molecular Profile of Long-Term Survival in Glioblastoma. *J. Neuropathol. Exp. Neurol.* **2020**, *79*, 1031–1037. [CrossRef]
61. Tykocki, T.; Eltayeb, M. Ten-year survival in glioblastoma. A systematic review. *J. Clin. Neurosci.* **2018**, *54*, 7–13. [CrossRef]
62. Di Nunno, V.; Franceschi, E.; Gatto, L.; Bartolini, S.; Brandes, A.A. Predictive markers of immune response in glioblastoma: Hopes and facts. *Future Oncol.* **2020**, *16*, 1053–1063. [CrossRef]
63. Franceschi, E.; Bartolotti, M.; Tosoni, A.; Bartolini, S.; Sturiale, C.; Fioravanti, A.; Pozzati, E.; Galzio, R.; Talacchi, A.; Volpin, L.; et al. The effect of re-operation on survival in patients with recurrent glioblastoma. *Anticancer Res.* **2015**, *35*, 1743–1748.
64. Franceschi, E.; Stupp, R.; van den Bent, M.J.; van Herpen, C.; Laigle Donadey, F.; Gorlia, T.; Hegi, M.; Lhermitte, B.; Strauss, L.C.; Allgeier, A.; et al. EORTC 26083 phase I/II trial of dasatinib in combination with CCNU in patients with recurrent glioblastoma. *Neuro Oncol.* **2012**, *14*, 1503–1510. [CrossRef] [PubMed]
65. Tosoni, A.; Franceschi, E.; Poggi, R.; Brandes, A.A. Relapsed Glioblastoma: Treatment Strategies for Initial and Subsequent Recurrences. *Curr. Treat. Opti. Oncol.* **2016**, *17*, 49. [CrossRef] [PubMed]
66. Franceschi, E.; Cavallo, G.; Lonardi, S.; Magrini, E.; Tosoni, A.; Grosso, D.; Scopece, L.; Blatt, V.; Urbini, B.; Pession, A.; et al. Gefitinib in patients with progressive high-grade gliomas: A multicentre phase II study by Gruppo Italiano Cooperativo di Neuro-Oncologia (GICNO). *Br. J. Cancer* **2007**, *96*, 1047–1051. [CrossRef]

67. Sepúlveda-Sánchez, J.M.; Vaz, M.; Balañá, C.; Gil-Gil, M.; Reynés, G.; Gallego, Ó.; Martínez-García, M.; Vicente, E.; Quindós, M.; Luque, R.; et al. Phase II trial of dacomitinib, a pan-human EGFR tyrosine kinase inhibitor, in recurrent glioblastoma patients with EGFR amplification. *Neuro Oncol.* **2017**, *19*, 1522–1531. [CrossRef] [PubMed]
68. Van den Bent, M.J.; Brandes, A.A.; Rampling, R.; Kouwenhoven, M.C.; Kros, J.M.; Carpentier, A.F.; Clement, P.M.; Frenay, M.; Campone, M.; Baurain, J.F.; et al. Randomized phase II trial of erlotinib versus temozolomide or carmustine in recurrent glioblastoma: EORTC brain tumor group study 26034. *J. Clin. Oncol.* **2009**, *27*, 1268–1274. [CrossRef]
69. Van Den Bent, M.; Eoli, M.; Sepulveda, J.M.; Smits, M.; Walenkamp, A.; Frenel, J.S.; Franceschi, E.; Clement, P.M.; Chinot, O.; De Vos, F.; et al. INTELLANCE 2/EORTC 1410 randomized phase II study of Depatux-M alone and with temozolomide vs. temozolomide or lomustine in recurrent EGFR amplified glioblastoma. *Neuro Oncol.* **2020**, *22*, 684–693. [CrossRef]
70. Hoogstrate, Y.; Vallentgoed, W.; Kros, J.M.; de Heer, I.; de Wit, M.; Eoli, M.; Sepulveda, J.M.; Walenkamp, A.M.E.; Frenel, J.S.; Franceschi, E.; et al. EGFR mutations are associated with response to depatux-m in combination with temozolomide and result in a receptor that is hypersensitive to ligand. *Neurooncol. Adv.* **2020**, *2*, vdz051. [CrossRef] [PubMed]
71. Brandes, A.A.; Bartolotti, M.; Tosoni, A.; Poggi, R.; Franceschi, E. Practical management of bevacizumab-related toxicities in glioblastoma. *Oncologist* **2015**, *20*, 166–175. [CrossRef] [PubMed]
72. Brandes, A.A.; Finocchiaro, G.; Zagonel, V.; Reni, M.; Fabi, A.; Caserta, C.; Tosoni, A.; Eoli, M.; Lombardi, G.; Clavarezza, M.; et al. Early tumour shrinkage as a survival predictor in patients with recurrent glioblastoma treated with bevacizumab in the AVAREG randomized phase II study. *Oncotarget* **2017**, *8*, 55575–55581. [CrossRef]
73. Brandes, A.A.; Gil-Gil, M.; Saran, F.; Carpentier, A.F.; Nowak, A.K.; Mason, W.; Zagonel, V.; Dubois, F.; Finocchiaro, G.; Fountzilas, G.; et al. A Randomized Phase II Trial (TAMIGA) Evaluating the Efficacy and Safety of Continuous Bevacizumab Through Multiple Lines of Treatment for Recurrent Glioblastoma. *Oncologist* **2019**, *24*, 521–528. [CrossRef] [PubMed]
74. Franceschi, E.; Lamberti, G.; Paccapelo, A.; Di Battista, M.; Genestreti, G.; Minichillo, S.; Mura, A.; Bartolini, S.; Agati, R.; Brandes, A.A. Third-line therapy in recurrent glioblastoma: Is it another chance for bevacizumab? *J. Neurooncol.* **2018**, *139*, 383–388. [CrossRef] [PubMed]
75. Friedman, H.S.; Prados, M.D.; Wen, P.Y.; Mikkelsen, T.; Schiff, D.; Abrey, L.E.; Yung, W.K.; Paleologos, N.; Nicholas, M.K.; Jensen, R.; et al. Bevacizumab alone and in combination with irinotecan in recurrent glioblastoma. *J. Clin. Oncol.* **2009**, *27*, 4733–4740. [CrossRef]
76. Reardon, D.A.; Desjardins, A.; Peters, K.B.; Gururangan, S.; Sampson, J.H.; McLendon, R.E.; Herndon, J.E., 2nd; Bulusu, A.; Threatt, S.; Friedman, A.H.; et al. Phase II study of carboplatin, irinotecan, and bevacizumab for bevacizumab naïve, recurrent glioblastoma. *J. Neurooncol.* **2012**, *107*, 155–164. [CrossRef]
77. Taal, W.; Oosterkamp, H.M.; Walenkamp, A.M.; Dubbink, H.J.; Beerepoot, L.V.; Hanse, M.C.; Buter, J.; Honkoop, A.H.; Boerman, D.; de Vos, F.Y.; et al. Single-agent bevacizumab or lomustine versus a combination of bevacizumab plus lomustine in patients with recurrent glioblastoma (BELOB trial): A randomised controlled phase 2 trial. *Lancet Oncol.* **2014**, *15*, 943–953. [CrossRef]
78. Vredenburgh, J.J.; Desjardins, A.; Herndon, J.E., 2nd; Dowell, J.M.; Reardon, D.A.; Quinn, J.A.; Rich, J.N.; Sathornsumetee, S.; Gururangan, S.; Wagner, M.; et al. Phase II trial of bevacizumab and irinotecan in recurrent malignant glioma. *Clin. Cancer Res.* **2007**, *13*, 1253–1259. [CrossRef]
79. Taylor, J.W.; Parikh, M.; Phillips, J.J.; James, C.D.; Molinaro, A.M.; Butowski, N.A.; Clarke, J.L.; Oberheim-Bush, N.A.; Chang, S.M.; Berger, M.S.; et al. Phase-2 trial of palbociclib in adult patients with recurrent RB1-positive glioblastoma. *J. Neurooncol.* **2018**, *140*, 477–483. [CrossRef] [PubMed]
80. Drilon, A.E.; DuBois, S.G.; Farago, A.F.; Geoerger, B.; Grilley-Olson, J.E.; Hong, D.S.; Sohal, D.; Tilburg, C.M.v.; Ziegler, D.S.; Ku, N.; et al. Activity of larotrectinib in TRK fusion cancer patients with brain metastases or primary central nervous system tumors. *J. Clin. Oncol.* **2019**, *37*, 2006. [CrossRef]
81. Schreck, K.C.; Grossman, S.A.; Pratilas, C.A. BRAF Mutations and the Utility of RAF and MEK Inhibitors in Primary Brain Tumors. *Cancers* **2019**, *11*, 1262. [CrossRef]
82. Kaley, T.; Touat, M.; Subbiah, V.; Hollebecque, A.; Rodon, J.; Lockhart, A.C.; Keedy, V.; Bielle, F.; Hofheinz, R.D.; Joly, F.; et al. BRAF Inhibition in BRAF(V600)-Mutant Gliomas: Results From the VE-BASKET Study. *J. Clin. Oncol.* **2018**, *36*, 3477–3484. [CrossRef] [PubMed]
83. Wen, P.; Stein, A.; van den Bent, M.; De Greve, J.; Dietrich, S.; De Vos, F.; von Bubnoff, N.; van Linde, M.; Lai, A.; Prager, G.; et al. ACTR-30. Updated Efficacy and Safety of Dabrafenib Plus Trametinib in Patients with Recurrent/Refractory Braf V600e–Mutated High-Grade Glioma (HGG) and Low-Grade Glioma (LGG). *Neuro Oncol.* **2019**, *21*, vi19–vi20. [CrossRef]
84. Cloughesy, T.F.; Mochizuki, A.Y.; Orpilla, J.R.; Hugo, W.; Lee, A.H.; Davidson, T.B.; Wang, A.C.; Ellingson, B.M.; Rytlewski, J.A.; Sanders, C.M.; et al. Neoadjuvant anti-PD-1 immunotherapy promotes a survival benefit with intratumoral and systemic immune responses in recurrent glioblastoma. *Nat. Med.* **2019**, *25*, 477–486. [CrossRef]
85. Reardon, D.A.; Desjardins, A.; Vredenburgh, J.J.; O'Rourke, D.M.; Tran, D.D.; Fink, K.L.; Nabors, L.B.; Li, G.; Bota, D.A.; Lukas, R.V.; et al. Rindopepimut with Bevacizumab for Patients with Relapsed EGFRvIII-Expressing Glioblastoma (ReACT): Results of a Double-Blind Randomized Phase II Trial. *Clin. Cancer Res.* **2020**, *26*, 1586–1594. [CrossRef] [PubMed]
86. Weller, M.; Butowski, N.; Tran, D.D.; Recht, L.D.; Lim, M.; Hirte, H.; Ashby, L.; Mechtler, L.; Goldlust, S.A.; Iwamoto, F. Rindopepimut with temozolomide for patients with newly diagnosed, EGFRvIII-expressing glioblastoma (ACT IV): A randomised, double-blind, international phase 3 trial. *Lancet Oncol.* **2017**, *18*, 1373–1385. [CrossRef]

87. Liau, L.M.; Ashkan, K.; Tran, D.D.; Campian, J.L.; Trusheim, J.E.; Cobbs, C.S.; Heth, J.A.; Salacz, M.; Taylor, S.; D'Andre, S.D.; et al. First results on survival from a large Phase 3 clinical trial of an autologous dendritic cell vaccine in newly diagnosed glioblastoma. *J. Transl. Med.* **2018**, *16*, 142. [CrossRef]
88. Winkfield, K.M. Improving access to cancer clinical trials by reducing the financial burden. *Cancer* **2020**, *126*, 14–16. [CrossRef]
89. Tosoni, A.; Gatto, L.; Franceschi, E.; Di Nunno, V.; Lodi, R.; Mura, A.; Di Battista, M.; Bartolini, S.; Brandes, A.A. Association between socioeconomic status and survival in glioblastoma: An Italian single-centre prospective observational study. *Eur. J. Cancer* **2021**, *145*, 171–178. [CrossRef] [PubMed]
90. Sharrocks, K.; Spicer, J.; Camidge, D.R.; Papa, S. The impact of socioeconomic status on access to cancer clinical trials. *Br. J. Cancer* **2014**, *111*, 1684–1687. [CrossRef] [PubMed]
91. Vanderbeek, A.M.; Ventz, S.; Rahman, R.; Fell, G.; Cloughesy, T.F.; Wen, P.Y.; Trippa, L.; Alexander, B.M. To randomize, or not to randomize, that is the question: Using data from prior clinical trials to guide future designs. *Neuro Oncol.* **2019**, *21*, 1239–1249. [CrossRef] [PubMed]
92. Trippa, L.; Lee, E.Q.; Wen, P.Y.; Batchelor, T.T.; Cloughesy, T.; Parmigiani, G.; Alexander, B.M. Bayesian adaptive randomized trial design for patients with recurrent glioblastoma. *J. Clin. Oncol.* **2012**, *30*, 3258–3263. [CrossRef]
93. Alexander, B.M.; Ba, S.; Berger, M.S.; Berry, D.A.; Cavenee, W.K.; Chang, S.M.; Cloughesy, T.F.; Jiang, T.; Khasraw, M.; Li, W.; et al. Adaptive Global Innovative Learning Environment for Glioblastoma: GBM AGILE. *Clin. Cancer Res.* **2018**, *24*, 737–743. [CrossRef]
94. Alexander, B.M.; Trippa, L.; Gaffey, S.; Arrillaga-Romany, I.C.; Lee, E.Q.; Rinne, M.L.; Ahluwalia, M.S.; Colman, H.; Fell, G.; Galanis, E.; et al. Individualized Screening Trial of Innovative Glioblastoma Therapy (INSIGhT): A Bayesian Adaptive Platform Trial to Develop Precision Medicines for Patients with Glioblastoma. *JCO Precis. Oncol.* **2019**, *3*. [CrossRef]
95. Alexander, B.M.; Trippa, L. Progression-free survival: Too much risk, not enough reward? *Neuro Oncol.* **2014**, *16*, 615–616. [CrossRef]
96. Trippa, L.; Wen, P.Y.; Parmigiani, G.; Berry, D.A.; Alexander, B.M. Combining progression-free survival and overall survival as a novel composite endpoint for glioblastoma trials. *Neuro Oncol.* **2015**, *17*, 1106–1113. [CrossRef]
97. Vogelbaum, M.A.; Krivosheya, D.; Borghei-Razavi, H.; Sanai, N.; Weller, M.; Wick, W.; Soffietti, R.; Reardon, D.A.; Aghi, M.K.; Galanis, E.; et al. Phase 0 and window of opportunity clinical trial design in neuro-oncology: A RANO review. *Neuro Oncol.* **2020**, *22*, 1568–1579. [CrossRef] [PubMed]
98. Wick, W.; Dettmer, S.; Berberich, A.; Kessler, T.; Karapanagiotou-Schenkel, I.; Wick, A.; Winkler, F.; Pfaff, E.; Brors, B.; Debus, J.; et al. N2M2 (NOA-20) phase I/II trial of molecularly matched targeted therapies plus radiotherapy in patients with newly diagnosed non-MGMT hypermethylated glioblastoma. *Neuro Oncol.* **2019**, *21*, 95–105. [CrossRef]
99. Brandes, A.A.; Franceschi, E. New agents and new end points for recurrent gliomas. *J. Clin. Oncol.* **2011**, *29*, e245–e246. [CrossRef] [PubMed]
100. Han, K.; Ren, M.; Wick, W.; Abrey, L.; Das, A.; Jin, J.; Reardon, D.A. Progression-free survival as a surrogate endpoint for overall survival in glioblastoma: A literature-based meta-analysis from 91 trials. *Neuro Oncol.* **2014**, *16*, 696–706. [CrossRef] [PubMed]
101. Franceschi, E.; Ermani, M.; Bartolini, S.; Bartolotti, M.; Poggi, R.; Tallini, G.; Marucci, G.; Fioravanti, A.; Tosoni, A.; Agati, R.; et al. Post progression survival in glioblastoma: Where are we? *J. Neurooncol.* **2015**, *121*, 399–404. [CrossRef]
102. Brandes, A.A.; Carpentier, A.F.; Kesari, S.; Sepulveda-Sanchez, J.M.; Wheeler, H.R.; Chinot, O.; Cher, L.; Steinbach, J.P.; Capper, D.; Specenier, P.; et al. A Phase II randomized study of galunisertib monotherapy or galunisertib plus lomustine compared with lomustine monotherapy in patients with recurrent glioblastoma. *Neuro Oncol.* **2016**, *18*, 1146–1156. [CrossRef]
103. Brandes, A.A.; Stupp, R.; Hau, P.; Lacombe, D.; Gorlia, T.; Tosoni, A.; Mirimanoff, R.O.; Kros, J.M.; van den Bent, M.J. EORTC study 26041-22041: Phase I/II study on concomitant and adjuvant temozolomide (TMZ) and radiotherapy (RT) with PTK787/ZK222584 (PTK/ZK) in newly diagnosed glioblastoma. *Eur. J. Cancer* **2010**, *46*, 348–354. [CrossRef]
104. Stupp, R.; Hegi, M.E.; Gorlia, T.; Erridge, S.C.; Perry, J.; Hong, Y.K.; Aldape, K.D.; Lhermitte, B.; Pietsch, T.; Grujicic, D.; et al. Cilengitide combined with standard treatment for patients with newly diagnosed glioblastoma with methylated MGMT promoter (CENTRIC EORTC 26071-22072 study): A multicentre, randomised, open-label, phase 3 trial. *Lancet Oncol.* **2014**, *15*, 1100–1108. [CrossRef]
105. Wick, W.; Gorlia, T.; Bady, P.; Platten, M.; van den Bent, M.J.; Taphoorn, M.J.; Steuve, J.; Brandes, A.A.; Hamou, M.F.; Wick, A.; et al. Phase II Study of Radiotherapy and Temsirolimus versus Radiochemotherapy with Temozolomide in Patients with Newly Diagnosed Glioblastoma without MGMT Promoter Hypermethylation (EORTC 26082). *Clin. Cancer Res.* **2016**, *22*, 4797–4806. [CrossRef]
106. Marenco-Hillembrand, L.; Wijesekera, O.; Suarez-Meade, P.; Mampre, D.; Jackson, C.; Peterson, J.; Trifiletti, D.; Hammack, J.; Ortiz, K.; Lesser, E.; et al. Trends in glioblastoma: Outcomes over time and type of intervention: A systematic evidence based analysis. *J. Neurooncol.* **2020**, *147*, 297–307. [CrossRef] [PubMed]
107. Delgado-López, P.D.; Riñones-Mena, E.; Corrales-García, E.M. Treatment-related changes in glioblastoma: A review on the controversies in response assessment criteria and the concepts of true progression, pseudoprogression, pseudoresponse and radionecrosis. *Clin. Transl. Oncol.* **2018**, *20*, 939–953. [CrossRef]
108. Ellingson, B.M.; Sampson, J.H.; Achrol, A.S.; Aghi, M.K.; Krystof Bankiewicz, K.; Wang, C.; Bexon, M.; Brem, S.; Brenner, A.J.; Chowdhary, S.; et al. Modified RANO (mRANO), iRANO, and standard RANO response to convection-enhanced delivery of IL4R-targeted immunotoxin MDNA55 in recurrent glioblastoma. *Clin. Cancer Res.* **2021**. [CrossRef] [PubMed]

109. Nayak, L.; DeAngelis, L.M.; Brandes, A.A.; Peereboom, D.M.; Galanis, E.; Lin, N.U.; Soffietti, R.; Macdonald, D.R.; Chamberlain, M.; Perry, J.; et al. The Neurologic Assessment in Neuro-Oncology (NANO) scale: A tool to assess neurologic function for integration into the Response Assessment in Neuro-Oncology (RANO) criteria. *Neuro Oncol.* **2017**, *19*, 625–635. [CrossRef] [PubMed]
110. Okada, H.; Weller, M.; Huang, R.; Finocchiaro, G.; Gilbert, M.R.; Wick, W.; Ellingson, B.M.; Hashimoto, N.; Pollack, I.F.; Brandes, A.A.; et al. Immunotherapy response assessment in neuro-oncology: A report of the RANO working group. *Lancet Oncol.* **2015**, *16*, e534–e542. [CrossRef]
111. Galldiks, N.; Niyazi, M.; Grosu, A.L.; Kocher, M.; Langen, K.J.; Law, I.; Minniti, G.; Kim, M.M.; Tsien, C.; Dhermain, F.; et al. Contribution of PET imaging to radiotherapy planning and monitoring in glioma patients—A report of the PET/RANO group. *Neuro Oncol.* **2021**. [CrossRef]
112. Holzgreve, A.; Albert, N.L.; Galldiks, N.; Suchorska, B. Use of PET Imaging in Neuro-Oncological Surgery. *Cancers* **2021**, *13*, 2093. [CrossRef]
113. Nakajo, K.; Uda, T.; Kawashima, T.; Terakawa, Y.; Ishibashi, K.; Tsuyuguchi, N.; Tanoue, Y.; Nagahama, A.; Uda, H.; Koh, S.; et al. Diagnostic Performance of [(11)C]Methionine Positron Emission Tomography in Newly Diagnosed and Untreated Glioma Based on the Revised World Health Organization 2016 Classification. *World Neurosurg.* **2021**, *148*, e471–e481. [CrossRef] [PubMed]
114. Chang, K.; Beers, A.L.; Bai, H.X.; Brown, J.M.; Ly, K.I.; Li, X.; Senders, J.T.; Kavouridis, V.K.; Boaro, A.; Su, C.; et al. Automatic assessment of glioma burden: A deep learning algorithm for fully automated volumetric and bidimensional measurement. *Neuro Oncol.* **2019**, *21*, 1412–1422. [CrossRef] [PubMed]
115. Kickingereder, P.; Isensee, F.; Tursunova, I.; Petersen, J.; Neuberger, U.; Bonekamp, D.; Brugnara, G.; Schell, M.; Kessler, T.; Foltyn, M.; et al. Automated quantitative tumour response assessment of MRI in neuro-oncology with artificial neural networks: A multicentre, retrospective study. *Lancet Oncol.* **2019**, *20*, 728–740. [CrossRef]
116. Rahman, R.; Trippa, L.; Fell, G.; Lee, E.Q.; Arrillaga-Romany, I.; Touat, M.; Drappatz, J.; Galanis, E.; Ahluwalia, M.S.; Colman, H.; et al. Evaluating the benefit of adaptive randomization in the CC-115 arm of the Individualized Screening Trial of Innovative Glioblastoma Therapy (INSIGhT): A phase II randomized Bayesian adaptive platform trial in newly diagnosed MGMT unmethylated glioblastoma. *J. Clin. Oncol.* **2021**, *39*, 2006. [CrossRef]
117. Lee, E.Q.; Trippa, L.; Fell, G.; Rahman, R.; Arrillaga-Romany, I.; Touat, M.; Drappatz, J.; Welch, M.R.; Galanis, E.; Ahluwalia, M.S.; et al. Preliminary results of the abemaciclib arm in the Individualized Screening Trial of Innovative Glioblastoma Therapy (INSIGhT): A phase II platform trial using Bayesian adaptive randomization. *J. Clin. Oncol.* **2021**, *39*, 2014. [CrossRef]

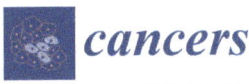

Review

Advances in Immunotherapy for Adult Glioblastoma

Chirayu R. Chokshi [1], Benjamin A. Brakel [1], Nazanin Tatari [1], Neil Savage [1], Sabra K. Salim [1], Chitra Venugopal [2] and Sheila K. Singh [1,2,*]

1 Department of Biochemistry and Biomedical Sciences, McMaster University, Hamilton, ON L8N 3Z5, Canada; chokshc@mcmaster.ca (C.R.C.); brakelb@mcmaster.ca (B.A.B.); tatarin@mcmaster.ca (N.T.); savagen@mcmaster.ca (N.S.); salims@mcmaster.ca (S.K.S.)
2 Department of Surgery, Faculty of Health Sciences, McMaster University, Hamilton, ON L8N 3Z5, Canada; venugop@mcmaster.ca
* Correspondence: ssingh@mcmaster.ca

Simple Summary: Therapy failure and disease recurrence are hallmarks of glioblastoma (GBM), the most common and lethal tumor in adults that originates in the brain. Despite aggressive standards of care, tumor recurrence is inevitable with no standardized second-line therapy. Recent clinical studies evaluating therapies that augment the anti-tumor immune response (i.e., immunotherapies) have yielded promising results in subsets of GBM patients. Here, we summarize clinical studies in the past decade that evaluate vaccines, immune checkpoint inhibitors and chimeric antigen receptor (CAR) T cells for treatment of GBM. Although immunotherapies have yet to return widespread efficacy for the majority of GBM patients, critical insights from completed and ongoing clinical trials are informing development of the next generation of therapies, with the goal to alleviate disease burden and extend patient survival.

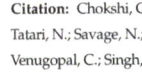

Citation: Chokshi, C.R.; Brakel, B.A.; Tatari, N.; Savage, N.; Salim, S.K.; Venugopal, C.; Singh, S.K. Advances in Immunotherapy for Adult Glioblastoma. *Cancers* **2021**, *13*, 3400. https://doi.org/10.3390/cancers13143400

Academic Editor: Stanley Stylli

Received: 9 June 2021
Accepted: 30 June 2021
Published: 7 July 2021

Publisher's Note: MDPI stays neutral with regard to jurisdictional claims in published maps and institutional affiliations.

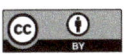

Copyright: © 2021 by the authors. Licensee MDPI, Basel, Switzerland. This article is an open access article distributed under the terms and conditions of the Creative Commons Attribution (CC BY) license (https://creativecommons.org/licenses/by/4.0/).

Abstract: Despite aggressive multimodal therapy, glioblastoma (GBM) remains the most common malignant primary brain tumor in adults. With the advent of therapies that revitalize the anti-tumor immune response, several immunotherapeutic modalities have been developed for treatment of GBM. In this review, we summarize recent clinical and preclinical efforts to evaluate vaccination strategies, immune checkpoint inhibitors (ICIs) and chimeric antigen receptor (CAR) T cells. Although these modalities have shown long-term tumor regression in subsets of treated patients, the underlying biology that may predict efficacy and inform therapy development is being actively investigated. Common to all therapeutic modalities are fundamental mechanisms of therapy evasion by tumor cells, including immense intratumoral heterogeneity, suppression of the tumor immune microenvironment and low mutational burden. These insights have led efforts to design rational combinatorial therapies that can reignite the anti-tumor immune response, effectively and specifically target tumor cells and reliably decrease tumor burden for GBM patients.

Keywords: glioblastoma; immunotherapy; vaccine; immune checkpoint inhibitors; chimeric antigen receptor (CAR) T cells

1. Introduction

Glioblastoma (GBM) remains the most aggressive and prevalent malignant primary brain tumor in adults [1]. Unchanged since 2005, patients undergo standard of care (SoC) that consists of gross total resection to remove the tumor bulk, followed by radiation therapy (RT) with concurrent and adjuvant chemotherapy with temozolomide (TMZ) [2,3]. Despite these aggressive therapeutic efforts, tumor relapse is inevitable, and patients face a median overall survival of 14.6 months and a 5-year survival rate of 5.5–6.8% [1,2,4]. A major contributor to treatment failure is intra-tumoral heterogeneity that gives rise to tumor cell populations distinct at the genomic, transcriptomic, proteomic and functional levels [5–9]. In addition to SoC, two therapeutics have received approval from the Food and

Drug Administration, including (1) an anti-vascular endothelial growth factor (VEGF) monoclonal antibody bevacizumab, and (2) tumor-treating fields that target proliferating tumor cells. However, these therapies have yet to be incorporated into SoC for GBM patients.

Emerging therapeutics for GBM have shifted towards reconfiguring the patient's immune system to generate an anti-tumor response. Here, we will summarize clinical findings and highlight promising preclinical studies of three major immunotherapeutic modalities designed to treat GBM, including vaccines, antibodies and chimeric antigen receptor (CAR) T cells (Figure 1). For a recent review of advances in oncolytic virotherapy for gliomas, refer to Rius-Rocabert et al. [10]. Given that resistance to SoC and disease relapse are inevitable for GBM patients, preclinical and clinical advancement of immunotherapeutic modalities, combined with recent insights into the tumor immune microenvironment, are poised to improve clinical outcomes for this patient population.

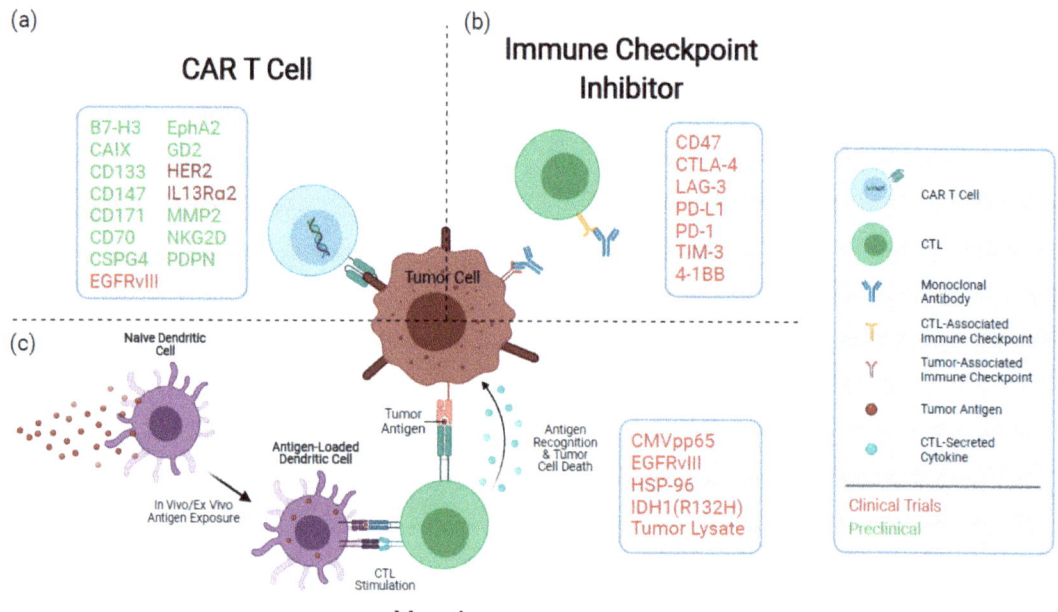

Figure 1. Overview of current immunotherapeutic modalities being investigated to treat GBM. (**a**) CAR T cells recognize antigens through a genetically engineered extracellular receptor which triggers intracellular T cell activation and degranulation upon antigen binding. (**b**) Inhibitors of immune checkpoint proteins prevent their attenuation of immune responses upon activation and exhaustion. (**c**) Vaccines expose antigen-presenting cells to tumoral antigens, stimulating a target-specific immune response. Boxes indicate therapeutic targets or mediators being pursued for each modality. CAR: chimeric antigen receptor; CTL: cytotoxic T lymphocyte.

2. Vaccines

Cancer vaccines function by exposing tumor-associated antigens to antigen-presenting cells (APCs), which activate immune effector cells to achieve an anti-cancer immune response. Several promising vaccines targeting both single and multiple antigens have shown varying degrees of clinical response (Table 1); however, vaccines for GBM have yet to translate to SoC. While GBM-specific targets are sparse, several have been identified that are expressed exclusively or enriched in tumor cells. Perhaps the most explored to date, epidermal growth factor receptor variant III (EGFRvIII) is a mutant version of the EGFR receptor specificically-expressed in GBM and has been targeted extensively through a variety of immunotherapeutic efforts, including vaccination. Similarly, the cytomegalovirus (CMV) tegument phosphoprotein 65 (pp65) and IDH1 (R132H)-mutant peptides are frequently and specifically expressed in GBM, in contrast to healthy brain tissues [11,12]. Vaccination strategies targeting these proteins have shown efficacy in clinical trials and often elicit strong immune responses; however, no targets identified to date are expressed on all GBM cells, likely allowing clonally driven recurrence to evade such treatments. In contrast, multi-targeted vaccines initiating an immune response to multiple tumor-associated antigens better address intratumoral heterogeneity; however, these treatments have shown limited clinical success.

Antigen presentation and the following activation and regulation of effector cells is another important process in achieving an effective immune response, which involves several proteins such as those mediating suppression of T cells, macrophages and other tumor-infiltrating lymphocytes. Current efforts acting on this front, such as antibodies against these suppressors, have shown preclinical promise but have fallen short in clinical trials. Additionally, success seems to vary greatly upon the combination of these inhibitors, underlining the importance of understanding and enhancing synergistic interactions among treatments.

Table 1. Summary of clinical trials for vaccines against GBM.

NCT Number	Treatment	Summary of Results	Indication	References
NCT00643097	EGFRvIII peptide vaccine + DI-TMZ	EGFRvIII-expressing cells eradicated and vaccine immunogenic, with DI-TMZ cohort having enhanced humoral response. Median overall survival of 23.6 months.	Primary GBM	Sampson et al. [13] Sampson et al. [14]
NCT00458601	EGFRvIII peptide vaccine + TMZ	Median overall survival of 21.8 months and 36-month survival of 26%. Anti-EGFRvIII antibodies increased ≥4-fold in 85% of patients with duration of treatment.	Primary GBM	Schuster et al. [15]
NCT01480479	EGFRvIII peptide vaccine + TMZ	Strong humoral responses; however, no survival advantage and loss of EGFRvIII expression upon recurrence.	Primary GBM	Weller et al. [16]
NCT01498328	EGFRvIII peptide vaccine + bevacizumab	24-month survival of 20% compared to 3% for controls.	Recurrent GBM	Reardon et al. [17]
NCT00639639	CMV pp65 DC vaccine + Td Toxoid + TMZ	Td toxoid pre-conditioning enhanced DC migration to the lymph nodes and improved survival. 3/6 Td toxoid patients were alive and progression-free at time of survival analysis (>36.6 months), while controls had median overall survival of 18.5 months.	Primary GBM	Mitchell et al. [18]
NCT00639639	CMV pp65 DC vaccine + DI-TMZ	Antigen-specific immune responses and median overall survival of 41.1 months in DI-TMZ cohort. A total of 36% survival 5 years from diagnosis, with four patients remaining progression-free at 59–64 months from diagnosis.	Primary GBM	Batich et al. [19]
NCT02366728	CMV pp65 DC vaccine + 111In-labeled DC vaccine + Td Toxoid + basiliximab	Ongoing, have reported increased DC migration to lymph nodes following Td toxoid pre-conditioning.	Primary GBM	Batich et al. [20]
NCT02454634	IDH1 peptide vaccine	A total of 93% vaccine-specific response rate, 84% survival >3 years.	High-grade glioma	Platten et al. [21]
NCT00045968	DCVax-L vaccine	Median overall survival of 23.1 months, with large group (n = 100) reaching 40.5 months.	Primary GBM	Liau et al. [22]
NCT00293423	HSPPC-96 peptide vaccine	Specific immune response in 11 of the 12 patients, responders had median overall survival of 11.8 months.	Recurrent GBM	Crane et al. [23] Bloch et al. [24]
NCT02122822	HSPPC-96 peptide vaccine + TMZ + radiotherapy	Median overall survival of 31.4 months. Patients with high tumor-specific immune responses had median overall survival of >40.5 months compared to 14.6 months for low responders.	Primary GBM	Ji et al. [25]
NCT00905060	HSPPC-96 vaccine + TMZ	Median overall survival of 23.8 months. Patients with low PD-L1 expression in myeloid cells had median overall survival of 44.7 months compared to 18 months for those with high expression.	Primary GBM	Bloch et al. [26]

2.1. Single-Target Vaccines

Several vaccines have been developed for GBM targeting a single, tumor-specific antigen. One such vaccine is rindopepimut, a peptide vaccine targeting EGFRvIII which has been identified as a tumor-specific mutant expressed in roughly one-third of GBM specimens [27]. This protein enhances GBM tumorigenicity [28,29] and is highly immunogenic [30], altogether providing a promising target for immunotherapy. Early preclinical studies have confirmed its immunogenicity and shown it to be effective in mice [31]; however, the protein's heterogeneous and unstable expression leaves room for EGFRvIII-negative tumor cells to drive therapy resistance and recurrence. A series of phase II rindopepimut trials, named "ACTIVATE, ACT II and ACT III," have shown promise (NCT00643097, NCT00458601), achieving median survival times between 22 and 26 months [13–15]. To validate these findings, a large phase III, trial termed "ACT IV", was completed with 371 patients (NCT01480479); however, no survival benefit was seen among vaccinated patients compared to controls, with median survivals of 20.1 and 20 months, respectively [16]. Interestingly, patients with significant residual disease received a greater benefit from the vaccine, perhaps due to a greater antigen load. Patients in the trial also showed strong humoral immune responses, suggesting resistance to the therapy was enabled at least in part by the heterogeneity of EGFRvIII expression. Indeed, those who underwent post-treatment biopsies of the recurrent tumor in both control and vaccinated groups showed loss of EGFRvIII expression in a majority of patients. This loss of expression highlights the limitations of single-target therapies in a heterogeneous tumor and underlines the importance combinatorial therapies will have in the future [32]. Additionally, the improved survival of the placebo group compared to historical controls was surprising, and future trials should account for this difference or change in control performance over time.

The complex interplay among therapies and the immune response must also be considered. For instance, rindopepimut was given along with TMZ, which induces lymphopenia [33]. While an accompanying increase in regulatory T cells suggests this may hinder the response to rindopepimut, previous findings have shown it can enhance it [14]. An additional study on rindopepimut was completed in 72 recurrent GBM patients in a phase II trial, termed "ReACT" (NCT01498328), combining the vaccine with bevacizumab, a monoclonal antibody against VEGF that has been shown to enhance immune responses [34]. The trial showed improvement upon the ACT IV trial, with 20% of treated patients surviving for 24 months compared to 3% for control-treated patients, in addition to a potential for rindopepimut to be combined with bevacizumab [17].

Another promising vaccination effort is the CMV dendritic cell (DC) vaccine. While rare in the healthy brain, viral proteins and nucleic acids of CMV are present in approximately 90% of GBM tumors [11]. The implications of CMV in tumor initiation and therapy resistance are not well understood; however, these viral antigens pose a potential immunotherapeutic target specific to cancerous cells. Of these antigens, CMV pp65 is highly expressed in glioma tumors and is the main target of current CMV vaccination strategies, as it elicits a strong cytotoxic T lymphocyte response following infection [35]. The CMV pp65 DC vaccine consists of autologous DCs pulsed with pp65 RNA fused in frame with the human Lysosomal Associated Membrane Protein (hLAMP) gene shown to enhance antigen processing [36]. A series of large phase II trials were recently completed with the vaccine in patients with newly diagnosed GBM following SoC treatment.

The initial "ATTAC" trial (NCT00639639) and subsequent "ATTAC-GM" trial (NCT00639639) both showed long-term survival in approximately one-third of patients. The initial trial also revealed that pre-conditioning with tetanus-diphtheria (Td) toxoid significantly increased DC migration to the lymph nodes, which correlated with increased survival, leading to half of the pre-conditioned patients remaining progression-free >36.6 months post diagnosis [18]. The second trial instead administered dose-intensified TMZ (DI-TMZ) with the vaccination, as DI-TMZ-induced lymphopenia has previously been shown to enhance both humoral and cellular immune responses [37]. While DI-TMZ increased immunosuppressive regulatory T cells, the group had a median survival of 41.1 months, greatly exceeding matched historical controls [19]. Excitingly, four patients remained progression-free at 59–64 months post-diagnosis, and overall, the trial showed the vaccine to be effective at targeting GBM based on the presence of CMV pp65. A subsequent phase II trial termed "ELEVATE" is ongoing to validate the benefit of Td toxoid pre-conditioning on DC migration and to evaluate synergy among vaccination, Td toxoid pre-conditioning and the anti-tumor antibody basiliximab (NCT02366728). To date, the trial has confirmed increased migration of DCs to the lymph nodes following pre-conditioning; however, analysis of other aims is not yet complete [20].

Vaccines have also been developed targeting the IDH1 subtype of gliomas, consisting of the IDH1 (R132H)-mutated peptide, which is present in <15% of GBM patients [12]. The vaccine was previously found to be effective in a mouse model transgenic for human MHC class I and II with IDH1 (R132H), showing MHC class II presentation of the epitope and mutation-specific T cell and antibody responses [38]. A phase I clinical trial termed "NOA-16" (NCT02454634) was recently completed for the vaccine delivered concurrently with topical imiquimod, a myeloid-activating TLR7 agonist. Results of the trial were extremely promising, with 93% of grade III-IV glioma patients showing a vaccine-specific immune response and 84% surviving >3 years [21]. A second phase II trial called "RESIST" is underway, adjuvating the vaccination with granulocyte-macrophage colony-stimulating factor (GM-CSF) in combination with TMZ and Td toxoid (NCT02193347).

2.2. Multi-Target Vaccines

To treat a heterogeneous disease such as GBM, targeting a single antigen can lead to clonal evolution and drive resistance. One way of overcoming this is by targeting multiple antigens concurrently. Interestingly, the greatest progress in therapeutic development has thus far been observed for single antigen-targeting vaccines, likely due to tumor-specific expression of these antigens. Regardless, the importance of targeting the molecular heterogeneity of GBM tumors is well established, and several multi-targeted GBM vaccines have shown promising results, such as personalized neoantigen-based vaccination strategies [39]. One such multi-targeted vaccine is DCVax-L, a personalized approach to peptide vaccination that uses autologous, or patient-derived, DCs pulsed with resected tumor lysate to target a variety of tumor antigens. In rat models, the vaccine was found to significantly increase survival and T cell infiltration [40], leading to several clinical trials. In a phase III trial (NCT00045968), a subset of patients (n = 232) were vaccinated and given concurrent TMZ, while all patients (n = 331) were given the vaccine upon tumor recurrence. The overall study population had a median survival of 23.1 months, with a large group (n = 100) having a particularly long median survival of 40.5 months unexplained by any prognostic factors, suggesting clinical efficacy related to vaccination [22]. A trial is now ongoing in patients who were previously ineligible due to post-chemoradiotherapy progression or insufficient vaccine production (NCT02146066). As an alternative approach to pulsing DCs with tumor lysate, DCs pulsed with a synthetic cocktail of tumor-associated antigens have shown promising preliminary results, with 5 of 16 vaccine-treated GBM patients surviving 6 years post-diagnosis [41,42].

Vaccines relying on heat shock proteins (HSP) are also being explored for GBM treatment. There have been several trials investigating HSP vaccines for glioma, which consist of HSPs and tumor-associated peptides. These vaccines primarily rely on tumor-derived HSP glycoprotein 96 (gp96), which binds tumor antigens forming the HSP protein complex-96 (HSPPC-96). This complex mediates presentation of antigens in antigen-presenting cells and can bind different peptides for a multi-targeted approach. An initial trial of a multi-peptide HSPPC-96 vaccine with TMZ (NCT00293423) confirmed strong peripheral and local immune responses specific to HSPPC-96-bound antigens in 11 of 12 treated patients [23]. These responders had a median survival of 11.8 months post-vaccination and surgery compared to 4 months for the single non-responding patient, and in the phase II portion of this trial, patients showed a median survival of 10.7 months, significantly exceeding controls [24]. Additionally, patients with pre-vaccination lymphopenia had decreased survival compared to those with higher lymphocyte counts, likely due to worsened immune function and thus decreased responses. Addressing this question and further validating effectiveness of this vaccine, another trial (NCT02122822) revealed those with strong tumor-specific immune responses indeed had longer median survival than those with weak responses (>40.5 months and 14.6 months, respectively), with the overall patient population reaching a median survival of 31.4 months and again exceeding controls [25].

Another phase II trial was recently completed with the HSPPC-96 vaccine and TMZ following SoC (NCT00905060), achieving a median survival of 23.8 months, further validating efficacy of this vaccine [26]. Interestingly, this trial found expression of the T cell-suppressing immune checkpoint PD-L1 in myeloid cells to be indicative of survival, with high expression leading to shorter survival as compared to patients with lower PD-L1 expression (18 months and 44.7 months, respectively). While a promising lead, no HSPPC-96 vaccines have been combined with anti-PD-L1 therapies to date. However, a trial is currently investigating the vaccine when combined with standard TMZ, radiotherapy and the antibody pembrolizumab targeting the PD-L1 receptor, which is ongoing (NCT03018288).

3. Antibodies Modulating the Tumor Immune Microenvironment

A complex system of stimulatory and inhibitory regulators functions to maintain immune homeostasis. An important part of this system is immune checkpoints, which regulate activation to avoid autoimmunity. Upon activation or exhaustion, several immune cells upregulate these inhibitory checkpoints, thus limiting the immune response. Cancer cells express immune checkpoint proteins as well, allowing them to suppress the anti-cancer immune response. As a result, antibodies against these checkpoints, known as immune checkpoint inhibitors (ICI), have shown success in several cancers such as melanoma and non-small-cell lung cancer [43], and several are being tested for GBM (Table 2). Of these antibodies, the greatest progress has been noted for ICIs blocking programmed cell death protein 1 (PD-1) and cytotoxic T lymphocyte antigen 4 (CTLA-4), which are expressed on T cells to inhibit T cell activation and killing of tumor cells [44,45].

Table 2. Summary of clinical trials for immune checkpoint inhibitors against GBM.

NCT Number	Treatment	Summary of Results	Indication	References
NCT02017717	Nivolumab (anti-PD-1) or bevacizumab	Median overall survival was around 10 months for both groups; 12-month survival rates were identical between treatments at 42%.	Recurrent GBM	Reardon et al. [46]
NCT02617589	Nivolumab + radiotherapy or TMZ + radiotherapy	No survival advantage over TMZ, median overall survival of 13.4 months for nivolumab cohort and 14.88 months for TMZ.	Primary GBM	No Reference
NCT02667587	Nivolumab + TMZ + radiotherapy	Nivolumab provided no survival advantage over placebo, trial still ongoing.	Primary GBM	Squibb et al. [47]
NCT02313272	Hypofractionated stereotactic irradiation + pembrolizumab (anti-PD-1) + bevacizumab	>50% patients had significant response; median overall survival of 13.5 months.	Recurrent high-grade glioma	Sahebjam et al. [48]
NCT02337491	Pembrolizumab or pembrolizumab + bevacizumab	Median overall survival of 8.8 months for pembrolizumab with bevacizumab, 10.3 months for pembrolizumab alone.	Recurrent GBM	Reardon et al. [49]
NCT02550249	Neoadjuvant nivolumab	Neoadjuvant nivolumab enhanced chemokine expression, TCR clonal diversity among TILs and immune cell infiltration of the tumor; however, median overall survival was only 7.3 months.	GBM	Schalper et al. [50]
NCT02336165	Durvalumab (anti-PD-L1) alone, with bevacizumab or with radiotherapy	Preliminary results of recurrent, bevacizumab-refractory cohort had 36% survival at 5.5 months. Trial still ongoing.	GBM	Reardon et al. [51]
NCT02658981	Anti-LAG-3 or anti-4-1BB alone or with anti-PD-1	Median overall survival of 8 months for anti-LAG-3, 7 months for anti-LAG-3, anti-PD-1 combination and 14 months for anti-4-1BB. Trial still ongoing.	Recurrent GBM	Lim et al. [52]

3.1. Immune Checkpoint Inhibitors

PD-1 targeting antibodies pembrolizumab and nivolumab have been approved to treat various solid tumors [43]; however, widespread clinical efficacy in GBM has yet to be achieved. Combination of an anti-PD-1 antibody and radiotherapy has shown preclinical success in vivo [53], leading to the phase III CheckMate 143 trial of nivolumab (NCT02017717) comparing it to the approved VEGF-A inhibitor bevacizumab in recurrent GBM. The trial results showed a median survival of around 10 months for both groups and identical 12-month survival rates of 42% [46]. Additionally, preliminary safety data of an earlier cohort of patients revealed high toxicity of a previously considered anti-PD-1/anti-CTLA-4 combination arm [54], leading to the discontinuation of this dual ICI therapy. Nivolumab has also been explored in other combinations such as the phase III CheckMate 498 trial (NCT02617589) delivered with radiotherapy, as compared to SoC (TMZ and radiotherapy); however, the trial showed no survival advantage of nivolumab treatment with similar median survivals around 14 months for both groups. Another phase III trial, CheckMate 548 (NCT02667587), is combining nivolumab, radiotherapy and TMZ. While still ongoing, an announcement was made that the trial failed to meet its primary endpoints of overall survival and progression-free survival [47].

Pembrolizumab is another anti-PD-1 antibody currently in trial for treatment of gliomas. In a phase I trial of 24 recurrent, high-grade glioma patients treated with pembrolizumab, bevacizumab and hypofractionated stereotactic irradiation (NCT02313272), more than half the patients achieved significant responses, and median survival was 13.5 months [48]. However, another phase I trial of pembrolizumab with bevacizumab compared to pembrolizumab alone in recurrent GBM patients (NCT02337491) showed a median survival of 8.8 months and 10.3 months, respectively [49]. The reduced survival upon lack of radiotherapy emphasizes the potential synergy of radiotherapy with anti-PD-1 therapies.

The interplay among chemotherapy and ICIs can also impact therapeutic efficacy, with preclinical studies showing that the order, timing and administration of chemotherapy relative to anti-PD-1 therapy drastically alter responsiveness of GBM tumors [55]. Additional efforts have been made to enhance the anti-tumor response, including neoadjuvant ICI administration prior to surgery, which has enhanced and prolonged the anti-tumor immune response and increased survival in other cancers [56,57]. A phase II trial using this approach with pembrolizumab in recurrent GBM patients showed increased survival with neoadjuvant and post-surgery adjuvant treatment, as compared to post-surgery adjuvant-only treatment (13.2 months and 6.3 months, respectively) [58]. Neoadjuvant administration also led to an upregulation of T cell- and interferon-γ-related gene expression and down-regulation of cell cycle-related genes. In a similar phase II trial (NCT02550249), neoadjuvant nivolumab was shown to enhance chemokine expression, T cell receptor (TCR) clonal diversity among tumor-infiltrating lymphocytes (TILs) and immune-cell infiltration in the tumor; however, median survival of treated patients was only 7.3 months [50]. Interestingly, two patients in the neoadjuvant cohort had complete surgical resection and remained disease-free for 33.3 and 28.5 months, which was not explainable by any recorded prognostic factors.

CTLA-4 (CD152) is another ICI that reduces CD28 co-stimulatory signaling by competitively binding to its natural ligands CD80 and CD86, suppressing T cell stimulation. Anti-CTLA-4 therapy has been approved for several cancers [43], extending survival of glioma-bearing mice [59], and in combination with anti-PD-1 therapy, shown eradication of tumors in a majority of mice [60]. Clinical trials have recently begun assessing anti-CTLA-4 therapies in treating gliomas (NCT02311920, NCT02829931), though no trials have been completed with glioma patients to date.

PD-L1, the ligand of PD-1 regularly expressed on APCs, is also expressed in cancer cells and mediates suppression of tumor-infiltrating T cells. Anti-PD-L1 antibodies have been approved in other cancers [43]; however, their efficacy in gliomas remains poor. An ongoing phase II trial is evaluating the anti-PD-L1 antibody durvalumab with radiotherapy and bevacizumab in GBM (NCT02336165), with preliminary results of the recurrent, bevacizumab-refractory cohort showing only 36% survival at 5.5 months [51].

Another phase I trial is looking at a different combination of ICIs, treating recurrent glioma patients with durvalumab and an anti-CTLA-4 antibody (NCT02794883); however, no updates have been given. Combinations of the anti-PD-L1 ICI avelumab are also being investigated, with ongoing phase II trials testing combinations with both hypofractionated radiation therapy (NCT02968940) and chemoradiotherapy (NCT03047473). Previous trials have found low expression of PD-L1 in GBM, with the CheckMate-143 trial finding only 10 of 37 patients with evaluable PD-L1 expression showing ≥10% [54]. This inherently limits any PD-L1 targeted therapies and may partially explain poor clinical outcomes thus far.

LAG-3 is another immune checkpoint receptor expressed on exhausted T cells that negatively regulates T cell responses. While anti-LAG-3 therapies have shown preclinical success [61], LAG-3 is expressed in a small percentage of tumor-infiltrating lymphocytes [62], thus limiting the potential impact of these therapies on stimulating the immune response. Regardless, a phase I trial evaluating the anti-LAG-3 antibody "BMS 986016" is underway, assessing its efficacy alone and in combination with the anti-PD-1 antibody nivolumab in recurrent GBM patients (NCT02658981). A recent update revealed a median survival of 8 months for the anti-LAG-3 group and 7 months for the anti-LAG-3, anti-PD-1 combination group. The trial also assessed an agonistic antibody targeting the 4-1BB (CD137) immune checkpoint protein. 4-1BB is a co-stimulatory receptor expressed by T cells upon activation, which augments activation signaling. The anti-4-1BB group had a promising median survival of 14 months [52]; however, while preclinical investigations support this therapy [63,64], further trials with anti-4-1BB antibodies are required.

TIM-3 is a receptor expressed on lymphocytes that can suppress the immune response by inducing T cell exhaustion, such that expression of TIM-3 in GBM has been linked with poor patient prognosis [65]. Anti-TIM-3 antibody therapy for GBM has shown success preclinically in combination with anti-PD-1 therapy and stereotactic radiosurgery (SRS). SRS drives the release of antigens from the tumor, enhancing the immune response, which is further stimulated by concurrent checkpoint inhibitors. While neither anti-TIM-3 nor SRS alone prolonged survival of GBM-bearing mice, combining the two increased median survival from 22 to 100 days, an effect similarly obtained using an anti-TIM-3 and anti-PD-1 combination [66]. When combining all three treatments, 100% of mice were alive 100 days post-engraftment, revealing great synergy and prompting a phase I trial of this combinational therapy, which is underway (NCT03961971).

3.2. Macrophage-Targeted Antibodies

Response to ICIs varies among tumor types and may depend on immune infiltrates such as TILs. Recently, mass cytometry and single-cell RNA sequencing of patient tumor specimens from various ICI-responding and non-responding cancers, such as GBM, revealed enrichment of CD73-high macrophages in GBM, which persist through anti-PD-1 treatment and limit ICI efficacy by inhibiting T cell infiltration [67]. Prevalence of these CD73-expressing macrophages correlated with a low response to ICIs, and genetic perturbation of CD73 in mice improved efficacy of anti-CTLA-4 and anti-PD-1 combination therapy, which correlated with greater T cell infiltration. These results show a promising and novel immunotherapeutic target to combine with existing ICIs.

CD47 is an enzyme that suppresses macrophage activation through binding the signal regulatory protein α (SIRPα). CD47 is overexpressed in many tumors [68], allowing cancer cells to avoid phagocytosis. Anti-CD47 antibodies have been developed to shift macrophages to an immunostimulatory phenotype, promoting an anti-tumor response [69] and effectively reducing growth of several tumors [70,71]. Preclinical studies of anti-CD47 therapies for glioma have shown that, while anti-CD47 therapy is sometimes effective at stimulating glioma cell phagocytosis [72], chemotherapy and radiotherapy are synergistic with treatment and may be required to enhance phagocytosis and extend survival in mice [73,74]. This enhanced phagocytosis also leads to increased antigen cross-presentation and T cell priming [74], and anti-CD47 therapies have shown synergy with autophagy inhibition [75,76], as well as other ICIs and tumor-specific antibodies [77]. The potential for synergistic co-therapies sophisticates treatment with anti-CD47 antibodies, and effective combinations should be compared prior to therapeutic development efforts.

4. Chimeric Antigen Receptor (CAR) T Cells

Chimeric antigen receptor (CAR) T cells represent an efficacious form of adoptive T cell therapy, in which peripheral T cells are genetically engineered to express a fusion receptor protein (i.e., CAR) that recognizes and targets a tumor-specific or -enriched antigen. Rapid and rational evolution of receptor design has transformed the first-generation CAR—composed of a ligand-binding domain, extracellular spacer, transmembrane domain and an intracellular signaling domain—that suffered from limited signaling strength to highly efficacious second- and third-generation CARs that incorporate one or more intracellular co-stimulatory domains, respectively, to initialize and sustain T cell signaling [78–81]. Irrespective of design principles, an antigen-bound CAR T cell activates a potent cytokine release and cytolytic degranulation response that kills antigen-expressing tumor cells and results in T cell proliferation [82]. CAR T cell therapy has been highly effective against hematological malignancies, achieving remission rates of up to 90% in patients with relapsed or refractory B cell malignancies with anti-CD19 CAR T cells [83]. However, widespread clinical responses of CAR T cells have yet to be seen for solid tumors, including GBM. Here, we summarize lessons learned from clinical evaluation of CAR T cell therapies in GBM patients, highlight promising preclinical candidates and discuss approaches to improving clinical efficacy.

Unlike hematological malignancies, CAR T cell therapy design and administration require unique considerations in the context of GBM, including factors such as intratumoral antigen heterogeneity, bypassing the blood–brain barrier (BBB) and exerting a potent anti-tumor response in a highly immunosuppressive microenvironment [84]. Two schools of thought have guided the delivery of CAR T cell therapy to the brain thus far, one which supports systemic intravenous administration, and the other prefers intracavitary or intraventricular dosing to bypass the BBB. Supported by reports of a dysregulated BBB in GBM patients [85,86], investigators evaluating CAR T cell therapies targeting EGFRvIII and HER2 preferred intravenous delivery of their modality [87,88]. Although no dose-limiting toxicities were observed for either modality when delivered intravenously, three grade 2–4 adverse events were possibly associated with HER2 CAR T cell therapy, including headache ($n = 1$) and seizure ($n = 2$). In contrast, intracavitary (or intratumoral) delivery of CAR T cells is not functionally restricted by the BBB. Using a reporter gene system, preliminary clinical evidence supports trafficking of intracerebrally administered anti-IL13Rα2 CAR T cells to the tumor region using [^{18}F]FHBG PET-based imaging [89]. Intracavitary treatment of GBM patients with anti-IL13Rα2 CAR T cells resulted in no dose-limiting toxicities [90,91]. However, similar to intravenous delivery of anti-EGFRvIII CAR T cells, two grade 3 adverse events were associated with the treatment, including headache ($n = 1$) and a neurologic event ($n = 1$). Unfortunately, an empirical and clinical comparison among CAR T cell delivery routes has yet to be performed for GBM.

To varying extents, clinical studies have evaluated CAR T cells for GBM targeting interleukin-13 receptor subunit alpha-2 (IL13Rα2), human epidermal growth factor receptor 2 (HER2) and EGFRvIII (Table 3), with follow-up studies targeting IL13Rα2 and HER2 underway. In addition, investigators have initiated clinical studies to evaluate CAR T cells targeting matrix metallopeptidase 2 (MMP2) [92], B7 family member B7-H3 [93–95], CD147 and NKG2-D type II integral membrane protein (NKG2D) [96,97]. Here, we outline clinical advances in CAR T cell therapies for the treatment of GBM.

Table 3. Summary of clinical trials for CAR T cells against GBM.

NCT Number	Treatment	Summary of Results	Indication	References
NCT00730613	IL13(E13Y)-CD3ζ CAR T cells (first generation)	Transient inflammation at tumor site and a significant decrease in IL13Rα2 expression post-treatment were observed. Two grade 3 adverse events were observed. A median survival of 11 months after tumor relapse was noted.	Recurrent GBM	Brown et al. [90]
NCT02208362	IL13(E13Y)-41BBζ CAR T cells (second generation)	A single patient with multifocal relapsed GBM was treated, resulting in 77–100% decrease in tumor burden and 7.5 months of progression-free survival. Increased presence of inflammatory cytokines at tumor site with no adverse events related to CAR T cell therapy.	Recurrent GBM	Brown et al. [91]
NCT01109095	HER2-CD28ζ CAR T cells (second generation)	No dose-limiting toxicity was observed and CAR T cells persisted for 12 months post-infusion. No significant increase in survival was noted, with a median overall survival of 11.1 months.	GBM	Ahmed et al. [98]
NCT02209376	EGFRvIII-41BBζ CAR T cells (second generation)	No dose-limiting toxicity was observed and EGFRvIII expression was reduced post-treatment. No significant increase in survival was noted, with a median overall survival of 8 months post-treatment.	Recurrent GBM	O'Rourke et al. [87]
NCT01454596	EGFRvIII-CD28-41BBζ CAR T cells (third generation)	At highest dose, 2 patients suffered dose-limiting toxicity. A median overall survival of 6.9 months was noted, with one patient alive at 59 months.	Recurrent GBM	Goff et al. [99]

4.1. IL13Rα2-Specific CAR T Cells

IL13Rα2 is a monomeric high-affinity receptor for interleukin 13 (IL13) that is enriched in GBM specimens compared to normal brain tissue [100,101]. In fact, IL13Rα2 expression correlates moderately with the mesenchymal signature [100], a subtype of GBM associated with greater proliferation, tumorigenicity and resistance to conventional chemoradiotherapy as compared to other subtypes [102,103]. Supported by these findings, IL13Rα2 CAR T cells were designed using a mutated IL13-zetakine binding domain (IL13.E13K.R109K), engineered to provide greater specificity for IL13Rα2 over IL13Rα1/IL4Rα and attached to a CD28 co-stimulation and CD3ζ signaling domain [104]. These IL13-zetakine CAR T cells were specifically and potently activated in the presence of IL13Rα2-expressing glioma cells, whereas no appreciable effect was seen in the absence of IL13Rα2 expression. Strikingly, a single intracranial injection of IL13-zetakine CAR T cells into mice with orthotopic glioma xenografts led to a robust decrease in tumor burden and increased median overall survival from 35 to 40 days in control mice to 88 days in IL13-zetakine CAR T cell-treated mice. These promising preclinical results led to the first-in-human pilot safety and feasibility study of IL13-zetakine CAR T cells in three patients with relapsed GBM [90]. In the study, IL13-zetakine CAR T cells were administered via an implanted reservoir/catheter system and led to treatment-induced inflammation at the tumor site. Although this treatment was well tolerated and led to decreased expression of IL13Rα2, two grade 3 headaches and a grade 3 neurologic event were observed following CAR T cell administration. A mean survival of 11 months after relapse was noted for these three patients, with one patient surviving 14 months.

Following this study, the group engineered second-generation IL13-targeted CAR T cells with a 4-1BB (CD137) co-stimulation domain and a mutated IgG4-Fc linker to improve anti-tumor potency and increase T cell persistence, while improving the safety profile [91,105]. These reengineered IL13BBζ-CAR T cells were administered to a patient with highly aggressive recurrent GBM with multifocal leptomeningeal disease and high IL13Rα2 expression. Although intracavitary infusions of IL13BBζ-CAR T cells did not cause any grade 3 or higher toxic effects and inhibited disease progression locally, distal non-resected tumors and new tumors progressed. Prompted by distant disease progression, IL13BBζ-CAR T cells were delivered via intraventricular infusions and led to dramatic reductions of all tumors after the fifth infusion, with a 77–100% decrease in tumor burden, a systemic anti-tumor inflammatory response and an absence of systemic toxic effects, allowing the patient to return to normal life and work activities. Unfortunately, disease recurrence was observed after 7.5 months with tumor formation in new locations and decreased expression of IL13Rα2, elucidating a common antigen loss response to targeted therapies and advocating for rational combinational or adjuvant therapies. Recently, preclinical efforts to improve IL13Rα2-directed CAR T cell therapy have included the incorporation of an IL13Rα2-specific single-chain variable fragment (scFv) [106], complementary IL15 expression to enhance T cell effector function [107], characterization of the tumor immune microenvironment following CAR T cell therapy [108] and optimal selection of T cell subsets for sustained CAR activity [109].

4.2. EGFRvIII-Specific CAR T Cells

Expressed heterogeneously in ~30% of GBM specimens [110], investigators have engineered and evaluated EGFRvIII-targeted CAR T cells in two in-human trials. A phase I study of EGFRvIII-targeted CAR T cells, previously tested in orthotopic xenograft models of EGFRvIII+ glioma for efficacy and specificity to EGFRvIII over EGFR [111,112], was conducted in 10 patients with EGFRvIII+ recurrent GBM to evaluate safety and feasibility as the primary endpoints [87]. Although no subjects experienced dose-limiting toxicities, including systemic cytokine release syndrome, tumor regression was not observed in any patients based on magnetic resonance (MR) imaging. A median overall survival of ~8 months was noted after CAR T cell infusion, with one long-term survivor exhibiting stable disease for >18 months. Of 10 treated patients, 7 underwent tumor resection post-infusion, and analysis of tumor tissue indicated a decrease or ablation of EGFRvIII expression. A second phase I clinical trial leveraged a third-generation EGFRvIII-targeted CAR with 4-1BB and CD38 co-stimulation domains to conduct a dose-escalation study in 18 patients with EGFRvIII+ GBM [99]. No dose-limiting toxicities were observed with EGFRvIII-targeted CAR T cells until the highest dose of $\geq 10^{10}$, at which point a patient developed acute dyspnea and experienced oxygen desaturation, eventually succumbing to severe hypotension. Despite efforts to increase CAR T cell persistence and tumor localization, no objective responses were noted using MR imaging, with 16 of 17 remaining patients showing signs of disease progression <3 months after infusion and a median survival of 6.9 months post-treatment. Interestingly, a single patient remained alive up to 59 months post-CAR therapy, and an additional two patients survived >1 year. In addition to further preclinical studies on third-generation anti-EGFRvIII CAR T cells by multiple groups [113–115], recent studies have augmented their approach to increase efficacy and decrease toxicity, including an approach to combine anti-EGFRvIII CAR T cells with anti-EGFR bispecific T cell-engager (BiTE) antibodies to treat EGFR-positive/EGFRvIII-negative GBM [116]. There are bispecific antibodies, such as BiTEs, that are synthetic antibody structures that bind to two separate epitopes, with intentions such as bridging tumor-immune cell interactions or increasing antibody specificity. An in-depth review of bispecific antibodies, including BiTEs, was recently presented by Lim et al. [117]. Moreover, investigators recently developed multi-antigen prime-and-kill synNotch-CAR T cells that use a dual receptor circuit, the first of which detects EGFRvIII or a brain-specific myelin oligodendrocyte glycoprotein to induce expression of CARs against EphA2 and IL13Rα2 [118]. In comparison to constitutively active anti-EGFRvIII/EphA2/IL13Rα2 CAR T cells, synNotch-CAR T cells showed greater anti-tumor efficacy without off-tumor toxicity.

4.3. HER2-Specific CAR T Cells

The human epidermal growth factor receptor 2 (HER2), originally discovered as a tumor-associated antigen in breast cancer, is a transmembrane glycoprotein with an intracellular tyrosine kinase domain [88]. HER2 is a sparsely expressed antigen in GBM, detected in up to 17% of specimens and indicative of poor prognosis [119,120]. With promising preclinical results of a second-generation anti-HER2 CAR engineered with a CD28 co-stimulatory domain [88], a clinical trial was undertaken to treat 17 patients with HER2-positive GBM with virus-specific anti-HER2 CAR T cells [98]. Although no dose-limiting toxicity was observed and CAR T cell persistence was noted up to 12 months post-infusion, no significant survival benefit was noted for treated patients with a median overall survival of 11.1 months.

5. Discussion

Immunotherapy has yet to significantly improve clinical outcomes for GBM patients, and clinical studies have been disappointing thus far. Here, we detailed clinical and pre-clinical advances in immune checkpoint blockade, vaccination strategies and emerging CAR T cell therapies for the treatment of GBM (Figure 1). Among the major hurdles to clinical efficacy are immense intratumoral heterogeneity [6,7], parallel modes of immunosuppression by tumor cells [121–123] and low mutational burden in GBM [124]. With these factors in mind, investigators and clinicians are shifting their focus to combinatorial and personalized treatment strategies to achieve synergistic effects, reduce treatment resistance and overcome immunosuppression.

Given their effectiveness in other cancers such as melanoma [125], ongoing clinical studies are combining ICIs with conventional chemoradiotherapy and experimental therapeutics to increase efficacy. A rational advancement of ICI therapy is co-targeting multiple immune checkpoints, with clinical trials initiated to test the following combinations in GBM: anti-CTLA4 and/or anti-PD-1 with TMZ in newly diagnosed GBM (NCT02311920), anti-CTLA-4 and anti-PD-L1 in recurrent GBM (NCT02794883), anti-LAG-3 and anti-PD-1 in recurrent GBM (NCT02658981), anti-IDO with anti-CTLA4 or anti-PD-1 in GBM (NCT02327078). In addition, hypofractionated stereotactic radiotherapy (NCT0289931, NCT02313272 and NCT02530502) and MRI-guided laser ablation (NCT02311582) are also being combined with ICI. As reviewed by Rius-Rocabert, Garcia-Romero, Garcia, Ayuso-Sacido and Nistal-Villan [10], oncolytic viruses are another form of immunotherapy that preferentially infect tumor cells, thereby activating the innate immune system and increasing T cell trafficking to the tumor bed. Based on promising preclinical data [126–128], clinical studies are evaluating a combination of adenovirus-based therapy DNX-2401 with anti-PD-1 blockade for recurrent GBM (NCT02798406). Furthermore, a preclinical study has confirmed the usefulness of an anti-PD-1 antibody at augmenting DC vaccination in glioma-bearing mice, showing a significant improvement in survival attributed to the strong T cell response enabled by ICI treatment [129]. Given that genetically engineered CAR T cells are exposed to the same immunosuppressive microenvironment as endogenous tumor-infiltrating lymphocytes, ICIs are being combined with CAR T cells to augment their performance. A phase I clinical trial is evaluating anti-IL13Rα2 CAR T cells as a single modality and in combination with ICIs Nivolumab and Ipilimumab (NCT04003649). Synergy among ICIs and other immunotherapeutic modalities will likely play a key role in advancing future therapies through addressing the immunosuppressive nature of the tumor.

Although CAR T cell therapy is a newer adaptation for GBM treatment, advancements to increase its clinical utility are rapidly progressing. Currently, 12 clinical trials are recruiting GBM patients to evaluate CAR T cell therapy against B7 family member B7-H3 (NCT04385173, NCT04077866), CD147, HER2 (NCT03389230), IL13Rα2 (NCT04003649, NCT04661384, NCT02208362), matrix metallopeptidase 2 (MMP2; NCT04214392) and NKG2D (NCT04717999). Furthermore, a recent clinical letter outlined the administration of B7-H3 CAR T cells to a 56-year-old woman with recurrent GBM, highlighting a potent but short-term anti-tumor response in situ, absent of grade 3 or higher toxicities associated with CAR T cell infusion [94]. Unfortunately, target antigen heterogeneity was predicted as the reason for treatment failure, as noted previously for CAR T cell therapy targeting EGFRvIII and IL13Rα2 [87,91]. Additionally, novel therapeutic targets for CAR T cell therapy are quickly emerging, including antigens such as the disialoganglioside GD2 [130], CD70 [131,132], CD133 [133], carbonic anhydrase IX (CAIX) [134], EphA2 [135,136], podoplanin (PDPN) [137], chondroitin sulfate proteoglycan 4 (CSPG4) [138,139] and adhesion molecule L1-CAM (CD171) [140]. Of these antigens, EphA2 is part of the EphR receptor tyrosine kinase family that coordinates positioning and patterning during early development [141]. Given that EphA2 is overexpressed in GBM specimens, especially in post-therapy GBM stem-like cells [142], anti-EphA2 CAR T cells [135,136] may be suited to target GBM at tumor recurrence. While current trials are focused on targeting single tumor-associated antigens, this increased repertoire of targets will allow multiple antigens to be targeted concurrently to overcome intertumoral heterogeneity. This approach has yielded fruitful results in preclinical glioma models, as shown by the development of tandem CAR T cells that bind HER2 and IL13Rα2 [143], as well as trivalent CAR T cells targeting HER2, IL13Rα2 and EphA2 [144]. In fact, these trivalent CAR T cells were able to eradicate nearly 100% of tumor cells from multiple GBM samples.

In addition to tumor-targeted CAR T cells and ICIs, modalities acting on other parts of the tumor immune microenvironment may play a vital role in achieving effective anti-tumor responses in a clinical setting. We summarized macrophage-targeted antibodies in Section 3.2 of this article. Another approach stems from a recent study that found natural killer cell function to be altered upon tumor infiltration, showing impairing lytic function as a possible mechanism of tumor immune evasion [145]. Strategies aimed at restoring natural killer cell activity against GBM are being investigated and have shown preclinical promise.

6. Conclusions

Emerging trends towards rational combinatorial therapies are likely to include a systemic reignition of the tumor immune microenvironment. The continued discovery of novel tumor-associated and tumor-specific antigens, paired with the improvement of therapeutic modalities to increase efficacy and reduce toxicity, are necessary for the clinical efficacy of immunotherapies. Overall, a combinatorial therapy delivered at various stages throughout SoC may reliably improve clinical outcomes in GBM patients.

Author Contributions: Conceptualization, S.K.S. (Sheila K. Singh), C.V., C.R.C. and B.A.B.; data curation, C.R.C. and B.A.B.; writing—original draft preparation, C.R.C. and B.A.B.; writing—review and editing, S.K.S. (Sheila K. Singh), C.V., C.R.C., B.A.B., N.T., N.S. and S.K.S. (Sabra K. Salim); visualization, B.A.B. and C.R.C.; supervision, S.K.S. (Sheila K. Singh); project administration, S.K.S. (Sheila K. Singh); funding acquisition, S.K.S. (Sheila K. Singh). All authors have read and agreed to the published version of the manuscript.

Funding: This research was funded by the Brain Tumor Foundation of Canada, BioCanRX, the McMaster University Department of Surgery, and Brain Cancer Canada.

Conflicts of Interest: S.K.S. is a consultant for and owns shares of Century Therapeutics Inc. This company, however, played no role in the design or writing of this review article.

References

1. Ostrom, Q.T.; Gittleman, H.; Xu, J.; Kromer, C.; Wolinsky, Y.; Kruchko, C.; Barnholtz-Sloan, J.S. CBTRUS Statistical Report: Primary Brain and Other Central Nervous System Tumors Diagnosed in the United States in 2009–2013. *Neuro-oncology* **2016**, *18*, v1–v75. [CrossRef]
2. Stupp, R.; Mason, W.P.; van den Bent, M.J.; Weller, M.; Fisher, B.; Taphoorn, M.J.; Belanger, K.; Brandes, A.A.; Marosi, C.; Bogdahn, U.; et al. Radiotherapy plus concomitant and adjuvant temozolomide for glioblastoma. *N. Engl. J. Med.* **2005**, *352*, 987–996. [CrossRef]
3. Lapointe, S.; Perry, A.; Butowski, N.A. Primary brain tumours in adults. *Lancet* **2018**, *392*, 432–446. [CrossRef]
4. Stupp, R.; Hegi, M.E.; Mason, W.P.; van den Bent, M.J.; Taphoorn, M.J.; Janzer, R.C.; Ludwin, S.K.; Allgeier, A.; Fisher, B.; Belanger, K.; et al. Effects of radiotherapy with concomitant and adjuvant temozolomide versus radiotherapy alone on survival in glioblastoma in a randomised phase III study: 5-year analysis of the EORTC-NCIC trial. *Lancet Oncol.* **2009**, *10*, 459–466. [CrossRef]
5. Kim, J.; Lee, I.H.; Cho, H.J.; Park, C.K.; Jung, Y.S.; Kim, Y.; Nam, S.H.; Kim, B.S.; Johnson, M.D.; Kong, D.S.; et al. Spatiotemporal Evolution of the Primary Glioblastoma Genome. *Cancer Cell* **2015**, *28*, 318–328. [CrossRef] [PubMed]
6. Neftel, C.; Laffy, J.; Filbin, M.G.; Hara, T.; Shore, M.E.; Rahme, G.J.; Richman, A.R.; Silverbush, D.; Shaw, M.L.; Hebert, C.M.; et al. An Integrative Model of Cellular States, Plasticity, and Genetics for Glioblastoma. *Cell* **2019**, *178*, 835–849.e821. [CrossRef]
7. Patel, A.P.; Tirosh, I.; Trombetta, J.J.; Shalek, A.K.; Gillespie, S.M.; Wakimoto, H.; Cahill, D.P.; Nahed, B.V.; Curry, W.T.; Martuza, R.L.; et al. Single-cell RNA-seq highlights intratumoral heterogeneity in primary glioblastoma. *Science* **2014**, *344*, 1396–1401. [CrossRef] [PubMed]
8. Wang, J.; Cazzato, E.; Ladewig, E.; Frattini, V.; Rosenbloom, D.I.; Zairis, S.; Abate, F.; Liu, Z.; Elliott, O.; Shin, Y.J.; et al. Clonal evolution of glioblastoma under therapy. *Nat. Genet.* **2016**, *48*, 768–776. [CrossRef]
9. Meyer, M.; Reimand, J.; Lan, X.; Head, R.; Zhu, X.; Kushida, M.; Bayani, J.; Pressey, J.C.; Lionel, A.C.; Clarke, I.D.; et al. Single cell-derived clonal analysis of human glioblastoma links functional and genomic heterogeneity. *Proc. Natl. Acad. Sci. USA* **2015**, *112*, 851–856. [CrossRef]
10. Rius-Rocabert, S.; Garcia-Romero, N.; Garcia, A.; Ayuso-Sacido, A.; Nistal-Villan, E. Oncolytic Virotherapy in Glioma Tumors. *Int. J. Mol. Sci.* **2020**, *21*, 7604. [CrossRef]
11. Mitchell, D.A.; Xie, W.; Schmittling, R.; Learn, C.; Friedman, A.; McLendon, R.E.; Sampson, J.H. Sensitive detection of human cytomegalovirus in tumors and peripheral blood of patients diagnosed with glioblastoma. *Neuro-oncology* **2008**, *10*, 10–18. [CrossRef]
12. Bleeker, F.E.; Lamba, S.; Leenstra, S.; Troost, D.; Hulsebos, T.; Vandertop, W.P.; Frattini, M.; Molinari, F.; Knowles, M.; Cerrato, A.; et al. IDH1 mutations at residue p.R132 (IDH1(R132)) occur frequently in high-grade gliomas but not in other solid tumors. *Hum. Mutat.* **2009**, *30*, 7–11. [CrossRef]
13. Sampson, J.H.; Heimberger, A.B.; Archer, G.E.; Aldape, K.D.; Friedman, A.H.; Friedman, H.S.; Gilbert, M.R.; Herndon, J.E., 2nd; McLendon, R.E.; Mitchell, D.A.; et al. Immunologic escape after prolonged progression-free survival with epidermal growth factor receptor variant III peptide vaccination in patients with newly diagnosed glioblastoma. *J. Clin. Oncol.* **2010**, *28*, 4722–4729. [CrossRef]
14. Sampson, J.H.; Aldape, K.D.; Archer, G.E.; Coan, A.; Desjardins, A.; Friedman, A.H.; Friedman, H.S.; Gilbert, M.R.; Herndon, J.E.; McLendon, R.E.; et al. Greater chemotherapy-induced lymphopenia enhances tumor-specific immune responses that eliminate EGFRvIII-expressing tumor cells in patients with glioblastoma. *Neuro-oncology* **2011**, *13*, 324–333. [CrossRef]
15. Schuster, J.; Lai, R.K.; Recht, L.D.; Reardon, D.A.; Paleologos, N.A.; Groves, M.D.; Mrugala, M.M.; Jensen, R.; Baehring, J.M.; Sloan, A.; et al. A phase II, multicenter trial of rindopepimut (CDX-110) in newly diagnosed glioblastoma: The ACT III study. *Neuro-oncology* **2015**, *17*, 854–861. [CrossRef] [PubMed]
16. Weller, M.; Butowski, N.; Tran, D.D.; Recht, L.D.; Lim, M.; Hirte, H.; Ashby, L.; Mechtler, L.; Goldlust, S.A.; Iwamoto, F.; et al. Rindopepimut with temozolomide for patients with newly diagnosed, EGFRvIII-expressing glioblastoma (ACT IV): A randomised, double-blind, international phase 3 trial. *Lancet Oncol.* **2017**, *18*, 1373–1385. [CrossRef]
17. Reardon, D.A.; Desjardins, A.; Vredenburgh, J.J.; O'Rourke, D.M.; Tran, D.D.; Fink, K.L.; Nabors, L.B.; Li, G.; Bota, D.A.; Lukas, R.V.; et al. Rindopepimut with Bevacizumab for Patients with Relapsed EGFRvIII-Expressing Glioblastoma (ReACT): Results of a Double-Blind Randomized Phase II Trial. *Clin. Cancer Res.* **2020**, *26*, 1586–1594. [CrossRef]
18. Mitchell, D.A.; Batich, K.A.; Gunn, M.D.; Huang, M.N.; Sanchez-Perez, L.; Nair, S.K.; Congdon, K.L.; Reap, E.A.; Archer, G.E.; Desjardins, A.; et al. Tetanus toxoid and CCL3 improve dendritic cell vaccines in mice and glioblastoma patients. *Nature* **2015**, *519*, 366–369. [CrossRef] [PubMed]
19. Batich, K.A.; Reap, E.A.; Archer, G.E.; Sanchez-Perez, L.; Nair, S.K.; Schmittling, R.J.; Norberg, P.; Xie, W.; Herndon, J.E., 2nd; Healy, P.; et al. Long-term Survival in Glioblastoma with Cytomegalovirus pp65-Targeted Vaccination. *Clin. Cancer Res.* **2017**, *23*, 1898–1909. [CrossRef]
20. Batich, K.A.; Mitchell, D.A.; Healy, P.; Herndon, J.E., 2nd; Sampson, J.H. Once, Twice, Three Times a Finding: Reproducibility of Dendritic Cell Vaccine Trials Targeting Cytomegalovirus in Glioblastoma. *Clin. Cancer Res.* **2020**, *26*, 5297–5303. [CrossRef]
21. Platten, M.; Bunse, L.; Wick, A.; Bunse, T.; Le Cornet, L.; Harting, I.; Sahm, F.; Sanghvi, K.; Tan, C.L.; Poschke, I.; et al. A vaccine targeting mutant IDH1 in newly diagnosed glioma. *Nature* **2021**, *592*, 463–468. [CrossRef]

22. Liau, L.M.; Ashkan, K.; Tran, D.D.; Campian, J.L.; Trusheim, J.E.; Cobbs, C.S.; Heth, J.A.; Salacz, M.; Taylor, S.; D'Andre, S.D.; et al. First results on survival from a large Phase 3 clinical trial of an autologous dendritic cell vaccine in newly diagnosed glioblastoma. *J. Transl. Med.* **2018**, *16*, 142. [CrossRef] [PubMed]
23. Crane, C.A.; Han, S.J.; Ahn, B.; Oehlke, J.; Kivett, V.; Fedoroff, A.; Butowski, N.; Chang, S.M.; Clarke, J.; Berger, M.S.; et al. Individual patient-specific immunity against high-grade glioma after vaccination with autologous tumor derived peptides bound to the 96 KD chaperone protein. *Clin. Cancer Res.* **2013**, *19*, 205–214. [CrossRef]
24. Bloch, O.; Crane, C.A.; Fuks, Y.; Kaur, R.; Aghi, M.K.; Berger, M.S.; Butowski, N.A.; Chang, S.M.; Clarke, J.L.; McDermott, M.W.; et al. Heat-shock protein peptide complex-96 vaccination for recurrent glioblastoma: A phase II, single-arm trial. *Neuro-oncology* **2014**, *16*, 274–279. [CrossRef] [PubMed]
25. Ji, N.; Zhang, Y.; Liu, Y.; Xie, J.; Wang, Y.; Hao, S.; Gao, Z. Heat shock protein peptide complex-96 vaccination for newly diagnosed glioblastoma: A phase I, single-arm trial. *JCI Insight* **2018**, *3*. [CrossRef]
26. Bloch, O.; Lim, M.; Sughrue, M.E.; Komotar, R.J.; Abrahams, J.M.; O'Rourke, D.M.; D'Ambrosio, A.; Bruce, J.N.; Parsa, A.T. Autologous Heat Shock Protein Peptide Vaccination for Newly Diagnosed Glioblastoma: Impact of Peripheral PD-L1 Expression on Response to Therapy. *Clin. Cancer Res.* **2017**, *23*, 3575–3584. [CrossRef]
27. Heimberger, A.B.; Hlatky, R.; Suki, D.; Yang, D.; Weinberg, J.; Gilbert, M.; Sawaya, R.; Aldape, K. Prognostic effect of epidermal growth factor receptor and EGFRvIII in glioblastoma multiforme patients. *Clin. Cancer Res. Off. J. Am. Assoc. Cancer Res.* **2005**, *11*, 1462–1466. [CrossRef] [PubMed]
28. Batra, S.K.; Castelino-Prabhu, S.; Wikstrand, C.J.; Zhu, X.; Humphrey, P.A.; Friedman, H.S.; Bigner, D.D. Epidermal growth factor ligand-independent, unregulated, cell-transforming potential of a naturally occurring human mutant EGFRvIII gene. *Cell Growth Differ.* **1995**, *6*, 1251–1259.
29. Nagane, M.; Coufal, F.; Lin, H.; Bogler, O.; Cavenee, W.K.; Huang, H.J. A common mutant epidermal growth factor receptor confers enhanced tumorigenicity on human glioblastoma cells by increasing proliferation and reducing apoptosis. *Cancer Res.* **1996**, *56*, 5079–5086.
30. Sampson, J.H.; Archer, G.E.; Mitchell, D.A.; Heimberger, A.B.; Herndon, J.E., 2nd; Lally-Goss, D.; McGehee-Norman, S.; Paolino, A.; Reardon, D.A.; Friedman, A.H.; et al. An epidermal growth factor receptor variant III-targeted vaccine is safe and immunogenic in patients with glioblastoma multiforme. *Mol. Cancer Ther.* **2009**, *8*, 2773–2779. [CrossRef]
31. Heimberger, A.B.; Crotty, L.E.; Archer, G.E.; Hess, K.R.; Wikstrand, C.J.; Friedman, A.H.; Friedman, H.S.; Bigner, D.D.; Sampson, J.H. Epidermal growth factor receptor VIII peptide vaccination is efficacious against established intracerebral tumors. *Clin Cancer Res.* **2003**, *9*, 4247–4254.
32. Schafer, N.; Gielen, G.H.; Rauschenbach, L.; Kebir, S.; Till, A.; Reinartz, R.; Simon, M.; Niehusmann, P.; Kleinschnitz, C.; Herrlinger, U.; et al. Longitudinal heterogeneity in glioblastoma: Moving targets in recurrent versus primary tumors. *J. Transl. Med.* **2019**, *17*, 96. [CrossRef]
33. Brock, C.S.; Newlands, E.S.; Wedge, S.R.; Bower, M.; Evans, H.; Colquhoun, I.; Roddie, M.; Glaser, M.; Brampton, M.H.; Rustin, G.J. Phase I trial of temozolomide using an extended continuous oral schedule. *Cancer Res.* **1998**, *58*, 4363–4367. [PubMed]
34. Mansfield, A.S.; Nevala, W.K.; Lieser, E.A.; Leontovich, A.A.; Markovic, S.N. The immunomodulatory effects of bevacizumab on systemic immunity in patients with metastatic melanoma. *Oncoimmunology* **2013**, *2*, e24436. [CrossRef] [PubMed]
35. Wills, M.R.; Carmichael, A.J.; Mynard, K.; Jin, X.; Weekes, M.P.; Plachter, B.; Sissons, J.G. The human cytotoxic T-lymphocyte (CTL) response to cytomegalovirus is dominated by structural protein pp65: Frequency, specificity, and T-cell receptor usage of pp65-specific CTL. *J. Virol.* **1996**, *70*, 7569–7579. [CrossRef] [PubMed]
36. Arruda, L.B.; Sim, D.; Chikhlikar, P.R.; Maciel, M., Jr.; Akasaki, K.; August, J.T.; Marques, E.T. Dendritic cell-lysosomal-associated membrane protein (LAMP) and LAMP-1-HIV-1 gag chimeras have distinct cellular trafficking pathways and prime T and B cell responses to a diverse repertoire of epitopes. *J. Immunol.* **2006**, *177*, 2265–2275. [CrossRef]
37. Mitchell, D.A.; Cui, X.; Schmittling, R.J.; Sanchez-Perez, L.; Snyder, D.J.; Congdon, K.L.; Archer, G.E.; Desjardins, A.; Friedman, A.H.; Friedman, H.S.; et al. Monoclonal antibody blockade of IL-2 receptor alpha during lymphopenia selectively depletes regulatory T cells in mice and humans. *Blood* **2011**, *118*, 3003–3012. [CrossRef]
38. Schumacher, T.; Bunse, L.; Pusch, S.; Sahm, F.; Wiestler, B.; Quandt, J.; Menn, O.; Osswald, M.; Oezen, I.; Ott, M.; et al. A vaccine targeting mutant IDH1 induces antitumour immunity. *Nature* **2014**, *512*, 324–327. [CrossRef]
39. Blass, E.; Ott, P.A. Advances in the development of personalized neoantigen-based therapeutic cancer vaccines. *Nat. Rev. Clin. Oncol.* **2021**, *18*, 215–229. [CrossRef]
40. Liau, L.M.; Black, K.L.; Prins, R.M.; Sykes, S.N.; DiPatre, P.L.; Cloughesy, T.F.; Becker, D.P.; Bronstein, J.M. Treatment of intracranial gliomas with bone marrow-derived dendritic cells pulsed with tumor antigens. *J. Neurosurg.* **1999**, *90*, 1115–1124. [CrossRef]
41. Mitsuya, K.; Akiyama, Y.; Iizuka, A.; Miyata, H.; Deguchi, S.; Hayashi, N.; Maeda, C.; Kondou, R.; Kanematsu, A.; Watanabe, K.; et al. Alpha-type-1 Polarized Dendritic Cell-based Vaccination in Newly Diagnosed High-grade Glioma: A Phase II Clinical Trial. *Anticancer. Res.* **2020**, *40*, 6473–6484. [CrossRef]
42. Akiyama, Y.; Oshita, C.; Kume, A.; Iizuka, A.; Miyata, H.; Komiyama, M.; Ashizawa, T.; Yagoto, M.; Abe, Y.; Mitsuya, K.; et al. alpha-type-1 polarized dendritic cell-based vaccination in recurrent high-grade glioma: A phase I clinical trial. *BMC Cancer* **2012**, *12*, 623. [CrossRef]
43. Vaddepally, R.K.; Kharel, P.; Pandey, R.; Garje, R.; Chandra, A.B. Review of Indications of FDA-Approved Immune Checkpoint Inhibitors per NCCN Guidelines with the Level of Evidence. *Cancers* **2020**, *12*, 738. [CrossRef]

44. Davidson, T.B.; Lee, A.; Hsu, M.; Sedighim, S.; Orpilla, J.; Treger, J.; Mastall, M.; Roesch, S.; Rapp, C.; Galvez, M.; et al. Expression of PD-1 by T Cells in Malignant Glioma Patients Reflects Exhaustion and Activation. *Clin. Cancer Res.* **2019**, *25*, 1913–1922. [CrossRef]
45. Contardi, E.; Palmisano, G.L.; Tazzari, P.L.; Martelli, A.M.; Fala, F.; Fabbi, M.; Kato, T.; Lucarelli, E.; Donati, D.; Polito, L.; et al. CTLA-4 is constitutively expressed on tumor cells and can trigger apoptosis upon ligand interaction. *Int. J. Cancer* **2005**, *117*, 538–550. [CrossRef]
46. Reardon, D.A.; Brandes, A.A.; Omuro, A.; Mulholland, P.; Lim, M.; Wick, A.; Baehring, J.; Ahluwalia, M.S.; Roth, P.; Bahr, O.; et al. Effect of Nivolumab vs Bevacizumab in Patients With Recurrent Glioblastoma: The CheckMate 143 Phase 3 Randomized Clinical Trial. *JAMA Oncol.* **2020**, *6*, 1003–1010. [CrossRef]
47. Bristol Myers Squibb Announces Update on Phase 3 CheckMate -548 Trial Evaluating Patients with Newly Diagnosed MGMT-Methylated Glioblastoma Multiforme. Available online: https://news.bms.com/news/corporate-financial/2020/Bristol-Myers-Squibb-Announces-Update-on-Phase-3-CheckMate--548-Trial-Evaluating-Patients-with-Newly-Diagnosed-MGMT-Methylated-Glioblastoma-Multiforme/default.aspx (accessed on 2 June 2021).
48. Sahebjam, S.; Forsyth, P.A.; Tran, N.D.; Arrington, J.A.; Macaulay, R.; Etame, A.B.; Walko, C.M.; Boyle, T.; Peguero, E.N.; Jaglal, M.; et al. Hypofractionated stereotactic re-irradiation with pembrolizumab and bevacizumab in patients with recurrent high-grade gliomas: Results from a phase I study. *Neuro-oncology* **2021**, *23*, 677–686. [CrossRef]
49. Reardon, D.A. Phase II study of pembrolizumab or pembrolizumab plus bevacizumab for recurrent glioblastoma (rGBM) patients. *J. Clin. Oncol.* **2006**, *36*. [CrossRef]
50. Schalper, K.A.; Rodriguez-Ruiz, M.E.; Diez-Valle, R.; Lopez-Janeiro, A.; Porciuncula, A.; Idoate, M.A.; Inoges, S.; de Andrea, C.; Lopez-Diaz de Cerio, A.; Tejada, S.; et al. Neoadjuvant nivolumab modifies the tumor immune microenvironment in resectable glioblastoma. *Nat. Med.* **2019**, *25*, 470–476. [CrossRef]
51. Reardon, D.A. Atim-12. Phase 2 study to evaluate the clinical efficacy and safety of medi4736 (durvalumab [dur]) in patients with bevacizumab (bev)-refractory recurrent glioblastoma (GBM). *Neuro-oncology* **2017**, *19*. [CrossRef]
52. Lim, M.; Ye, X.; Piotrowski, A.F.; Desai, A.S.; Ahluwalia, M.S.; Walbert, T.; Fisher, J.D.; Desideri, S.; Belcaid, Z.; Jackson, C.; et al. Updated phase I trial of anti-LAG-3 or anti-CD137 alone and in combination with anti-PD-1 in patients with recurrent GBM. *J. Clin. Oncol.* **2019**, *37*, 2017. [CrossRef]
53. Zeng, J.; See, A.P.; Phallen, J.; Jackson, C.M.; Belcaid, Z.; Ruzevick, J.; Durham, N.; Meyer, C.; Harris, T.J.; Albesiano, E.; et al. Anti-PD-1 blockade and stereotactic radiation produce long-term survival in mice with intracranial gliomas. *Int. J. Radiat. Oncol. Biol. Phys.* **2013**, *86*, 343–349. [CrossRef]
54. Omuro, A.; Vlahovic, G.; Lim, M.; Sahebjam, S.; Baehring, J.; Cloughesy, T.; Voloschin, A.; Ramkissoon, S.H.; Ligon, K.L.; Latek, R.; et al. Nivolumab with or without ipilimumab in patients with recurrent glioblastoma: Results from exploratory phase I cohorts of CheckMate 143. *Neuro-oncology* **2018**, *20*, 674–686. [CrossRef]
55. Mathios, D.; Kim, J.E.; Mangraviti, A.; Phallen, J.; Park, C.K.; Jackson, C.M.; Garzon-Muvdi, T.; Kim, E.; Theodros, D.; Polanczyk, M.; et al. Anti-PD-1 antitumor immunity is enhanced by local and abrogated by systemic chemotherapy in GBM. *Sci. Transl. Med.* **2016**, *8*, 370ra180. [CrossRef]
56. Liu, J.; Blake, S.J.; Yong, M.C.; Harjunpaa, H.; Ngiow, S.F.; Takeda, K.; Young, A.; O'Donnell, J.S.; Allen, S.; Smyth, M.J.; et al. Improved Efficacy of Neoadjuvant Compared to Adjuvant Immunotherapy to Eradicate Metastatic Disease. *Cancer Discov.* **2016**, *6*, 1382–1399. [CrossRef]
57. Blank, C.U.; Rozeman, E.A.; Fanchi, L.F.; Sikorska, K.; van de Wiel, B.; Kvistborg, P.; Krijgsman, O.; van den Braber, M.; Philips, D.; Broeks, A.; et al. Neoadjuvant versus adjuvant ipilimumab plus nivolumab in macroscopic stage III melanoma. *Nat. Med.* **2018**, *24*, 1655–1661. [CrossRef]
58. Cloughesy, T.F.; Mochizuki, A.Y.; Orpilla, J.R.; Hugo, W.; Lee, A.H.; Davidson, T.B.; Wang, A.C.; Ellingson, B.M.; Rytlewski, J.A.; Sanders, C.M.; et al. Neoadjuvant anti-PD-1 immunotherapy promotes a survival benefit with intratumoral and systemic immune responses in recurrent glioblastoma. *Nat. Med.* **2019**, *25*, 477–486. [CrossRef]
59. Fecci, P.E.; Ochiai, H.; Mitchell, D.A.; Grossi, P.M.; Sweeney, A.E.; Archer, G.E.; Cummings, T.; Allison, J.P.; Bigner, D.D.; Sampson, J.H. Systemic CTLA-4 blockade ameliorates glioma-induced changes to the CD4+ T cell compartment without affecting regulatory T-cell function. *Clin. Cancer Res.* **2007**, *13*, 2158–2167. [CrossRef]
60. Reardon, D.A.; Gokhale, P.C.; Klein, S.R.; Ligon, K.L.; Rodig, S.J.; Ramkissoon, S.H.; Jones, K.L.; Conway, A.S.; Liao, X.; Zhou, J.; et al. Glioblastoma Eradication Following Immune Checkpoint Blockade in an Orthotopic, Immunocompetent Model. *Cancer Immunol. Res.* **2016**, *4*, 124–135. [CrossRef]
61. Harris-Bookman, S.; Mathios, D.; Martin, A.M.; Xia, Y.; Kim, E.; Xu, H.; Belcaid, Z.; Polanczyk, M.; Barberi, T.; Theodros, D.; et al. Expression of LAG-3 and efficacy of combination treatment with anti-LAG-3 and anti-PD-1 monoclonal antibodies in glioblastoma. *Int. J. Cancer* **2018**, *143*, 3201–3208. [CrossRef]
62. Mair, M.J.; Kiesel, B.; Feldmann, K.; Widhalm, G.; Dieckmann, K.; Wohrer, A.; Mullauer, L.; Preusser, M.; Berghoff, A.S. LAG-3 expression in the inflammatory microenvironment of glioma. *J. Neurooncol.* **2021**, *152*, 533–539. [CrossRef]
63. Kuhnol, C.; Herbarth, M.; Foll, J.; Staege, M.S.; Kramm, C. CD137 stimulation and p38 MAPK inhibition improve reactivity in an in vitro model of glioblastoma immunotherapy. *Cancer Immunol. Immunother.* **2013**, *62*, 1797–1809. [CrossRef]
64. Newcomb, E.W.; Lukyanov, Y.; Kawashima, N.; Alonso-Basanta, M.; Wang, S.C.; Liu, M.; Jure-Kunkel, M.; Zagzag, D.; Demaria, S.; Formenti, S.C. Radiotherapy enhances antitumor effect of anti-CD137 therapy in a mouse Glioma model. *Radiat. Res.* **2010**, *173*, 426–432. [CrossRef]

65. Zhang, J.; Sai, K.; Wang, X.L.; Ye, S.Q.; Liang, L.J.; Zhou, Y.; Chen, Z.J.; Hu, W.M.; Liu, J.M. Tim-3 Expression and MGMT Methylation Status Association With Survival in Glioblastoma. *Front. Pharmacol.* **2020**, *11*, 584652. [CrossRef]
66. Kim, J.E.; Patel, M.A.; Mangraviti, A.; Kim, E.S.; Theodros, D.; Velarde, E.; Liu, A.; Sankey, E.W.; Tam, A.; Xu, H.; et al. Combination Therapy with Anti-PD-1, Anti-TIM-3, and Focal Radiation Results in Regression of Murine Gliomas. *Clin. Cancer Res.* **2017**, *23*, 124–136. [CrossRef]
67. Goswami, S.; Walle, T.; Cornish, A.E.; Basu, S.; Anandhan, S.; Fernandez, I.; Vence, L.; Blando, J.; Zhao, H.; Yadav, S.S.; et al. Immune profiling of human tumors identifies CD73 as a combinatorial target in glioblastoma. *Nat. Med.* **2020**, *26*, 39–46. [CrossRef] [PubMed]
68. Willingham, S.B.; Volkmer, J.P.; Gentles, A.J.; Sahoo, D.; Dalerba, P.; Mitra, S.S.; Wang, J.; Contreras-Trujillo, H.; Martin, R.; Cohen, J.D.; et al. The CD47-signal regulatory protein alpha (SIRPa) interaction is a therapeutic target for human solid tumors. *Proc. Natl. Acad. Sci. USA* **2012**, *109*, 6662–6667. [CrossRef]
69. Zhang, M.; Hutter, G.; Kahn, S.A.; Azad, T.D.; Gholamin, S.; Xu, C.Y.; Liu, J.; Achrol, A.S.; Richard, C.; Sommerkamp, P.; et al. Anti-CD47 Treatment Stimulates Phagocytosis of Glioblastoma by M1 and M2 Polarized Macrophages and Promotes M1 Polarized Macrophages In Vivo. *PLoS ONE* **2016**, *11*, e0153550. [CrossRef] [PubMed]
70. Zhang, X.; Fan, J.; Wang, S.; Li, Y.; Wang, Y.; Li, S.; Luan, J.; Wang, Z.; Song, P.; Chen, Q.; et al. Targeting CD47 and Autophagy Elicited Enhanced Antitumor Effects in Non-Small Cell Lung Cancer. *Cancer Immunol. Res.* **2017**, *5*, 363–375. [CrossRef] [PubMed]
71. Edris, B.; Weiskopf, K.; Volkmer, A.K.; Volkmer, J.P.; Willingham, S.B.; Contreras-Trujillo, H.; Liu, J.; Majeti, R.; West, R.B.; Fletcher, J.A.; et al. Antibody therapy targeting the CD47 protein is effective in a model of aggressive metastatic leiomyosarcoma. *Proc. Natl. Acad. Sci. USA* **2012**, *109*, 6656–6661. [CrossRef]
72. Li, F.; Lv, B.; Liu, Y.; Hua, T.; Han, J.; Sun, C.; Xu, L.; Zhang, Z.; Feng, Z.; Cai, Y.; et al. Blocking the CD47-SIRPalpha axis by delivery of anti-CD47 antibody induces antitumor effects in glioma and glioma stem cells. *Oncoimmunology* **2018**, *7*, e1391973. [CrossRef] [PubMed]
73. Gholamin, S.; Youssef, O.A.; Rafat, M.; Esparza, R.; Kahn, S.; Shahin, M.; Giaccia, A.J.; Graves, E.E.; Weissman, I.; Mitra, S.; et al. Irradiation or temozolomide chemotherapy enhances anti-CD47 treatment of glioblastoma. *Innate. Immun.* **2020**, *26*, 130–137. [CrossRef] [PubMed]
74. von Roemeling, C.A.; Wang, Y.; Qie, Y.; Yuan, H.; Zhao, H.; Liu, X.; Yang, Z.; Yang, M.; Deng, W.; Bruno, K.A.; et al. Therapeutic modulation of phagocytosis in glioblastoma can activate both innate and adaptive antitumour immunity. *Nat. Commun.* **2020**, *11*, 1508. [CrossRef] [PubMed]
75. Zhang, X.; Chen, W.; Fan, J.; Wang, S.; Xian, Z.; Luan, J.; Li, Y.; Wang, Y.; Nan, Y.; Luo, M.; et al. Disrupting CD47-SIRPalpha axis alone or combined with autophagy depletion for the therapy of glioblastoma. *Carcinogenesis* **2018**, *39*, 689–699. [CrossRef]
76. Zhang, X.; Wang, S.; Nan, Y.; Fan, J.; Chen, W.; Luan, J.; Wang, Y.; Liang, Y.; Li, S.; Tian, W.; et al. Inhibition of autophagy potentiated the anti-tumor effects of VEGF and CD47 bispecific therapy in glioblastoma. *Appl. Microbiol. Biotechnol.* **2018**, *102*, 6503–6513. [CrossRef]
77. Sockolosky, J.T.; Dougan, M.; Ingram, J.R.; Ho, C.C.; Kauke, M.J.; Almo, S.C.; Ploegh, H.L.; Garcia, K.C. Durable antitumor responses to CD47 blockade require adaptive immune stimulation. *Proc. Natl. Acad. Sci. USA* **2016**, *113*, E2646–E2654. [CrossRef]
78. Sadelain, M.; Brentjens, R.; Riviere, I. The basic principles of chimeric antigen receptor design. *Cancer Discov.* **2013**, *3*, 388–398. [CrossRef]
79. Finney, H.M.; Lawson, A.D.; Bebbington, C.R.; Weir, A.N. Chimeric receptors providing both primary and costimulatory signaling in T cells from a single gene product. *J. Immunol.* **1998**, *161*, 2791–2797. [PubMed]
80. Finney, H.M.; Akbar, A.N.; Lawson, A.D. Activation of resting human primary T cells with chimeric receptors: Costimulation from CD28, inducible costimulator, CD134, and CD137 in series with signals from the TCR zeta chain. *J. Immunol.* **2004**, *172*, 104–113. [CrossRef]
81. Imai, C.; Mihara, K.; Andreansky, M.; Nicholson, I.C.; Pui, C.H.; Geiger, T.L.; Campana, D. Chimeric receptors with 4-1BB signaling capacity provoke potent cytotoxicity against acute lymphoblastic leukemia. *Leukemia* **2004**, *18*, 676–684. [CrossRef]
82. Hombach, A.; Wieczarkowiecz, A.; Marquardt, T.; Heuser, C.; Usai, L.; Pohl, C.; Seliger, B.; Abken, H. Tumor-specific T cell activation by recombinant immunoreceptors: CD3 zeta signaling and CD28 costimulation are simultaneously required for efficient IL-2 secretion and can be integrated into one combined CD28/CD3 zeta signaling receptor molecule. *J. Immunol.* **2001**, *167*, 6123–6131. [CrossRef]
83. Maude, S.L.; Frey, N.; Shaw, P.A.; Aplenc, R.; Barrett, D.M.; Bunin, N.J.; Chew, A.; Gonzalez, V.E.; Zheng, Z.; Lacey, S.F.; et al. Chimeric antigen receptor T cells for sustained remissions in leukemia. *N. Engl. J. Med.* **2014**, *371*, 1507–1517. [CrossRef]
84. Bagley, S.J.; Desai, A.S.; Linette, G.P.; June, C.H.; O'Rourke, D.M. CAR T-cell therapy for glioblastoma: Recent clinical advances and future challenges. *Neuro-oncology* **2018**, *20*, 1429–1438. [CrossRef]
85. Sarkaria, J.N.; Hu, L.S.; Parney, I.F.; Pafundi, D.H.; Brinkmann, D.H.; Laack, N.N.; Giannini, C.; Burns, T.C.; Kizilbash, S.H.; Laramy, J.K.; et al. Is the blood-brain barrier really disrupted in all glioblastomas? A critical assessment of existing clinical data. *Neuro-oncology* **2018**, *20*, 184–191. [CrossRef] [PubMed]
86. Watkins, S.; Robel, S.; Kimbrough, I.F.; Robert, S.M.; Ellis-Davies, G.; Sontheimer, H. Disruption of astrocyte-vascular coupling and the blood-brain barrier by invading glioma cells. *Nat. Commun.* **2014**, *5*, 4196. [CrossRef]

87. O'Rourke, D.M.; Nasrallah, M.P.; Desai, A.; Melenhorst, J.J.; Mansfield, K.; Morrissette, J.J.D.; Martinez-Lage, M.; Brem, S.; Maloney, E.; Shen, A.; et al. A single dose of peripherally infused EGFRvIII-directed CAR T cells mediates antigen loss and induces adaptive resistance in patients with recurrent glioblastoma. *Sci. Transl. Med.* 2017, 9. [CrossRef] [PubMed]
88. Ahmed, N.; Salsman, V.S.; Kew, Y.; Shaffer, D.; Powell, S.; Zhang, Y.J.; Grossman, R.G.; Heslop, H.E.; Gottschalk, S. HER2-specific T cells target primary glioblastoma stem cells and induce regression of autologous experimental tumors. *Clin. Cancer Res. Off. J. Am. Assoc. Cancer Res.* 2010, 16, 474–485. [CrossRef] [PubMed]
89. Keu, K.V.; Witney, T.H.; Yaghoubi, S.; Rosenberg, J.; Kurien, A.; Magnusson, R.; Williams, J.; Habte, F.; Wagner, J.R.; Forman, S.; et al. Reporter gene imaging of targeted T cell immunotherapy in recurrent glioma. *Sci. Transl. Med.* 2017, 9. [CrossRef]
90. Brown, C.E.; Badie, B.; Barish, M.E.; Weng, L.; Ostberg, J.R.; Chang, W.C.; Naranjo, A.; Starr, R.; Wagner, J.; Wright, C.; et al. Bioactivity and Safety of IL13Ralpha2-Redirected Chimeric Antigen Receptor CD8+ T Cells in Patients with Recurrent Glioblastoma. *Clin. Cancer Res. Off. J. Am. Assoc. Cancer Res.* 2015, 21, 4062–4072. [CrossRef] [PubMed]
91. Brown, C.E.; Alizadeh, D.; Starr, R.; Weng, L.; Wagner, J.R.; Naranjo, A.; Ostberg, J.R.; Blanchard, M.S.; Kilpatrick, J.; Simpson, J.; et al. Regression of Glioblastoma after Chimeric Antigen Receptor T-Cell Therapy. *N. Engl. J. Med.* 2016, 375, 2561–2569. [CrossRef] [PubMed]
92. Wang, D.; Starr, R.; Chang, W.C.; Aguilar, B.; Alizadeh, D.; Wright, S.L.; Yang, X.; Brito, A.; Sarkissian, A.; Ostberg, J.R.; et al. Chlorotoxin-directed CAR T cells for specific and effective targeting of glioblastoma. *Sci. Transl. Med.* 2020, 12. [CrossRef]
93. Tang, X.; Zhao, S.; Zhang, Y.; Wang, Y.; Zhang, Z.; Yang, M.; Zhu, Y.; Zhang, G.; Guo, G.; Tong, A.; et al. B7-H3 as a Novel CAR-T Therapeutic Target for Glioblastoma. *Mol. Ther. Oncolytics* 2019, 14, 279–287. [CrossRef]
94. Tang, X.; Wang, Y.; Huang, J.; Zhang, Z.; Liu, F.; Xu, J.; Guo, G.; Wang, W.; Tong, A.; Zhou, L. Administration of B7-H3 targeted chimeric antigen receptor-T cells induce regression of glioblastoma. *Signal Transduct. Target. Ther.* 2021, 6, 125. [CrossRef]
95. Nehama, D.; Di Ianni, N.; Musio, S.; Du, H.; Patane, M.; Pollo, B.; Finocchiaro, G.; Park, J.J.H.; Dunn, D.E.; Edwards, D.S.; et al. B7-H3-redirected chimeric antigen receptor T cells target glioblastoma and neurospheres. *EBioMedicine* 2019, 47, 33–43. [CrossRef] [PubMed]
96. Zhang, Y.; Li, X.; Zhang, J.; Mao, L. Novel cellular immunotherapy using NKG2D CAR-T for the treatment of cervical cancer. *Biomed. Pharmacother. Biomed. Pharmacother.* 2020, 131, 110562. [CrossRef]
97. Yang, D.; Sun, B.; Dai, H.; Li, W.; Shi, L.; Zhang, P.; Li, S.; Zhao, X. T cells expressing NKG2D chimeric antigen receptors efficiently eliminate glioblastoma and cancer stem cells. *J. Immunother. Cancer* 2019, 7, 171. [CrossRef] [PubMed]
98. Ahmed, N.; Brawley, V.; Hegde, M.; Bielamowicz, K.; Kalra, M.; Landi, D.; Robertson, C.; Gray, T.L.; Diouf, O.; Wakefield, A.; et al. HER2-Specific Chimeric Antigen Receptor-Modified Virus-Specific T Cells for Progressive Glioblastoma: A Phase 1 Dose-Escalation Trial. *JAMA Oncol.* 2017, 3, 1094–1101. [CrossRef] [PubMed]
99. Goff, S.L.; Morgan, R.A.; Yang, J.C.; Sherry, R.M.; Robbins, P.F.; Restifo, N.P.; Feldman, S.A.; Lu, Y.C.; Lu, L.; Zheng, Z.; et al. Pilot Trial of Adoptive Transfer of Chimeric Antigen Receptor-transduced T Cells Targeting EGFRvIII in Patients With Glioblastoma. *J. Immunother.* 2019, 42, 126–135. [CrossRef]
100. Brown, C.E.; Warden, C.D.; Starr, R.; Deng, X.; Badie, B.; Yuan, Y.C.; Forman, S.J.; Barish, M.E. Glioma IL13Ralpha2 is associated with mesenchymal signature gene expression and poor patient prognosis. *PLoS ONE* 2013, 8, e77769. [CrossRef]
101. Debinski, W.; Gibo, D.M.; Hulet, S.W.; Connor, J.R.; Gillespie, G.Y. Receptor for interleukin 13 is a marker and therapeutic target for human high-grade gliomas. *Clin. Cancer Res. Off. J. Am. Assoc. Cancer Res.* 1999, 5, 985–990.
102. Bhat, K.P.L.; Balasubramaniyan, V.; Vaillant, B.; Ezhilarasan, R.; Hummelink, K.; Hollingsworth, F.; Wani, K.; Heathcock, L.; James, J.D.; Goodman, L.D.; et al. Mesenchymal differentiation mediated by NF-kappaB promotes radiation resistance in glioblastoma. *Cancer Cell* 2013, 24, 331–346. [CrossRef]
103. Wang, Q.; Hu, B.; Hu, X.; Kim, H.; Squatrito, M.; Scarpace, L.; de Carvalho, A.C.; Lyu, S.; Li, P.; Li, Y.; et al. Tumor Evolution of Glioma-Intrinsic Gene Expression Subtypes Associates with Immunological Changes in the Microenvironment. *Cancer Cell* 2018, 33, 152. [CrossRef]
104. Kong, S.; Sengupta, S.; Tyler, B.; Bais, A.J.; Ma, Q.; Doucette, S.; Zhou, J.; Sahin, A.; Carter, B.S.; Brem, H.; et al. Suppression of human glioma xenografts with second-generation IL13R-specific chimeric antigen receptor-modified T cells. *Clin. Cancer Res. Off. J. Am. Assoc. Cancer Res.* 2012, 18, 5949–5960. [CrossRef] [PubMed]
105. Brown, C.E.; Aguilar, B.; Starr, R.; Yang, X.; Chang, W.C.; Weng, L.; Chang, B.; Sarkissian, A.; Brito, A.; Sanchez, J.F.; et al. Optimization of IL13Ralpha2-Targeted Chimeric Antigen Receptor T Cells for Improved Anti-tumor Efficacy against Glioblastoma. *Mol. Ther. J. Am. Soc. Gene Ther.* 2018, 26, 31–44. [CrossRef] [PubMed]
106. Krenciute, G.; Krebs, S.; Torres, D.; Wu, M.F.; Liu, H.; Dotti, G.; Li, X.N.; Lesniak, M.S.; Balyasnikova, I.V.; Gottschalk, S. Characterization and Functional Analysis of scFv-based Chimeric Antigen Receptors to Redirect T Cells to IL13Ralpha2-positive Glioma. *Mol. Ther. J. Am. Soc. Gene Ther.* 2016, 24, 354–363. [CrossRef]
107. Krenciute, G.; Prinzing, B.L.; Yi, Z.; Wu, M.F.; Liu, H.; Dotti, G.; Balyasnikova, I.V.; Gottschalk, S. Transgenic Expression of IL15 Improves Antiglioma Activity of IL13Ralpha2-CAR T Cells but Results in Antigen Loss Variants. *Cancer Immunol. Res.* 2017, 5, 571–581. [CrossRef] [PubMed]
108. Pituch, K.C.; Miska, J.; Krenciute, G.; Panek, W.K.; Li, G.; Rodriguez-Cruz, T.; Wu, M.; Han, Y.; Lesniak, M.S.; Gottschalk, S.; et al. Adoptive Transfer of IL13Ralpha2-Specific Chimeric Antigen Receptor T Cells Creates a Pro-inflammatory Environment in Glioblastoma. *Mol. Ther. J. Am. Soc. Gene Ther.* 2018, 26, 986–995. [CrossRef]

109. Wang, D.; Aguilar, B.; Starr, R.; Alizadeh, D.; Brito, A.; Sarkissian, A.; Ostberg, J.R.; Forman, S.J.; Brown, C.E. Glioblastoma-targeted CD4+ CAR T cells mediate superior antitumor activity. *JCI Insight* **2018**, *3*. [CrossRef] [PubMed]
110. Padfield, E.; Ellis, H.P.; Kurian, K.M. Current Therapeutic Advances Targeting EGFR and EGFRvIII in Glioblastoma. *Front. Oncol.* **2015**, *5*, 5. [CrossRef]
111. Johnson, L.A.; Scholler, J.; Ohkuri, T.; Kosaka, A.; Patel, P.R.; McGettigan, S.E.; Nace, A.K.; Dentchev, T.; Thekkat, P.; Loew, A.; et al. Rational development and characterization of humanized anti-EGFR variant III chimeric antigen receptor T cells for glioblastoma. *Sci. Transl. Med.* **2015**, *7*, 275ra222. [CrossRef] [PubMed]
112. Ohno, M.; Ohkuri, T.; Kosaka, A.; Tanahashi, K.; June, C.H.; Natsume, A.; Okada, H. Expression of miR-17-92 enhances anti-tumor activity of T-cells transduced with the anti-EGFRvIII chimeric antigen receptor in mice bearing human GBM xenografts. *J. Immunother. Cancer* **2013**, *1*, 21. [CrossRef] [PubMed]
113. Choi, B.D.; Suryadevara, C.M.; Gedeon, P.C.; Herndon, J.E., 2nd; Sanchez-Perez, L.; Bigner, D.D.; Sampson, J.H. Intracerebral delivery of a third generation EGFRvIII-specific chimeric antigen receptor is efficacious against human glioma. *J. Clin. Neurosci. Off. J. Neurosurg. Soc. Australas.* **2014**, *21*, 189–190. [CrossRef]
114. Sampson, J.H.; Choi, B.D.; Sanchez-Perez, L.; Suryadevara, C.M.; Snyder, D.J.; Flores, C.T.; Schmittling, R.J.; Nair, S.K.; Reap, E.A.; Norberg, P.K.; et al. EGFRvIII mCAR-modified T-cell therapy cures mice with established intracerebral glioma and generates host immunity against tumor-antigen loss. *Clin. Cancer Res. Off. J. Am. Assoc. Cancer Res.* **2014**, *20*, 972–984. [CrossRef]
115. Miao, H.; Choi, B.D.; Suryadevara, C.M.; Sanchez-Perez, L.; Yang, S.; De Leon, G.; Sayour, E.J.; McLendon, R.; Herndon, J.E., 2nd; Healy, P.; et al. EGFRvIII-specific chimeric antigen receptor T cells migrate to and kill tumor deposits infiltrating the brain parenchyma in an invasive xenograft model of glioblastoma. *PLoS ONE* **2014**, *9*, e94281. [CrossRef]
116. Choi, B.D.; Yu, X.; Castano, A.P.; Bouffard, A.A.; Schmidts, A.; Larson, R.C.; Bailey, S.R.; Boroughs, A.C.; Frigault, M.J.; Leick, M.B.; et al. CAR-T cells secreting BiTEs circumvent antigen escape without detectable toxicity. *Nat. Biotechnol.* **2019**, *37*, 1049–1058. [CrossRef] [PubMed]
117. Lim, S.M.; Pyo, K.H.; Soo, R.A.; Cho, B.C. The promise of bispecific antibodies: Clinical applications and challenges. *Cancer Treat. Rev.* **2021**, *99*, 102240. [CrossRef] [PubMed]
118. Choe, J.H.; Watchmaker, P.B.; Simic, M.S.; Gilbert, R.D.; Li, A.W.; Krasnow, N.A.; Downey, K.M.; Yu, W.; Carrera, D.A.; Celli, A.; et al. SynNotch-CAR T cells overcome challenges of specificity, heterogeneity, and persistence in treating glioblastoma. *Sci. Transl. Med.* **2021**, *13*. [CrossRef] [PubMed]
119. Haynik, D.M.; Roma, A.A.; Prayson, R.A. HER-2/neu expression in glioblastoma multiforme. *Appl. Immunohistochem. Mol. Morphol.* **2007**, *15*, 56–58. [CrossRef]
120. Koka, V.; Potti, A.; Forseen, S.E.; Pervez, H.; Fraiman, G.N.; Koch, M.; Levitt, R. Role of Her-2/neu overexpression and clinical determinants of early mortality in glioblastoma multiforme. *Am. J. Clin. Oncol.* **2003**, *26*, 332–335. [CrossRef]
121. Jackson, C.M.; Choi, J.; Lim, M. Mechanisms of immunotherapy resistance: Lessons from glioblastoma. *Nat. Immunol.* **2019**, *20*, 1100–1109. [CrossRef] [PubMed]
122. Wang, X.; Lu, J.; Guo, G.; Yu, J. Immunotherapy for recurrent glioblastoma: Practical insights and challenging prospects. *Cell Death Dis.* **2021**, *12*, 299. [CrossRef] [PubMed]
123. Yu, M.W.; Quail, D.F. Immunotherapy for Glioblastoma: Current Progress and Challenge. *Front. Immunol.* **2021**, *12*, 676301. [CrossRef] [PubMed]
124. Hodges, T.R.; Ott, M.; Xiu, J.; Gatalica, Z.; Swensen, J.; Zhou, S.; Huse, J.T.; de Groot, J.; Li, S.; Overwijk, W.W.; et al. Mutational burden, immune checkpoint expression, and mismatch repair in glioma: Implications for immune checkpoint immunotherapy. *Neuro-oncology* **2017**, *19*, 1047–1057. [CrossRef]
125. Wei, S.C.; Duffy, C.R.; Allison, J.P. Fundamental Mechanisms of Immune Checkpoint Blockade Therapy. *Cancer Discov.* **2018**, *8*, 1069–1086. [CrossRef] [PubMed]
126. Cockle, J.V.; Rajani, K.; Zaidi, S.; Kottke, T.; Thompson, J.; Diaz, R.M.; Shim, K.; Peterson, T.; Parney, I.F.; Short, S.; et al. Combination viroimmunotherapy with checkpoint inhibition to treat glioma, based on location-specific tumor profiling. *Neuro-oncology* **2016**, *18*, 518–527. [CrossRef]
127. Jiang, H.; Rivera-Molina, Y.; Gomez-Manzano, C.; Clise-Dwyer, K.; Bover, L.; Vence, L.M.; Yuan, Y.; Lang, F.F.; Toniatti, C.; Hossain, M.B.; et al. Oncolytic Adenovirus and Tumor-Targeting Immune Modulatory Therapy Improve Autologous Cancer Vaccination. *Cancer Res.* **2017**, *77*, 3894–3907. [CrossRef]
128. Chen, C.Y.; Hutzen, B.; Wedekind, M.F.; Cripe, T.P. Oncolytic virus and PD-1/PD-L1 blockade combination therapy. *Oncolytic Virother.* **2018**, *7*, 65–77. [CrossRef]
129. Antonios, J.P.; Soto, H.; Everson, R.G.; Orpilla, J.; Moughon, D.; Shin, N.; Sedighim, S.; Yong, W.H.; Li, G.; Cloughesy, T.F.; et al. PD-1 blockade enhances the vaccination-induced immune response in glioma. *JCI Insight* **2016**, *1*. [CrossRef]
130. Murty, S.; Haile, S.T.; Beinat, C.; Aalipour, A.; Alam, I.S.; Murty, T.; Shaffer, T.M.; Patel, C.B.; Graves, E.E.; Mackall, C.L.; et al. Intravital imaging reveals synergistic effect of CAR T-cells and radiation therapy in a preclinical immunocompetent glioblastoma model. *Oncoimmunology* **2020**, *9*, 1757360. [CrossRef]
131. Yang, M.; Tang, X.; Zhang, Z.; Gu, L.; Wei, H.; Zhao, S.; Zhong, K.; Mu, M.; Huang, C.; Jiang, C.; et al. Tandem CAR-T cells targeting CD70 and B7-H3 exhibit potent preclinical activity against multiple solid tumors. *Theranostics* **2020**, *10*, 7622–7634. [CrossRef]
132. Jin, L.; Ge, H.; Long, Y.; Yang, C.; Chang, Y.E.; Mu, L.; Sayour, E.J.; De Leon, G.; Wang, Q.J.; Yang, J.C.; et al. CD70, a novel target of CAR T-cell therapy for gliomas. *Neuro-oncology* **2018**, *20*, 55–65. [CrossRef] [PubMed]

133. Vora, P.; Venugopal, C.; Salim, S.K.; Tatari, N.; Bakhshinyan, D.; Singh, M.; Seyfrid, M.; Upreti, D.; Rentas, S.; Wong, N.; et al. The Rational Development of CD133-Targeting Immunotherapies for Glioblastoma. *Cell Stem Cell* **2020**, *26*, 832–844.e836. [CrossRef] [PubMed]
134. Cui, J.; Zhang, Q.; Song, Q.; Wang, H.; Dmitriev, P.; Sun, M.Y.; Cao, X.; Wang, Y.; Guo, L.; Indig, I.H.; et al. Targeting hypoxia downstream signaling protein, CAIX, for CAR T-cell therapy against glioblastoma. *Neuro-oncology* **2019**, *21*, 1436–1446. [CrossRef]
135. Yi, Z.; Prinzing, B.L.; Cao, F.; Gottschalk, S.; Krenciute, G. Optimizing EphA2-CAR T Cells for the Adoptive Immunotherapy of Glioma. *Mol. Ther. Methods Clin. Dev.* **2018**, *9*, 70–80. [CrossRef] [PubMed]
136. Chow, K.K.; Naik, S.; Kakarla, S.; Brawley, V.S.; Shaffer, D.R.; Yi, Z.; Rainusso, N.; Wu, M.F.; Liu, H.; Kew, Y.; et al. T cells redirected to EphA2 for the immunotherapy of glioblastoma. *Mol. Ther. J. Am. Soc. Gene Ther.* **2013**, *21*, 629–637. [CrossRef]
137. Shiina, S.; Ohno, M.; Ohka, F.; Kuramitsu, S.; Yamamichi, A.; Kato, A.; Motomura, K.; Tanahashi, K.; Yamamoto, T.; Watanabe, R.; et al. CAR T Cells Targeting Podoplanin Reduce Orthotopic Glioblastomas in Mouse Brains. *Cancer Immunol. Res.* **2016**, *4*, 259–268. [CrossRef] [PubMed]
138. Beard, R.E.; Zheng, Z.; Lagisetty, K.H.; Burns, W.R.; Tran, E.; Hewitt, S.M.; Abate-Daga, D.; Rosati, S.F.; Fine, H.A.; Ferrone, S.; et al. Multiple chimeric antigen receptors successfully target chondroitin sulfate proteoglycan 4 in several different cancer histologies and cancer stem cells. *J. Immunother. Cancer* **2014**, *2*, 25. [CrossRef]
139. Geldres, C.; Savoldo, B.; Hoyos, V.; Caruana, I.; Zhang, M.; Yvon, E.; Del Vecchio, M.; Creighton, C.J.; Ittmann, M.; Ferrone, S.; et al. T lymphocytes redirected against the chondroitin sulfate proteoglycan-4 control the growth of multiple solid tumors both in vitro and in vivo. *Clin. Cancer Res. Off. J. Am. Assoc. Cancer Res.* **2014**, *20*, 962–971. [CrossRef]
140. Hong, H.; Stastny, M.; Brown, C.; Chang, W.C.; Ostberg, J.R.; Forman, S.J.; Jensen, M.C. Diverse solid tumors expressing a restricted epitope of L1-CAM can be targeted by chimeric antigen receptor redirected T lymphocytes. *J. Immunother.* **2014**, *37*, 93–104. [CrossRef]
141. Pasquale, E.B. Eph-ephrin bidirectional signaling in physiology and disease. *Cell* **2008**, *133*, 38–52. [CrossRef]
142. Qazi, M.A.; Vora, P.; Venugopal, C.; Adams, J.; Singh, M.; Hu, A.; Gorelik, M.; Subapanditha, M.K.; Savage, N.; Yang, J.; et al. Cotargeting Ephrin Receptor Tyrosine Kinases A2 and A3 in Cancer Stem Cells Reduces Growth of Recurrent Glioblastoma. *Cancer Res.* **2018**, *78*, 5023–5037. [CrossRef]
143. Hegde, M.; Mukherjee, M.; Grada, Z.; Pignata, A.; Landi, D.; Navai, S.A.; Wakefield, A.; Fousek, K.; Bielamowicz, K.; Chow, K.K.; et al. Tandem CAR T cells targeting HER2 and IL13Ralpha2 mitigate tumor antigen escape. *J. Clin. Investig.* **2016**, *126*, 3036–3052. [CrossRef] [PubMed]
144. Bielamowicz, K.; Fousek, K.; Byrd, T.T.; Samaha, H.; Mukherjee, M.; Aware, N.; Wu, M.F.; Orange, J.S.; Sumazin, P.; Man, T.K.; et al. Trivalent CAR T cells overcome interpatient antigenic variability in glioblastoma. *Neuro-oncology* **2018**, *20*, 506–518. [CrossRef] [PubMed]
145. Shaim, H.; Shanley, M.; Basar, R.; Daher, M.; Gumin, J.; Zamler, D.B.; Uprety, N.; Wang, F.; Huang, Y.; Gabrusiewicz, K.; et al. Targeting the alphav integrin-TGF-beta axis improves natural killer cell function against glioblastoma stem cells. *J. Clin. Investig.* **2021**. [CrossRef] [PubMed]

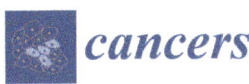

Article

Anti-Cancer Activities of Thyrointegrin $\alpha_v\beta_3$ Antagonist Mono- and Bis-Triazole Tetraiodothyroacetic Acid Conjugated via Polyethylene Glycols in Glioblastoma

Kavitha Godugu, Mehdi Rajabi and Shaker A. Mousa *

The Pharmaceutical Research Institute, Albany College of Pharmacy and Health Sciences, Rensselaer, NY 12208, USA; Kavitha.Godugu@acphs.edu (K.G.); m.rajabi.s@gmail.com (M.R.)
* Correspondence: shaker.mousa@acphs.edu; Tel.: +1-518-694-7397; Fax: +1-518-694-7567

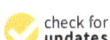

Citation: Godugu, K.; Rajabi, M.; Mousa, S.A. Anti-Cancer Activities of Thyrointegrin $\alpha_v\beta_3$ Antagonist Mono- and Bis-Triazole Tetraiodothyroacetic Acid Conjugated via Polyethylene Glycols in Glioblastoma. *Cancers* **2021**, *13*, 2780. https://doi.org/10.3390/cancers13112780

Academic Editor: Stanley Stylli

Received: 17 May 2021
Accepted: 31 May 2021
Published: 3 June 2021

Publisher's Note: MDPI stays neutral with regard to jurisdictional claims in published maps and institutional affiliations.

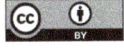

Copyright: © 2021 by the authors. Licensee MDPI, Basel, Switzerland. This article is an open access article distributed under the terms and conditions of the Creative Commons Attribution (CC BY) license (https://creativecommons.org/licenses/by/4.0/).

Simple Summary: Different Triazole Tetrac (TAT) thyrointegrin $\alpha v\beta 3$ antagonists exhibited optimal therapeutic efficacy against U87 or primary glioblastoma cells. TAT containing molecules bind with high affinity to the integrin $\alpha v\beta 3$ and plasma protein Transthyretin (TTR), which facilitate transport across the blood brain barrier. Biological studies showed that decreasing the PEG linker size (1600 versus 4000) or having mono-TAT versus bi-TAT had no significant impact on their $\alpha v\beta 3$ binding affinity, anti-angiogenesis, and overall anti-cancer efficacy.

Abstract: Integrin $\alpha v\beta 3$ receptors are overexpressed in different tumors and their associated neovascularization and hence, represent a potential cancer target. We previously synthesized a high affinity thyrointegrin $\alpha v\beta 3$, P_{4000}-bi-TAT (tetrac derivative), with potent anticancer properties. However, the long polydisperse PEG conjugate showed large scaleup and analytical/bioanalytical issues. Hence, in the present study, we synthesized a mono versus bi-triazole tetrac with discrete monodisperse PEG, which provided improvement in scaleup and bioanalysis. In the present study, we compared binding affinity and anticancer activates with a smaller PEG size (P_{1600}-bi-TAT, Compound **2**) and the removal of one TAT molecule (P_{1600}-m-TAT, Compound **3**) versus P_{4000}-bi-TAT, Compound **1**. The results of the selectivity and affinity of TATs showed greater affinity to integrin $\alpha v\beta 3$. The xenograft weights and tumor cell viabilities were decreased by >90% at all doses compared to the control (ON Treatment, *** $p < 0.001$) in cells treated with Compounds **1**, **2**, and **3** in U87-Luc-treated mice. The in vivo luminescent signals of U87-luc cells reflect the proliferation and distribution of tumor cells in the animals and the maximum intensity corresponding to the maximum tumor cells that the animals could tolerate. We found that the three thyrointegrin $\alpha v\beta 3$ antagonists exhibited optimal therapeutic efficacy against U87 or primary glioblastoma cells. Biological studies showed that decreasing the PEG linker size (1600 vs. 4000) or having mono-TAT or bi-TAT had no significant impact on their $\alpha v\beta 3$ binding affinity, anti-angiogenesis, or overall anti-cancer efficacy.

Keywords: anticancer; glioblastoma; anti-angiogenesis; thyrointegrin $\alpha v\beta 3$; PEG; triazole tetrac; P-bi-TAT; P-m-TAT; tetrac

1. Introduction

Glioblastoma multiforme (GBM) is the most aggressive brain tumor with a high mortality rate [1,2]. Due to the severity of the disease, patients survive an average of only 12 months, and most do not survive beyond two years. Standard treatments of surgery, radiation, and conventional chemotherapy can increase the five-year survival rate to 5–8% [3,4]. Overall survival has been improved in clinical trial populations within the last few years from 12 months to 16 months. However, tumor heterogenicity and resistance mechanisms are expressed by GBM, which limits the effectiveness of therapeutic interventions.

Integrin αvβ3, a heterodimeric cell surface adhesion membrane receptor, is overexpressed in GBM at the tumor margins (invasive regions) and tumor-relevant blood vessels [5]. It has a high affinity for the protein components of the extracellular matrix (ECM) and plays an important role in cell invasion and motility, allowing for crosstalk between the cell and the surrounding stroma as well as with adjacent vascular growth factor receptors. The arginine–glycine–aspartate (RGD) recognition site on integrins αvβ3 is involved in ECM protein interactions and may activate signal transduction pathways. Thus, integrin αvβ3 plays a pleiotropic role in GBM, and the RGD domain is a therapeutic target for antitumor products, which has allowed for the development of various RGD-based antagonists, conjugates, and nanoparticles [6,7].

The extracellular domain of integrin αvβ3 bears a novel small molecule binding site that exclusively recognizes thyroid hormones and thyroid hormone analogs [8,9]. These analogs include tetraiodothyroacetic acid (tetrac), a deaminated derivative of l-thyroxine (T4), and a "thyrointegrin" antagonist that displaces l-triiodothyronine (T3) and T4 from the thyroid hormone analog receptor site on integrin αvβ3 and also initiates a number of intracellular actions via the integrin in the absence of T4 [9–11]. Our several previous studies showed that the nano-diamino-tetrac, (NDAT) based on poly(lactic-co-glycolic acid) (PLGA) that is conjugated to tetrac, have improved activity compared to tetrac alone at the integrin in terms of reduced cancer cell proliferation and induced apoptosis. These anticancer actions primarily reflect changes in the transcription of specific genes [12–14].

We recently synthesized a high affinity thyrointegrin αvβ3 antagonist, P-bi-TAT, a tetrac-based inhibitor with a triazole moiety on the outer ring of tetrac and covalently conjugated to a polymer via poly(ethylene glycol) (PEG, P) PEGylation (Compound 1, Figure 1A). Thus, Compound 1 is a dimer, or bis triazole tetrac (TAT); P-bi-TAT has two tetrac molecules covalently bound via triazoles to PEG_{4000} (MW = 4000). It is effective against xenografts of human GBM. PEG modification affords a long-circulating property by evading macrophage-mediated uptake and removal from the systemic circulation. A PEG spacer allows the ligand to remain in the systemic circulation and provides flexibility to the attached ligand for efficient interaction with its target [11]. In spite of high binding to the αvβ3 receptor and favorable anticancer effects, these long polydisperse PEG conjugates of the molecule showed analysis issues in quality control and bioanalytical assays and also difficulty in its synthesis and scalability. Hence, in order to overcome these above issues, we synthesized a smaller PEG with a molecular weight of 1600 (Compound 2, Figure 1B) and removed one TAT molecule of P-bi-TAT to form a mono-TAT agent, the P-m-TAT molecule (Compound 3, Figure 1C), retaining the excellent solubility and potency of Compound 1.

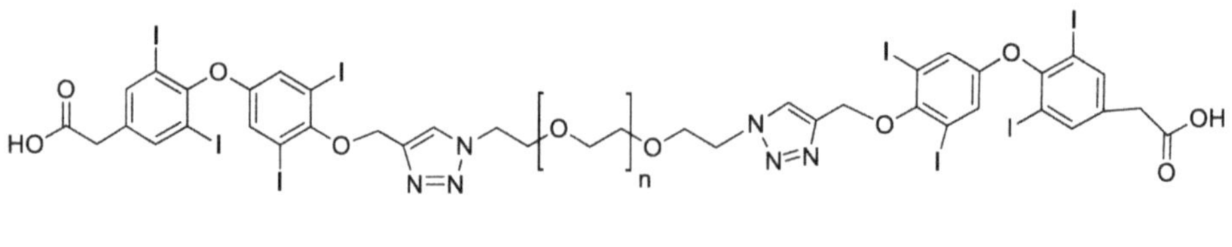

A & B (Compound 1, n ~ 90 and Compound 2, n = 35, respectively).

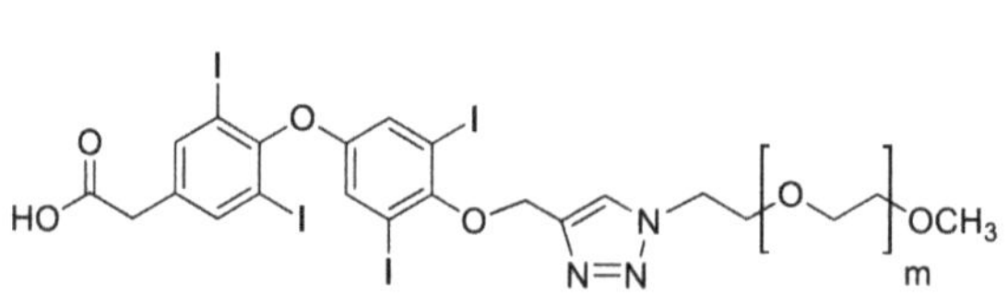

C (Compound 3, n = 35).

Figure 1. Schematic structures of (**A**) P_{4000}-bi-TAT (Compound 1), (**B**) P_{1600}-bi-TAT (Compound 2), and (**C**) P_{1600}-m-TAT (Compound 3). In the structure, 'n' and 'm' indicate the PEG size. (**A**,**B**) differ in PEG size, with a molecular weight of 4000 (n ~ 90) and 1600 (n = 35), respectively.

In this study, we tested the hypothesis that decreasing the PEG size from 4000 to 1600 MW and removing one TAT molecule of P-bi-TAT would improve its binding affinity and therapeutic value. An integrin $\alpha v \beta 3$ binding assay was used to explore the binding modes of P_{4000}-bi-TAT (Compound **1**), P_{1600}-bi-TAT (Compound **2**), and P_{1600}-m-TAT (Compound **3**), and we further evaluated their therapeutic efficacies using U87 glioma cells.

2. Materials and Methods

P_{4000}-bi-TAT (Compound **1**), P_{1600}-bi-TAT (Compound **2**), and P_{1600}-m-TAT (Compound **3**) were synthesized in our laboratory according to our previously described method [11]. Dulbecco's Modified Eagle Medium (DMEM), fetal bovine serum (FBS), penicillin, streptomycin, trypsin/EDTA, and bovine serum albumin (BSA) were purchased from Sigma-Aldrich (St. Louis, MO, USA). The human glioblastoma U87-luc cells U87-luc cells were from ATCC (Manassas, VA, USA), and the human primary GBM cells 052814, 021913, and 101,813 were a generous gift from the University at Pittsburgh Medical Center (Department of Neurosurgery). Purified $\alpha v \beta 3$ and anti-$\alpha v \beta 3$ conjugated with biotin were obtained from Bioss Inc. (Woburn, MA, USA), the streptavidin—HRP conjugates were from Thermo Fisher Scientific (Grand Island, NY, USA), the fibrinogen was from Millipore Sigma (Burlington, MA, USA), and the 3,3′,5,5′-tetramethylbbenzidine (TMB) and TMB-stop solution were from ABCAM Inc (Cambridge, MA, USA).

2.1. Binding Affinity of Compounds to Integrins Purified $\alpha v \beta 3$ (1 µg/mL)

The binding affinity of Compounds **1**, **2**, and **3** to purified $\alpha v \beta 3$ was measured using previously described methods with slight modifications [12,15–17]. Fibrinogen was coated to polystyrene microtiter plate wells and incubated at 4 °C overnight, and then the wells were blocked with 3% BSA for 2 h at room temperature. The wells were washed with Buffer A (50 mM Tris/HCl, 100 mM NaCl, 1 mM $CaCl_2$, 1 mM $MgCl_2$, 1% BSA) three times. Integrins $\alpha v \beta 1$, $\alpha v \beta 3$, $\alpha v \beta 5$, $\alpha v \beta 6$, IIb$\beta 3$, and $\alpha 5 \beta 1$ (ACRO Biosystems, Newark, DE, USA) and increasing concentrations of the compounds were added and incubated for 2 h at room temperature, and then the wells were washed three times with Buffer A and incubated with a streptavidin–HRP conjugate (1:1000 in Buffer A) for 1 h at room temperature. Finally, the wells were washed three times with Buffer A, and 100 µL peroxidase substrate TMB was added, and the reaction was terminated after 30 min with 50 µL of 450 nm of stop solution for TMB. The absorbance was determined at 450 nm with a Microplate Reader (Bio-Rad, Hercules, CA, USA). The best-fit 50% inhibitory concentration (IC_{50}) values for the different compounds were calculated by fitting the data with nonlinear regression using GraphPad Prism (GraphPad, San Diego, CA, USA).

2.2. Cell Culture

The human glioblastoma U87-luc and primary GBM cells were obtained from ATCC (Manassas, PA, USA) and a generous gift from University of Pittsburgh Medical Center (Pittsburgh, PA, USA) and were grown in Dulbecco's Modified Eagle's Medium (DMEM) supplemented with 10% fetal bovine serum, 10% penicillin, and 1% streptomycin. The cells were cultured at 37 °C to sub-confluence and treated with 0.25% (w/v) trypsin/ethylenediaminetetraacetic acid (EDTA) to induce cell release from the flask. The cells were washed with a culture medium that was free of phenol red and fetal bovine serum, and then counted.

2.3. Cell Proliferation Assay

The glioblastoma cells (U87-luc) and primary cells GBM 101813, GBM 021,913 were seeded in 96-well plates (0.5 million cells per well) and treated with Compounds **1**, **2**, and **3** at 5 concentrations (1, 3, 10, 30, and 100 µM). At the end of the experiments, the cell cultures were supplemented with MTT reagent (3-(4,5-dimethylthiazol-2-yl)-2,5-diphenyltetrazolium bromide) and incubated for an additional 4 h. Then, dimethyl sulfoxide (0.1% DMSO) was added to the cell culture to dissolve the formazan crystals and incubated for 10 min at room temperature. The absorbance rate of the cell cultures was read at 570 nm by using a Microplate Reader. All the reactions were performed in triplicate. The measured data of the cellular proliferation were calculated using the viability values of the untreated control cells (100%).

2.4. Chorioallantoic Membrane Assay (CAM)

Neovascularization was examined in the CAM model, as previously described [18–21]. We purchased 10-day-old chick embryos purchased from Charles River Avian Vaccine Services (Norwich, CT, USA) and incubated them at 37 °C with 55% relative humidity. A hypodermic needle was used to make a small hole in the shells at the air sacs, and a second hole was made on the broadside of the eggs, directly over an avascular portion of the embryonic membrane that was identified by candling. A false air sac was created beneath the second hole by the application of negative pressure at the first hole, causing the CAM to separate the shell. A window of approximately 1.0 cm^2 was cut in the shell over the dropped CAM using a small craft grinding wheel (Dermal, Division of Emerson Electric Co. Racine, WI, USA), allowing for direct access to the underlying membrane. b-FGF (10 ng/CAM) was used as a standard proangiogenic agent, and sterile disks of No. 1 filter paper (Whatman International, Kent, UK) were pretreated with 1 µg/CAM of Compounds **1**, **2**, and **3**, air-dried under sterile conditions and placed on the CAMs.

2.5. Microscopic Analysis of CAM Sections

After incubation at 37 °C with 55% relative humidity for 3 days, the CAM tissue directly beneath each filter disk was resected from each CAM sample. The tissues were washed three times with PBS, placed in 35 mm Petri dishes (Nalge Nunc, Rochester, NY, USA), and examined under SV6 stereomicroscope (Carl Zeiss, Thornwood, NY, USA) at ×50 magnification. Digital images of the CAM sections exposed to the treatment filters were collected using a 3-CCD color video camera system (Toshiba America, New York, NY, USA), and analyzed with Image-Pro software (Media Cybernetics, Silver Spring, MD, USA). The number of vessel branch points contained in a circular region equal to the area of each filter disk were counted. There was 1 image counted in each CAM preparation, and findings from 8 CAM preparations per each treatment condition. The results are presented as the mean ± SD of new branch points in the collected samples from each treatment condition.

2.6. Animals

Immunodeficient female NCr nude homozygous mice aged 5–6 weeks and weighing 20–25 g were purchased from Taconic Biosciences, Inc (Germantown, NY, USA). All animal studies were conducted at the animal facility of the Veteran Affairs Medical Center (Albany, NY, USA) in accordance with the approved institutional guidelines for humane animal treatment and according to the current guidelines. The mice were kept under specific pathogen-free conditions and housed under controlled conditions of temperature (20–24 °C) and humidity (60–70%) and a 12 h light/dark cycle with ad libitum access to water and food. The mice were allowed to acclimatize for 5 days before the study.

2.7. Glioblastoma Xenografts

For the subcutaneous (s.c.) glioma tumor model, the study was conducted as diagrammed in Figure 2. U87-luc cells were harvested, suspended in 100 µL of DMEM with 50% Matrigel® (Pasadena, TX, USA) and 2×10^6 cells were implanted s.c. dorsally in each flank to achieve two independent tumors per animal. Immediately prior to the initiation of treatments, the animals were randomized into treatment groups (5 animals/group) by tumor volume measurements with Vernier calipers. Treatments began after the detection of a palpable tumor mass (4–5 days post-implantation). Because these compounds had different percentages of the active tetrac portion (s) of the molecule relative to the full molecule, we dosed the compounds at equivalent moles/kg triazole tetrac (TAT) levels rather than mg/kg of the intact compound. Thus, compounds were dosed at 0.354 µmol/kg, 1.06 µmol/kg, and 3.54 µmol/kg TAT. The treatments were the control (PBS), Compound **1** (0.354, 1.06, 3.54 mg/kg), Compound **2** (0.354, 1.06, 3.54 mg/kg), and Compound **3** (0.354, 1.06, 3.54 mg/kg). The agents were administered daily, s.c., for 21 days (ON Treatment), and in another set of animals, the compounds were administrated daily for 21 days, followed by 21 days of discontinuation (ON Treatment + OFF Treatment). The animals were then humanely sacrificed, and the tumors were harvested. The tumor weights and the cell viabilities (bioluminescent signal intensity) were measured.

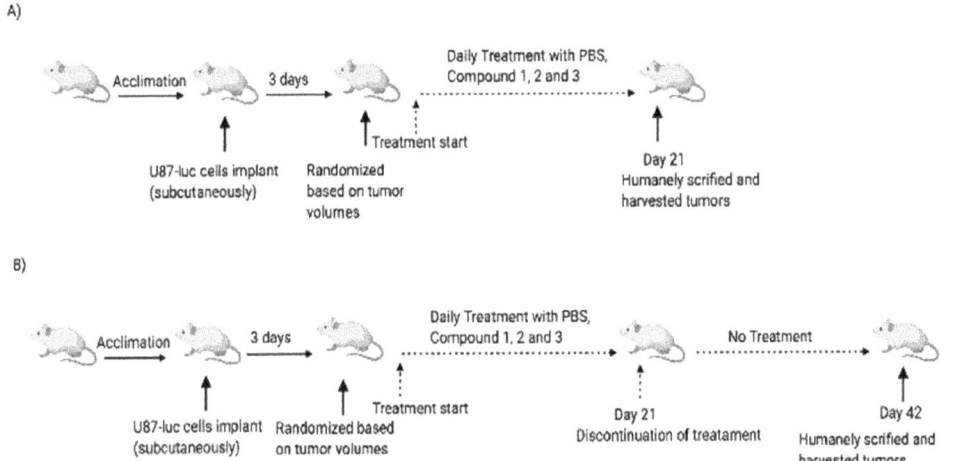

Figure 2. Protocol for subcutaneous administration of compounds in mice with U87-luc xenografts. (**A**) ON Treatment: the compounds were administered daily, s.c. for 21 days, and (**B**) ON + OFF Treatment: the compounds were administrated daily for 21 days followed by 21 days of discontinuation. At the end of the study, the animals were humanely sacrificed, and the tumors were harvested.

2.8. Tumor Volume and Weight

The tumor widths and lengths were measured with calipers at 3-day intervals during the ON and ON + OFF studies, and the volumes were calculated using the standard formula $W \times L^2/2$. The tumor weights measured were of harvested lesions following animal sacrifice.

2.9. Bioluminescence

The mice were injected s.c. with 50 µL D-luciferin (30 mg/mL). They were anesthetized using isoflurane, and post-luciferin administration mice were imaged in an in vivo imaging system (Xenogen-IVIS spectrum, PerkinElmer Inc., Waltham, MA, USA). Photographic and luminescence images were taken at a constant exposure time. Xenogen IVIS Living Image software (version 3.2) was used to quantify non-saturated bioluminescence in regions of interest (ROI). Bioluminescence was quantified as photons/s for each ROI. Ex vivo tumor imaging was performed to confirm the signal intensity in the tumors after the termination of the study.

2.10. Histopathology

The tumors were fixed in 10% formalin, placed in cassettes, and dehydrated using an automated tissue processor. The processed tissues were embedded in paraffin wax and the blocks were trimmed and sectioned to about a $5 \times 5 \times 4$ µm size using a microtome. The tissue sections were mounted on glass slides using a hot plate and subsequently treated in the order of 100%, 90%, and 70% ethanol for 2 min. Finally, the tissue sections were rinsed with water, stained with Harris's hematoxylin and eosin (H&E), and examined under a light microscope.

2.11. Statistical Analysis

Statistical analysis was performed with GraphPad Prism 7 software. Data are presented as the mean ± SD. For comparison between two or more sets of data, ANOVA was used. * $p < 0.05$, ** $p < 0.01$, and *** $p < 0.001$ were considered statistically significant.

3. Results

3.1. Binding Affinity of Compounds to Integrins

To evaluate the specificity and selectivity of TATs to integrins, we investigated for the subtypes $\alpha v \beta 1$, $\alpha v \beta 3$, $\alpha v \beta 5$, $\alpha v \beta 6$, IIb$\beta 3$, $\alpha 5 \beta 1$, and $\alpha v \beta 3$ in an integrin–ligand binding assay. The lowest IC$_{50}$ values of Compounds **1**, **2**, and **3** were 0.14, 0.23, and 0.36 nM, respectively, were observed for $\alpha v \beta 3$ (Figure 3). No significant changes in IC$_{50}$ values were observed for Compounds **2** and **3** when compared to Compound **1**.

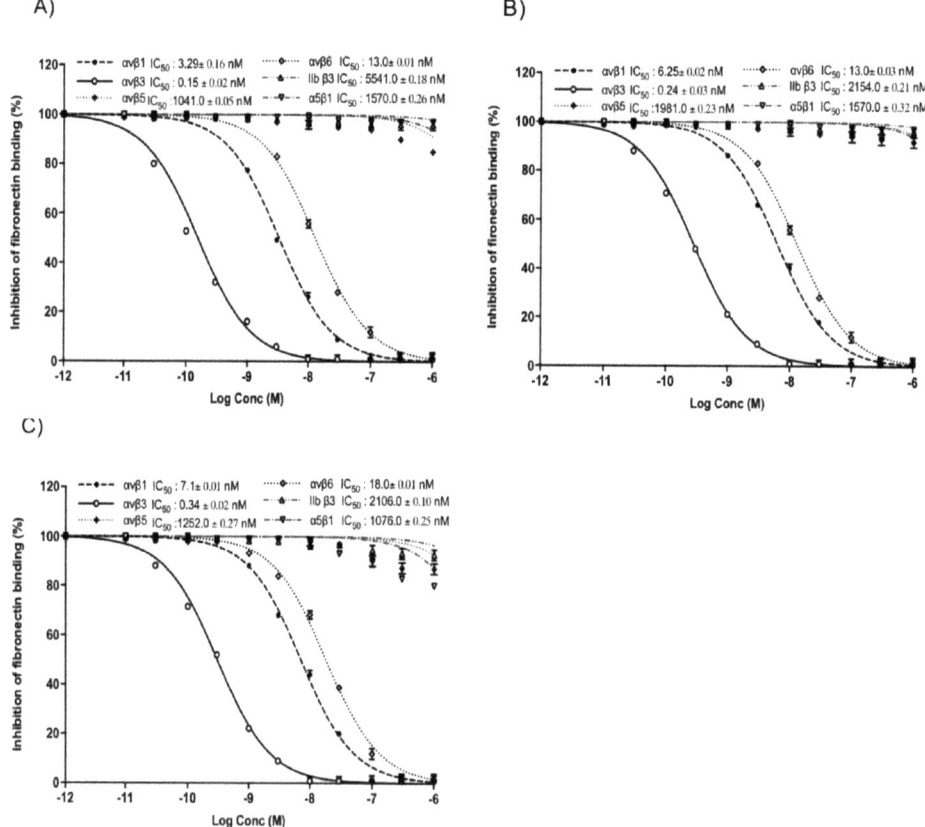

Figure 3. Binding affinity of TATs for the integrins $\alpha v \beta 1$, $\alpha v \beta 3$, $\alpha v \beta 5$, $\alpha v \beta 6$, IIb$\beta 3$, $\alpha 5 \beta 1$, and $\alpha v \beta 3$. (**A**) Compound **1**, (**B**) Compound **2**, (**C**) Compound **3**. Dose-response curve (mean IC$_{50}$ (nM) ± SD) of three independent experiments. x-axis show Log Concentrations from −12 to −6.

Integrins are adhesion receptors that play an essential role in cell–cell communications. $\alpha v \beta 3$ is an attractive target for therapeutic intervention because of its presence in many types of cancer cells and their neovasculature, which plays a key role in tumor growth, tumor angiogenesis, and metastasis.

3.2. Effect of TATs on Cell Proliferation of U87-Luc Cells

To compare the in vitro anticancer activity of the three TATs, an MTT assay was used. As shown in Figure 4, we evaluated the effects of these compounds on the growth of human glioblastoma U87-luc cell lines and primary cells (GBM 101813, GBM 021913). In the MTT assay, the U87-luc cell line showed decreases in proliferation of 56%, 59%, and 58% at 24 h, and 42%, 44%, and 43% at 48 h, with 100 µM of Compounds **1**, **2**, and **3**, respectively compared to the untreated cells (Figure 4C,D). For the GBM 101813, cells with 100 µM of Compounds **1**, **2**, and **3** showed decreases in proliferation of 52%, 54%, and 55% at 24 h, and 41%, 43%, and 45% at 48 h, respectively (Figure 4C,D). Further, GBM 021913 showed decreases in cell proliferation of 54%, 57%, and 57% at 24 h, and 48%, 52%, and 50% with 100 µM of Compounds **1**, **2**, and **3** compared to the untreated cells (Figure 4E,F).

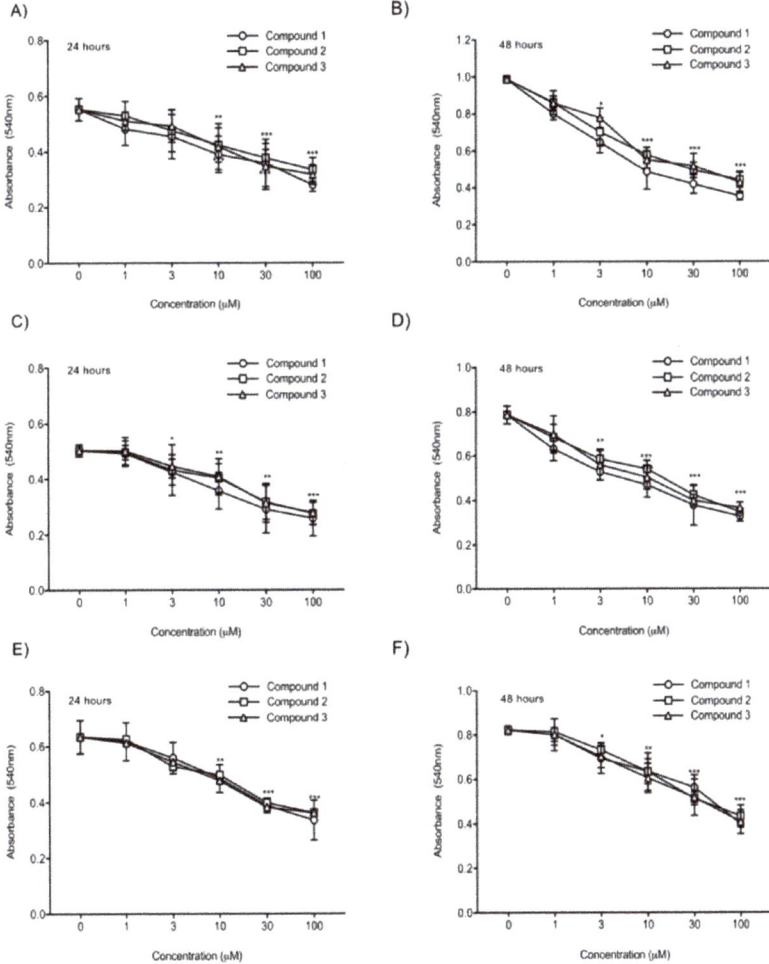

Figure 4. Cell proliferation assay. U87-luc and primary (GBM 101813, GBM 021913) cells were incubated with Compounds **1**, **2**, and **3** at different concentrations (1, 3, 10, 30, and 100 µM) for 24 h and 48 h and were measured with MTT assay. (**A,B**) U87-luc; (**C,D**) GBM 101813; (**E,F**) GBM 021913. Values are presented as the mean ± S.D of three independent experiments. *** $p < 0.001$, ** $p < 0.01$, * $p < 0.05$ compared to the control (PBS).

3.3. Anti-Angiogenesis Efficacy of TATs

To compare the anti-angiogenic efficacy of the three TATs, a CAM assay was used. As shown in Figure 5, a basic fibroblast growth factor (FGF2 or b-FGF) was used to stimulate angiogenesis, and then the compounds were administrated. Compounds **1**, **2**, and **3** showed maximum inhibition of the number of vessel branch points (angiogenesis) at 1 µg/CAM. No statistically significant changes in the percentages of inhibition of angiogenesis were observed between the three TATs. The TAT molecules also showed maximum inhibition of angiogenesis in the presence of different growth factors (VEGF, HGF, and in combination).

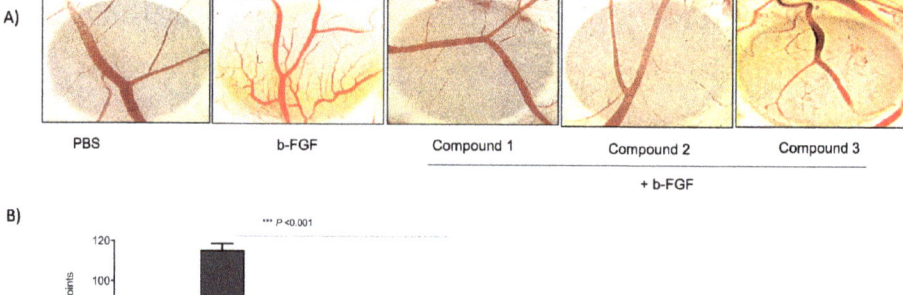

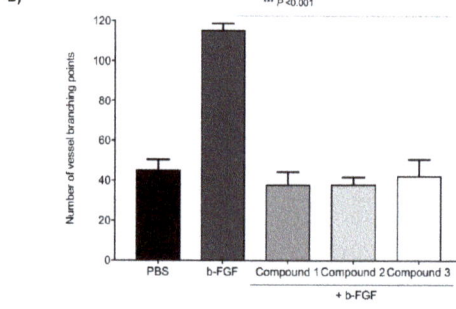

Figure 5. Inhibition of angiogenesis in chick chorioallantoic membrane (CAM). With the development of small new blood vessels, typical neovascularization was visible with CAM assay. (**A**) Images represent the inhibition of the b-FGF (10 ng/CAM)-induced angiogenesis by Compounds **1**, **2**, and **3** at 1 µg/CAM. (**B**) Data illustrate the decrease of compounds. Values are presented as the mean ± S.D *** $p < 0.001$, compared to the control.

3.4. Antitumor Effect

With the intent to study the in vivo antitumor efficacies of Compounds **1**, **2**, and **3** on tumor growth, U87-luc glioblastoma cells were implanted in each flank of the animals, and then the mice were treated daily for 21 days with Compounds **1**, **2**, and **3**. The tumor volumes significantly decreased when treated with Compounds **1**, **2**, and **3** at 0.354, 1.06, and 3.54 µmole/kg, respectively, compared to the controls (Figure 6). All the treatments at 0.354, 1.06, and 3.54 µmole/kg significantly reduced the tumor weight after daily treatment for 21 days. The xenograft weights and tumor cell viabilities decreased by >90% with all doses (ON Treatment, *** $p < 0.001$) compared to the control (Figure 7A). In the second group, Compound **1**-treated mice, the xenografts were observed for an additional 21 days with no further treatment (ON Treatment + OFF Treatment). There was no re-growth of tumors in these groups of animals and the absence of cell viability persisted (Figure 7B). Similar results were obtained from mice treated daily with Compounds **2** and **3** for 21 days (ON Treatment) and another group treated daily for 21 days followed by discontinuation for 21 days (ON + OFF Treatment).

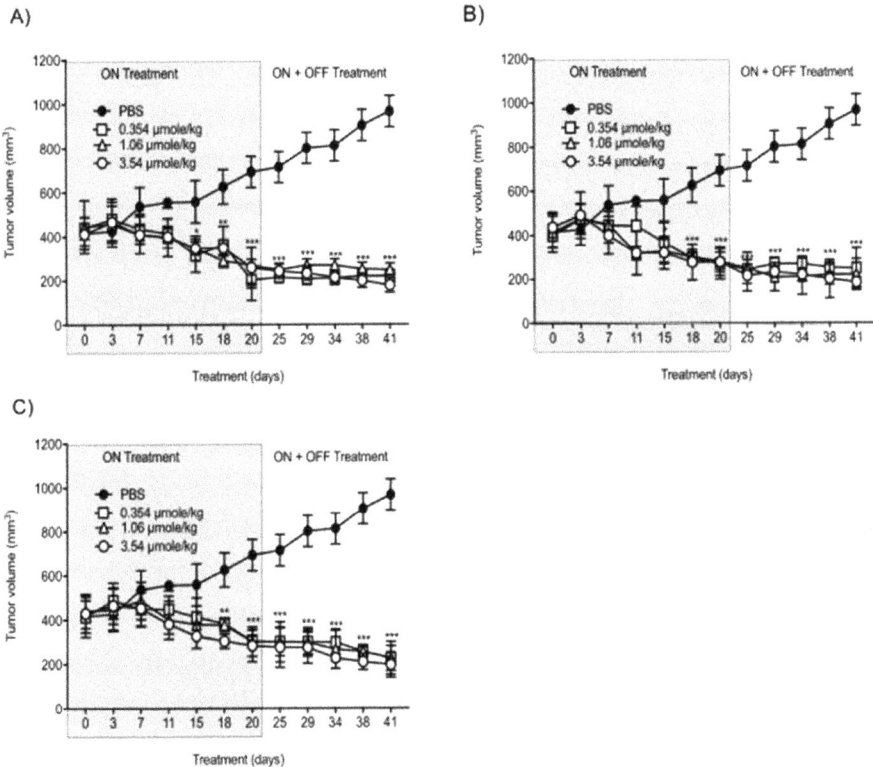

Figure 6. Anti-cancer effects of Compounds **1**, **2**, and **3** on tumor volumes. (**A**) Compound **1**; (**B**) Compound **2**; (**C**) Compound **3**. U87-luc glioblastoma cells implanted mice were treated daily with Compounds **1**, **2**, and **3** (ON Treatment) for 21 days, and in the second group, the xenografts were observed for an additional 21 days with no further treatment (ON Treatment + OFF Treatment). Values are presented as the mean tumor volume (mm^3) ± S.D. *** $p < 0.001$, ** $p < 0.01$, * $p < 0.05$, compared to the control.

The in vivo luminescent signals of viable cancer cells were quantified (photons/second) for the different groups using a Xenogen-IVIS Spectrum. A statistically significant ($p < 0.001$) decrease of viable U87-Luc cells was observed in groups treated with TATs compared to the control. No significant differences were observed when comparing the treated groups (Figure 7C,D).

Further, the histological sections obtained from the U87 xenografts were used to evaluate the antagonist treatments on cell proliferation. A large necrotic area was observed in the tumor masses from all doses of the treatment groups. However, there was no significant difference between the three antagonist treatments (Figure 8).

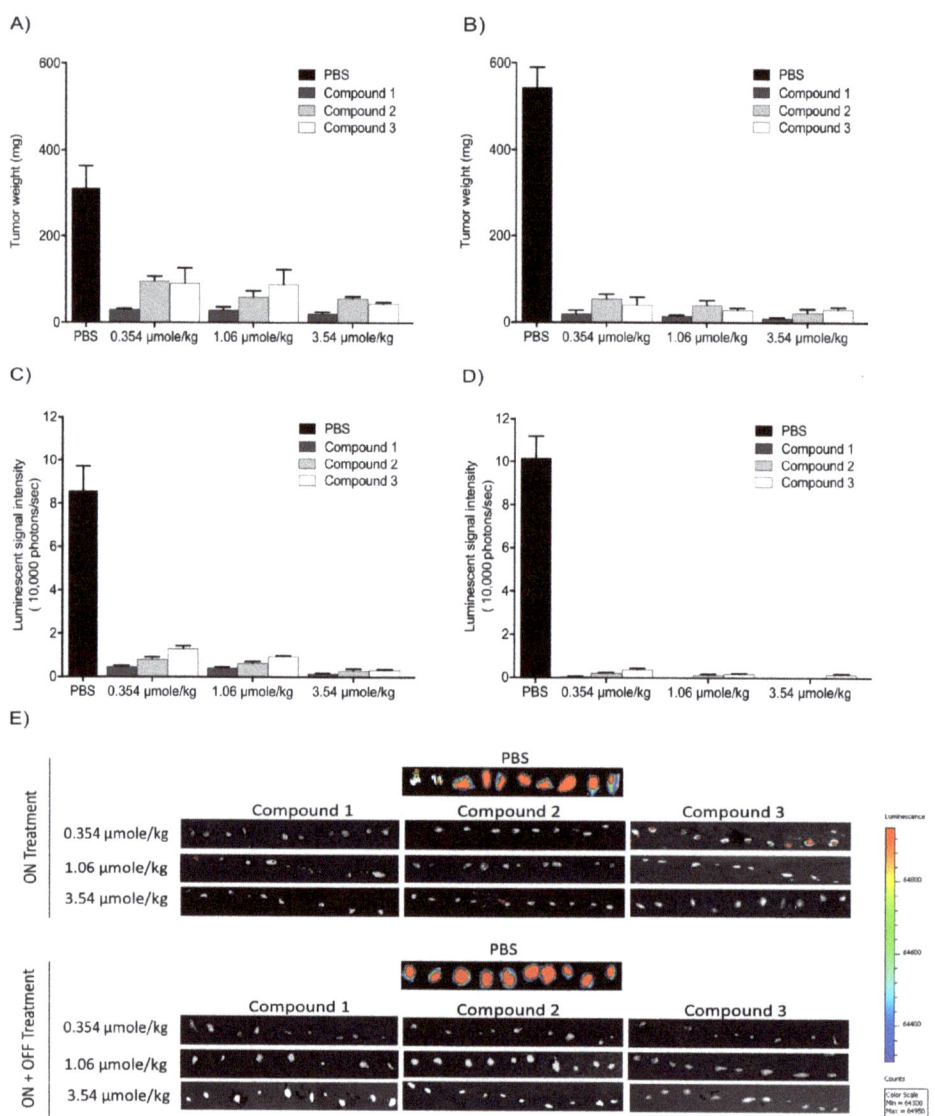

Figure 7. Antitumor effects of Compounds **1**, **2**, and **3** on xenografts. (**A**,**B**) Tumor weight; (**C**,**D**) luminescence signals in xenografts; (**E**) representative IVIS images of luminescent signals in tumors. Values are presented as the mean ± S.D.

3.5. Transthyretin (TTR) Binding Assay

Further, we tested the ability of TTR binding using competitive fluorescence binding assay. FITC-T_4 and TTR were mixed in a 96-well plate and incubated with different concentrations of Compounds **1**, **2**, and **3**, and the intensity of fluorescence was measured at 518 nm. The IC_{50} values of Compounds **1**, **2**, and **3** were 5.5 nm, 5.6 nm, and 4.8 nm, respectively (Figure 9).

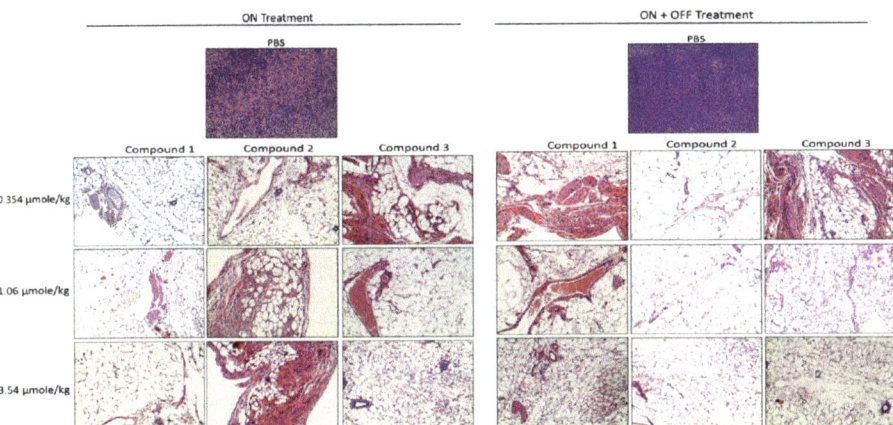

Figure 8. Histopathological images of H&E staining of glioblastoma xenografts in nude mice treated with Compounds 1, 2, and 3. The scale bar is 10×. Complete infiltration with the malignant cells ~100% was observed in the controls. In the treatment groups, necrosis, and hyalinization > 90% were observed.

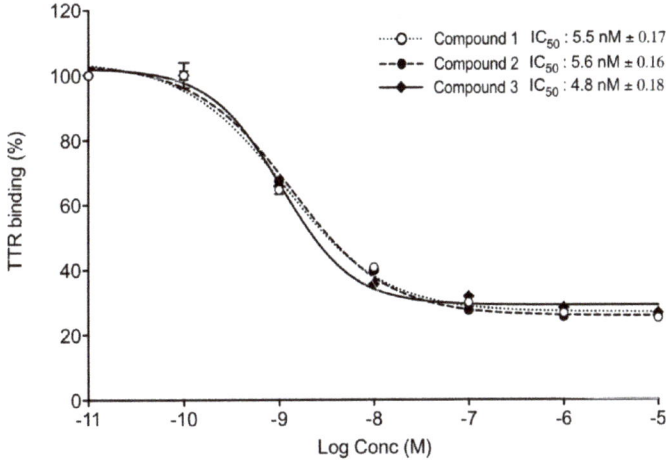

Figure 9. TTR binding assay. TTR and FITC-T_4 were mixed and incubated with different concentrations of Compounds **1**, **2**, and **3**. Competitive fluorescence binding curves (mean $IC_{50} \pm SD$) of three independent experiments. x-axis shows Log Concentrations from -11 to -5.

4. Discussion

The integrin $\alpha v\beta 3$ plays a critical role in glioblastoma-associated biological processes, making it an important target for the development of novel targeted ligands. GBM is a thyroid hormone-dependent tumor, and this effect was mediated via non-genomic actions of the cell-surface receptor on integrin $\alpha v\beta 3$ [22]. Although various integrin ligands have been reported, most of them are universal ligands for multiple integrin receptors and show a limited binding affinity for integrin $\alpha v\beta 3$. A number of in vitro and in vivo studies have supported the role of thyroid hormones (L-thyroxine, T4; 3,5,3′-triido-L-thyronine, T3) in the proliferation of tumor cells. In the present study, we compared the therapeutic efficacy of the two integrin $\alpha v\beta 3$ antagonists, the monomer P-m-TAT (Compound **3**) and P-bi-TAT dimer, (Compound **2**) with P-bi-TAT dimer (Compound **1**). Recently, we showed that the incorporation of a triazole group and PEG molecules within P-bi-TAT (Compound **1**), and without any change to the carboxylic acid group, significantly increased the integrin binding affinity compared to the tetrac [11]. Our group previously compared the potency of NDAT in in vitro and in vivo studies using U87 glioblastoma cells [12]. The chain length of PEG that restricts the nuclear translation of the thyromimetic tetrac within the molecule as well the improved solubility in an aqueous buffer for subcutaneous injection has to be greater than 1200 Dalton, which is why we used PEGs between 1600–4000 Daltons [5,11].

In the past decade, our studies have shown the $\alpha v \beta 3$-dependent antiproliferative, anti-angiogenic, and anticancer properties of agonist thyroid hormones (T4, T3) by tetrac in various cancer types. In the present study, the inhibition of U87 cell growth by TATs was comparable at a higher drug concentration (100 μM), but there was increased sensitivity to P-bi-TAT (Compound 1) at a lower drug concentration of the used agents. Cody et al., 2007 showed that unmodified tetrac may penetrate cells and can interact with the thyroid hormone nuclear receptor to where it is a low potency agonist (thyromimetic) [23]. On the other hand, P-bi-TAT (Compound 1) does not gain access to the cell nucleus and shows a more robust antiproliferative effect. It has been well documented that increasing PEG substitution can lower the binding affinities of different therapeutics [24–27].

In earlier in vitro studies, we showed that three rodent glioma cell lines proliferated in response to thyroid hormone, which is blocked by tetrac [11]. Beyond antiproliferation at the level of the tumor cell, a second important facet of the properties of $\alpha v \beta 3$ antagonists is that they have anticancer efficacy by multiple mechanisms. Here, the in vivo antitumor efficacies of the $\alpha v \beta 3$ antagonists were evaluated in U87-luc glioblastoma tumor-bearing nude mice, and the compounds significantly reduced tumor volumes and impaired tumor growth in a dose-dependent manner by suppressing angiogenesis (ON Treatment). In the second group of treated mice, the xenografts were observed for an additional 21 days with no further treatment (ON + OFF Treatment). No regrowth of tumors was observed, and the absence of cell viability persisted. One explanation for these observed effects is that tetrac impairs tumor growth by blocking angiogenesis and by impairing the endothelial cell function rather than by impeding tumor cell growth directly. We have ascribed conventional pro-apoptotic activity to tetrac that would account for the progressive decrease in tumor volume that occurred over 21 days of treatment.

Previously, our group formulated a polymeric nanoparticle, NDAT, against a variety of xenografts. Chemical changes to the tetrac molecule at the outer ring hydroxyl by adding a triazole and PEG molecule did not allow the agent to gain access to the cell interior and thus, the tetrac that is ether-bonded to the PLGA particle via the outer ring hydroxyl can act only at the integrin receptor, where it is exclusively an antagonist and not at the nuclear receptor for thyroid hormone. Further, the histopathological sections represent that the extensive necrosis induced in the tumor mass is present in all treated tumors, causing apoptosis.

The following are limitations of the study: GBM tumor implants were xenografted versus orthotopically implanted in the brain to allow for an extended investigation of the effect of TAT treatment for up to 3 weeks in one group, and in another group, the TAT treatment for up to 3 weeks was followed by 3 weeks off treatment to examine the impact on tumor re-growth or relapse. A total of 6 weeks (3 weeks ON treatment + 3 weeks OFF) was the maximum duration that the implanted animals had minimal pain and distress, and significant pain and distress developed beyond that duration.

We have also developed satisfactory evidence that TATs cross the blood–brain barrier. The luminescent signals of the single molecular target on $\alpha v \beta 3$, the target that, when activated by chemically modified tetrac, regulates a network of intracellular signaling pathways and plasma membrane functions, and further, controls specific gene transcription and cell surface vascular growth factor receptor functions that are highly relevant to cancer and cancer-linked angiogenesis. Previous studies showed that $\alpha v \beta 3$ antagonists' multivalency results in increased binding affinity, which then improved targeted therapeutic delivery [11,28,29]. However, despite many studies over years, there are no reports that have demonstrated improved therapeutic effectiveness of dimer αvβ3 antagonists over monomer αvβ3 antagonists.

The CENTRIC phase 3 trial, a multicenter, randomized, open-label, phase 3 trial that assessed cilengitide in addition to the standard of care treatment against newly diagnosed GBM, which failed to improve survival [30]. Therefore, the role of integrins as a target for glioblastoma can be debated. The failure of cilengitide, as pointed out above, is mainly due to the kinetics and the fact that cilengitide acts as a partial agonist; αvβ3 integrin is activated when cilengitide concentration declines because of its fast off-rate from the αvβ3 integrin and its stability and short half-life [31]. In contrast, our TAT derivatives are pure antagonists, stable along with a fast on-rate and a slow off-rate of binding to the αvβ3 integrin.

5. Conclusions

In conclusion, we found that the three TATs integrin αvβ3 antagonists showed no significant differences among them in their binding affinities to the αvβ3 receptor. Furthermore, the biological studies showed that decreasing PEG linker sizes and mono-TAT versus bi-TAT molecules resulted in no significant change in antitumor efficacy against glioblastoma.

Author Contributions: K.G. conducted all biological studies in the manuscript (formal analysis, methodology, data curation, software, M.R. synthesized the different TAT molecules used in the study, and S.A.M. designed, conceptualization, supervision, and wrote the article. All authors have read and agreed to the published version of the manuscript.

Funding: Funding was received from both NanoPharmaceuticals LLC, Rensselaer, NY, USA and from the Pharmaceutical Research Institute (PRI) at Albany College of Pharmacy and Health Sciences.

Institutional Review Board Statement: Human studies are N/A.

Data Availability Statement: The data presented in this study are available on request from the corresponding author.

Conflicts of Interest: S.A.M. is the founder and the inventor of patents assigned to NanoPharmaceuticals LLC, which is developing anti-cancer drugs. The remaining authors declare that the research was conducted in the absence of any commercial or financial relationships that could be construed as a potential conflict of interest.

Animal Studies

All studies were conducted in accordance with guidelines under IACUC animal protocol approved by the VA Medical Center, Albany, NY, USA.

References

1. Dong, Z.; Cui, H. The Emerging Roles of RNA Modifications in Glioblastoma. *Cancers* **2020**, *12*, 736. [CrossRef]
2. Yang, J.; Shi, Z.; Liu, R.; Wu, Y.; Zhang, X. Combined-therapeutic strategies synergistically potentiate glioblastoma multiforme treatment via nanotechnology. *Theranostics* **2020**, *10*, 3223–3239. [CrossRef]
3. Auffinger, B.; Spencer, D.; Pytel, P.; Ahmed, A.U.; Lesniak, M.S. The role of glioma stem cells in chemotherapy resistance and glioblastoma multiforme recurrence. *Expert Rev. Neurother.* **2015**, *15*, 741–752. [CrossRef]
4. Ibarra, L.E.; Vilchez, M.L.; Caverzán, M.D.; Sanabria, L.N.M. Understanding the glioblastoma tumor biology to optimize photodynamic therapy: From molecular to cellular events. *J. Neurosci. Res.* **2021**, *99*, 1024–1047. [CrossRef] [PubMed]
5. Davis, P.J.; Mousa, S.A.; Lin, H.-Y. Nongenomic Actions of Thyroid Hormone: The Integrin Component. *Physiol. Rev.* **2021**, *101*, 319–352. [CrossRef]
6. Fu, S.; Xu, X.; Ma, Y.; Zhang, S.; Zhang, S. RGD peptide-based non-viral gene delivery vectors targeting integrin αvβ3 for cancer therapy. *J. Drug Target.* **2019**, *27*, 1–11. [CrossRef] [PubMed]
7. Sun, C.-C.; Qu, X.-J.; Gao, Z.-H. Arginine-Glycine-Aspartate–Binding Integrins as Therapeutic and Diagnostic Targets. *Am. J. Ther.* **2016**, *23*, e198–e207. [CrossRef]
8. Davis, P.J.; Glinsky, G.V.; Lin, H.-Y.; Mousa, S.A. Actions of Thyroid Hormone Analogues on Chemokines. *J. Immunol. Res.* **2016**, *2016*, 1–7. [CrossRef] [PubMed]
9. Davis, P.J.; Tang, H.-Y.; Hercbergs, A.; Lin, H.-Y.; Keating, K.A.; Mousa, S.A. Bioactivity of Thyroid Hormone Analogs at Cancer Cells. *Front. Endocrinol.* **2018**, *9*, 739. [CrossRef]

10. Mousa, S.A.; Glinsky, G.V.; Lin, H.-Y.; Ashur-Fabian, O.; Hercbergs, A.; Keating, K.A.; Davis, P.J. Contributions of Thyroid Hormone to Cancer Metastasis. *Biomedicines* **2018**, *6*, 89. [CrossRef]
11. Rajabi, M.; Godugu, K.; Sudha, T.; Bharali, D.J.; Mousa, S.A. Triazole Modified Tetraiodothyroacetic Acid Conjugated to Polyethylene Glycol: High Affinity Thyrointegrin alphavbeta3 Antagonist with Potent Anticancer Activities in Glioblastoma Multiforme. *Bioconjug. Chem.* **2019**, *30*, 3087–3097. [CrossRef] [PubMed]
12. Li, W.; Yalcin, M.; Bharali, D.J.; Lin, Q.; Godugu, K.; Fujioka, K.; Keating, K.A.; Mousa, S.A. Pharmacokinetics, Biodistribution, and Anti-Angiogenesis Efficacy of Diamino Propane Tetraiodothyroacetic Acid-conjugated Biodegradable Polymeric Nanoparticle. *Sci. Rep.* **2019**, *9*, 9006. [CrossRef] [PubMed]
13. Ho, Y.; Wu, C.-Y.; Chin, Y.-T.; Li, Z.-L.; Pan, Y.-S.; Huang, T.-Y.; Su, P.-Y.; Lee, S.-Y.; Crawford, D.R.; Su, K.-W.; et al. NDAT suppresses pro-inflammatory gene expression to enhance resveratrol-induced anti-proliferation in oral cancer cells. *Food Chem. Toxicol.* **2020**, *136*, 111092. [CrossRef] [PubMed]
14. Huang, T.-Y.; Chang, T.-C.; Chin, Y.-T.; Pan, Y.-S.; Chang, W.-J.; Liu, F.-C.; Hastuti, E.D.; Chiu, S.-J.; Wang, S.-H.; Changou, C.A.; et al. NDAT Targets PI3K-Mediated PD-L1 Upregulation to Reduce Proliferation in Gefitinib-Resistant Colorectal Cancer. *Cells* **2020**, *9*, 1830. [CrossRef]
15. Kouns, W.; Hadvary, P.; Haering, P.; Steiner, B. Conformational modulation of purified glycoprotein (GP) IIb-IIIa allows proteolytic generation of active fragments from either active or inactive GPIIb-IIIa. *J. Biol. Chem.* **1992**, *267*, 18844–18851. [CrossRef]
16. Hay, B.A.; Godugu, K.; Darwish, N.H.E.; Fujioka, K.; Sudha, T.; Karakus, O.O.; Mousa, S.A. New Thyrointegrin $\alpha_v\beta_3$ Antagonist with a Scalable Synthesis, Brain Penetration, and Potent Activity against Glioblastoma Multiforme. *J. Med. Chem.* **2021**, *64*, 6300–6309. [CrossRef]
17. Kapp, T.G.; Rechenmacher, F.; Neubauer, S.; Maltsev, O.V.; Cavalcanti-Adam, E.A.; Zarka, R.; Reuning, U.; Notni, J.; Wester, H.-J.; Mas-Moruno, C.; et al. A Comprehensive Evaluation of the Activity and Selectivity Profile of Ligands for RGD-binding Integrins. *Sci. Rep.* **2017**, *7*, 39805. [CrossRef]
18. Davis, F.B.; Mousa, S.A.; O'Connor, L.; Mohamed, S.; Lin, H.-Y.; Cao, H.J.; Davis, P.J. Proangiogenic Action of Thyroid Hormone Is Fibroblast Growth Factor–Dependent and Is Initiated at the Cell Surface. *Circ. Res.* **2004**, *94*, 1500–1506. [CrossRef]
19. Mousa, S.A.; O'Connor, L.J.; Bergh, J.J.; Davis, F.B.; Scanlan, T.S.; Davis, P.J. The Proangiogenic Action of Thyroid Hormone Analogue GC-1 Is Initiated at an Integrin. *J. Cardiovasc. Pharmacol.* **2005**, *46*, 356–360. [CrossRef]
20. Mousa, D.S.; El-Far, A.H.; Saddiq, A.A.; Sudha, T.; Mousa, S.A. Nanoformulated Bioactive Compounds Derived from Different Natural Products Combat Pancreatic Cancer Cell Proliferation. *Int. J. Nanomed.* **2020**, *15*, 2259–2268. [CrossRef]
21. Stryker, Z.I.; Rajabi, M.; Davis, P.J.; Mousa, S.A. Evaluation of Angiogenesis Assays. *Biomedicines* **2019**, *7*, 37. [CrossRef] [PubMed]
22. Hercbergs, A.A.; Goyal, L.K.; Suh, J.H.; Lee, S.; Reddy, C.A.; Cohen, B.H.; Stevens, G.H.; Reddy, S.K.; Peereboom, D.M.; Elson, P.J.; et al. Propylthiouracil-induced chemical hypothyroidism with high-dose tamoxifen prolongs survival in recurrent high grade glioma: A phase I/II study. *Anticancer Res.* **2003**, *23*, 617–626.
23. Cody, V.; Davis, P.J.; Davis, F.B. Molecular modeling of the thyroid hormone interactions with $\alpha v\beta 3$ integrin. *Steroids* **2007**, *72*, 165–170. [CrossRef]
24. Li, W.; Zhan, P.; De Clercq, E.; Lou, H.; Liu, X. Current drug research on PEGylation with small molecular agents. *Prog. Polym. Sci.* **2013**, *38*, 421–444. [CrossRef]
25. Zaghmi, A.; Mendez-Villuendas, E.; Greschner, A.; Liu, J.; de Haan, H.; Gauthier, M. Mechanisms of activity loss for a multi-PEGylated protein by experiment and simulation. *Mater. Today Chem.* **2019**, *12*, 121–131. [CrossRef]
26. Baumann, A.; Tuerck, D.; Prabhu, S.; Dickmann, L.; Sims, J. Pharmacokinetics, metabolism and distribution of PEGs and PEGylated proteins: Quo vadis? *Drug Discov. Today* **2014**, *19*, 1623–1631. [CrossRef] [PubMed]
27. Han, Y.; Yuan, Z.; Zhang, P.; Jiang, S. Zwitterlation mitigates protein bioactivity loss in vitro over PEGylation. *Chem. Sci.* **2018**, *9*, 8561–8566. [CrossRef]
28. Davis, P.J.; Lin, H.-Y.; Thangirala, S.; Yalcin, M.; Tang, H.-Y.; Hercbergs, A.; Leith, J.T.; Luidens, M.K.; Ashur-Fabian, O.; Incerpi, S.; et al. Nanotetrac targets integrin $\alpha v \beta 3$ on tumor cells to disorder cell defense pathways and block angiogenesis. *OncoTargets Ther.* **2014**, *7*, 1619–1624. [CrossRef] [PubMed]
29. Coskun, M.D.; Sudha, T.; Bharali, D.J.; Celikler, S.; Davis, P.J.; Mousa, S.A. $\alpha v \beta 3$ Integrin Antagonists Enhance Chemotherapy Response in an Orthotopic Pancreatic Cancer Model. *Front. Pharmacol.* **2020**, *11*, 95. [CrossRef]
30. Stupp, R.; Hegi, M.E.; Gorlia, T.; Erridge, S.C.; Perry, J.; Hong, Y.-K.; Aldape, K.D.; Lhermitte, B.; Pietsch, T.; Grujicic, D.; et al. Cilengitide combined with standard treatment for patients with newly diagnosed glioblastoma with methylated MGMT promoter (CENTRIC EORTC 26071-22072 study): A multicenter, randomised, open-label, phase 3 trial. *Lancet Oncol.* **2014**, *15*, 1100–1108. [CrossRef]
31. Li, J.; Fukase, Y.; Shang, Y.; Zou, W.; Muñoz-Félix, J.M.; Buitrago, L.; van Agthoven, J.; Zhang, Y.; Hara, R.; Tanaka, Y.; et al. Novel Pure alphaV beta3 Integrin Antagonists That Do Not Induce Receptor Extension, Prime the Receptor, or Enhance Angiogenesis at Low Concentrations. *ACS Pharmacol. Transl. Sci.* **2019**, *2*, 387–401. [CrossRef] [PubMed]

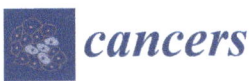

Article

CK2 Activity Mediates the Aggressive Molecular Signature of Glioblastoma Multiforme by Inducing Nerve/Glial Antigen (NG)2 Expression

Beate M. Schmitt [1], Anne S. Boewe [1], Claudia Götz [2], Stephan E. Philipp [3], Steffi Urbschat [4], Joachim Oertel [4], Michael D. Menger [1], Matthias W. Laschke [1] and Emmanuel Ampofo [1,*]

[1] Institute for Clinical & Experimental Surgery, Saarland University, 66421 Homburg, Germany; beate.schmitt@uks.eu (B.M.S.); anne.boewe@uks.eu (A.S.B.); michael.menger@uks.eu (M.D.M.); matthias.laschke@uks.eu (M.W.L.)

[2] Medical Biochemistry and Molecular Biology, Saarland University, 66421 Homburg, Germany; claudia.goetz@uks.eu

[3] Experimental and Clinical Pharmacology and Toxicology, Center for Molecular Signaling (PZMS), Saarland University, 66421 Homburg, Germany; stephan.philipp@uks.eu

[4] Department of Neurosurgery, Faculty of Medicine, Saarland University, 66421 Homburg, Germany; steffi.urbschat@uks.eu (S.U.); joachim.oertel@uks.eu (J.O.)

* Correspondence: emmanuel.ampofo@uks.eu

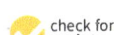

Citation: Schmitt, B.M.; Boewe, A.S.; Götz, C.; Philipp, S.E.; Urbschat, S.; Oertel, J.; Menger, M.D.; Laschke, M.W.; Ampofo, E. CK2 Activity Mediates the Aggressive Molecular Signature of Glioblastoma Multiforme by Inducing Nerve/Glial Antigen (NG)2 Expression. *Cancers* **2021**, *13*, 1678. https://doi.org/10.3390/cancers13071678

Academic Editor: Stanley Stylli

Received: 11 March 2021
Accepted: 25 March 2021
Published: 2 April 2021

Publisher's Note: MDPI stays neutral with regard to jurisdictional claims in published maps and institutional affiliations.

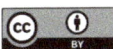

Copyright: © 2021 by the authors. Licensee MDPI, Basel, Switzerland. This article is an open access article distributed under the terms and conditions of the Creative Commons Attribution (CC BY) license (https://creativecommons.org/licenses/by/4.0/).

Simple Summary: Glioblastoma multiforme (GBM) is the most common and lethal primary malignant cancer of the central nervous system with a median patient survival of ~15 months. It has been reported that particularly nerve/glial antigen (NG)2-positive GBM is associated with an aggressive clinical phenotype and poor prognosis. Based on our latest findings, that protein kinase CK2 is a crucial regulator of NG2 expression in pericytes, we investigated the effect of CK2 inhibition by CX-4945 as well as CK2 KO on NG2 expression in human GBM cells. We found that CK2 inhibition suppresses proliferation and migration of different NG2-positive GBM cells. In silico analyses revealed a positive correlation between the mRNA expression of the two proteins. Moreover, we verified the decreased expression of NG2 in patient-derived GBM cells after CX-4945 treatment. These novel insights into the molecular signaling of NG2-positive GBM demonstrate that CX-4945 may represent a promising drug for future GBM therapy.

Abstract: Nerve/glial antigen (NG)2 expression crucially determines the aggressiveness of glioblastoma multiforme (GBM). Recent evidence suggests that protein kinase CK2 regulates NG2 expression. Therefore, we investigated in the present study whether CK2 inhibition suppresses proliferation and migration of NG2-positive GBM cells. For this purpose, CK2 activity was suppressed in the NG2-positive cell lines A1207 and U87 by the pharmacological inhibitor CX-4945 and CRISPR/Cas9-mediated knockout of CK2α. As shown by quantitative real-time PCR, luciferase-reporter assays, flow cytometry and western blot, this significantly reduced NG2 gene and protein expression when compared to vehicle-treated and wild type controls. In addition, CK2 inhibition markedly reduced NG2-dependent A1207 and U87 cell proliferation and migration. The Cancer Genome Atlas (TCGA)-based data further revealed not only a high expression of both NG2 and CK2 in GBM but also a positive correlation between the mRNA expression of the two proteins. Finally, we verified a decreased NG2 expression after CX-4945 treatment in patient-derived GBM cells. These findings indicate that the inhibition of CK2 represents a promising approach to suppress the aggressive molecular signature of NG2-positive GBM cells. Therefore, CX-4945 may be a suitable drug for the future treatment of NG2-positive GBM.

Keywords: glioblastoma multiforme; GBM; nerve/glial antigen 2; NG2; CK2; CX-4945; proliferation; migration; CRISPR/Cas9

1. Introduction

CK2 is a ubiquitously expressed, constitutively active serine/threonine kinase consisting of two catalytic CK2α- or CK2α'- and two non-catalytic CK2β-subunits [1]. With more than 500 substrates, CK2 is involved in various biological processes and estimated to be responsible for up to 10% of the human phosphoproteome [2,3]. CK2 exerts oncogenic activity, because its overexpression promotes tumor development and progression via the activation of proliferation and inhibition of apoptosis [4–6]. Hence, a broad spectrum of CK2 inhibitors have been developed as potential anti-cancer drugs, including CIGB-300 [7], 4,5,6,7-tetrabromobenzotriazole (TBB) [8] and CX-4945 [9].

Nerve/glial antigen (NG)2 is a type-1 transmembrane proteoglycan with a core of 290 kDa that is expressed in pericytes and different progenitor cells under physiological conditions [10]. The extracellular domain of the proteoglycan is able to bind components of the extracellular matrix (ECM) [11] as well as to interact with integrin β1, platelet-derived growth factor (PDGF)α and fibroblast growth factor (FGF)2 [12]. These interactions trigger different signaling pathways, including extracellular signal-regulated kinases (ERK)1/2 and focal adhesion kinase (FAK) [13,14]. This, in turn, activates cell proliferation, cell motility, inflammation and angiogenesis [15–18]. Recently, we have identified CK2 as a novel regulator of NG2-dependent signaling pathways [19]. Our results revealed that inhibition of CK2 suppresses NG2 expression in pericytes, which reduces their angiogenic activity [19].

Besides its expression in normal tissue, NG2 is also expressed in distinct tumors, including glioblastoma multiforme (GBM). GBM is categorized as grade IV glioma and associated with a poor outcome, as reflected by a median survival of less than 15 months from the day of diagnosis [5,20,21]. Although considerable efforts have been made in GBM research, effective therapeutic approaches for the treatment of this cancer type are still missing [21]. This is due to the fact that GBM expresses various genes promoting proliferation, invasion as well as drug resistance of tumor cells [5,21,22]. Several studies reported that particularly NG2-positive GBM is associated with an aggressive clinical phenotype and poor prognosis [11,23–25], which is why the proteoglycan is described as a potential therapeutic target.

Based on these findings, we hypothesize that CK2 inhibition suppresses proliferation and migration of NG2-positive GBM cells. To test this, we investigated the effect of pharmacological CK2 inhibition with CX-4945 as well as CK2α knockout (KO) on NG2 expression, cell proliferation and migration in human NG2-positive GBM cell lines. The Cancer Genome Atlas (TCGA)-based data from human gliomas were used to study the mRNA expression of CK2 and NG2 as well as the correlation between the two proteins. Finally, we assessed the expression of NG2 in patient-derived GBM cells, which were treated with CX-4945.

2. Results

2.1. CK2 Inhibition Reduces NG2 Expression in Human GBM Cell Lines

First, we investigated the effect of CK2 inhibition on NG2 protein expression in the NG2-positive human GBM cell lines A1207 and U87. For this purpose, the cells were treated with the CK2 inhibitor CX-4945 (10 µM) for 72 h and the expression of different proteins was assessed by western blot and flow cytometry. We found that all CK2 subunits are expressed in A1207 and U87 cells (Figure 1A and Figures S1 and S2). Of note, the expression of CK2α was more pronounced when compared to that of CK2α' (Figure 1A and Figure S1). In addition, we detected a significantly reduced phosphorylation of the CK2 specific phosphorylation site serine 129 of Akt (pAkt^{S129}) in CX-4945-treated cells. This confirms the efficiency of the CK2 inhibitor (Figure 1A–C and Figures S3 and S4). Moreover, CX-4945 significantly reduced the NG2 expression in the two cell lines when compared to controls (Figure 1A,D–G and Figures S5 and S6). To exclude that the herein observed effects of CX-4945 are independent of CK2 inhibition, we additionally generated CK2α KO in A1207 and U87 cells by means of the CRISPR/Cas9 system. CK2α was completely absent in KO cells. The protein expression of CK2β was markedly reduced (Figure 1H and Figures S7–S12). This observation has already been reported for other cell lines and can be explained by the instability of free CK2β subunits [26]. As expected, the loss of CK2α resulted in a markedly reduced phosphorylation of Akt^{S129} and expression of NG2 (Figure 1H–N and Figures S13–S20). These results were verified by western blot analyses of additional CK2α KO clones (Figure S21A,B). Moreover, we noticed a decreased phosphorylation of FAK in CK2α KO cells when compared to wild type cells (Figure 1O,P and Figures S22–S24).

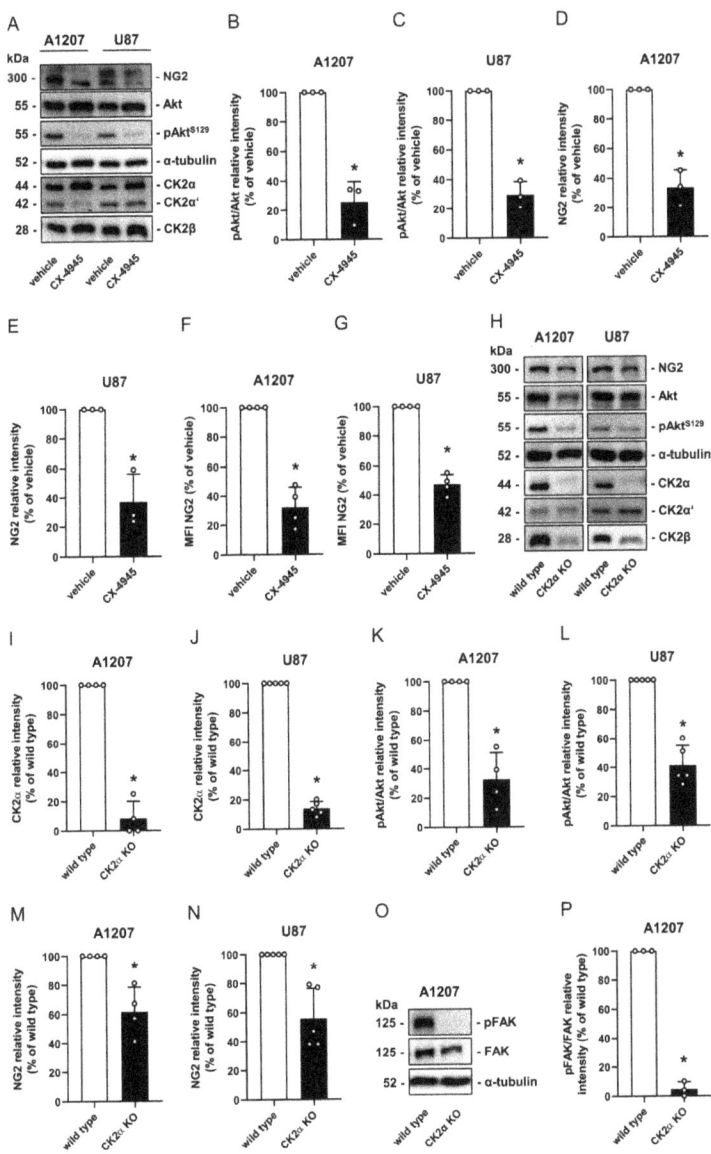

Figure 1. CK2 inhibition reduces NG2 expression in human GBM cell lines. (**A**) A1207 and U87 cells

were treated with vehicle (DMSO) or CX-4945 (10 µM) for 72 h. The cells were lysed and the expression of NG2, Akt, pAkt^{S129}, CK2α, CK2α', CK2β and α-tubulin (as loading control) was analyzed by western blot. (**B–E**) A1207 and U87 cells were treated as described in (**A**) and the expression of pAkt/Akt (**B,C**) and NG2 (**D,E**) was quantitatively analyzed. Vehicle-treated cells were set 100%. Mean ± SD. * $p < 0.05$ vs. vehicle ($n = 3$). (**F,G**) A1207 and U87 cells were treated as described in (**A**), scratched and the mean fluorescence intensity (MFI) of NG2-positive cells was assessed by flow cytometry. The MFI of vehicle-treated cells was set 100%. Mean ± SD. * $p < 0.05$ vs. vehicle ($n = 4$). (**H**) A1207 and U87 wild type and CK2α KO cells were lysed and the expression of NG2, Akt, pAkt^{S129}, CK2α, CK2α', CK2β and α-tubulin (as loading control) was analyzed by western blot. (**I–N**) A1207 and U87 cells were treated as described in (**H**) and the expression of CK2α (**I,J**), pAkt/Akt (**K,L**) and NG2 (**M,N**) was quantitatively assessed. Wild type cells were set 100%. Mean ± SD. * $p < 0.05$ vs. wild type (A1207: $n = 4$; U87: $n = 5$). (**O**) A1207 wild type and CK2α KO cells were lysed and the expression of FAK, pFAK and α-tubulin (as loading control) was analyzed by western blot. (**P**) A1207 wild type and CK2α KO cells were lysed and the expression of pFAK/FAK was quantitatively assessed. Wild type cells were set 100%. Mean ± SD. * $p < 0.05$ vs. wild type ($n = 3$).

2.2. CK2 Inhibition Reduces NG2 Gene Expression in Human GBM Cell Lines

Recently, we have identified a 114-bp fragment (NG2$^{P1.2.4.1}$) close to the NG2 start codon as a CK2-dependent active promoter region in human pericytes [19]. Therefore, we investigated whether the activity of NG2$^{P1.2.4.1}$ is also affected by CK2 inhibition in GBM cells. To test this, A1207 CK2α KO and wild type cells were transfected with pGL4-NG2$^{P1.2.4.1}$ reporter construct and the luciferase activity was measured (Figure 2A). In addition, A1207 cells transfected with pGL4-NG2$^{P1.2.4.1}$ reporter construct were treated with CX-4945 or vehicle and subsequently analyzed by luciferase assay (Figure 2B). In line with our previous results, we detected a reduced transcriptional activity of NG2$^{P1.2.4.1}$ after CK2 inhibition (Figure 2A,B). Additional quantitative real-time PCR (qRT-PCR) analyses showed a reduced NG2 mRNA expression in CX-4945-treated A1207 and U87 cells when compared to controls (Figure 2C,D). We further performed cycloheximide experiments to study the stability of the NG2 protein. Flow cytometric analyses clearly demonstrated that CX-4945 does not affect the stability of the protein (Figure 2E,F).

2.3. CK2 Inhibition Suppresses the Proliferation of Human GBM Cell Lines

In the next set of experiments, we assessed the proliferation of NG2-positive GBM cell lines after CX-4945 treatment. Water-soluble tetrazolium (WST)-1 assay revealed a significantly reduced mitochondrial activity in A1207 and U87 cells after CX-4945 treatment when compared to vehicle-treated controls (Figure 3A,B). Additional flow cytometric analyses of Bromodeoxyuridine (BrdU) incorporation, growth curves and scratch assays of CX-4945-and vehicle-treated cells confirmed the anti-proliferative effect of CK2 inhibition (Figure 3C–J). Of note, lactate dehydrogenase (LDH) assays showed that this effect is not caused by cytotoxicity of 10 µM CX-4945 (Figure 3K,L).

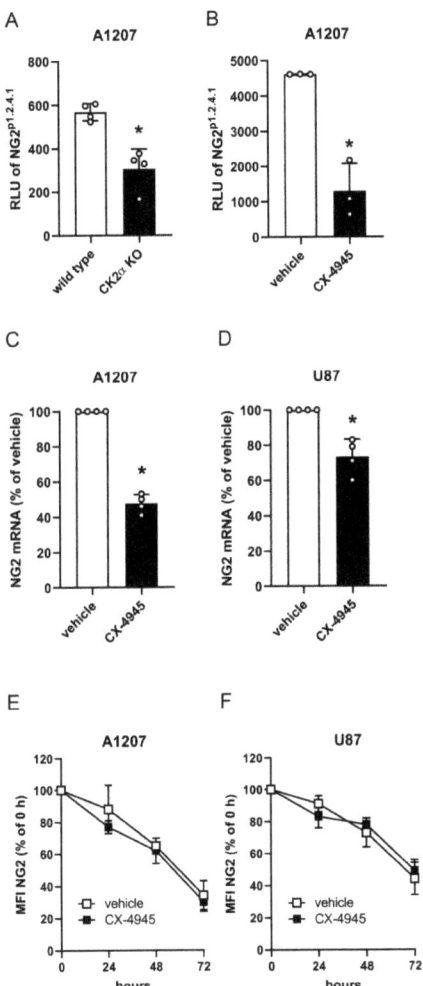

Figure 2. CK2 inhibition reduces NG2 gene expression in human GBM cell lines. (**A**) A1207 wild type and CK2α KO cells were transfected with pGL4-NG2P$^{p1.2.4.1}$, cultivated for 24 h, lysed and the transcriptional activity was detected by a luciferase assay. Relative luciferase units (RLU) of wild type cells were used as control. Mean ± SD. * $p < 0.05$ vs. wild type ($n = 4$). (**B**) A1207 cells were transfected with pGL4-NG2P$^{p1.2.4.1}$ for 24 h, treated with vehicle (DMSO) or CX-4945 (10 μM) and analyzed by a luciferase assay. RLU of vehicle-treated cells were used as control. Mean ± SD. * $p < 0.05$ vs. vehicle ($n = 3$). (**C,D**) A1207 and U87 cells were treated with vehicle (DMSO) or CX-4945 (10 μM) for 72 h, harvested and total RNA was isolated. The relative gene expression of NG2 was examined by qRT-PCR normalized to GAPDH. Vehicle-treated cells were set 100%. Mean ± SD. * $p < 0.05$ vs. vehicle ($n = 4$). (**E,F**) A1207 and U87 cells were treated with vehicle (DMSO) or CX-4945 (10 μM) in the presence of cycloheximide. The cells were scratched after 0 h, 24 h, 48 h and 72 h and the MFI of NG2-positive cells was assessed by flow cytometry. MFI of cells at 0 h was set 100%. Mean ± SD ($n = 4$).

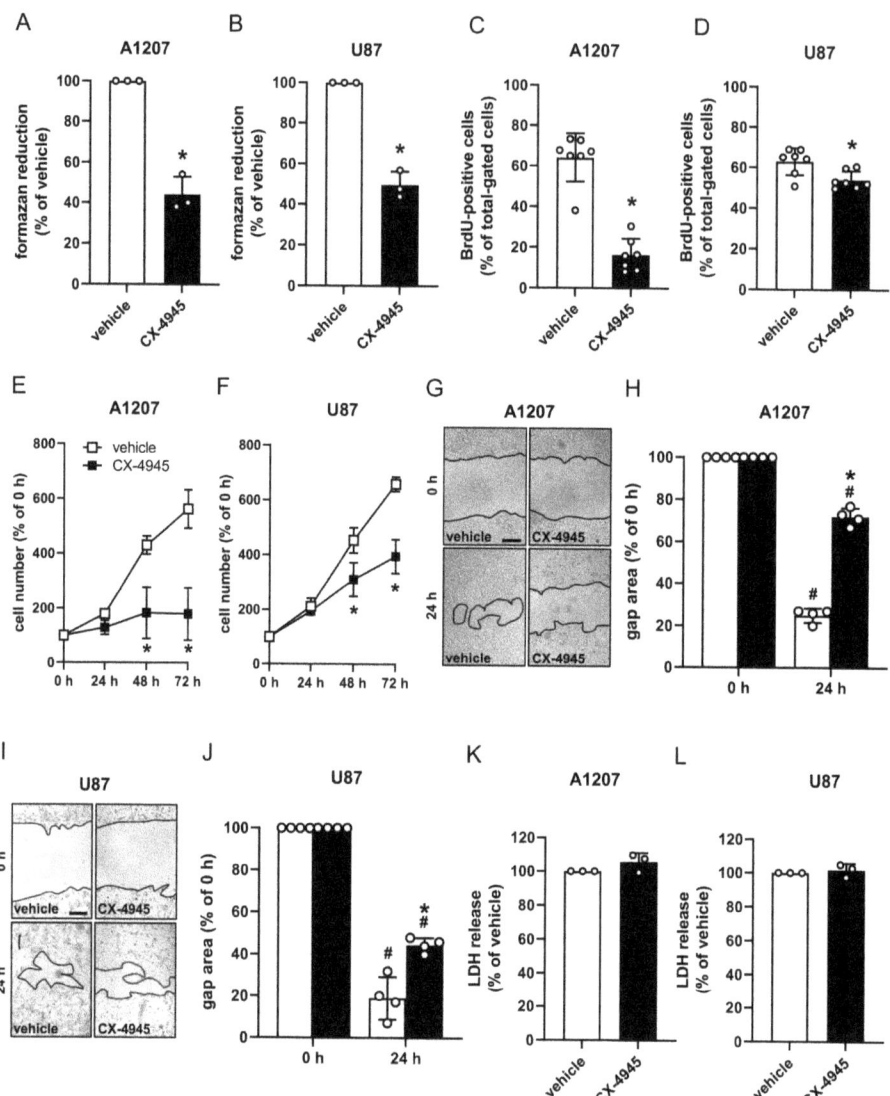

Figure 3. CK2 inhibition suppresses the proliferation of human GBM cell lines. (**A,B**) A1207 and U87 cells were treated with vehicle (DMSO) or CX-4945 (10 µM) for 72 h and the mitochondrial activity was analyzed by WST-1 assays. Vehicle-treated cells were set 100%. Mean ± SD. * $p < 0.05$ vs. vehicle ($n = 3$). (**C,D**) A1207 and U87 cells were treated as described in (**A,B**) and the MFI of BrdU-positive cells (% of total gated cells) was assessed by flow cytometry. Vehicle-treated cells were used as control. Mean ± SD. Mean ± SD. * $p < 0.05$ vs. vehicle ($n = 7$). (**E,F**) A1207 and U87 cells were seeded in a 24-well plate, cultivated for 24 h and subsequently treated with vehicle (DMSO) or CX-4945 (10 µM). The cell number was determined at 0 h, 24 h, 48 h and 72 h after treatment. The cell number at 0 h was set 100%. Mean ± SD. * $p < 0.05$ vs. vehicle ($n = 4$). (**G–J**) A1207 and U87 cells were cultivated and treated as described in (**E,F**) and analyzed by scratch assays (scale bars in G and I: 200 µm). The gap area was measured after 0 h and 24 h. The gap area at 0 h was set 100%. Mean ± SD. * $p < 0.05$ vs. vehicle at 24 h; # $p < 0.05$ vs. 0 h ($n = 4$). (**K,L**) A1207 and U87 cells were treated as described in (**A,B**) and the cytotoxicity of CX-4945 was assessed by LDH assays. Vehicle-treated cells were used as control and set 100% ($n = 3$).

2.4. CK2 Inhibition Reduces the Migratory Capacity of NG2-Positive GBM Cell Lines

NG2 promotes cell migration via its binding to the ECM [11,23,24]. To study the impact of CK2 on NG2-dependent cell migration, we performed a panel of transwell assays. As expected, silencing of NG2 in A1207 cells markedly reduced the number of migrated cells (Figure 4A–C). Furthermore, CK2 inhibition with CX-4945 also reduced the migratory capacity of A1207 cells (Figure 4D,E). To verify that CK2 mediates cell migration via NG2, we overexpressed NG2 in A1207 cells (Figure 4F and Figures S25–S27), which were subsequently treated with CX-4945. We found that overexpression of NG2 partially rescued the reduced migratory capacity of CX-4945-treated cells (Figure 4G,H).

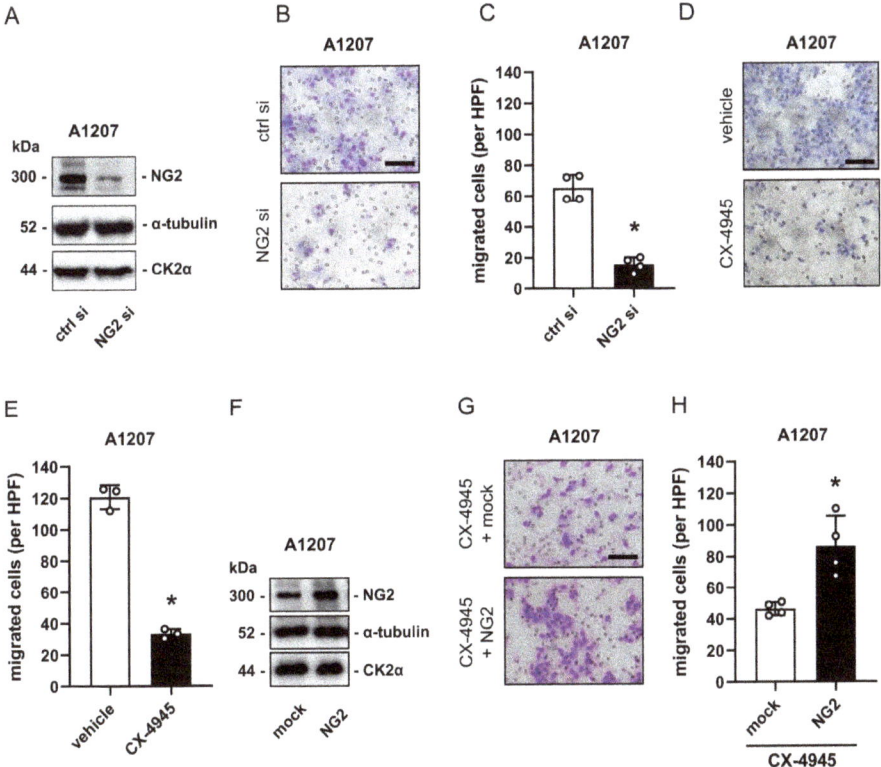

Figure 4. CK2 inhibition reduces the migratory capacity of NG2-positive GBM cell lines. (**A**) A1207 cells were transfected with ctrl si or NG2 si for 72 h. The cells were harvested, lysed and the expression of NG2, CK2α and α-tubulin (as loading control) was analyzed by western blot. (**B**) A1207 cells were treated as described in (**A**), detached and their migration was assessed by transwell assays (scale bar: 50 µm). (**C**) A1207 cells were treated as described in (**A**) and the migration was quantitatively assessed. Ctrl si-transfected cells were used as control. Mean ± SD. * $p < 0.05$ vs. ctrl si ($n = 4$). (**D**) A1207 cells were treated with vehicle (DMSO) or CX-4945 (10 µM) for 72 h, detached and their migration was assessed by transwell assays (scale bar: 50 µm). (**E**) A1207 cells were treated as described in (**D**) and migration was quantitatively assessed. Vehicle-treated cells were used as control. Mean ± SD. * $p < 0.05$ vs. vehicle ($n = 4$). (**F**) A1207 were transfected with mock (pEF6 vector) or NG2 plasmid and incubated for 48 h. Expression of NG2, CK2α and α-tubulin (as loading control) was analyzed by western blot. (**G**) A1207 cells were transfected as described in (**F**), treated with CX-4945 for 24 h, detached and their migration was assessed by transwell assays (scale bar: 50 µm). (**H**) A1207 cells were transfected and treated as described in (**G**) and migration was quantitatively assessed. Mock-transfected cells were used as control. Mean ± SD. * $p < 0.05$ vs. mock ($n = 4$).

2.5. CK2 and NG2 mRNA Expression Positively Correlate in Human GBM

Next, we assessed the gene expression of CK2 subunits and NG2 in different human gliomas (grade I–IV) based on TCGA data. These analyses showed that the mRNA expression of NG2 is significantly elevated in GBM compared to lower grade gliomas (Figure 5A). Of interest, the mRNA expression of CK2α, CK2α' and CK2β was also significantly higher in GBM (Figure 5B–D). We noticed positive correlations between all CK2 subunits and NG2 in GBM (Figure 5E–G). Particularly, we detected a strong positive correlation between CK2α and NG2, as indicated by a Spearman's correlation coefficient of r = 0.54 ($p < 0.0001$). These findings support our in vitro results showing that CK2 is involved in NG2 expression.

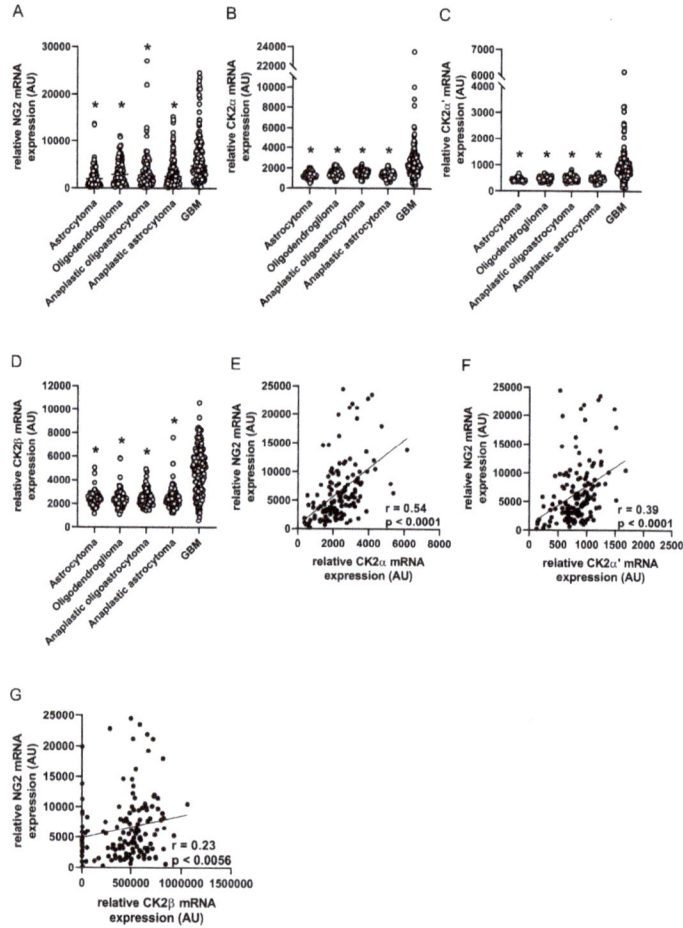

Figure 5. CK2 and NG2 mRNA expression positively correlate in human GBM. (**A–D**) The relative mRNA expression (TCGA-based data; arbitrary units (AU)) of NG2 (**A**), CK2α (**B**), CK2α' (**C**) and CK2β (**D**) was analyzed in human astrocytoma (grade I-II), oligodendroglioma (grade II), anaplastic oligoastrocytoma and astrocytoma (grade III) as well as in GBM (grade IV). * $p < 0.05$ vs. GBM (n = 682). (**E–G**) Spearman correlations of NG2 mRNA expression (AU) with CK2α (**E**), CK2α' (**F**) and CK2β (**G**) mRNA expression (TCGA-based data, AU, n = 141).

2.6. CK2 Inhibition Reduces NG2 Expression in Patient-Derived GBM Cells

Finally, we investigated the effect of CX-4945 on NG2 expression in patient-derived GBM cells. The herein analyzed cells (T8399, T8478, T8475 and T8470) originated from primary GBM grade IV, as indicated by a lack of the *IDH1* mutation R132H [27]. Of note, NG2 and the two catalytic CK2α and α' subunits were expressed in all patient-derived cells. Although the expression of these proteins markedly differed between the cells of individual patients, CX-4945 treatment reduced the CK2-dependent phosphorylation of Akt^{S129} as well as NG2 expression in all patient-derived cells (Figure 6A–D and Figures S28–S37).

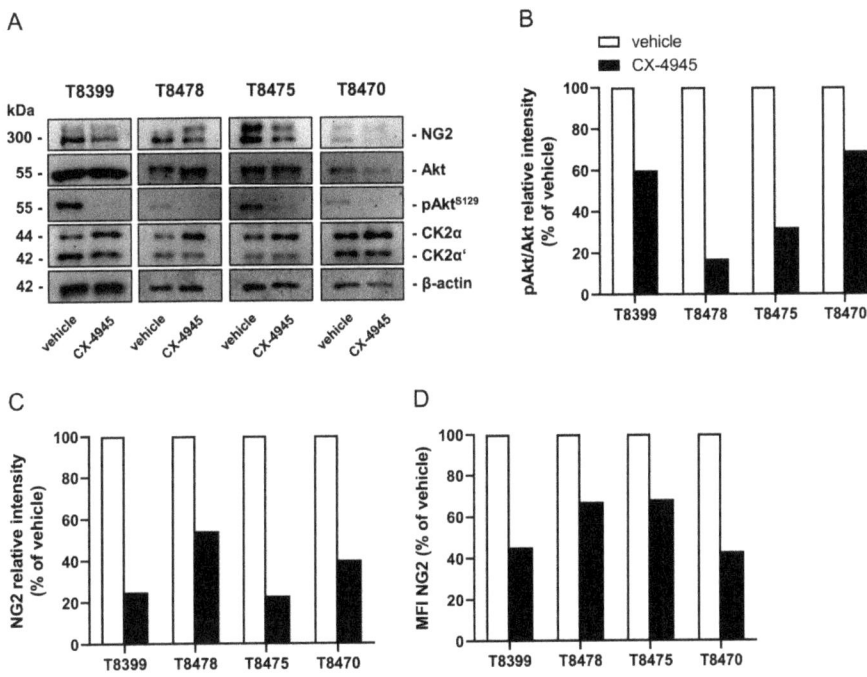

Figure 6. CK2 inhibition reduces NG2 expression in patient-derived GBM cells. (**A**) Patient-derived GBM cells (T8399, T8478, T8475 and T8470) were treated with vehicle (DMSO) or CX-4945 (10 µM) for 72 h. Subsequently, the cells were lysed and the expression of NG2, Akt, pAkt^{S129}, CK2α, CK2α' and β-actin (as loading control) was analyzed by western blot. (**B**,**C**) The cells were treated as described in (A) and the expression of pAkt/Akt (**B**) and NG2 (**C**) was quantitatively analyzed. Vehicle-treated cells were set 100%. (**D**) Patient-derived GBM cells (T8399, T8478, T8475 and T8470) were treated with vehicle (DMSO) or CX-4945 (10 µM) for 72 h, scratched and the MFI of NG2-positive cells was assessed by flow cytometry. Vehicle-treated cells were set 100%.

3. Discussion

In the present study, we hypothesized that CK2 inhibition suppresses proliferation and migration of NG2-positive GBM cells. Of interest, we found that the pharmacological inhibition as well as CK2α KO in NG2-postive GBM cell lines significantly reduces NG2 expression. Gene regulatory analyses further demonstrated that this is due to a diminished gene expression of NG2. Moreover, we detected a markedly decreased NG2-dependent cell proliferation and migration after CK2 inhibition. TCGA-based data revealed that both NG2 and CK2 are highly expressed in GBM. In addition, we observed a positive correlation between the mRNA expression of CK2α and NG2. Finally, we verified the decrease of NG2 expression after CX-4945 treatment in patient-derived GBM cells. This indicates that the oncogenic activity of CK2 mediates the aggressive molecular signature of GBM by inducing NG2 expression.

The overexpression of CK2 in various tumor types suppresses apoptosis while promoting cell proliferation and migration by dysregulating signaling pathways, such as nuclear factor kappa (NFk)B and phosphoinositide 3-kinase (PI3K)/Akt. Given these central functions of CK2 in tumorigenesis, it is not surprising that a broad spectrum of CK2 inhibitors has been developed, culminating in the synthesis of CX-4945. This compound is the most specific CK2 inhibitor to date and has a high bioavailability [28]. Of note, CX-4945 has the ability to cross the blood-brain-barrier and, thus, may be suitable in the treatment of brain tumors, including GBM [29,30].

GBM is the most common and lethal primary malignant cancer of the central nervous system with a median patient survival of ~15 months from the day of diagnosis [1]. Investigating the molecular mechanisms of CK2 in GBM development and progression, the group of Benveniste demonstrated that this kinase is required for the activation of pro-survival pathways, such as Januskinase/Signal Transducers and Activators of Transcription (JAK/STAT) and PI3K/AKT [31,32]. Moreover, it is well known that GBM often exhibits a striking cellular heterogeneity [20,33,34]. For instance, it has been shown that NG2-positive cells are associated with an aggressive clinical phenotype and poor prognosis [11,23-25]. We herein found that the inhibition of CK2 significantly reduces NG2 gene expression in the GBM cell lines A1207 and U87. For this purpose, CX-4945 was used to suppress CK2 activity. To identify suitable, non-toxic concentrations of this inhibitor, GBM cells were treated with 2.5 µM, 5 µM and 10 µM CX-4945 over 24 h, 48 h and 72 h, and both cell proliferation and cytotoxicity were determined. We found that none of the tested concentrations is cytotoxic. However, only 10 µM CX-4945 for 72 h lowered cell proliferation more than 50%. More importantly, 10 µM CX-4945 was the most efficient concentration for the reduction of NG2 expression. Based on these findings, we decided to use 10 µM CX-4945 to study the effects on NG2 expression and NG2-dependent cellular functions. To exclude that the herein observed reduced NG2 expression is due to unspecific effects of CX-4945 and, thus, CK2-independent, we additionally generated CK2α KO cell lines showing that the loss of CK2 activity significantly reduces NG2 expression. The analysis of the gene regulatory mechanism revealed that this is caused by a decreased transcriptional activity of a 114 bp fragment close to the NG2 start codon. This region harbors a binding site for the transcription factor SP1, which can activate or repress gene expression [35]. It has been reported that posttranslational modifications of SP1, including phosphorylation, affect GBM cell proliferation and invasion [36,37]. Of note, CK2 phosphorylates SP1 and inhibition of this kinase increases its DNA binding capacity [38,39]. Hence, it is tempting to speculate that CK2 regulates NG2 gene expression via SP1-dependent phosphorylation in GBM cells.

Various posttranslational modifications of the NG2 core protein, resulting in higher molecular forms, have been identified. For instance, the group of Stallcup showed that NG2 is phosphorylated at threonine 2256 by protein kinase C and threonine 2314 by ERK1/2, which promotes cell proliferation and cell motility [40]. Moreover, high molecular forms of NG2 caused by glycosylation are observed. However, the nature of this glycosylation and its biological significance is still unknown [41,42]. In this study, we detected higher molecular forms of NG2 by western blot, which are partially reduced after CK2 inhibition. Hence, we cannot exclude that CK2 additionally reduces the NG2 protein level by phosphorylation of the proteoglycan or by inhibition of glycosyltransferases.

In GBM, NG2 is involved in cell proliferation, migration and invasion via a wide range of molecular interactions [24]. The proteoglycan promotes cell proliferation and motility by binding to integrin β1, PDGFα and FGF2 [12]. In addition, the invasive and migratory activity of NG2-positive GBM cells is stimulated by the interaction with ECM proteins [11]. In line with these findings, we could show that CK2 inhibition reduces the migration of NG2-positive GBM cell lines. It is well known that CK2 regulates cell migration via various signaling pathways [31,32]. To verify that the herein observed anti-migratory effect is mediated by NG2, we performed additional rescue experiments. Our results clearly demonstrate the importance of NG2 in CK2-dependent migration of GBM cells, as shown by an improved migratory ability of NG2-overexpressing cells after CK2 inhibition.

FAK mediates integrin- and growth factor-induced signaling transduction resulting in the activation of proliferative pathways. Kim et al. [43] reported that CX-4945 is capable of reducing TGF-β1-induced FAK phosphorylation. Furthermore, silencing of NG2 decreases the activity of FAK, resulting in a diminished cell proliferation [44]. In our study, we observed a diminished phosphorylation of FAK in CK2α KO cells. Therefore, it is tempting to speculate that the reduced proliferation of NG2-positive, CX-4945-treated GBM cells may be caused by a disturbed NG2/FAK signaling.

Recently, Al-Mayhani et al. [23] reported that NG2-positive cells from GBM patient tumor samples proliferate faster than NG2-negative ones. On the other hand, it has been shown that NG2 promotes the vascularization of GBM [45]. This indicates that NG2 is not only involved in tumor cell proliferation but also in angiogenesis. We previously found that CK2 inhibition reduces the NG2-dependent angiogenic activity of human pericytes [19]. Therefore, we suggest that CX-4945 is a promising compound for the treatment of NG2-positive GBM, because it targets both the vascular and tumor compartment.

We further analyzed the mRNA expression pattern of NG2, CK2α, CK2α' and CK2β in different gliomas using TCGA-based data. As previously reported [24,46], we found the highest expression of NG2 in GBM when compared to other gliomas. The expression of the CK2 subunits was also remarkably higher in GBM. The correlation between NG2 and CK2 mRNA revealed that all CK2 subunits were positively correlated with NG2. Of note, the strongest correlation was observed between CK2α and NG2. This may be explained by the fact that CK2α and CK2α' exert tissue-specific functions, because of their partially different substrates [26]. We herein detected an increased expression of CK2α when compared to CK2α' in NG2-positive GBM cells. This indicates that CK2α may have a superior function in the regulation of NG2 expression when compared to CK2α'.

Overexpression of NG2 has not been reported to be a result of genetic aberrations, such as gene amplifications or chromosome translocation, in GBM [47]. Moreover, there are no mutations known in the NG2 gene leading to gain or loss of function. In contrast, genome-wide copy number variation analyses in GBM demonstrated that chromosome 20 harbors frequent gains in gene dosage, which may be driven by several oncogenic targets [48]. Of note, the CK2α gene is located on chromosome 20 and it has been reported that CK2 expression is required for the activation of survival pathways, including the JAK/STAT, NFκB and PI3K/AKT pathways in GBM [32]. Hence, it can be assumed that the gains in CK2α gene dosage may be a crucial oncogenic driver during gliomagenesis.

Finally, we assessed the effect of CK2 inhibition on patient-derived NG2-positive GBM cells. This is of major importance, as recent evidence suggests that classically established cell lines from different tumors, including GBM, do not fully reflect the genotypes and phenotypes of primary tumors [49]. Notably, we also detected a decreased NG2 expression after CX-4945 treatment in patient-derived cells, demonstrating that our cell line-based results on CK2/NG2-interaction in GBM are robust and reproducible in clinical samples. CX-4945 is currently tested in phase I and II clinical trials for the treatment of different cancer types, including cholangiocarcinoma (NCT02128282), multiple myeloma (NCT01199718) and medulloblastoma (NCT03904862). Therefore, we suggest that treatment of NG2-positive GBM with this compound represents a promising therapeutic approach, which should be clinically evaluated in the near future.

4. Materials and Methods

4.1. Chemical and Biological Reagents

Roswell Park Memorial Institute (RPMI) 1640 medium, Dulbecco's Modified Eagle's Medium (DMEM), Lipofectamine3000 reagent, Opti-MEM Reduced Serum Medium (Gibco), fetal calf serum (FCS), penicillin-streptomycin and small interfering RNA (siRNA) duplexes directed against NG2 (ID: 146.147) were from Thermo Fisher Scientific (Karlsruhe,

Germany). Cycloheximide was from Sigma-Aldrich (Taufkirchen, Germany). Bovine serum albumin (BSA) was from Santa Cruz Biotechnology (Heidelberg, Germany). CX-4945 was from ActivateScientific (Prien, Germany). BrdU was from Roche (Mannheim, Germany). Cell lysis reagent QIAzol and HiPerFect transfection reagent were from Qiagen (Hilden, Germany). The qScriber cDNA Synthesis Kit and ORA SEE qPCR Green ROX L Mix were from HighQu (Kraichtal, Germany). The NG2-plasmid (pEF6-CSPG4-myc-his) was from addgene (Watertown, MA, USA). Luciferase Assay System was from Promega (Walldorf, Germany).

4.2. Antibodies

Anti-NG2 antibody (sc-166251) and anti-CK2β antibody (E9) were from Santa Cruz Biotechnology. Anti-β-actin antibody (66009) and anti-α-tubulin antibody (66031) were from Proteintech Germany GMBH (St. Leon-Rot, Germany). The anti-Akt1/2/3 antibody (11E7), anti-FAK antibody (3285) and anti-pFAK antibody (3283) were from Cell Signaling (Frankfurt am Main, Germany). Anti-CK2α antibody and anti-CK2α' antibody were generated as described previously [50]. Anti-pAKT antibody (EPR6150) was from Abcam (Cambridge, UK). Peroxidase-labeled anti-mouse antibody (NIF 825) and peroxidase-labeled anti-rabbit antibody (NIF 824) were from GE healthcare (Freiburg, Germany). Anti-chondroitin sulfate proteoglycan 4 (NG2) (562415) was from BD Biosciences (Heidelberg, Germany) and the BrdU antibody (BU20A) was from eBioscience Fisher Scientific (Schwerte, Germany).

4.3. Cell Culture

The human GBM cell lines A1207 (SymbioTec GmbH, Saarbrücken, Germany) and U87 (ATCC, Manassas, VA, USA) were cultivated in RPMI or DMEM supplemented with 10% FCS and penicillin-streptomycin at 37 °C under a humidified 95%/5% (vol/vol) mixture of air and CO_2. The cells were passaged at a split ratio of 1:3 after reaching confluence.

Primary GBM cells (T8399, T8478, T8475 and T8470) were obtained from the tumor tissue of patients undergoing surgery at the Department of Neurosurgery (Saarland University), as previously described in detail [51]. Briefly, tumor samples were mechanically processed and the resulting cell suspension was cultured in DMEM supplemented with 10% FCS, 1% non-essential amino acids and 1% penicillin-streptomycin at 37 °C and 5% CO_2. The medium was changed twice a week and the cells were used at passage 0 to 2. The study was approved by the local German ethical board (Ethikkommission der Ärztekammer des Saarlandes, Saarbrücken, Germany, General Medical Council of the State Saarland, NO 93/16).

4.4. WST-1 Assay

A WST-1 assay (Roche) was used to determine the mitochondrial activity of A1207 and U87 cells as a parameter of cell viability, as described previously in detail [52].

4.5. LDH Assay

A LDH assay (Cytotoxicity Detection KitPLUS, Roche) was used to evaluate the cytotoxic effects of CX-4945 on A1207 and U87 cells, as previously described in detail [52].

4.6. Generation of CK2α KO Cells by CRISPR-Cas9

All-in-one plasmid expressing Cas9-Dasher green fluorescent protein (GFP) and the two single guide RNAs (sgRNA) (pD 1401-AD: CMV-Cas9N-2A-GFP, Cas9-ElecD) to target CK2α were from ATUM (Newark, CA, USA). The sgRNA guide sequences targeting CK2α were: 5'-CCTGGATTATTGTCACAGCA-3' and 5'-GGTGGGATGAACGGGTCAGAA-3'. The CK2α KO was performed as previously described in detail [53]. Briefly, cells were transfected with the all-in-one plasmid by means of Lipofectamine3000 according to the manufacturer's instructions. Forty-eight hours after transfection, single GFP-positive cells were separated by fluorescence-activated cell sorting (MoFlo XDP Cell Sorter (Beckman

Coulter GmbH, Krefeld, Germany) and expanded to obtain individual clones. CK2α KO was verified by western blot analysis.

4.7. Reporter Gene Assay

The transcriptional activity of the NG2 promoter fragment NG2P[1.2.4.1] was assessed by reporter gene assays according to the manufacturer's instructions (Promega). Briefly, A1207 cells were transfected with pGL4 or pGL4-NG2P[1.2.4.1] reporter vectors by Lipofectamine3000 for 24 h. The cells were lysed and the luciferase activity was detected by a luminescence plate reader.

4.8. NG2 Silencing and NG2 Overexpression

For NG2 silencing, A1207 cells were transfected using HiPerFect transfection reagent for 72 h with 20 nM control siRNA or NG2 siRNA: sense 5′-GCUAUUUAACAUGGUGCUGtt-3′ and antisense 5′-CAGCACCAUGUUAAAUAGCtt-3′. For NG2 overexpression, the cells were transfected with a ctrl-plasmid (mock) or pEF6-CSPG4-myc-his using Lipofectamine3000 reagent for 48 h. Subsequently, the cells were harvested and used for flow cytometry or western blot analyses.

4.9. Scratch Assay

The migratory capacity of A1207 and U87 cells was assessed by means of scratch assays. The cells were seeded in a 24-well plate and cultivated until confluence. Subsequently, the cell monolayer was scratched with a pipette tip and then washed twice with phosphate-buffered saline (PBS) to remove non-adherent cells. Phase-contrast light microscopic images were taken immediately (0 h) and 24 h after scratching. The gap area was determined by means of ImageJ software (U.S. National Institutes of Health (NIH), Bethesda, MD, USA).

4.10. Growth Curves

A1207 and U87 cells were seeded in a 24-well plate and cultivated for 16 h. Thereafter, the cells were treated with vehicle or CX-4945 (10 μM) for 24 h, 48 h and 72 h. Then, the cells were detached, centrifuged and suspended with fresh culture medium. Ten μL of the suspended cells were stained with trypan blue solution (0.4%) and counted by a LUNA Automated Cell Counter according to the manufacturer's protocol.

4.11. Transwell Migration Assay

The migratory activity of A1207 cells was analyzed using 24-well chemotaxis chambers and polyvinylpyrrolidone-coated polycarbonate filters with a pore size of 8 μm (BD Biosciences). The filters were incubated overnight (37 °C, 5% CO_2) in RPMI without any supplements, medium was removed and 750 μL culture medium supplemented with 5% FCS was added to each of the lower wells. The upper wells were filled with 200 μL RPMI (0.1% FCS) containing 2.0×10^5 treated cells. Non-migrated cells were removed from the upper surface of the filters by cotton swabs after 5 h of cultivation. Migrated cells, which adhere to the lower surface, were fixed with methanol and stained with Dade Diff-Quick (Dade Diagnostika GmbH, München, Germany). Migrated cells were counted in 20 microscopic high-power fields (HPF) at 200× magnification (BZ-8000; Keyence, Osaka, Japan).

4.12. Western Blot Analysis

The separation of whole cell extracts was performed through a 7.5% or 12.5% SDS polyacrylamide gels, which were transferred onto a polyvinylidene difluoride (PVDF) membranes. The membranes were blocked with 5% BSA in Tris-buffered saline TBS (0.1% Tween20) for 1 h and subsequently incubated with the primary antibodies (anti-pAkt, anti-Akt, anti-pFAK, FAK, anti-CK2α, anti-CK2α′, anti-CK2β, anti-NG2, anti-β-actin and anti-α-tubulin; 1:500) in TBS (0.1% Tween20, 1% BSA) overnight (4 °C). The membrane was incubated with a peroxidase-coupled secondary antibody (anti-rabbit 1:1500 or anti-mouse

1:2000) for 1 h and washed with TBS (0.1% Tween20, 1% BSA). The expression of the proteins was visualized by luminol-enhanced chemiluminescence (ECL; GE Healthcare).

4.13. Flow Cytometry

Cells were washed with PBS (4 °C) and harvested by scratching. Subsequently, the cells were incubated with a phycoerythrin (PE)-labeled primary anti-NG2 antibody for 1 h at room temperature. Afterwards, the cells were washed in PBS and the MFI of 3000 cells was analyzed by a FACSLyrics flow cytometer (BD).

Cell proliferation was assessed by a BrdU-assay according to the manufacturer's protocol (Thermo Scientific). Briefly, A1207 and U87 cells were incubated with BrdU. After 10 h, the cells were washed, fixed and permeabilized. Incorporated BrdU was detected by using a BrdU antibody. The MFI of 3000 cells was analyzed in the FL-1 and FL-2 channel by a FACSLyrics flow cytometer.

4.14. Gene Expression Analysis

QIAzol lysis reagent was used to isolate total RNA and cDNA was transcribed by means of a qScriber cDNA Synthesis Kit. The amount of mRNA was determined by qRT-PCR using ORA SEE qPCR Green ROX L Mix according to the manufacturer's instructions. Primers (NG2 forward 5′-GGCTGTCAAAACCAGGGTAA-3′ and reverse 5′-AGAGGGCAAGGAGAAGGAAG-3′; GAPDH forward 5′-CCACCCATGGCAAATTCC-3′ and reverse 5′-ACTCCACGACGTACTCAG-3′) were used at a concentration of 500 nM. Data collection and analyses were performed by a MiniOpticon Real-Time PCR Detection System and the $2^{-\Delta\Delta Ct}$ method.

4.15. TCGA Data-Based Analyses

We used two TCGA datasets (Firehose Legacy (Brain Lower Grade Glioma) and Cell 2013 (Glioblastoma)) from cBioPortal (http://cbioportal.org, accessed on 10 November 2020). This platform is an open-access resource for interactive analyses of multidimensional cancer genomics datasets [54,55], to analyze the mRNA expression of NG2, CK2α, CK2α' and CK2β in different human gliomas (human astrocytoma (grade I-II), oligodendroglioma (grade II), anaplastic oligoastrocytoma and astrocytoma (grade III) as well as in GBM (grade IV)). Moreover, we used RNA Seq V2 RSEM-based data from the TCGA dataset (Cell 2013 (Glioblastoma)) to analyze the correlations between NG2 and CK2 subunits.

4.16. Statistical Analysis

All data were tested for normal distribution and equal variance. Differences between two groups were assessed by the unpaired Student's *t*-test. To detect differences between multiple groups, one-way ANOVA was applied. This was followed by the Tukey post-hoc test, including the correction of the α-error according to Bonferroni probabilities. The association between NG2 and CK2 subunits was analyzed using the Spearman's correlation method. Statistics were performed by GraphPad Prism (version 8). All values are given as mean ± SD. Statistical significance was accepted for $p < 0.05$.

5. Conclusions

The expression of NG2 in GBM is associated with an aggressive clinical phenotype and poor prognosis. In the present study, we identified the protein kinase CK2 as a novel regulator of NG2 expression in GBM. We could demonstrate that inhibition of this kinase by CX-4945 as well as CK2 knockout significantly decreases the expression of NG2, resulting in a reduced proliferation and migration of GBM cells. In silico, analyses showed a positive correlation between CK2 and NG2 in TCGA-based data. More importantly, we detected a reduced NG2 expression after CX-4945 treatment in patient-derived GBM cells. In conclusion, inhibition of CK2 activity may represent a promising approach for NG2-positive GBM therapy.

Supplementary Materials: The following are available online at https://www.mdpi.com/article/10.3390/cancers13071678/s1, Figures S1–S20, S22–S37 are original uncropped Western blots from Figures 1, 4 and 6. Figure S21: (A and B) A1207 (A) and U87 (B) wild type and CK2α KO cells were lysed and the expression of NG2, Akt, pAkt^{S129}, CK2α, CK2α', CK2β and α-tubulin (as loading control) was analyzed by Western blot.

Author Contributions: B.M.S., A.S.B. and E.A. conceived and designed the experiments; B.M.S., A.S.B., C.G., S.U., J.O. and S.E.P. performed the experiments; B.M.S., A.S.B. and E.A. analyzed the data; E.A., S.U., M.W.L., J.O. and M.D.M. contributed to the reagents/materials/analysis tools; B.M.S., M.W.L., M.D.M. and E.A. wrote the paper. All authors have read and agreed to the published version of the manuscript.

Funding: The study was supported by HOMFORexzellenz 2016/2017.

Institutional Review Board Statement: The study was approved by the local German ethical board (Ethikkommission der Ärztekammer des Saarlandes, Saarbrücken, Germany, General Medical Council of the State Saarland, NO 93/16).

Informed Consent Statement: Informed consent was obtained from all subjects involved in the study.

Data Availability Statement: Data are contained within the article or supplementary materials.

Acknowledgments: The authors are grateful for the excellent technical assistance of Caroline Bickelmann.

Conflicts of Interest: The authors declare no conflict of interest.

References

1. Castello, J.; Ragnauth, A.; Friedman, E.; Rebholz, H. CK2-An Emerging Target for Neurological and Psychiatric Disorders. *Pharmaceuticals* **2017**, *10*, 7. [CrossRef]
2. Nunez de Villavicencio-Diaz, T.; Rabalski, A.J.; Litchfield, D.W. Protein Kinase CK2: Intricate Relationships within Regulatory Cellular Networks. *Pharmaceuticals* **2017**, *10*, 27. [CrossRef]
3. Salvi, M.; Sarno, S.; Cesaro, L.; Nakamura, H.; Pinna, L.A. Extraordinary pleiotropy of protein kinase CK2 revealed by weblogo phosphoproteome analysis. *Biochim. Biophys. Acta* **2009**, *1793*, 847–859. [CrossRef]
4. Ampofo, E.; Nalbach, L.; Menger, M.D.; Montenarh, M.; Gotz, C. Protein Kinase CK2-A Putative Target for the Therapy of Diabetes Mellitus? *Int. J. Mol. Sci.* **2019**, *20*, 4398. [CrossRef]
5. De Gooijer, M.C.; Guillen Navarro, M.; Bernards, R.; Wurdinger, T.; van Tellingen, O. An Experimenter's Guide to Glioblastoma Invasion Pathways. *Trends Mol. Med.* **2018**, *24*, 763–780. [CrossRef]
6. Ferrer-Font, L.; Villamanan, L.; Arias-Ramos, N.; Vilardell, J.; Plana, M.; Ruzzene, M.; Pinna, L.A.; Itarte, E.; Arus, C.; Candiota, A.P. Targeting Protein Kinase CK2: Evaluating CX-4945 Potential for GL261 Glioblastoma Therapy in Immunocompetent Mice. *Pharmaceuticals* **2017**, *10*, 24. [CrossRef]
7. Perea, S.E.; Baladron, I.; Garcia, Y.; Perera, Y.; Lopez, A.; Soriano, J.L.; Batista, N.; Palau, A.; Hernandez, I.; Farina, H.; et al. CIGB-300, a synthetic peptide-based drug that targets the CK2 phosphoacceptor domain. Translational and clinical research. *Mol. Cell Biochem.* **2011**, *356*, 45–50. [CrossRef]
8. Ruzzene, M.; Penzo, D.; Pinna, L.A. Protein kinase CK2 inhibitor 4,5,6,7-tetrabromobenzotriazole (TBB) induces apoptosis and caspase-dependent degradation of haematopoietic lineage cell-specific protein 1 (HS1) in Jurkat cells. *Biochem. J.* **2002**, *364*, 41–47. [CrossRef]
9. Siddiqui-Jain, A.; Drygin, D.; Streiner, N.; Chua, P.; Pierre, F.; O'Brien, S.E.; Bliesath, J.; Omori, M.; Huser, N.; Ho, C.; et al. CX-4945, an orally bioavailable selective inhibitor of protein kinase CK2, inhibits prosurvival and angiogenic signaling and exhibits antitumor efficacy. *Cancer Res.* **2010**, *70*, 10288–10298. [CrossRef]
10. Ampofo, E.; Schmitt, B.M.; Menger, M.D.; Laschke, M.W. The regulatory mechanisms of NG2/CSPG4 expression. *Cell. Mol. Biol. Lett.* **2017**, *22*, 4. [CrossRef]
11. Burg, M.A.; Nishiyama, A.; Stallcup, W.B. A central segment of the NG2 proteoglycan is critical for the ability of glioma cells to bind and migrate toward type VI collagen. *Exp. Cell Res.* **1997**, *235*, 254–264. [CrossRef]
12. Stallcup, W.B.; Huang, F.J. A role for the NG2 proteoglycan in glioma progression. *Cell Adh. Migr.* **2008**, *2*, 192–201. [CrossRef]
13. Stallcup, W.B. NG2 Proteoglycan Enhances Brain Tumor Progression by Promoting Beta-1 Integrin Activation in both Cis and Trans Orientations. *Cancers* **2017**, *9*, 31. [CrossRef]
14. Schmitt, B.M.; Laschke, M.W.; Rossler, O.G.; Huang, W.; Scheller, A.; Menger, M.D.; Ampofo, E. Nerve/glial antigen (NG) 2 is a crucial regulator of intercellular adhesion molecule (ICAM)-1 expression. *Biochim. Biophys. Acta Mol. Cell Res.* **2018**, *1865*, 57–66. [CrossRef] [PubMed]
15. Ferrara, G.; Errede, M.; Girolamo, F.; Morando, S.; Ivaldi, F.; Panini, N.; Bendotti, C.; Perris, R.; Furlan, R.; Virgintino, D.; et al. NG2, a common denominator for neuroinflammation, blood-brain barrier alteration, and oligodendrocyte precursor response in EAE, plays a role in dendritic cell activation. *Acta Neuropathol.* **2016**, *132*, 23–42. [CrossRef]

16. Fukushi, J.; Makagiansar, I.T.; Stallcup, W.B. NG2 proteoglycan promotes endothelial cell motility and angiogenesis via engagement of galectin-3 and alpha3beta1 integrin. *Mol. Biol. Cell* **2004**, *15*, 3580–3590. [CrossRef]
17. Ozerdem, U.; Stallcup, W.B. Pathological angiogenesis is reduced by targeting pericytes via the NG2 proteoglycan. *Angiogenesis* **2004**, *7*, 269–276. [CrossRef]
18. Rivera, Z.; Ferrone, S.; Wang, X.; Jube, S.; Yang, H.; Pass, H.I.; Kanodia, S.; Gaudino, G.; Carbone, M. CSPG4 as a target of antibody-based immunotherapy for malignant mesothelioma. *Clin. Cancer Res.* **2012**, *18*, 5352–5363. [CrossRef]
19. Schmitt, B.M.; Boewe, A.S.; Becker, V.; Nalbach, L.; Gu, Y.; Gotz, C.; Menger, M.D.; Laschke, M.W.; Ampofo, E. Protein Kinase CK2 Regulates Nerve/Glial Antigen (NG)2-Mediated Angiogenic Activity of Human Pericytes. *Cells* **2020**, *9*, 1546. [CrossRef]
20. Friedmann-Morvinski, D. Glioblastoma heterogeneity and cancer cell plasticity. *Crit. Rev. Oncog.* **2014**, *19*, 327–336. [CrossRef]
21. Rajaratnam, V.; Islam, M.M.; Yang, M.; Slaby, R.; Ramirez, H.M.; Mirza, S.P. Glioblastoma: Pathogenesis and Current Status of Chemotherapy and Other Novel Treatments. *Cancers* **2020**, *12*, 937. [CrossRef]
22. Schaff, L.R.; Yan, D.; Thyparambil, S.; Tian, Y.; Cecchi, F.; Rosenblum, M.; Reiner, A.S.; Panageas, K.S.; Hembrough, T.; Lin, A.L. Characterization of MGMT and EGFR protein expression in glioblastoma and association with survival. *J. Neurooncol.* **2020**, *146*, 163–170. [CrossRef]
23. Al-Mayhani, M.T.; Grenfell, R.; Narita, M.; Piccirillo, S.; Kenney-Herbert, E.; Fawcett, J.W.; Collins, V.P.; Ichimura, K.; Watts, C. NG2 expression in glioblastoma identifies an actively proliferating population with an aggressive molecular signature. *Neuro. Oncol.* **2011**, *13*, 830–845. [CrossRef]
24. Schiffer, D.; Mellai, M.; Boldorini, R.; Bisogno, I.; Grifoni, S.; Corona, C.; Bertero, L.; Cassoni, P.; Casalone, C.; Annovazzi, L. The Significance of Chondroitin Sulfate Proteoglycan 4 (CSPG4) in Human Gliomas. *Int. J. Mol. Sci.* **2018**, *19*, 2724. [CrossRef]
25. Tsidulko, A.Y.; Kazanskaya, G.M.; Kostromskaya, D.V.; Aidagulova, S.V.; Kiselev, R.S.; Volkov, A.M.; Kobozev, V.V.; Gaitan, A.S.; Krivoshapkin, A.L.; Grigorieva, E.V. Prognostic relevance of NG2/CSPG4, CD44 and Ki-67 in patients with glioblastoma. *Tumour Biol.* **2017**, *39*. [CrossRef]
26. Salizzato, V.; Zanin, S.; Borgo, C.; Lidron, E.; Salvi, M.; Rizzuto, R.; Pallafacchina, G.; Donella-Deana, A. Protein kinase CK2 subunits exert specific and coordinated functions in skeletal muscle differentiation and fusogenic activity. *FASEB J.* **2019**, *33*, 10648–10667. [CrossRef]
27. Parsons, D.W.; Jones, S.; Zhang, X.; Lin, J.C.; Leary, R.J.; Angenendt, P.; Mankoo, P.; Carter, H.; Siu, I.M.; Gallia, G.L.; et al. An integrated genomic analysis of human glioblastoma multiforme. *Science* **2008**, *321*, 1807–1812. [CrossRef]
28. Chon, H.J.; Bae, K.J.; Lee, Y.; Kim, J. The casein kinase 2 inhibitor, CX-4945, as an anti-cancer drug in treatment of human hematological malignancies. *Front. Pharmacol.* **2015**, *6*, 70. [CrossRef]
29. Liu, X.; Chen, J.; Li, W.; Hang, C.; Dai, Y. Inhibition of Casein Kinase II by CX-4945, But Not Yes-associated protein (YAP) by Verteporfin, Enhances the Antitumor Efficacy of Temozolomide in Glioblastoma. *Transl. Oncol.* **2020**, *13*, 70–78. [CrossRef]
30. Nitta, R.T.; Gholamin, S.; Feroze, A.H.; Agarwal, M.; Cheshier, S.H.; Mitra, S.S.; Li, G. Casein kinase 2alpha regulates glioblastoma brain tumor-initiating cell growth through the beta-catenin pathway. *Oncogene* **2015**, *34*, 3688–3699. [CrossRef]
31. Rowse, A.L.; Gibson, S.A.; Meares, G.P.; Rajbhandari, R.; Nozell, S.E.; Dees, K.J.; Hjelmeland, A.B.; McFarland, B.C.; Benveniste, E.N. Protein kinase CK2 is important for the function of glioblastoma brain tumor initiating cells. *J. Neurooncol.* **2017**, *132*, 219–229. [CrossRef]
32. Zheng, Y.; McFarland, B.C.; Drygin, D.; Yu, H.; Bellis, S.L.; Kim, H.; Bredel, M.; Benveniste, E.N. Targeting protein kinase CK2 suppresses prosurvival signaling pathways and growth of glioblastoma. *Clin. Cancer Res.* **2013**, *19*, 6484–6494. [CrossRef]
33. Qazi, M.A.; Vora, P.; Venugopal, C.; Sidhu, S.S.; Moffat, J.; Swanton, C.; Singh, S.K. Intratumoral heterogeneity: Pathways to treatment resistance and relapse in human glioblastoma. *Ann. Oncol.* **2017**, *28*, 1448–1456. [CrossRef]
34. Vartanian, A.; Singh, S.K.; Agnihotri, S.; Jalali, S.; Burrell, K.; Aldape, K.D.; Zadeh, G. GBM's multifaceted landscape: Highlighting regional and microenvironmental heterogeneity. *Neuro. Oncol.* **2014**, *16*, 1167–1175. [CrossRef]
35. O'Connor, L.; Gilmour, J.; Bonifer, C. The Role of the Ubiquitously Expressed Transcription Factor Sp1 in Tissue-specific Transcriptional Regulation and in Disease. *Yale J. Biol. Med.* **2016**, *89*, 513–525.
36. Kambe, A.; Yoshioka, H.; Kamitani, H.; Watanabe, T.; Baek, S.J.; Eling, T.E. The cyclooxygenase inhibitor sulindac sulfide inhibits EP4 expression and suppresses the growth of glioblastoma cells. *Cancer Prev. Res.* **2009**, *2*, 1088–1099. [CrossRef]
37. Park, M.H.; Ahn, B.H.; Hong, Y.K.; Min do, S. Overexpression of phospholipase D enhances matrix metalloproteinase-2 expression and glioma cell invasion via protein kinase C and protein kinase A/NF-kappaB/Sp1-mediated signaling pathways. *Carcinogenesis* **2009**, *30*, 356–365. [CrossRef]
38. Armstrong, S.A.; Barry, D.A.; Leggett, R.W.; Mueller, C.R. Casein kinase II-mediated phosphorylation of the C terminus of Sp1 decreases its DNA binding activity. *J. Biol. Chem.* **1997**, *272*, 13489–13495. [CrossRef]
39. Zhang, S.; Kim, K.H. Protein kinase CK2 down-regulates glucose-activated expression of the acetyl-CoA carboxylase gene. *Arch. Biochem. Biophys.* **1997**, *338*, 227–232. [CrossRef]
40. Makagiansar, I.T.; Williams, S.; Mustelin, T.; Stallcup, W.B. Differential phosphorylation of NG2 proteoglycan by ERK and PKCalpha helps balance cell proliferation and migration. *J. Cell Biol.* **2007**, *178*, 155–165. [CrossRef]
41. Girolamo, F.; Dallatomasina, A.; Rizzi, M.; Errede, M.; Walchli, T.; Mucignat, M.T.; Frei, K.; Roncali, L.; Perris, R.; Virgintino, D. Diversified expression of NG2/CSPG4 isoforms in glioblastoma and human foetal brain identifies pericyte subsets. *PLoS ONE* **2013**, *8*, e84883. [CrossRef] [PubMed]

42. Muir, E.M.; Fyfe, I.; Gardiner, S.; Li, L.; Warren, P.; Fawcett, J.W.; Keynes, R.J.; Rogers, J.H. Modification of N-glycosylation sites allows secretion of bacterial chondroitinase ABC from mammalian cells. *J. Biotechnol.* **2010**, *145*, 103–110. [CrossRef] [PubMed]
43. Kim, J.; Hwan Kim, S. CK2 inhibitor CX-4945 blocks TGF-beta1-induced epithelial-to-mesenchymal transition in A549 human lung adenocarcinoma cells. *PLoS ONE* **2013**, *8*, e74342.
44. You, W.K.; Yotsumoto, F.; Sakimura, K.; Adams, R.H.; Stallcup, W.B. NG2 proteoglycan promotes tumor vascularization via integrin-dependent effects on pericyte function. *Angiogenesis* **2014**, *17*, 61–76. [CrossRef] [PubMed]
45. Wang, J.; Svendsen, A.; Kmiecik, J.; Immervoll, H.; Skaftnesmo, K.O.; Planaguma, J.; Reed, R.K.; Bjerkvig, R.; Miletic, H.; Enger, P.O.; et al. Targeting the NG2/CSPG4 proteoglycan retards tumour growth and angiogenesis in preclinical models of GBM and melanoma. *PLoS ONE* **2011**, *6*, e23062. [CrossRef] [PubMed]
46. Wade, A.; Robinson, A.E.; Engler, J.R.; Petritsch, C.; James, C.D.; Phillips, J.J. Proteoglycans and their roles in brain cancer. *FEBS J.* **2013**, *280*, 2399–2417. [CrossRef] [PubMed]
47. Ilieva, K.M.; Cheung, A.; Mele, S.; Chiaruttini, G.; Crescioli, S.; Griffin, M.; Nakamura, M.; Spicer, J.F.; Tsoka, S.; Lacy, K.E.; et al. Chondroitin Sulfate Proteoglycan 4 and Its Potential As an Antibody Immunotherapy Target across Different Tumor Types. *Front. Immunol.* **2017**, *8*, 1911. [CrossRef]
48. Bredel, M.; Scholtens, D.M.; Harsh, G.R.; Bredel, C.; Chandler, J.P.; Renfrow, J.J.; Yadav, A.K.; Vogel, H.; Scheck, A.C.; Tibshirani, R.; et al. A network model of a cooperative genetic landscape in brain tumors. *JAMA* **2009**, *302*, 261–275. [CrossRef]
49. Seidel, S.; Garvalov, B.K.; Acker, T. Isolation and culture of primary glioblastoma cells from human tumor specimens. *Methods Mol. Biol.* **2015**, *1235*, 263–275.
50. Faust, M.; Schuster, N.; Montenarh, M. Specific binding of protein kinase CK2 catalytic subunits to tubulin. *FEBS Lett.* **1999**, *462*, 51–56. [CrossRef]
51. Lerner, C.; Ketter, R.; Linsler, S.; Henn, W.; Oertel, J.; Urbschat, S. Establishment of a molecular cytogenetic analysis for native tumor tissue of meningiomas-suitable for clinical application. *Mol. Cytogenet.* **2014**, *7*, 12. [CrossRef]
52. Ampofo, E.; Rudzitis-Auth, J.; Dahmke, I.N.; Rossler, O.G.; Thiel, G.; Montenarh, M.; Menger, M.D.; Laschke, M.W. Inhibition of protein kinase CK2 suppresses tumor necrosis factor (TNF)-alpha-induced leukocyte-endothelial cell interaction. *Biochim. Biophys. Acta* **2015**, *1852*, 2123–2136. [CrossRef]
53. Borgo, C.; Franchin, C.; Scalco, S.; Bosello-Travain, V.; Donella-Deana, A.; Arrigoni, G.; Salvi, M.; Pinna, L.A. Generation and quantitative proteomics analysis of CK2alpha/alpha'((−/−)) cells. *Sci. Rep.* **2017**, *7*, 42409. [CrossRef]
54. Cerami, E.; Gao, J.; Dogrusoz, U.; Gross, B.E.; Sumer, S.O.; Aksoy, B.A.; Jacobsen, A.; Byrne, C.J.; Heuer, M.L.; Larsson, E.; et al. The cBio cancer genomics portal: An open platform for exploring multidimensional cancer genomics data. *Cancer Discov.* **2012**, *2*, 401–404. [CrossRef]
55. Gao, J.; Aksoy, B.A.; Dogrusoz, U.; Dresdner, G.; Gross, B.; Sumer, S.O.; Sun, Y.; Jacobsen, A.; Sinha, R.; Larsson, E.; et al. Integrative analysis of complex cancer genomics and clinical profiles using the cBioPortal. *Sci. Signal.* **2013**, *6*, pl1. [CrossRef]

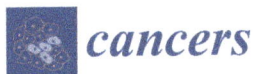

Review

Viral Vectors as Gene Therapy Agents for Treatment of Glioblastoma

Oleg Mozhei [1,*], Anja G. Teschemacher [2] and Sergey Kasparov [1,2,*]

1. School of Life Sciences, Immanuel Kant Baltic Federal University, 236041 Kaliningrad, Russia
2. School of Physiology, Neuroscience and Pharmacology, University of Bristol, Bristol BS8 1TD, UK; anja.teschemacher@bristol.ac.uk
* Correspondence: omozhei@gmail.com (O.M.); Sergey.Kasparov@Bristol.ac.uk (S.K.)

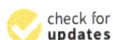

Received: 21 October 2020; Accepted: 7 December 2020; Published: 11 December 2020

Simple Summary: Glioblastoma is the most malignant cancer of the brain and current therapeutic strategies are clearly inadequate. In addition to surgical intervention, conventional drugs and ratio-therapy, scientists are looking at approaches based on gene therapy with genetically modified viruses. In this review we give a snapshot of the current state of play in this field of research and the available information about the clinical trials. We make some suggestions as to what opportunities could be explored further and hope that this review will stimulate discussion and conception of new life saving strategies.

Abstract: In this review, we scrutinize the idea of using viral vectors either as cytotoxic agents or gene delivery tools for treatment of glioblastoma multiforme (GBM) in light of the experience that our laboratory has accumulated over ~20 years when using similar vectors in experimental neuroscience. We review molecular strategies and current clinical trials and argue that approaches which are based on targeting a specific biochemical pathway or a characteristic mutation are inherently prone to failure because of the high genomic instability and clonal selection characteristics of GBM. For the same reasons, attempts to develop a viral system which selectively transduces only GBM cells are also unlikely to be universally successful. One of the common gene therapy approaches is to use cytotoxic viruses which replicate and cause preferential lysis of the GBM cells. This strategy, in addition to its reliance on the specific biochemical makeup of the GBM cells, bears a risk of necrotic cell death accompanied by release of large quantities of pro-inflammatory molecules. On the other hand, engaging the immune system in the anti-GBM response seems to be a potential avenue to explore further. We suggest that a plausible strategy is to focus on viral vectors which efficiently transduce brain cells via a non-selective, ubiquitous mechanism and which target (ideally irreversibly) processes that are critical only for dividing tumor cells and are dispensable for quiescent brain cells.

Keywords: gene therapy; glioblastoma; glioma; viral vectors

1. Introduction

Glioblastoma multiforme (GBM) is a highly malignant primary brain cancer of predominantly astrocytic origin [1]. The main features of GBM that lead to malignancy and high mortality are its high resistance to DNA-damaging drugs, including the only Food and Drug Administration FDA-approved alkylating agent temozolomide (TMZ), which is achieved by O6-methylguanine-DNA methyltransferase overexpression, moderate response to radiation, genomic instability and powerful clonal selection. A particularly grave feature of GBM is its high invasiveness.

New insights into the genomic landscape of GBM revealed typical mutations in an array of genes, including *TERT, PTEN, IDH1, IDH2, TP53, ATRX, PIK3CA, PIK3R1, NF1, H3F3A, CDKN2A, EGFR,*

PDGFRA, MET, CDK4, CDK6, MDM2, MDM4 [2]. Traditionally, based largely on neuroanatomical considerations, gliomas were subdivided into four grades. Glioblastoma is the most malignant (grade IV) glioma [3].

The introduction by the World Health Organisation (WHO), in 2016, of the "integrated" classification based on histology and genetics was developed in the hope of improving diagnostic accuracy, patient management and prognosis of the response to treatments [4]. However, as of today, most of the treatment algorithms are not based on molecular histological characteristics and are essentially universal, consisting of maximal surgical resection, followed by radiotherapy and chemotherapy with TMZ, followed by TMZ, known as the "Stupp protocol" [5,6].

Unfortunately, even this aggressive treatment has low efficiency, with survival rates remaining between 12 and 15 months and the 3-year survival rate only at about 15%. Despite introduction of newer treatments, such as Carmustine wafers, the monoclonal antibody bevacizumab and cyclin-dependent kinases (CDK) inhibitors, GBM is still an essentially incurable disease, resulting in a patient death rate of more than 95% within five years of diagnosis.

Even though classic metastases are exceedingly rare in GBM, its cells have a tendency to migrate into the parenchyma and eventually spread extensively throughout the brain. For this reason, already upon primary diagnosis, some patients have infiltration in more than one part of the brain, with tumor cells moving across the corpus callosum or through the walls of the ventricles. In cases such as those, surgery may be performed only for the sake of decompression but has little effect on the overall progression of the disease. The only feasible option to pursue, then, is systemic pharmacotherapy and radiotherapy. However, GBM presents formidable challenges for traditional drug design. Movement of drugs across the blood–brain barrier (BBB) is a significant problem because it depends on too many factors (charge, molecular weight and conformation, hydrophobicity, presence of specific transporters, vascularization of the tumor, etc.). Moreover, the relationship between these factors and drug transfer across the BBB is non-linear. It is estimated that less than 2% of small-molecule drugs and no large-molecule drugs or nucleic acid-based constructs can reach the brain because of the BBB [7]. Insufficient saturation of brain tissue with anti-cancer drugs allows GBM cells to benefit from the selection of the most aggressive and drug-resistant subclones. In addition, tumors engage various efflux transport systems (for instance, ATP-binding cassette sub-family B member 1 (*ABCB1*) gene, which extrude drugs from cancer cells) [8]. The other well-known mechanism of tumor defense is expression of high levels of the DNA repair enzyme O6-methylguanine-DNA methyltransferase, mentioned above [9].

However, upon initial diagnosis, GBM tumors frequently appear relatively well-localized and surgically accessible. Nevertheless, due to the infiltration, tumors almost inevitably reoccur after resection, typically originating from sites adjacent to the surgical cavity. Surgeons are limited in their actions because GBM often grows near critical regions of the brain (major nerve tracts, essential centers and large blood vessels). Damage to those areas is too risky and may cause severe disabilities or even be lethal. In cases of well-localized and relatively superficial primary GBM, the key task is, therefore, the prevention of infiltration around the surgical cavity. Here is the scope for locally delivered therapies, such as slow-release formulations of anti-cancer drugs [10], photodynamic therapy [11] or viral vectors, which are the topic of this review.

2. Molecular Strategies for Viral Gene Therapy of the GBM

For patients with well-localized primary GBM, one could envisage a strategy where after the de-bulking surgery, the adjacent parenchyma is infiltrated by viral gene therapy vectors which selectively destroy the GBM cells. In a more dramatic scenario, a viral gene therapy tool could be injected systemically, selectively affecting tumor cells in the whole of the CNS and eliminate them. Attempts to develop gene therapy with the aid of viral vectors have been under development for some time, and below, we summarize some of the main strategies and their outcomes.

1. Oncolytic viruses which destroy tumor cells were amongst the first vectors which were tested in patients. The rationale for this approach was based on pre-clinical data demonstrating that some strains of various viruses replicate well only in tumor cell lines. It was then suggested that it is possible to selectively destroy cancer cells in situ, with minimal impact on normal cells. In clinical studies, either wild-type or genetically engineered viruses were used; the specificity of the latter was enhanced by targeted changes in their genomes. It needs to be stressed that oncolytic viruses are able to destroy any cells which they invade and, unless tightly controlled by an additional mechanism, might cause excessive tumor necrosis and dangerous brain oedema [12,13]. While several viral progenitors have been used (see Section 2.1 below), the first oncolytic viruses were wild-type viruses, followed by second generations of genetically modified viruses and third-generation vectors equipped with transgenes to further induce therapeutic effects [12].

2. Suicide gene therapy is based on heterologous expression of *Escherichia coli* or yeast cytosine deaminase or *Herpes simplex* virus thymidine kinase in the cancer cells [14]. Cytosine deaminase converts the prodrug 5-Fluorocytosine (5-FC) to a toxic 5-Fluorouracil (5-FU) metabolite, whereas thymidine kinase (HSV-tk) converts ganciclovir to ganciclovir monophosphate, which, in turn, is converted to toxic ganciclovir triphosphate by tumor cells' enzymes. This leads to damage and lysis of transgene-expressing cells and those surrounding them (so-called bystander effect).

3. Immunomodulatory vectors aim to engage a strong immune response against the GBM cells. This can be achieved by expression of strong antigens on tumor cells' surface or by the production of factors which stimulate and attract the immune cells.

4. Introduction of anti-oncogenes and tumor suppressors in cancer cells aims to decrease proliferation, stimulate differentiation or induce apoptosis by a dominant gain-of-function effect.

To achieve maximum efficiency, some approaches can be combined. For example, an oncolytic effect may accompany release of immunomodulatory proteins expressed by genes delivered with a viral vector.

2.1. Viral Vector Types Proposed for Gene Therapy of GBM

The effectiveness of gene therapy tools is a function of virus biology, mechanism of action, specificity and replication competency. If the viral genome is partially deleted to prevent replication, this clears room for the delivery of the therapeutic genes. If, however, the virus is allowed to replicate, it will cause cytopathic effects, lysis and new virions will proceed to infect other cells. There are currently over 20 viral vectors that have been used in clinical trials for gene therapy of GBM, as summarized in Table 1. Figure 1 describes the selection criteria.

Table 1. Comparison of key features of viral vectors proposed for treatment of GBM.

Name	Structure of Vector	Mechanism of Action	Specificity	Replication Competent
DNX2401	Ad5	Lytic viral cycle in targeted cells	Replicate in cells defective in the Rb/p16 tumor suppressor pathway and expressing integrins $\alpha v \beta 3$ and $\alpha v \beta 5$	±
DNX2440	Ad5	Lytic viral cycle in targeted cells and immunomodulatory effect	Replicate in cells defective in the Rb/p16 tumor suppressor pathway and expressing integrins $\alpha v \beta 3$ and $\alpha v \beta 5$	±
ONYX-015	chimeric Ad2 and Ad5	Lytic viral cycle in targeted cells	Replicate in tumor cells with altered p53 pathway	±
Ad-hCMV-TK	Ad5	Converts harmless ganciclovir to toxic product in transduced cells	Transduce CAR-expressing cells. CMV-dependent expression mechanism	−
ADV/HSV-tk	Ad5	Converts harmless ganciclovir to toxic product in transduced cells	Transduce CAR-expressing cells. RSV-dependent expression mechanism	−

Table 1. Cont.

Name	Structure of Vector	Mechanism of Action	Specificity	Replication Competent
Ad-hCMV-Flt3L	Ad5	Immunomodulatory effect by stimulating both the proliferation of dendritic cells (DCs) and their migration to the tumor site	Transduce CAR expressing cells	−
Ad-RTS-hIL12	Ad5	Immunomodulatory effect by activation of immune system via IL-12 release	Transduce CAR-expressing cells	−
Ad.hIFN-β	Ad5	Immunomodulatory effect by activation of immune system via human Interferon-β release	Transduce CAR-expressing cells	−
VB-111	Ad5	Decrease excessive angiogenesis via inhibition of endothelial cells	Transduce CAR-expressing cells, promotor initializes transcription only in endothelial cells undergoing angiogenesis	−
HSV 1716	HSV-1	Lytic viral cycle in targeted cells and indirect T cell-mediated cell death	Replication in PKR-deficient cells	±
G207	HSV-1	Lytic viral cycle in targeted cells and indirect T cell-mediated cell death	Replication in PKR-deficient and fast dividing cells	±
C134	HSV-1	Lytic viral cycle in targeted cells and indirect T cell-mediated cell death	Replication in PKR-deficient and fast dividing cells	±
rQNestin34.5v.2	HSV-1	Lytic viral cycle in targeted cells and indirect T-cell mediated cell death	Replication in PKR-deficient, Nestin-positive and fast dividing cells	±
M032-HSV-1	HSV-1	Lytic viral cycle in targeted cells, indirect T-cell mediated cell death and immune system stimulation via IL12 release	Replication in PKR-defective and fast dividing cells	±
Pelareorep (Reolysin)	Wild-type reovirus	Lytic viral cycle in targeted cells	Replication in ras-positive cells	+
ParvOryx	Wild-type parvovirus	Lytic viral cycle in targeted cells	Replication in fast dividing cells	+
NDV-HUJ	Wild-type HUJ strain of Newcastle disease virus	Livin-mediated apoptosis	Replication in fast dividing cells, apoptosis of livin-positive cells	+
PVSRIPO	Recombinant poliovirus type 1	Lytic viral cycle in targeted cells	Replication restricted to CD155-expressing non-neuronal cells	+
Toca 511	Recombinant Gammaretrovirus	CD-mediated prodrug conversion to cytotoxic drug in transduced cells	Replication in fast dividing cells	+
TG6002	Recombinant vaccinia virus	Lytic viral cycle in targeted cells, CD-mediated prodrug conversion	Replication in cells expressing ribonucleotide reductase	+
MV-CEA	Recombinant measles virus	Lytic viral cycle in targeted cells	Transduce CD46-expressing cells	+

In relation to the ability to replicate, + denotes replication competent vectors, − stands for replication incompetent ones and ± for conditionally replication competent vectors. CAR-chimeric antigen receptor; CMV–cytomegalovirus; RSV-rous sarcoma virus; PKR-protein kinase R; HUJ-Hebrew University, Jerusalem; CD-cytosine deaminase.

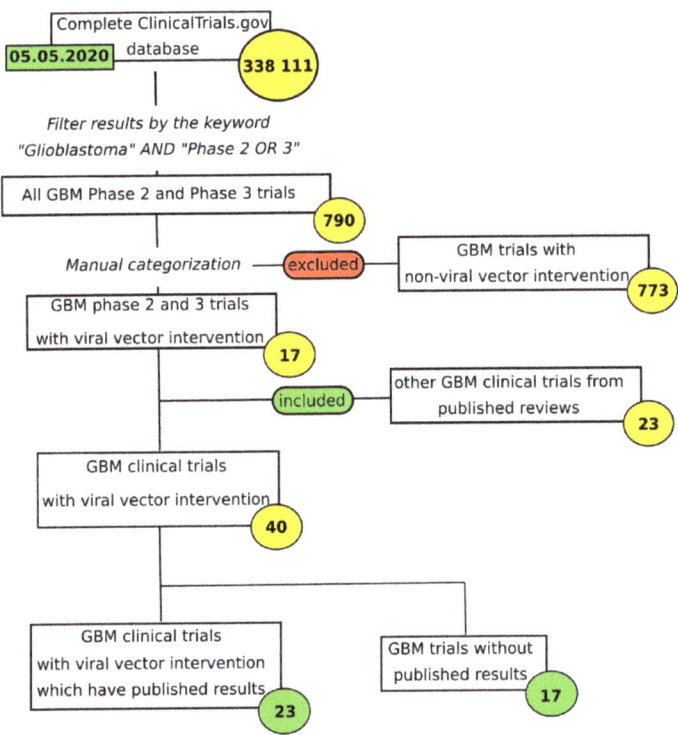

Figure 1. Selection and inclusion criteria for review of glioblastoma multiforme (GBM)-targeting viral vector trials.

2.2. Adenovirus-Based Vectors

Adenovirus (Ad) is a double-stranded DNA virus (Baltimore Classification class I [15]) without an envelope [16]. There are at least 57 serotypes of human Ad, Ad1–Ad57, in seven species, A–G [17]. The human Ad genome contains five early transcription units (E1A, E1B, E2, E3 and E4), four intermediate and one late transcription unit [17]. Main modification of Ad genome are shown in Figure 2. Viral entry is coxsackie-adenovirus receptor (CAR)-dependent. One of the crucial steps in the adenoviral replication cycle is interaction of the *E1A* gene product with E2F-Rb or E2F-DP1 transcription complexes to force the infected cell into the S phase since it is helps the virus to use the cellular DNA replication machinery to replicate its own genome [18]. These processes can be altered to achieve increased selectivity towards GBM and will be discussed later. Most Ad vectors originate from Ad5 (Species C). Non-replicating Ads are widely used as experimental gene delivery tools, while replicating Ads have been engineered to be tumor-specific agents. The conventional strategy to achieve replication deficiency is to delete *E1* and *E3* genes. The genomes of such vectors, after entering the target cell nucleus, remain as additional DNA elements not integrated into the chromosomes (i.e., episomal). This has major implications for their fate in the cancer, as well as in any other dividing cells, because after a few divisions, episomes which do not replicate are diluted and expression drops rapidly.

The strategies for targeting Ad vectors to GBM include (1) use of tumor-specific promoters; (2) deletion of critical viral genes which are supplied by tumor cells in trans; (3) modification of the viral capsid to enable selective entry into GBM cells.

ONYX-015 was the first oncolytic Ad vector to be described [19]. This is a recombinant selectively replication-competent chimeric Ad2 and Ad5 vector [17]. ONYX-015 lacks the *E1B* gene. The normal function of the protein encoded by *E1B* is to inactivate p53 protein in infected cells. Thus, ONYX-015 was expected to replicate only in p53-deficient cells [20], but later, it was found that ONYX replication is not, in fact, p53-dependent [21,22].

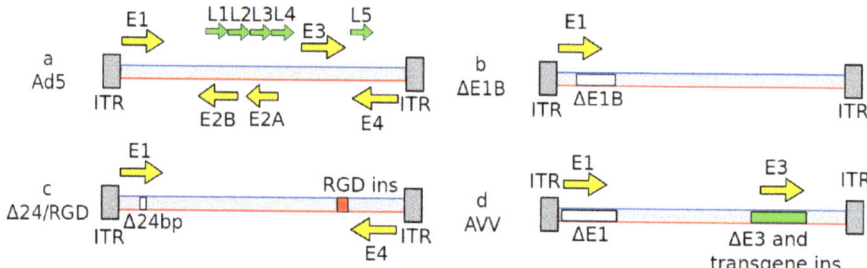

Figure 2. Schematic of the genome structures of adenovirus type 5 (Ad5) and Ad5-based vectors. (**a**) Wild-type Ad5 virus. Arrows indicate transcriptional units. ITR—Inverted terminal repeat. (**b**) In the ONYX-015 adenoviral vector, the *E1B* gene is deleted. (**c**) DNX-2401 adenoviral vector structure. Δ24 bp indicates 24 base pairs' deletion in the Rb-binding domain of the E1A gene; RGD ins indicates an insertion of an additional peptide sequence in the Ad fiber-encoding part of the genome. (**d**) Adenoviral vectors, often referred as AVVs in the literature, are replication-incompetent viral particles produced by deleting *E1* and *E3* genes and inserting a desired transgene. Such vectors are widely used in experimental neuroscience for gene delivery by various groups, including ourselves [23–25].

DNX2401 (Delta-24-RGD) is a recombinant serotype 5 strain Ad [26]. This oncolytic vector has two modifications in its genome that make it selectively replication-competent in cells defective in the Rb/p16 tumor suppressor pathway. The first modification is the 24-bp deletion (bp 923–946) in the Rb-binding domain of the *E1A* gene [26]. Under normal circumstances, viral E1A proteins promote cells towards a mitotic state by releasing E2F transcriptional factors from the block by Rb proteins. The unstable version of the *E1A* gene in DNX2401 cannot bind to E2F-Rb or E2F-DP1 transcription complexes and release E1A. This prevents replication in cells with a normal Rb/p16 tumor suppressor pathway. GBM often have defective Rb/p16 tumor suppressor pathways, which makes it possible for viruses to replicate selectively in GBM cells because cells are free from the Rb/p16 block anyway. Most cancer cells lack, or poorly express, CAR receptors required for adenovirus binding and internalization. To circumvent this problem, the second modification, an additional RGD peptide sequence in the HI loop of the Ad fiber, allows the virus to bind to cells expressing integrins $\alpha v \beta 3$ and $\alpha v \beta 5$ which are found on the surface of most cancer cells, including glioma and GBM [26,27].

DNX-2440 (Delta-24-RGDOX) is an immunomodulatory recombinant selectively replication-competent serotype 5 strain Ad-encoding OX40 ligand (OX40L) driven by the cytomegalovirus (CMV) promoter. The protein is able to activate T cells via interaction with its receptor on the surface of T lymphocytes [28,29].

AVV-CMV-HSV-tk (Ad-hCMV-TK) uses the suicide gene strategy and is a recombinant replication-defective serotype 5 Ad with *Herpes simplex virus thymidine kinase (HSV-tk)* gene under the transcriptional control of the CMV promoter [30]. CMV is often referred to as ubiquitously and constitutively active. However, experimental neuroscience demonstrated that this is, in fact, not the case, since CMV-bearing viral vectors effectively drive expression only in some cell types in the normal rodent brain and expression may be transient [31]. It follows that the brain cells have mechanisms to silence CMV and this may very well apply to the clones within GBM.

AVV-RSV-HSV-tk (ADV/HSV-tk) is a similar suicide gene virus but expresses *HSV-tk* under control of Rous sarcoma virus long-terminal-repeat promoter (RSV) [32]. The RSV promoter is considered a strong constitutive promoter, similar to CMV. RSV, in comparison with CMV, exhibits a lag phase prior to the onset of viral DNA replication and has a somewhat different profile of tissue-specific expression, although it is not entirely clear whether this confers an advantage in this case [33].

Ad-hCMV-Flt3L is a recombinant replication-deficient serotype 5 Ad for CMV promoter-driven expression of human fms-like tyrosine kinase 3 ligand (Flt3L). Flt3L is a hematopoietic growth factor and ligand for the Flt3 tyrosine kinase receptor, which is expressed on the surface of dendritic cells (DCs). The transgene provides an immunomodulatory effect by stimulating both the proliferation of dendritic cells and their migration to the tumor site. The vector is usually used with other conventional drugs for eliciting a stronger response to GBM via release of Flt3L from destroyed cells [34].

Ad-RTS-hIL12 also aims at immunomodulation. It is a recombinant replication-deficient serotype 5 Ad-encoding human pro-inflammatory interleukin-12 (IL-12: hIL indicates human origin of the gene) gene under control of RheoSwitch Therapeutic System (RTS) promoter. RTS is an artificial veledimex-inducible promoter that leads to uniform and long-term release of interleukin-12 in the tumor area after a single vector injection. This system is based on recruiting transcription factor to a synthetic promoter via Gal4–Gal4-binding site interactions [35]. The cassette consists of Gal4-EcR fusion protein sequence, internal ribosome entry site (IRES) linker and *VP16-RXR fusion protein* gene and is driven by *human ubiquitin C* gene promoter (Figure 3). Upstream, there is a customizable promoter with Gal4 binding sites to which these fusion proteins are recruited and the target gene is transcribed [35]. IL-12 activates the immune system, which may result in immune-mediated tumor cell lysis and inhibition of cancer cell proliferation [36].

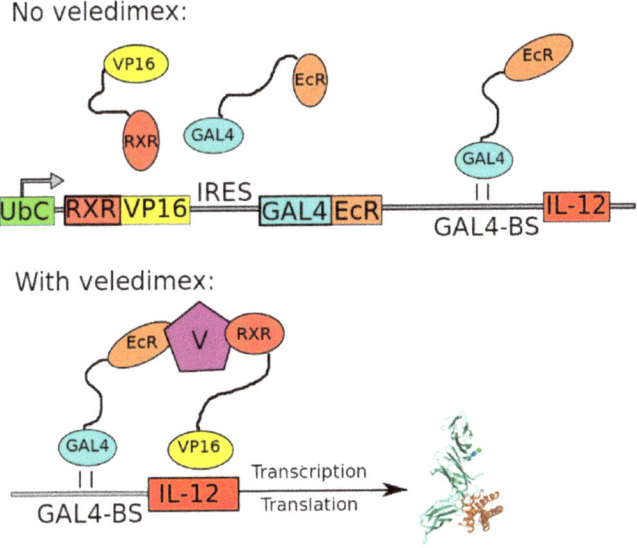

Figure 3. Schematic representation of *RTS* gene switch cassettes. Upon administration of veledimex, RXR-VP16 and GAL4-EcR proteins dimerize and activate transgene expression. The GAL4 domain recognizes unique specific binding sites (GAL4-BS) while VP16 acts as a powerful activation of transcription in mammalian cells. The protein 3D structure was adopted from Yoon et al. [37].

Ad.hIFN-β is another immunomodulating replication-defective serotype 5 Ad-encoding human *Interferon-β (IFN-β)* gene under control of CMV promoter [38]. Interferon-β (IFN-β) is a pleiotropic cytokine with anti-tumor activity which demonstrated promising outcomes in some clinical trials [39]. However, overall efficacy was limited and transient mainly because of high-dose toxicity (myelosuppression, transaminitis, neurotoxicity, including seizures, etc.) [38]. To overcome this limitation, Ad.hIFN-β was developed to drive synthesis of Interferon-β in cancer cells. A schematic representation of the genome is shown in Figure 2.

VB-111 is recombinant replication-defective serotype 5 Ad-encoding Fas-TNFR-1 gene under control of pre-proendothelin-1 promoter. The promoter was chosen with the aim of achieving selectivity to endothelial cells undergoing angiogenesis. Cell apoptosis is induced when circulating TNF-α interacts with the Fas-TNFR-1 receptor [40]. The expected outcome is the prevention of vascularization and, therefore, metabolic insult to the tumor.

As mentioned above, replication-incompetent Ad vectors stay episomal in the transduced cells and are not propagated when the cell divides. This leads to a rapid dilution of the viral genomes in any dividing cells, such as GBM. In this respect, replication-competent viruses, such as ONYX-015, are different because they replicate in the affected cells. The downside of this strategy is the lack of control over the spread of the virus and infection of the healthy cells, which then, inevitably, become targets for 5FC. In addition, release of the activated, toxic products of pro-drugs non-selectively kills adjacent cells (the "bystander effect").

2.3. Herpes Simplex Virus-Based Vectors

Herpes simplex virus (HSV) is an enveloped double-stranded DNA virus (Class I according to the Baltimore classification [15]). HSV can target both dividing and non-dividing cells and has broad tropism but predominantly infects neurons. Herpes viruses are classified into subfamilies, and for gene therapy applications, HSV-1 is used. The genome of HSV-1 is ~150 kbp long and can, therefore, potentially carry a substantial payload (Figure 4). During the viral life cycle, HSV-1 remains episomal as a circular DNA molecule [41].

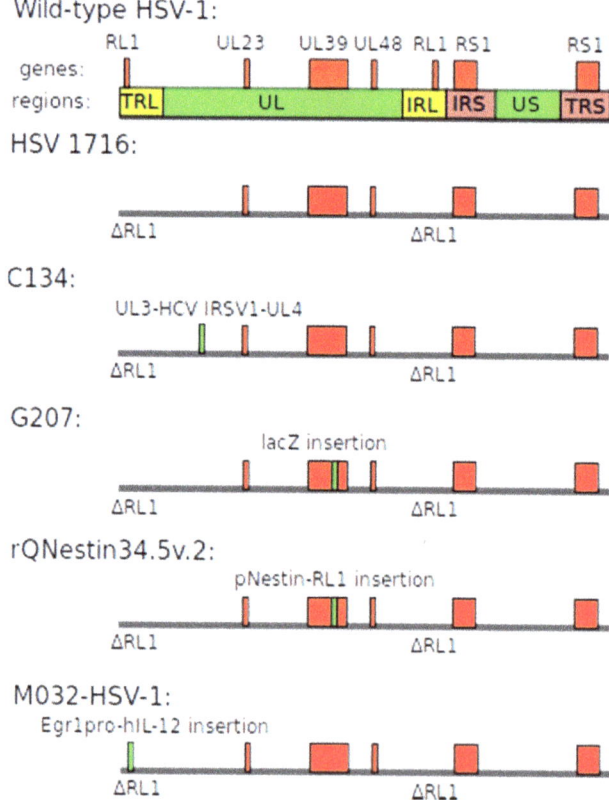

Figure 4. Schematic of the *Herpes simplex* virus 1 (HSV-1)-based vectors. The genome of wild-type HSV-1 can be divided into six regions which contain specific genes. Information about specific vectors is provided in the text.

The RL1 gene (also known as γ34.5), one of the essential genes for replication, can be used to modulate specificity. During viral replication, the host cellular defense system typically responds with translational arrest and reduction in the global synthesis of viral and cellular proteins [42]. This process is facilitated by phosphorylation of the translation initiation factor eIF2α by protein kinase R (PKR). *RL1* gene encodes The Infected Cell Protein 34.5 (ICP34.5), also known as Neurovirulence factor ICP34.5. This multifunctional protein binds and retargets the host phosphatase PP1α to eIF2α, thus reversing the phosphorylation and the shutdown of the protein synthesis [43]. Mutated ICP34.5 is unable to counteract PKR action, which, theoretically, should protect healthy cells. Since in tumors, the PKR pathway is often inhibited, lack of ICP34.5 function does not limit viral replication and should result in selective replication of this mutated HSV-1 in such cancer cells.

The other important HSV-1 gene is UL39, which encodes the large subunit of ribonucleotide reductase, also known as ICP6. The ribonucleotide reductase complex converts ribonucleotides to deoxyribonucleotides needed for viral DNA replication. The host ribonucleotide reductase enzyme is highly active only in mitotic cells. Thus, UL39-defective HSV-1 UL39 cannot replicate efficiently in non-dividing cells [44]. Specific examples are given below.

HSV 1716 is an oncolytic recombinant replication-competent HSV-1. Deletions in both copies of the *RL1* gene (see above) were made with the aim to permit replication only in PKR-defective tumor cells [45].

C134 is an oncolytic HSV-1. In this virus, *RL1* genes are deleted and human cytomegalovirus (HCMV) *IRS1* gene was inserted between *UL3* and *UL4* genes [46]. The *IRS1* gene enhances replication in fast dividing tumor cells [46]. The exact molecular mechanism of action of IRS1 protein is still not known.

G207 is an oncolytic recombinant replication-competent HSV-1 which has two modifications to increase specificity towards GBM cells: deletions in both copies of the *RL1* gene to target PKR-defective cancer cells and disruption of *UL39* gene to eliminate the possibility to replicate in non-dividing normal cells. During the lytic phase, the vector causes direct cytopathic effect and indirect T cell-mediated cell death [47].

rQNestin34.5v.2 is a recombinant HSV-1 also devoid of *UL39* and all *RL1* genes. Lack of *RL1* gene should limit replication in normal cells via the mechanism explained above. Instead, this vector carries one copy of *RL1* gene under transcriptional control of the nestin promoter, which is frequently upregulated in gliomas [48]. Thus, nestin promoter is expected to drive expression of functional ICP34.5 selectively in glioma cells, resulting in a cytopathic effect. It is worth noting that the selectivity of this promoter is not widely known and that nestin is also expressed in normal brain cells [49].

M032-HSV-1 is a combined (oncolytic and immunomodulatory) replication-competent HSV-1. The virus has deletions of both copies of the *R1* (γ34.5) gene and inserted *interleukin-12 (IL-12)* gene [50]. Deletions limit replication to PKR-defective tumor cells. In addition, interleukin-12 promotes an immune response against surviving tumor cells and decreases angiogenesis.

2.4. Vectors Based on other Viral Backgrounds

Pelareorep (Reolysin) is a human wild-type reovirus [51,52]. Reovirus is a non-enveloped double-stranded RNA virus (Class III according to the Baltimore Classification [15]). It causes mild infections in humans—for instance, gastroenteritis. Reoviruses can be used as oncolytic agents because they replicate predominantly in cells where the Ras pathway is highly active, as is typical for many cancers [53]. Specific examples are provided in Tables 1 and 2.

Newcastle disease virus (NDV) is a single-stranded enveloped RNA virus whose natural host is poultry. It has been shown that the virus can induce apoptosis in melanoma cultures overexpressing a protein called Livin, encoded by the BIRC7 gene. This protein belongs to a family of anti-apoptotic proteins which are commonly overexpressed by tumors and it has been demonstrated that melanoma tumor cells that do not express Livin are relatively resistant to the virus [54]. Attempts have been made to use it against GBM [54]. NDV-HUJ is a wild-type oncolytic HUJ strain of Newcastle disease virus.

ParvOryx, or H-1PV, is an oncolytic wild-type parvovirus, a small single-stranded DNA virus (Class II according to the Baltimore classification [15]) without an envelope. In nature, this is a rodent virus, but H-1PV is able to infect cells of other species, including humans. Replication of H-1PV greatly depends on the activity of the host enzymes expressed during the S-phase, making it selectively replication-competent in fast dividing cancer cells [55].

PVSRIPO is a poliovirus type 1 (Sabin type) viral vector with its cognate internal ribosome entry site (IRES) replaced with that of human rhinovirus type 2. The vector binds to CD155 (poliovirus receptor, PVR or NECL5), internalizes and eventually causes tumor cell lysis [56]. The exchange of the IRES should, in theory, restrict replication in cells of neuronal origin [56].

Toca 511 is a replicating gamma-retrovirus which carries a *yeast cytosine deaminase (CD)* gene. Administration of 5-FC leads to generation of toxic 5-FU by CD [57]. As a result, tumor cells infected by this virus should die and release 5-FU, which can cause the bystander effect [58]. The vector has specificity for replicating cells, and replication in non-malignant cells in vivo is reportedly insignificant [59].

TG6002—recombinant vaccinia viral vector, also encoding the suicide gene *CD* [60]. Vaccinia virus is a 190-kbp dsDNA-enveloped virus which causes small pox [61]. To increase safety and specificity to fast dividing cells, the *J2R* gene (encoding thymidine kinase) and the *I4L* gene (encoding the large subunit of the ribonucleotide reductase) were deleted [61].

MV-CEA is a recombinant Edmonston strain of measles virus, expressing a soluble extracellular N-terminal domain of human carcinoembryonic antigen (CEA) [62]. Internalization is mediated through CD46 binding, leading to formation of syncytium and cell lysis [62]. The expressed CEA is expected to stimulate the immune system to recognize and destroy targeted cells.

2.5. Evaluating Vector Efficacy

The main goal of patient treatment is to increase life expectancy and improve the quality of life. Unfortunately, GBMs are a very heterogeneous group of diseases. Even morphologically-similar tumors can have different driver mutations and responses to treatment, which makes it impossible to directly compare the results of clinical trials. It should be noted that regional features of healthcare systems and even personal experiences of the attending physician can introduce bias. Moreover, previous treatment changes the tumor makeup due to clonal selection, which must be taken into account.

For the purpose of this review, we have stratified studies into three types.

1. Dose-escalating studies to assess the maximum acceptable dosage of the gene therapy vector. In accordance with the possible side effects of the administration of viral vectors, these studies are not carried out on healthy volunteers.

2. Comparison of the new therapy with existing ones when used in patients with recurrent or progressive GBM. In such patients, the prior therapy has led to the emergence of resistance and more aggressive clones, thereby diminishing the potential benefit of TMZ and justifying the application of a new therapeutic regime.

3. Comparison of the new treatment with standard treatment in patients with newly diagnosed GBM. If a therapy has shown effectiveness against TMZ-resistant GBM, it is advisable to study it in new cases as an alternative (or even replacement) to standard treatment.

We also deliberately include the date on which the study record was first available on ClinicalTrials.gov [63]. This makes it possible to identify viral vectors which have been discontinued for various reasons (including insufficient efficacy) from those that are still in ongoing trials but without published results yet (Table 2).

Table 2. Clinical trials using viral vectors.

Vector	A Unique Identification Code Given to Clinical Study Registered on ClinicalTrials.gov	Study Date	Study Type (Safety/Trials in Recurrent GBM/Trials in Newly Diagnosed GBM)	Results/Comments
DNX2401	NCT00805376	2008	Dose-escalation study in recurrent GBM	Reported in 2018: DNX-2401 is safe, improves clinical outcome. Post-treatment histology examination of biopsy revealed sites of necrosis in GBM [64].
-	NCT01582516	2012	Dose-escalation study in recurrent GBM	No posted results.
-	NCT01956734	2013	Safety and efficacy study in recurrent GBM DNX2401 + TMZ vs. TMZ alone	Reported in 2017: The safety objective of the trial was achieved with no severe toxicities related to DNX-2401 [65].
-	NCT02197169	2014	Safety and efficacy study in recurrent GBM, DNX2401 + IFN vs. DMX2401 alone	Reported in 2017: DNX-2401 was well tolerated as monotherapy. The addition of interferon did not improve survival [66].
-	NCT02798406	2016	Safety and efficacy study in recurrent GBM, DNX2401 + pembrolizumab	No posted results.
DNX2440	NCT03714334	2018	Safety and efficacy study in recurrent GBM, DNX2440 alone	No posted results.
ONYX-015	Was not registered at ClinicalTrials.gov	-	Dose-escalation study	Reported in 2004: None of the 24 patients experienced serious adverse events related to ONYX-015 [67].
ADV/HSV-tk	NCT00589875	2008	Study of AdV-tk + valacyclovir Gene therapy in combination with standard radiation therapy for malignant glioma	Reported in 2016: Addition of ADV/HSV-tk to SoC improves outcome [68].
-	NCT00870181	2009	Safety and efficacy of intravenous-administered ADV/HSV-tk in recurrent GBM vs. surgery or systemic chemotherapy or palliative care	Reported in 2016: ADV/HSV-tk is safe and can provide benefits [69].
-	NCT03603405	2018	Safety and efficacy study of standard treatment + ADV/HSV-tk in newly diagnosed GBM	No results posted.
-	NCT03596086	2018	Safety and efficacy of ADV/HSV-tk in recurrent GBM	No results posted.
Ad-hCMV-Flt3L + 4. Ad-hCMV-TK (combination)	NCT01811992	2013	Dose-escalation study in newly diagnosed GBM + standard treatment	Reported in 2019: Examination of tumor samples reveals increase in the infiltration of inflammatory cells. Preliminary data suggest that virotherapy can improve outcomes [70].

Table 2. Cont.

Vector	A Unique Identification Code Given to Clinical Study Registered on ClinicalTrials.gov	Study Date	Study Type (Safety/Trials in Recurrent GBM/Trials in Newly Diagnosed GBM)	Results/Comments
Ad-RTS-hIL12	NCT02026271	2014	Safety and tolerability of a single tumor injection of Ad-RTS-hIL-12 given with oral veledimex (the activator of RTS promoter) in patients with recurrent or progressive GBM	Reported in 2019: The clinical trial demonstrated tolerability of veledimex-induced hIL-12 expression [71].
-	NCT04006119	2019	Safety and efficacy of intratumoral Ad-RTS-hIL-12 and oral veledimex in combination with cemiplimab-rwlc in patients with recurrent or progressive GBM	No results posted.
Ad.hIFN-β	Was not registered	-	Dose-escalation study	Reported in 2008: The most common adverse events were considered by the investigator as being unrelated to treatment [38].
VB-111	NCT01260506	2010	Dose-escalation study of VB-111 in combination with bevacizumab in recurrent GBM.	Reported in 2013: VB-111 was safe and well tolerated in patients with recurrent GBM with repeat doses of up to 1×10^{13} VPs. Tumor responses were seen [72].
-	NCT02511405	2015	Comparison of VB-111 plus bevacizumab to bevacizumab in patients with recurrent GBM	Reported in 2020: Upfront concomitant administration of VB-111 and bevacizumab failed to improve outcomes [73].
HSV 1716	Was not registered	-	Safety and feasibility of intratumoral administration of HSV1716	Reported in 2000: HSV1716 is safe when injected into sites around the post-resection tumor cavity [74].
-	Was not registered	-	Efficacy of HSV1716	Reported in 2002: HSV1716 replicates in HGG without causing toxicity [75].
-	Was not registered	-	Efficacy of HSV1716	Reported in 2004: Study demonstrates that HSV1716 injections can provide benefits [76].
G207	Was not registered	-	Dose-escalation study	Reported in 2000: No viral-related toxicity; evidence of antitumor activity. While adverse events were noted in some patients, no toxicity or serious adverse events could unequivocally be ascribed to G207 [77].
-	NCT00028158	2001	Dose-escalation study. Doses 1E9, 3E9 and 1E10 pfu were tested	Reported in 2009: No encephalitis; evidence of antitumor activity and viral replication [78].

Table 2. Cont.

Vector	A Unique Identification Code Given to Clinical Study Registered on ClinicalTrials.gov	Study Date	Study Type (Safety/Trials in Recurrent GBM/Trials in Newly Diagnosed GBM)	Results/Comments
-	NCT00157703	2005	De-escalation study. First patients received the highest dose (1E10 pfu). and if excessive toxicity had occurred, the dose would be reduced for the following patients	As reported in 2014: Treatment was well tolerated with signs of improving outcomes [79].
C134	NCT03657576	2018	Dose-escalation study in recurrent/progressive GBM, anaplastic astrocytoma, or gliosarcoma	No results posted.
rQNestin34.5v.2	NCT03152318	2017	Dose-escalation study of in patients with recurrent GBM	No results posted.
M032-HSV-1	NCT02062827	2014	Dose escalation in recurrent/progressive GBM, anaplastic astrocytoma or gliosarcoma	No results posted.
Pelareorep (Reolysin)	NCT02444546	2015	Dose-escalation study of Pelareorep in combination with sargramostim in recurrent/progressive GBM	No results posted.
-	NCT00528684	2007	Dose-escalation study of Pelareorep in recurrent GBM	Reported in 2008: The intratumoral administration of the genetically unmodified reovirus was well tolerated using these doses and schedule in patients with recurrent GBM [80].
ParvOryx	NCT01301430	2011	Dose-escalation study of ParvOryx in patients with progressive or recurrent GBM	Reported in 2012 and 2017: No dose-limiting toxicity was reported but clinical response did not depend on the dose or mode of ParvOryx administration. No statistical confirmation of efficacy [81,82].
NDV-HUJ	Was not registered	-	Dose-escalation study of NDV-HUJ	Reported in 2006: Toxicity was minimal with Grade I/II constitutional fever being seen in five patients. Maximum tolerated dose was not achieved [83].
-	NCT01174537	2010	Safety and efficacy of single dose intravenously administered	No results posted.
PVSRIPO	NCT02986178	2016	Safety and efficacy of single dose PVSRIPO administered intratumorally in patients with recurrent GBM	No results posted.

Table 2. *Cont.*

Vector	A Unique Identification Code Given to Clinical Study Registered on ClinicalTrials.gov	Study Date	Study Type (Safety/Trials in Recurrent GBM/Trials in Newly Diagnosed GBM)	Results/Comments
-	NCT03973879	2019	Safety and efficacy of single dose PVSRIPO administered intratumorally with atezolizumab treatment in patients with recurrent GBM	Withdrawn.
-	NCT01491893	2011	Dose-escalation study of PVSRIPO administered intratumorally in patients with recurrent GBM	Reported in 2018: Intratumoral infusion of PVSRIPO in patients with recurrent WHO grade IV malignant glioma confirmed the absence of neurovirulent potential [84].
Toca 511	NCT04105374	2019	Toca 511, Toca FC and standard of care vs. standard of care in newly diagnosed GBM	Withdrawn.
-	NCT02414165	2015	Toca 511/Toca FC vs. Lomustine, Temozolomide, or Bevacizumab in recurrent GBM	Reported in 2020: administration of Toca 511 and Toca FC, compared with SoC, did not improve overall survival (11.10 months vs. 12.22 months, respectively) or other end points [85].
-	NCT01470794	2011	Dose-escalation study of Toca 511/Toca FC administered by injections into resection cavity wall in patients with recurrent GBM	Reported in 2016, 2016, 2018: Toca 511/Toca FC is safe and can provide durable complete response in some patients [86–88].
-	NCT01156584	2010	Dose-escalation study of Toca 511/Toca FC administered by intratumoral injections in patients with recurrent GBM	Reported in 2015, 2016:Safe and well tolerated [87–89].
-	NCT01985256	2013	Dose-escalation study of Toca 511/Toca FC administered by intravenously in patients with recurrent GBM	Reported in 2016: Injections were well tolerated [87].
TG6002	NCT03294486	2017	Dose-escalation study of TG6002 in patients with recurrent GBM	No results posted.
MV-CEA	NCT00390299	2006	Dose-escalation study of MV-CEA in patients with recurrent GBM	No results posted.

GBM—glioblastoma multiforme; TMZ—temozolomide; IFN—interferon; SoC—standard of care; RTS—RheoSwitch Therapeutic System; VPs—vector particles; HGG—high grade glioma; pfu—plaque forming unit; WHO—world health organization.

3. Discussion

The search for a gene therapy solution is driven by the abysmal prognosis currently typical for GBM. As of today, many different ideas have been proposed and tested, some of which are summarized above. However, so far, no obvious breakthrough is evident.

Of the many studies listed in Table 2 and other parts of this review, we have selected two, both using Ad, which have led to interesting results and were published recently. They pursue different strategies and are interesting to compare.

Lang et al. reported the outcome of the trial of DNX 2401 (Delta-24-RGD) on 25 patients without surgical resection and 12 patients where the vector was first injected into the tumor via an implanted catheter, which was followed by surgical removal of the tumor 14 days later and multiple intramural injections of DNX 2401 [64]. Viral loads varied between cases between 10^7 and 3×10^{10} viral particles (vp) in 1 mL volumes. The paper mentions that 3×10^{10} vp in 1 mL was the highest concentration of Ad which could be manufactured, which is close to the experience of our laboratory. In the group treated with a single intratumoral injection of DNX 2401 (no surgery), tumor reduction occurred in 18 of 25 patients (72%). The median survival time in that group was only 9.5 months, regardless of the vector dose, which does not look to be a major success; however, five patients (20%) from this group survived for more than 3 years, which is rather striking given that they were all initially enrolled as recurrent cases with previous history of drug treatments and resistance. Obviously, all patients also received therapies other than DNX 2401. Some limited spread of the vector outside of the brain was detected and anti-Ad5 antibodies appeared in a significant number of patients in both cohorts. In histological specimens, various signs of immune response and inflammatory infiltration as well as viral cell death were evident. The incidence of side effects was very high—for example, 68% experienced headaches, 32% experienced hemiparesis, and 24% convulsions—but the authors argue that they were mainly disease- and not treatment-related. Overall, the paper shows clearly that DNX 2401 can induce an oncolytic effect accompanied by an immune response. This study can, perhaps, be seen as one of the fairly successful preliminary trials which relies on the concept of conditionally replicating oncolytic viruses. From the available information, it seems that the control provided by the requirement for the defective Rb/p16 pathway, as characteristic for many tumors, is sufficiently tight, and the spread of the virus was obviously not too fast and was limited to the locality of injection, rather than becoming generalized encephalitis, which is encouraging news. It is a pity that the integrity of Rb/p16 was not assessed in the patients' biopsies—perhaps that could help to predict the efficacy of the treatment. It would also be important to confirm directly that DNX 2401 is still able to infect the GBM cells after the tumor is given time to undergo clonal selection as it typically happens with GBM. Can GBM cells escape by downregulating the binding sites for the RGD motif, incorporated in this gene therapy agent? It will be very interesting to watch further developments in this dimension.

Recently, the results of NCT02026271 (ClinicalTrials.gov Identifier), which uses Ad–RTS–hIL-12, were published [71]. It is interesting to analyze the approach used in that study in more detail since it highlights many problems facing the field. As mentioned above, Ad–RTS–hIL-12 is a replication-incompetent AVV with a promoter, controllable by a small-molecule drug veledimex (VDX), allowing drug-induced production of interleukin-12 (IL-12) by the cells where AVV genomes are active. The study mainly focused on the demonstration of the ability to induce IL-12 production by VDX and the safety of this treatment. Patients enrolled were all already previously treated with various regimes and, obviously, represented a really tough challenge. After surgical resection of the bulk, AVVs were injected into one spot in white matter as a single injection of 50 µL containing 2×10^{11} viral particles, which corresponds to the titer of 10^{13} vp/mL, which our laboratory was never able to achieve and seems to be an extremely concentrated AVV stock administered in a very small volume (compare to the previously mentioned paper [70]). The drug treatment lasted for 14 days. During that period, the drug clearly induced production of IL-12, which spilled over into the systemic circulation, and various signs of inflammatory response were visible in the patients; luckily, they were easily reversible by VDX discontinuation. Interestingly, patients treated with 20 mg VDX seemed to survive better than both those treated with lower and higher doses, the latter probably being a sign of a negative effect of excessive immunostimulation. Over the 30-month observation period, 30 of 31 enrolled patients died, which can hardly be considered a therapeutic success. Nevertheless, the authors successfully demonstrated infiltration of the tumor by the immune cells, indicating that, at least mechanistically, they achieved the expected result. Considering the results of this study, as reasoned above, non-replicating AVV genomes are inevitably diluted in dividing tumor cells. Since the whole protocol lasted for 14 days, this could be the only period when there was enough active transgene in the remaining GBM cells. Unfortunately, in the paper, there is no information on the presence of the viral genomes in the post-mortem samples. This issue, i.e., survival of the transcriptionally active adenoviral genomes in the GBM, is both interesting and important but we do not have the answer yet. It would be very interesting to know whether VDX could effectively trigger a wave of IL-12 production 3–5 months after the transduction. The other question is whether the cells producing IL-12 were mainly the GBM cells or other cells in the vicinity of the injection track. Overall, this strategy is in progress and seems to critically depend on the ability to quickly destroy the infiltrating GBM cells while the AVV are still functional.

What are the limitations, and can they be overcome, at least theoretically? The first point to consider is that of infection or transduction efficiency and stability of transgene expression. Viral vectors must be able to very efficiently enter the target cells and introduce any transgene cargo into their nuclei. Viral vectors have been extensively used in biomedical research and neuroscience for the last 20 years and there is a wealth of information about many of the vectors, similar to those used in human trials. For example, the internalization mechanism of species C adenoviruses is based on their interaction with CAR and Integrin $\alpha v \beta 5$ proteins on the surface of the target cells [90], PVSRIPO requires CD155 [56], MV-CEA cell entry is based on interaction with CD46 [62], and so forth. We argue that this makes strategies involving adenoviral and similar vectors, which require specific GBM surface proteins for entry, vulnerable to the common mechanism of tumor defense based on downregulation of the relevant proteins and consecutive clonal selection and expansion. Ad has been used in vitro by many groups, including ourselves, in experimental neuroscience for transgene expression in both neurons and glia [91,92]. In vivo, however, these vectors clearly prefer astrocytes over all other cell types in the brain [25,92], and thus, unmodified Ad cannot be seen as a universally efficient delivery tool, irrespective of the putative origin of the GBM. In some Ad-derived gene therapy vectors, such as DNX 2410, a specific modification of the fiber H-loop should enable them to bind to specific integrins expressed by many tumor cells, but this mechanism is vulnerable to downregulation of the target integrins. The obvious differences in transductional tropism between adeno- and lentiviral vectors in rodent CNS were demonstrated long ago [93]. It was noted that vesicular stomatitis virus G-protein (VSVG)-pseudotyped lentiviruses which do not utilize a specific receptor-dependent entry pathway have a much wider transduction potential. In our laboratory, VSVG-pseudotyped HIV-derived lentivirus was used to transduce six patient-derived GBM cell lines with an apparent 100% success rate (unpublished observations). We suggest that the requirement for a specific interaction partner protein on the target cells is a limitation of vectors used for gene therapy of GBM because these can be easily eliminated by selection, making tumor cells resistant. Could lentivirus be a route to explore? Another fundamental issue is the possible silencing of exogenous expression cassettes. In experimental neuroscience, this was noted a long time ago for a commonly used promoter CMV, which is incorporated in several viral vectors listed here [31,94]. The mechanisms of CMV-mediated transgene silencing are not well understood but could be based on RNA interference or methylation of the viral promoters by cell defense machinery [95,96]. Additionally, as mentioned above, replication-incompetent vectors which stay episomal fail to propagate to the progeny of the cells they invade, which means that unless the infected GBM cells die immediately, they will eliminate viral genomes by dilution after a few divisions.

The next important point is the mechanism of action of viral gene therapy. Oncolytic viruses use the natural feature of viruses to multiply and destroy cells. Obviously, such processes, if uncontrolled, will be lethal, as exemplified above by Reolysin or C134. Various mechanisms of transcriptional control are used to enable replication predominantly in fast dividing cells. However, if this strategy is really successful and, thus, leads to a powerful cytopathic effect, rapid destruction of GBM in clinical settings can cause brain edema with subsequent impairment of vital functions and even death. Specificity of viral gene therapy is a fundamental problem. For cytopathic viruses, this solely relies on the dependence of their replication on factors highly expressed by tumor cells. However, GBM cells, even within the same tumor, are heterogenous [97]. Is it even possible to find a ubiquitous driver/controller of viral replication in the pool of diverse GBM cells? At this point, such a possibility remains to be demonstrated. So far, the selectivity of the published vectors is obviously not sufficient to fully prevent destruction of normal brain cells. With some vectors, such damage can be inflicted by the conversion of pro-drugs into toxic specimens which are then released—the so-called bystander effect. This problem is particularly relevant to the brain, where elimination, dilution and biodegradation of these harmful molecules might be slower than in the periphery. An added problem introduced by replicating vectors is the release of viral particles into the bloodstream, leading to an inevitable immune response.

The success of viral gene therapy critically depends on the physical access of the virus to the GBM cells. Shall they be injected into the brain at the time of surgery or administered using some other means? It would be ideal to inject the virus into the bloodstream because it could reach all GBM cells which are spread within the parenchyma, but can this be done? Outside of the field of neuro-oncology, the best current example of an attempt to achieve generalized expression in the human brain with an i.v.-injected viral vector is Zolgensma (AVXS-101), an adeno-associated viral vector carrying the SMN1 transgene [98]. However, in humans, this virus has to be delivered before 2 years of age, when the blood–brain barrier is still not completely mature, and large doses are used, requiring administration of steroids to prevent a severe immune response [99]. This is in stark contrast with multiple studies in mice where a brain-wide expression has been achieved with some strains of adeno-associated virus injected i.v. [100]. Adeno-associated viruses are extremely small and definitely have the best chances of reaching the CNS when their concentration in the bloodstream is high enough, but they do not seem to have any tropism to GBM in addition to the fact that the adult human BBB is probably completely impermeable to them. Moreover, after a single application into the bloodstream, a strong antibody response is inevitable, making this a "single shot only" strategy. It is therefore unlikely that we will see successful targeting of disseminated GBM with any type of currently available viral vector applied via the bloodstream.

To summarize, the attempts to develop an efficient gene therapy for GBM with viral vectors face the following fundamental problems.

(a) Vectors relying on a specific mechanism of internalization are unlikely to be successful because of the extreme instability of GBM genomes, the multitude of clones in the same tumor and the ease of clonal selection of resistant cells to which the virus will have no access. It follows that using less specific mechanisms of viral entry might be a winning strategy.

(b) GBM cells divide, and some do it at a very high pace. In such cells, non-integrating viral genomes will be rapidly diluted and probably become inefficient, unless they cause immediate death of the cell. The ability to silence transgenes adds to this problem. The only way to ensure downwards transmission of the transgene is the use of integrating vectors, such as lentiviruses.

(c) Specificity of the effect is one of the key requirements and we have listed, above, some of the strategies used to limit the impact to GBM cells vs. the rest of the brain. So far, many of these strategies have been demonstrated to work in vitro and sometimes even in GBM-bearing mice in vivo. Whether a sufficiently reliable and universal strategy can be found for clinical application remains to be seen. We hypothesize that one avenue to explore is to try to suppress the mitotic apparatus, since healthy cells in the postnatal human brain rarely or never divide.

(d) Injection in the bloodstream is unlikely to be successful. We are therefore left with a necessity to infiltrate with viral gene therapeutics the areas of the putative GBM growth during the debulking surgery or, possibly, by stereotaxis at a later stage.

We hope that this review will allow readers to get a feel for the current options for the viral gene therapy of GBM and initiate a discussion about its future directions. We suggest that a more plausible strategy might be to focus on viruses which enter via a non-selective, ubiquitous mechanism. We hypothesize that it might be possible to irreversibly block processes critical for dividing tumor cells which are dispensable for quiescent healthy brain cells. Mitosis is a highly specialized stage of a cell's life and depends on a range of proteins which are expressed in non-dividing cells at low levels. This idea may be illustrated by the current attempts to target, for example, cyclin-dependent kinases with inhibitors. The key difference is that the peripheral cells—for example, in the bone marrow—should not be affected and inhibited by a virus which is delivered into the brain parenchyma. Hence, the issue of systemic toxicity could become less critical.

As stated in the beginning, this review reflects the view of the experimentalist neuroscientists and, hopefully, might stimulate a discussion leading to new discoveries in the field of neuro-oncology.

4. Conclusions

Viral gene therapy of GBM is a promising field but several major hurdles need to be overcome for it to become an accepted part of the currently available portfolio of therapeutic interventions. As yet, some potentially encouraging results have been obtained with a conditionally replicating oncolytic Ad, but the fundamental challenge of tumor resistance via downregulation of the proteins, critical for viral proliferation remains to be overcome. Obviously not all the options have been yet explored and we hope to see new types of vectors entering clinical trials in years to come.

Author Contributions: All authors have read and agreed to the published version of the manuscript.

Funding: O.M. was funded by the 5/100 Programme from the Russian Government to Baltic Federal University, Kaliningrad, Russian Federation and The Fellowship of the President of the Russian Federation. A.G.T. was funded by the British Heart Foundation (PG/18/8/33540). S.K. and A.G.T. were funded by the British Heart Foundation (RG/14/4/39736).

Conflicts of Interest: The authors declare no conflict of interest.

References

1. Jiang, Y.; Uhrbom, L. On the origin of glioma. *Upsala J. Med. Sci.* **2012**, *117*, 113–121. [CrossRef] [PubMed]
2. Reifenberger, G.; Wirsching, H.-G.; Knobbe-Thomsen, G.R.C.B.; Weller, H.-G.W.M. Advances in the molecular genetics of gliomas—Implications for classification and therapy. *Nat. Rev. Clin. Oncol.* **2017**, *14*, 434–452. [CrossRef] [PubMed]
3. Louis, D.N.; Ohgaki, H.; Wiestler, O.D.; Cavenee, W.K.; Burger, P.C.; Jouvet, A.; Scheithauer, B.W.; Kleihues, P. The 2007 WHO Classification of Tumours of the Central Nervous System. *Acta Neuropathol.* **2007**, *114*, 97–109. [CrossRef]
4. Louis, D.N.; Perry, A.; Reifenberger, G.; Von Deimling, A.; Figarella-Branger, D.; Cavenee, W.K.; Ohgaki, H.; Wiestler, O.D.; Kleihues, P.; Ellison, D.W. The 2016 World Health Organization Classification of Tumors of the Central Nervous System: A summary. *Acta Neuropathol.* **2016**, *131*, 803–820. [CrossRef]
5. Stupp, R.; Mason, W.P.; van den Bent, M.J.; Weller, M.; Fisher, B.; Taphoorn, M.J.B.; Belanger, K.; Brandes, A.A.; Marosi, C.; Bogdahn, U.; et al. Radiotherapy plus Concomitant and Adjuvant Temozolomide for Glioblastoma. *N. Engl. J. Med.* **2005**, *352*, 987–996. [CrossRef]
6. Stupp, R.; Hegi, M.E.; Mason, W.P.; Bent, M.J.V.D.; Taphoorn, M.J.B.; Janzer, R.C.; Ludwin, S.K.; Allgeier, A.; Fisher, B.; Belanger, K.; et al. Effects of radiotherapy with concomitant and adjuvant temozolomide versus radiotherapy alone on survival in glioblastoma in a randomised phase III study: 5-year analysis of the EORTC-NCIC trial. *Lancet Oncol.* **2009**, *10*, 459–466. [CrossRef]
7. Pardridge, W.M. The blood-brain barrier: Bottleneck in brain drug development. *NeuroRX* **2005**, *2*, 3–14. [CrossRef]
8. Schaich, M.; Kestel, L.; Pfirrmann, M.; Robel, K.; Illmer, T.; Kramer, M.; Dill, C.; Ehninger, G.; Schackert, G.; Krex, D. A MDR1 (ABCB1) gene single nucleotide polymorphism predicts outcome of temozolomide treatment in glioblastoma patients. *Ann. Oncol.* **2009**, *20*, 175–181. [CrossRef]
9. Hegi, M.E.; Diserens, A.-C.; Gorlia, T.; Hamou, M.-F.; De Tribolet, N.; Weller, M.; Kros, J.M.; Hainfellner, J.A.; Mason, W.; Mariani, L.; et al. MGMT Gene Silencing and Benefit from Temozolomide in Glioblastoma. *N. Engl. J. Med.* **2005**, *352*, 997–1003. [CrossRef]
10. Chowdhary, S.A.; Ryken, T.; Newton, H.B. Survival outcomes and safety of carmustine wafers in the treatment of high-grade gliomas: A meta-analysis. *J. Neuro Oncol.* **2015**, *122*, 367–382. [CrossRef]

11. Vasilev, A.; Sofi, R.; Tong, L.; Teschemacher, A.G.; Kasparov, S. In Search of a Breakthrough Therapy for Glioblastoma Multiforme. *Neuroglia* **2018**, *1*, 292–310. [CrossRef]
12. Liu, T.-C.; Galanis, E.; Kirn, D.H. Clinical trial results with oncolytic virotherapy: A century of promise, a decade of progress. *Nat. Clin. Pract. Oncol.* **2007**, *4*, 101–117. [CrossRef] [PubMed]
13. Choi, A.H.; O'Leary, M.P.; Fong, Y.; Chen, N.G. From Benchtop to Bedside: A Review of Oncolytic Virotherapy. *Biomedicines* **2016**, *4*, 18. [CrossRef] [PubMed]
14. Zarogoulidis, P.; Darwiche, K.; Sakkas, A.; Yarmus, L.; Huang, H.; Li, Q.; Freitag, L.; Zarogoulidis, K.; Malecki, M. Suicide Gene Therapy for Cancer—Current Strategies. *J. Genet. Syndr. Gene Ther.* **2013**, *4*, 16849. [CrossRef] [PubMed]
15. International Committee on Taxonomy of Viruses (ICTV). Available online: http://www.ictvonline.org/ (accessed on 15 October 2020).
16. Harrach, B. Adenoviruses: General Features. In *Encyclopedia of Virology*; Elsevier Ltd.: Amsterdam, The Netherlands, 2014; pp. 1–9.
17. Knipe, D.M.; Howley, P.M. *Fields Virology*; Lippincott Williams & Wilkins: Philadelphia, PA, USA, 2013.
18. Pelka, P.; Miller, M.S.; Cecchini, M.; Yousef, A.F.; Bowdish, D.M.E.; Dick, F.; Whyte, P.; Mymryk, J.S. Adenovirus E1A Directly Targets the E2F/DP-1 Complex. *J. Virol.* **2011**, *85*, 8841–8851. [CrossRef] [PubMed]
19. Wold, W.S.M.; Toth, K. Adenovirus Vectors for Gene Therapy, Vaccination and Cancer Gene Therapy. *Curr. Gene Ther.* **2014**, *13*, 421–433. [CrossRef]
20. Ganly, I.; Kirn, D.; Eckhardt, G.; I Rodriguez, G.; Soutar, D.S.; Otto, R.; Robertson, A.G.; Park, O.; Gulley, M.L.; Heise, C.; et al. A phase I study of Onyx-015, an E1B attenuated adenovirus, administered intratumorally to patients with recurrent head and neck cancer. *Clin. Cancer Res.* **2000**, *6*, 798–806.
21. Rothmann, T.; Hengstermann, A.; Whitaker, N.J.; Scheffner, M.; Hausen, H.Z. Replication of ONYX-015, a Potential Anticancer Adenovirus, Is Independent of p53 Status in Tumor Cells. *J. Virol.* **1998**, *72*, 9470–9478. [CrossRef]
22. Edwards, S.; Dix, B.R.; Myers, C.J.; Dobson-Le, D.; Huschtscha, L.; Hibma, M.; Royds, J.; Braithwaite, A.W. Evidence that Replication of the Antitumor Adenovirus ONYX-015 Is Not Controlled by the p53 and p14ARF Tumor Suppressor Genes. *J. Virol.* **2002**, *76*, 12483–12490. [CrossRef]
23. Marina, N.; Christie, I.N.; Korsak, A.; Doronin, M.; Brazhe, A.; Hosford, P.S.; Wells, J.A.; Sheikhbahaei, S.; Humoud, I.; Paton, J.F.R.; et al. Astrocytes monitor cerebral perfusion and control systemic circulation to maintain brain blood flow. *Nat. Commun.* **2020**, *11*, 1–9. [CrossRef]
24. Wong, L.; Polson, J.W.; Murphy, D.; Paton, J.F.R.; Kasparov, S. Genetic and pharmacological dissection of pathways involved in the angiotensin II-mediated depression of baroreflex function. *FASEB J.* **2002**, *16*, 1595–1601. [CrossRef] [PubMed]
25. Gourine, A.V.; Kasymov, V.; Marina, N.; Tang, F.; Figueiredo, M.F.; Lane, S.; Teschemacher, A.G.; Spyer, K.M.; Deisseroth, K.; Kasparov, S. Astrocytes Control Breathing Through pH-Dependent Release of ATP. *Science* **2010**, *329*, 571–576. [CrossRef] [PubMed]
26. Fueyo-margareto, J.; Manzano-gomez, C.; Conrad, C.; Lang, F.; Yung, W.A.; Tufaro, F. Treatment of Brain Cancer with Oncolytic Adenovirus. WIPO Patent No. WO 2014/204814 A1, 24 December 2014.
27. Philbrick, B.; Adamson, C. DNX-2401: An investigational drug for the treatment of recurrent glioblastoma. *Expert Opin. Investig. Drugs* **2019**, *28*, 1041–1049. [CrossRef] [PubMed]
28. Jiang, H.; Shin, D.H.; Nguyen, T.T.; Fueyo, J.; Fan, X.; Henry, V.; Carrillo, C.C.; Yi, Y.; Alonso, M.M.; Collier, T.L.; et al. Localized Treatment with Oncolytic Adenovirus Delta-24-RGDOX Induces Systemic Immunity against Disseminated Subcutaneous and Intracranial Melanomas. *Clin. Cancer Res.* **2019**, *25*, 6801–6814. [CrossRef] [PubMed]
29. Tufaro, F.; Fueyo-Margareto, J.; Gomez-Manzano, C.; Conrad, C.; Yung, A.W.; Jiang, H. Adenovirus Expressing Immune Cell Stimulatory Receptor Agonist(s). WIPO Patent No. WO 2015/077624 Al, 28 May 2015.
30. Smitt, P.S.; Driesse, M.; Wolbers, J.; Kros, M.; Avezaat, C. Treatment of relapsed malignant glioma with an adenoviral vector containing the herpes simplex thymidine kinase gene followed by ganciclovir. *Mol. Ther.* **2003**, *7*, 851–858. [CrossRef]
31. Kasparov, S. Suitability of hCMV for viral gene expression in the brain. *Nat. Methods* **2007**, *4*, 379. [CrossRef]
32. Germano, I.M.; Fable, J.; Gultekin, S.H.; Silvers, A. Adenovirus/herpes simplex-thymidine kinase/ganciclovir complex: Preliminary results of a phase I trial in patients with recurrent malignant gliomas. *J. Neuro-Oncol.* **2003**, *65*, 279–289. [CrossRef]

33. Smith, R.L.; Traul, D.L.; Schaack, J.; Clayton, G.H.; Staley, K.J.; Wilcox, C.L. Characterization of Promoter Function and Cell-Type-Specific Expression from Viral Vectors in the Nervous System. *J. Virol.* **2000**, *74*, 11254–11261. [CrossRef]
34. Lowenstein, P.; Castro, M.G. Evolutionary basis of a new gene- and immune-therapeutic approach for the treatment of malignant brain tumors: From mice to clinical trials for glioma patients. *Clin. Immunol.* **2018**, *189*, 43–51. [CrossRef]
35. Vilaboa, N.; Boellmann, F.; Voellmy, R.W. Gene Switches for Deliberate Regulation of Transgene Expression: Recent Advances in System Development and Uses. *J. Genet. Syndr. Gene Ther.* **2011**, *2*. [CrossRef]
36. Barrett, J.A.; Cai, H.; Miao, J.; Khare, P.D.; Gonzalez, P.; Dalsing-Hernandez, J.; Sharma, G.; Chan, T.; Cooper, L.J.; Lebel, F. Regulated intratumoral expression of IL-12 using a RheoSwitch Therapeutic System® (RTS®) gene switch as gene therapy for the treatment of glioma. *Cancer Gene Ther.* **2018**, *25*, 106–116. [CrossRef] [PubMed]
37. Yoon, C.; Johnston, S.C.; Tang, J.; Stahl, M.; Tobin, J.F.; Somers, W.S. Charged residues dominate a unique interlocking topography in the heterodimeric cytokine interleukin-12. *EMBO J.* **2000**, *19*, 3530–3541. [CrossRef] [PubMed]
38. Chiocca, E.A.; Smith, K.M.; McKinney, B.; Palmer, C.; Rosenfeld, S.; Lillehei, K.; Hamilton, A.; DeMasters, B.K.; Judy, K.; Kirn, D. A Phase I Trial of Ad.hIFN-β Gene Therapy for Glioma. *Mol. Ther.* **2008**, *16*, 618–626. [CrossRef] [PubMed]
39. Yung, W.K.; Prados, M.; Levin, V.A.; Fetell, M.R.; Bennett, J.; Mahaley, M.S.; Salcman, M.; Etcubanas, E. Intravenous Recombinant Interferon beta in Patients With Recurrent Malignant Gliomas: A Phase I/II Study. *J. Clin. Oncol.* **1991**, *9*, 1945–1949. [CrossRef]
40. Breitbart, E.; Leubitz, A.; Feige, E.; Penson, R. Treatment Methods Using Adenovirus. WIPO Patent No. WO 2014/060848 A2, 24 April 2014.
41. Artusi, S.; Miyagawa, Y.; Goins, W.F.; Cohen, J.B.; Glorioso, J.C. Herpes Simplex Virus Vectors for Gene Transfer to the Central Nervous System. *Diseases* **2018**, *6*, 74. [CrossRef]
42. Gale, M.; Katze, M.G. Molecular Mechanisms of Interferon Resistance Mediated by Viral-Directed Inhibition of PKR, the Interferon-Induced Protein Kinase. *Pharmacol. Ther.* **1998**, *78*, 29–46. [CrossRef]
43. Cheng, G.; Gross, M.; Brett, M.-E.; He, B. AlaArg Motif in the Carboxyl Terminus of the γ134.5 Protein of Herpes Simplex Virus Type 1 Is Required for the Formation of a High-Molecular-Weight Complex That Dephosphorylates eIF-2α. *J. Virol.* **2001**, *75*, 3666–3674. [CrossRef]
44. Mostafa, H.H.; Thompson, T.W.; Konen, A.J.; Haenchen, S.D.; Hilliard, J.G.; Macdonald, S.J.; Morrison, L.A.; Davido, D.J. Herpes Simplex Virus 1 Mutant with Point Mutations inUL39Is Impaired for Acute Viral Replication in Mice, Establishment of Latency, and Explant-Induced Reactivation. *J. Virol.* **2018**, *92*, 1–12. [CrossRef]
45. Streby, K.A.; Geller, J.I.; Currier, M.A.; Warren, P.S.; Racadio, J.M.; Towbin, A.J.; Vaughan, M.R.; Triplet, M.; Ott-Napier, K.; Dishman, D.J.; et al. Intratumoral Injection of HSV1716, an Oncolytic Herpes Virus, Is Safe and Shows Evidence of Immune Response and Viral Replication in Young Cancer Patients. *Clin. Cancer Res.* **2017**, *23*, 3566–3574. [CrossRef]
46. Cassady, K.A.; Bauer, D.F.; Roth, J.; Chambers, M.R.; Shoeb, T.; Coleman, J.; Prichard, M.; Gillespie, G.Y.; Markert, J.M. Pre-clinical Assessment of C134, a Chimeric Oncolytic Herpes Simplex Virus, in Mice and Non-human Primates. *Mol. Ther. Oncolytics* **2017**, *5*, 1–10. [CrossRef]
47. Cinatl, J.; Michaelis, M.; Driever, P.H.; Činátl, J.; Hraběta, J.; Suhan, T.; Doerr, H.W.; Vogel, J.-U. Multimutated Herpes Simplex Virus G207 Is a Potent Inhibitor of Angiogenesis1. *Neoplasia* **2004**, *6*, 725–735. [CrossRef] [PubMed]
48. Chiocca, E.A.; Nakashima, H.; Kasai, K.; Fernandez, S.A.; Oglesbee, M. Preclinical Toxicology of rQNestin34.5v.2: An Oncolytic Herpes Virus with Transcriptional Regulation of the ICP34.5 Neurovirulence Gene. *Mol. Ther. Methods Clin. Dev.* **2020**, *17*, 871–893. [CrossRef] [PubMed]
49. Matsuda, Y.; Yoshimura, H.; Suzuki, T.; Ishiwata, T. Nestin: Neural Stem/Progenitor Cell Marker in Brain Tumors. In *Evolution of the Molecular Biology of Brain Tumors and the Therapeutic Implications*; IntechOpen: London, UK, 2013.
50. Peters, C.; Rabkin, S.D. Designing herpes viruses as oncolytics. *Mol. Ther. Oncolytics* **2015**, *2*, 15010. [CrossRef]
51. Strong, J.E.; Coffey, M.C.; Tang, D.; Sabinin, P.; Lee, P.W. The molecular basis of viral oncolysis: Usurpation of the Ras signaling pathway by reovirus. *EMBO J.* **1998**, *17*, 3351–3362. [CrossRef]

52. Werner, K. Use of a Virus Regimen for the Treatment of Diseases. WIPO Patent No. PCT/EP2009/003074, 12 November 2009.
53. Biederer, C.; Ries, S.; Brandts, C.H.; McCormick, F. Replication-selective viruses for cancer therapy. *J. Mol. Med.* **2001**, *80*, 163–175. [CrossRef]
54. Lazar, I.; Yaacov, B.; Shiloach, T.; Eliahoo, E.; Kadouri, L.; Lotem, M.; Perlman, R.; Zakay-Rones, Z.; Panet, A.; Ben-Yehuda, D. The Oncolytic Activity of Newcastle Disease Virus NDV-HUJ on Chemoresistant Primary Melanoma Cells Is Dependent on the Proapoptotic Activity of the Inhibitor of Apoptosis Protein Livin. *J. Virol.* **2009**, *84*, 639–646. [CrossRef]
55. Marchini, A.; Bonifati, S.; Scott, E.M.; Angelova, A.L.; Rommelaere, J. Oncolytic parvoviruses: From basic virology to clinical applications. *Virol. J.* **2015**, *12*, 1–16. [CrossRef]
56. Merrill, M.K.; Bernhardt, G.; Sampson, J.H.; Wikstrand, C.J.; Bigner, D.D.; Gromeier, M. Poliovirus receptor CD155-targeted oncolysis of glioma. *Neuro Oncol.* **2004**, *6*, 208–217. [CrossRef]
57. Perez, O.D.; Logg, C.R.; Hiraoka, K.; Diago, O.; Burnett, R.; Inagaki, A.; Jolson, D.; Amundson, K.; Buckley, T.; Lohse, D.; et al. Design and Selection of Toca 511 for Clinical Use: Modified Retroviral Replicating Vector With Improved Stability and Gene Expression. *Mol. Ther.* **2012**, *20*, 1689–1698. [CrossRef]
58. Hogan, D.J.; Zhu, J.-J.; Diago, O.R.; Gammon, D.K.; Haghighi, A.; Lu, G.; Das, A.; Gruber, H.E.; Jolly, D.J.; Ostertag, D. Molecular Analyses Support the Safety and Activity of Retroviral Replicating Vector Toca 511 in Patients. *Clin. Cancer Res.* **2018**, *24*, 4680–4693. [CrossRef]
59. Huang, T.T.; Hlavaty, J.; Ostertag, D.; Espinoza, F.L.; Martin, B.; Petznek, H.; Rodriguez-Aguirre, M.; E Ibanez, C.; Kasahara, N.; Gunzburg, W.; et al. Toca 511 gene transfer and 5-fluorocytosine in combination with temozolomide demonstrates synergistic therapeutic efficacy in a temozolomide-sensitive glioblastoma model. *Cancer Gene Ther.* **2013**, *20*, 544–551. [CrossRef] [PubMed]
60. Foloppe, J.; Kempf, J.; Futin, N.; Kintz, J.; Cordier, P.; Pichon, C.; Findeli, A.; Vorburger, F.; Quemeneur, E.; Erbs, P. The Enhanced Tumor Specificity of TG6002, an Armed Oncolytic Vaccinia Virus Deleted in Two Genes Involved in Nucleotide Metabolism. *Mol. Ther. Oncolytics* **2019**, *14*, 1–14. [CrossRef] [PubMed]
61. E Hruby, D. Vaccinia virus vectors: New strategies for producing recombinant vaccines. *Clin. Microbiol. Rev.* **1990**, *3*, 153–170. [CrossRef] [PubMed]
62. Blechacz, B.; Splinter, P.L.; Greiner, S.; Myers, R.; Peng, K.-W.; Federspiel, M.J.; Russell, S.J.; LaRusso, N.F. Engineered measles virus as a novel oncolytic viral therapy system for hepatocellular carcinoma. *Hepatology* **2006**, *44*, 1465–1477. [CrossRef] [PubMed]
63. A Database of Privately and Publicly Funded Clinical Studies Conducted Around the World (ClinicalTrials.com Database). Available online: https://clinicaltrials.gov/ (accessed on 5 November 2020).
64. Lang, F.F.; Conrad, C.; Gomez-Manzano, C.; Yung, W.A.; Sawaya, R.; Weinberg, J.S.; Prabhu, S.S.; Rao, G.; Fuller, G.N.; Aldape, K.D.; et al. Phase I Study of DNX-2401 (Delta-24-RGD) Oncolytic Adenovirus: Replication and Immunotherapeutic Effects in Recurrent Malignant Glioma. *J. Clin. Oncol.* **2018**, *36*, 1419–1427. [CrossRef]
65. Alonso, M.M.; García-Moure, M.; Gonzalez-Huarriz, M.; Marigil, M.; Hernandez-Alcoceba, R.; Buñales, M.; Hervás, S.; Gallego, J.; Gomez-Manzano, C.; Fueyo, J.; et al. Abstract CT027: Oncolytic virus DNX-2401 with a short course of temozolomide for glioblastoma at first recurrence: Clinical data and prognostic biomarkers. In Proceedings of the AACR Annual Meeting 2017, Washington, DC, USA, 1–5 April 2017. [CrossRef]
66. Regeneron. Phase 1b open-label randomized study of the oncolytic adenovirus DNX- 2401 administered with or without interferon gamma for recurrent glioblastoma. *J. Clin. Oncol.* **2017**, *35*, 3008. [CrossRef]
67. Chiocca, E.A.; Abbed, K.M.; Tatter, S.; Louis, D.N.; Hochberg, F.H.; Barker, F.; Kracher, J.; Grossman, S.A.; Fisher, J.D.; Carson, K.; et al. A Phase I Open-Label, Dose-Escalation, Multi-Institutional Trial of Injection with an E1B-Attenuated Adenovirus, ONYX-015, into the Peritumoral Region of Recurrent Malignant Gliomas, in the Adjuvant Setting. *Mol. Ther.* **2004**, *10*, 958–966. [CrossRef]
68. Wheeler, L.A.; Manzanera, A.G.; Bell, S.D.; Cavaliere, R.; McGregor, J.M.; Grecula, J.C.; Newton, H.B.; Lo, S.S.; Badie, B.; Portnow, J.; et al. Phase II multicenter study of gene-mediated cytotoxic immunotherapy as adjuvant to surgical resection for newly diagnosed malignant glioma. *Neuro-oncology* **2016**, *18*, 1137–1145. [CrossRef]
69. Ji, N.; Weng, D.; Liu, C.; Gu, Z.; Chen, S.; Guo, Y.; Fan, Z.; Wang, X.; Chen, J.; Zhao, Y.; et al. Adenovirus-mediated delivery of herpes simplex virus thymidine kinase administration improves outcome of recurrent high-grade glioma. *Oncotarget* **2015**, *7*, 4369–4378. [CrossRef]

70. Lowenstein, P.R.; A Orringer, D.; Sagher, O.; Heth, J.; Hervey-Jumper, S.L.; Mammoser, A.G.; Junck, L.; Leung, D.; Umemura, Y.; Lawrence, T.S.; et al. First-in-human phase I trial of the combination of two adenoviral vectors expressing HSV1-TK and FLT3L for the treatment of newly diagnosed resectable malignant glioma: Initial results from the therapeutic reprogramming of the brain immune system. *J. Clin. Oncol.* **2019**, *37*, 2019. [CrossRef]
71. Chiocca, E.A.; Yu, J.S.; Lukas, R.V.; Solomon, I.H.; Ligon, K.L.; Nakashima, H.; Triggs, D.A.; Reardon, D.A.; Wen, P.; Stopa, B.M.; et al. Regulatable interleukin-12 gene therapy in patients with recurrent high-grade glioma: Results of a phase 1 trial. *Sci. Transl. Med.* **2019**, *11*, eaaw5680. [CrossRef] [PubMed]
72. Brenner, A.J.; Cohen, Y.; Vredenburgh, J.J.; Peters, K.B.; Breitbart, E.; Bangio, L.; Sher, N.; Harats, D.; Wen, P.Y. Phase I/II dose-escalation study of VB-111, an antiangiogenic gene therapy, in patients with recurrent glioblastoma multiforme. *J. Clin. Oncol.* **2013**. [CrossRef]
73. Cloughesy, T.; Brenner, A.; De Groot, J.F.; A Butowski, N.; Zach, L.; Campian, J.L.; Ellingson, B.M.; Freedman, L.S.; Cohen, Y.C.; Lowenton-Spier, N.; et al. A randomized controlled phase III study of VB-111 combined with bevacizumab vs bevacizumab monotherapy in patients with recurrent glioblastoma (GLOBE). *Neuro Oncol.* **2019**, *22*, 705–717. [CrossRef] [PubMed]
74. Rampling, R.; Cruickshank, G.; Papanastassiou, V.; Nicoll, J.A.R.; Hadley, D.M.; Brennan, D.C.; Petty, R.; MacLean, A.; Harland, J.; A McKie, E.; et al. Toxicity evaluation of replication-competent herpes simplex virus (ICP 34.5 null mutant 1716) in patients with recurrent malignant glioma. *Gene Ther.* **2000**, *7*, 859–866. [CrossRef]
75. Papanastassiou, V.; Rampling, R.; Fraser, M.; Petty, R.; Hadley, D.; Nicoll, J.; Harland, J.; Mabbs, R.; Brown, M. The potential for efficacy of the modified (ICP 34.5−) herpes simplex virus HSV1716 following intratumoural injection into human malignant glioma: A proof of principle study. *Gene Ther.* **2002**, *9*, 398–406. [CrossRef]
76. Harrow, S.; Papanastassiou, V.; Harland, J.; Mabbs, R.; Petty, R.D.; Fraser, M.J.; Hadley, D.M.; Patterson, J.; Brown, S.M.; Rampling, R. HSV1716 injection into the brain adjacent to tumour following surgical resection of high-grade glioma: Safety data and long-term survival. *Gene Ther.* **2004**, *11*, 1648–1658. [CrossRef]
77. Markert, J.M.; Medlock, M.D.; Rabkin, S.D.; Gillespie, G.Y.; Todo, T.; Hunter, W.D.; A Palmer, C.; Feigenbaum, F.; Tornatore, C.; Tufaro, F.; et al. Conditionally replicating herpes simplex virus mutant, G207 for the treatment of malignant glioma: Results of a phase I trial. *Gene Ther.* **2000**, *7*, 867–874. [CrossRef]
78. Markert, J.M.; Liechty, P.G.; Wang, W.; Gaston, S.; Braz, E.; Karrasch, M.; Nabors, L.B.; Markiewicz, M.; Lakeman, A.D.; A Palmer, C.; et al. Phase Ib Trial of Mutant Herpes Simplex Virus G207 Inoculated Pre-and Post-tumor Resection for Recurrent GBM. *Mol. Ther.* **2009**, *17*, 199–207. [CrossRef]
79. Markert, J.M.; Razdan, S.N.; Kuo, H.-C.; Cantor, A.; Knoll, A.; Karrasch, M.; Nabors, L.B.; Markiewicz, M.; Agee, B.S.; Coleman, J.M.; et al. A Phase 1 Trial of Oncolytic HSV-1, G207, Given in Combination With Radiation for Recurrent GBM Demonstrates Safety and Radiographic Responses. *Mol. Ther.* **2014**, *22*, 1048–1055. [CrossRef]
80. A Forsyth, P.; Roldán, G.; George, D.J.; Wallace, C.; Palmer, C.A.; Morris, D.; Cairncross, G.; Matthews, M.V.; Markert, J.M.; Gillespie, Y.; et al. A Phase I Trial of Intratumoral Administration of Reovirus in Patients with Histologically Confirmed Recurrent Malignant Gliomas. *Mol. Ther.* **2008**, *16*, 627–632. [CrossRef]
81. Geletneky, K.; Hajda, J.; Angelova, A.L.; Leuchs, B.; Capper, D.; Bartsch, A.J.; Neumann, J.-O.; Schöning, T.; Hüsing, J.; Beelte, B.; et al. Oncolytic H-1 Parvovirus Shows Safety and Signs of Immunogenic Activity in a First Phase I/IIa Glioblastoma Trial. *Mol. Ther.* **2017**, *25*, 2620–2634. [CrossRef] [PubMed]
82. Geletneky, K.; Hüsing, J.; Rommelaere, J.; Schlehofer, J.; Leuchs, B.; Dahm, M.; Krebs, O.; Doeberitz, M.V.K.; Huber, B.; Hajda, J. Phase I/IIa study of intratumoral/intracerebral or intravenous/intracerebral administration of Parvovirus H-1 (ParvOryx) in patients with progressive primary or recurrent glioblastoma multiforme: ParvOryx01 protocol. *BMC Cancer* **2012**, *12*, 99. [CrossRef] [PubMed]
83. Freeman, A.I.; Zakay-Rones, Z.; Gomori, J.M.; Linetsky, E.; Rasooly, L.; Greenbaum, E.; Rozenman-Yair, S.; Panet, A.; Libson, E.; Irving, C.S.; et al. Phase I/II Trial of Intravenous NDV-HUJ Oncolytic Virus in Recurrent Glioblastoma Multiforme. *Mol. Ther.* **2006**, *13*, 221–228. [CrossRef] [PubMed]
84. Desjardins, A.; Gromeier, M.; Ii, J.E.H.; Beaubier, N.; Bolognesi, D.P.; Friedman, A.H.; Friedman, H.S.; McSherry, F.; Muscat, A.; Nair, S.; et al. Recurrent Glioblastoma Treated with Recombinant Poliovirus. *N. Engl. J. Med.* **2018**, *379*, 150–161. [CrossRef] [PubMed]
85. Cloughesy, T.F.; Petrecca, K.; Walbert, T.; Butowski, N.; Salacz, M.; Perry, J.; Damek, D.; Bota, D.; Bettegowda, C.; Zhu, J.-J.; et al. Effect of Vocimagene Amiretrorepvec in Combination With Flucytosine vs Standard of Care on Survival Following Tumor Resection in Patients With Recurrent High-Grade Glioma: A Randomized Clinical Trial. *JAMA Oncol.* **2020**, *33612*. [CrossRef]

86. Cloughesy, T.F.; Landolfi, J.; Hogan, D.J.; Bloomfield, S.; Carter, B.; Chen, C.C.; Elder, J.B.; Kalkanis, S.N.; Kesari, S.; Lai, A.; et al. Phase 1 trial of vocimagene amiretrorepvec and 5-fluorocytosine for recurrent high-grade glioma. *Sci. Transl. Med.* **2016**, *8*, 341ra75. [CrossRef]
87. Jolly, D.J.; Robbins, J.M.; Ostertag, D.; Ibañez, C.; Kasahara, N.; Gruber, H.; Kalkanis, S.N.; Vogelbaum, M.; Aghi, M.K.; Cloughesy, T.; et al. 61. Ascending Dose Trials of a Retroviral Replicating Vector (Toca 511) in Patients with Recurrent High-Grade Glioma: Clinical Update, Molecular Analyses, and Proposed Mechanism of Action. *Mol. Ther.* **2016**, *24*, S27. [CrossRef]
88. Cloughesy, T.; Landolfi, J.; A Vogelbaum, M.; Ostertag, D.; Elder, J.B.; Bloomfield, S.; Carter, B.; Chen, C.C.; Kalkanis, S.N.; Kesari, S.; et al. Durable complete responses in some recurrent high-grade glioma patients treated with Toca 511 + Toca FC. *Neuro-Oncology* **2018**, *20*, 1383–1392. [CrossRef]
89. Kalkanis, S.N.; Aghi, M.K.; Cloughsy, T.F.; Kaptain, G.; Portnow, J.; Vogelbaum, M.A.; Kesari, S.; Mikkelsen, T.; Elder, J.B.; Chen, C.C.; et al. DDEL-06 Preliminary Safety of Toca 511, a Retroviral Replicating Vector, in Patients with Recurrent High Grade Glioma across Three Separate Phase 1 Studies. *Neuro Oncol.* **2015**, *17*, v74. [CrossRef]
90. Lyle, C.; McCormick, F. Integrin αvβ5 is a primary receptor for adenovirus in CAR-negative cells. *Virol. J.* **2010**, *7*, 148. [CrossRef]
91. Suzuki, K.; Tsunekawa, Y.; Hernandez-Benitez, R.; Wu, J.; Zhu, J.; Kim, E.J.; Hatanaka, F.; Yamamoto, M.; Araoka, T.; Li, Z.; et al. In vivo genome editing via CRISPR/Cas9 mediated homology-independent targeted integration. *Nature* **2016**, *540*, 144–149. [CrossRef] [PubMed]
92. Tang, F.; Lane, S.; Korsak, A.; Paton, J.F.R.; Gourine, A.V.; Kasparov, S.; Teschemacher, A.G. Lactate-mediated glia-neuronal signalling in the mammalian brain. *Nat. Commun.* **2014**, *5*, 3284. [CrossRef] [PubMed]
93. Duale, H.; Kasparov, S.; Paton, J.F.R.; Teschemacher, A.G. Differences in transductional tropism of adenoviral and lentiviral vectors in the rat brainstem. *Exp. Physiol.* **2005**, *90*, 71–78. [CrossRef] [PubMed]
94. Liu, B.; Paton, J.F.R.; Kasparov, S. Viral vectors based on bidirectional cell-specific mammalian promoters and transcriptional amplification strategy for use in vitro and in vivo. *BMC Biotechnol.* **2008**, *8*, 49. [CrossRef] [PubMed]
95. Hsu, C.-C.; Li, H.-P.; Hung, Y.-H.; Leu, Y.-W.; Wu, W.-H.; Wang, F.-S.; Lee, K.-D.; Chang, P.-J.; Wu, C.-S.; Lu, Y.-J.; et al. Targeted methylation of CMV and E1A viral promoters. *Biochem. Biophys. Res. Commun.* **2010**, *402*, 228–234. [CrossRef]
96. Wang, X.; Xu, Z.; Tian, Z.; Zhang, X.; Xu, D.; Li, Q.; Zhang, J.; Wang, T. The EF-1α promoter maintains high-level transgene expression from episomal vectors in transfected CHO-K1 cells. *J. Cell. Mol. Med.* **2017**, *21*, 3044–3054. [CrossRef]
97. Friedmann-Morvinski, D. Glioblastoma Heterogeneity and Cancer Cell Plasticity. *Crit. Rev. Oncog.* **2014**, *19*, 327–336. [CrossRef]
98. Sharma, P.; Khuc, K. Summary Basis for Regulatory Action. 2018. Available online: https://www.fda.gov/media/125157/download (accessed on 10 October 2020).
99. Al-Zaidy, S.A.; Mendell, J.R. From Clinical Trials to Clinical Practice: Practical Considerations for Gene Replacement Therapy in SMA Type 1. *Pediatr. Neurol.* **2019**, *100*, 3–11. [CrossRef]
100. Chan, K.Y.; Jang, M.J.; Yoo, B.B.; Greenbaum, A.; Ravi, N.; Wu, W.-L.; Sánchez-Guardado, L.; Lois, C.; Mazmanian, S.K.; E Deverman, B.; et al. Engineered AAVs for efficient noninvasive gene delivery to the central and peripheral nervous systems. *Nat. Neurosci.* **2017**, *20*, 1172–1179. [CrossRef]

Publisher's Note: MDPI stays neutral with regard to jurisdictional claims in published maps and institutional affiliations.

© 2020 by the authors. Licensee MDPI, Basel, Switzerland. This article is an open access article distributed under the terms and conditions of the Creative Commons Attribution (CC BY) license (http://creativecommons.org/licenses/by/4.0/).

Review

Nanomedicine: A Useful Tool against Glioma Stem Cells

Elia Bozzato [1], Chiara Bastiancich [2] and Véronique Préat [1,*]

1 Advanced Drug Delivery and Biomaterials, Louvain Drug Research Institute, Université Catholique de Louvain, 1200 Brussels, Belgium; elia.bozzato@uclouvain.be
2 Institute Neurophysiopathol, INP, CNRS, Aix-Marseille University, 13005 Marseille, France; chiara.bastiancich@univ-amu.fr
* Correspondence: veronique.preat@uclouvain.be

Simple Summary: Glioblastoma is one of the deadliest brain cancers, and despite the efforts made in the last few years, the life expectancy of patients is still low. In most cases, even with the best treatments available, the tumor will eventually return. One of the main causes of this appears to be a fraction of cancer cells that are known as glioma stem cells. They have different characteristics than normal cancer cells, and some drugs can eliminate them. However, using such drugs is not always safe or effective, and nanomedicine can have improved effects as well as additional benefits. This review focuses on the nanomedicine strategies that have been employed in the last 5 years and their relative advantages, which make nanomedicine a promising approach for the eradication of glioma stem cells.

Abstract: The standard of care therapy of glioblastoma (GBM) includes invasive surgical resection, followed by radiotherapy and concomitant chemotherapy. However, this therapy has limited success, and the prognosis for GBM patients is very poor. Although many factors may contribute to the failure of current treatments, one of the main causes of GBM recurrences are glioma stem cells (GSCs). This review focuses on nanomedicine strategies that have been developed to eliminate GSCs and the benefits that they have brought to the fight against cancer. The first section describes the characteristics of GSCs and the chemotherapeutic strategies that have been used to selectively kill them. The second section outlines the nano-based delivery systems that have been developed to act against GSCs by dividing them into nontargeted and targeted nanocarriers. We also highlight the advantages of nanomedicine compared to conventional chemotherapy and examine the different targeting strategies that have been employed. The results achieved thus far are encouraging for the pursuit of effective strategies for the eradication of GSCs.

Keywords: glioblastoma; brain tumor; nanomedicine; cancer stem cell; targeted therapy

1. Introduction

Glioblastoma (GBM) is a grade IV astrocytoma, and the prognosis for GBM patients is very poor. Currently, the standard of care therapy includes surgical resection of the main tumor mass, followed by radiotherapy and concomitant chemotherapy with oral temozolomide (TMZ) [1]. However, this therapy has limited success due to the intrinsic characteristics of the tumor, such as the tumor heterogenicity, development of chemoresistance, and presence of glioma stem cells (GSCs). These factors lead to tumor recurrences. Recently, the overall survival of GBM patients has slightly increased from 16.0 months to 20.9 months with the additional application of tumor-treating fields to the standard of care therapy [2]. Nevertheless, despite this significant improvement, GBM still remains an unmet medical need, and successful long-term therapies urgently need to be found.

GBM is characterized by resistance to treatment and high intertumor and intratumor phenotypic and genetic heterogeneity [3]. Many advances have been made in the past decade to uncover the genetic diversity of GBM and the clone-specific functional profile, showing that even within the same tumor, the combination of various molecular subclasses could be found (e.g., [4–6]). This diversity also indicates the presence of GSCs, which are defined as a quiescent subpopulation of cancer cells with high self-renewing abilities that are able to recreate a tumor after transplantation [7]. Even though the precise cell of origin of GBM is still a controversial issue, as some experts contend that it arises from a subpopulation of neural stem cells, while others argue that it arises from the transformation of more differentiated astrocytes [8], it is now recognized that presence of GSCs and crosstalk with their supportive niche contributes to tumor malignancy [9]. Moreover, they are responsible for the onset of tumor recurrence, and therefore, are a promising therapeutic target to prevent GBM relapse. Several publications have recently highlighted how GSC location at the invasive margins, heterogeneity, and dynamism (transcriptional, epigenetic, and metabolic) can play an important role in the response to surgery, radiotherapy, and chemotherapy (e.g., [10,11]). A review from Liu et al. [12] evaluates the potential involvement of brain tumor stem cells in postoperative stem cell niches and their role in tumor relapse, and their input should be considered for the development of adapted nanomedicines. Indeed, while it is true that most nanomedicines are intended for a post-surgical application, most studies report their efficacy on preclinical models designed to treat established GBM. This overlooks the fact that surgical resection of brain tumors can create an environment that can stimulate the proliferation of residual tumor cells (GSCs, tumor microtubes, and infiltrating GBM cells), leading to tumor recurrences. Here, we would like to highlight how nanomedicines can be used to overcome some of the limitations of conventional chemotherapies targeting GSCs, thus representing a promising approach for GBM therapy.

2. Glioma Stem Cells

Due to their dormant state, GSCs are intrinsically resistant to conventional chemotherapeutics that act on rapidly proliferating cancer cells, such as alkylating agents, antimetabolites, and mitotic inhibitors. Furthermore, they can actively resist chemo- or radiotherapy by the activation of checkpoint mechanisms, in order to recover efficiently from the genotoxicity induced by the therapy. Another mechanism of resistance for GSCs is the expression of drug efflux mechanisms (ABC transporters) to protect the cells from xenogeneic molecules [13]. Autophagy, which is required for stemness maintenance, not only in normal tissue stem cells but also in GSCs, has been shown to contribute to therapy resistance [14]. Moreover, the Notch signaling pathway is involved in the resistance of GSCs to radiotherapy. The inhibition of this pathway through γ-secretase inhibitors is able to induce radiosensitivity by targeting the subpopulation of cells that bears the GSC marker CD133 [15].

GSCs are also characterized by specific pathways that are implied in the conservation of stemness characteristics or in tumor formation. The Notch pathway can inhibit cell differentiation and therefore maintain the stem-like properties of GSCs [16]. In patient-derived GSCs taken from the periphery of the tumor, Hu and collaborators demonstrated that Notch promotes self-renewal and inhibits differentiation [17]. In recurrent GBM samples, CD133, Notch, and VEGF expression was higher after radiotherapy and chemotherapy, and after a second surgery and treatment with bevacizumab, the overall survival was significantly longer for Notch-negative patients [18]. Furthermore, cells from the interface region are $CD133^+/Notch1^+$, and there is a positive-feedback loop between NOTCH1 and SOX2 [19]. The aberrant activation of Wnt signaling causes the transcription of c-Myc and other target genes leading to tumor formation [20]. It also participates in the maintenance of stemness characteristics by regulating the expression of PLAGL2 (pleiomorphic adenoma gene-like 2) that is able to suppress the differentiation of GSCs [21]. Finally, the Sonic Hedgehog (Shh) pathway is essential for cell survival and sustained growth of the tumor. In fact, it regulates the expression of stemness genes in glioma GSCs [22].

GSCs can be isolated from cancer cells and tissue stem cells using specific intracellular or extracellular markers (Figure 1), although functional validation should also be employed to assess the stem cell characteristics (self-renewal and tumor formation) [8]. The most common marker is CD133 or Prominin-1, a transmembrane glycoprotein that is also expressed by human neural stem cells [23]. However, evidence also suggests the existence of CD133⁻ GSCs [24], and therefore, a single marker cannot automatically identify GSCs. Other common markers are A2B5, a glycolipid found on the cell surface of oligodendrocyte progenitors; stage-specific embryonic antigen-1 (SSEA-1, also known as CD15) an embryonic antigen with a carbohydrate structure; and Nestin, a filament protein that is also expressed by neural progenitor cells [25]. Additionally, high ALDH-1 (aldehyde dehydrogenase 1) activity and the high extrusion of xenobiotics through ABC transporters are two functional markers that have been associated with GSCs [25].

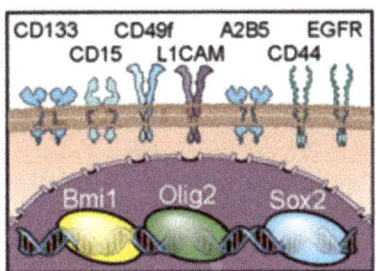

Figure 1. Intracellular and extracellular glioma stem cell (GSC) markers. Adapted from [26].

The metabolism of GSCs is very plastic. In fact, the dependence on oxidative or nonoxidative metabolism is heterogeneous throughout the tumor. Fast-dividing cells rely more on anaerobic glycolysis [27], creating the Warburg effect as an adaptation metabolism for their rapid growth. In an acidic environment, GSCs can undergo mesenchymal differentiation, resulting in an increase of therapy resistance [28]. On the other hand, slowly proliferating cells are more dependent on oxidative phosphorylation (OXPHOS) and lipid oxidation, and GSCs in particular can metabolize various substrates, making it difficult to find a pharmacological target [10]. GSCs have been reported to have lower glucose consumption than normal GBM cells [10]. However, depending on their microenvironment, they are able to adapt to nutrient and stress conditions by increasing their glycolytic activity [10]. In fact, GSCs can also upregulate high-affinity transporters, such as GLUT3, to obtain sufficient nutrients and support their rapid metabolism [10].

GSCs can adapt and are able to interact with different niches. For example, GSCs that are located at the perivascular niche are in contact with the endothelium that secretes ligands that bind to the transmembrane Notch receptor on GSCs, leading to the activation of the Notch pathway and supporting GSC self-renewal. In exchange, GSCs can transdifferentiate into pericytes to contribute to the vascular structure, thus promoting tumor growth [26]. GSCs can also interact with immune cells through their metabolism. They can regulate the microenvironment and generate stress for immune cells, thus creating a globally suppressive tumor microenvironment that allows for immune escape and tumor progression [10]. In return, macrophages, which are the most represented type of tumor-infiltrating cell, participate to the regulation of GSC metabolism by increasing their fatty acids synthesis and trafficking, thus promoting lipid oxidation, which is one of the main metabolic pathway of GSCs [10]. Moreover, through the secretion of interleukin 10 (IL-10) and transforming growth factor beta (TGF-β), GSCs are able to suppress the tumor-associated microglia, generating an M2 immunosuppressive phenotype [26]. Furthermore, GSCs are able to regulate immune cells directly, causing the activation of regulatory T cells, the inhibition of cytotoxic T cell proliferation, and the induction of cytotoxic T cell apoptosis [29,30].

GSCs however are not a static, discreet cell subpopulation; their stemness is rather a dynamic and reversible state. There is considerable evidence that EMT (epithelial to mesenchymal transition) is involved in the dynamism of GSCs [31], and that various factors can stimulate or revert this transition [32–34]. Furthermore, based on their location in the tumor, they can have different characteristics and exert different functions: while GSCs in the core hypoxic regions support proliferation and therapy resistance, GSCs from the outer invasive region are enriched for their invasive potential and promote tumor recurrence after resection [11].

3. Chemotherapy against GSCs

Despite the high number of researchers and clinicians investigating GBM, treatment options for this tumor have remained nearly unchanged for the last 15 years [35]. Some progress has been made in the field of personalized therapy, thanks to the ChemoID assay, which consists of a viability test on GSCs and bulk tumor cells from freshly resected samples, in order to identify the most effective drug or combination of drugs. Patients were therefore treated with the selected drugs, and 12 out of 14 cases had complete or at least partial response to the therapy [36]. In order to better relate to intra-tumor heterogeneity, this same approach could be used on samples obtained from different tumor regions from each patient. After the viability assay on GSCs from each sample, the patient could be treated with the combination of drugs that demonstrated cytotoxicity in the different regions. However, the study from Ranjan et al. [36] suggests that, along with chemotherapy directed against GBM cells, combination therapies also targeting GSCs could be necessary. The possible approaches that can be adopted in order to eliminate GSCs are represented in Figure 2.

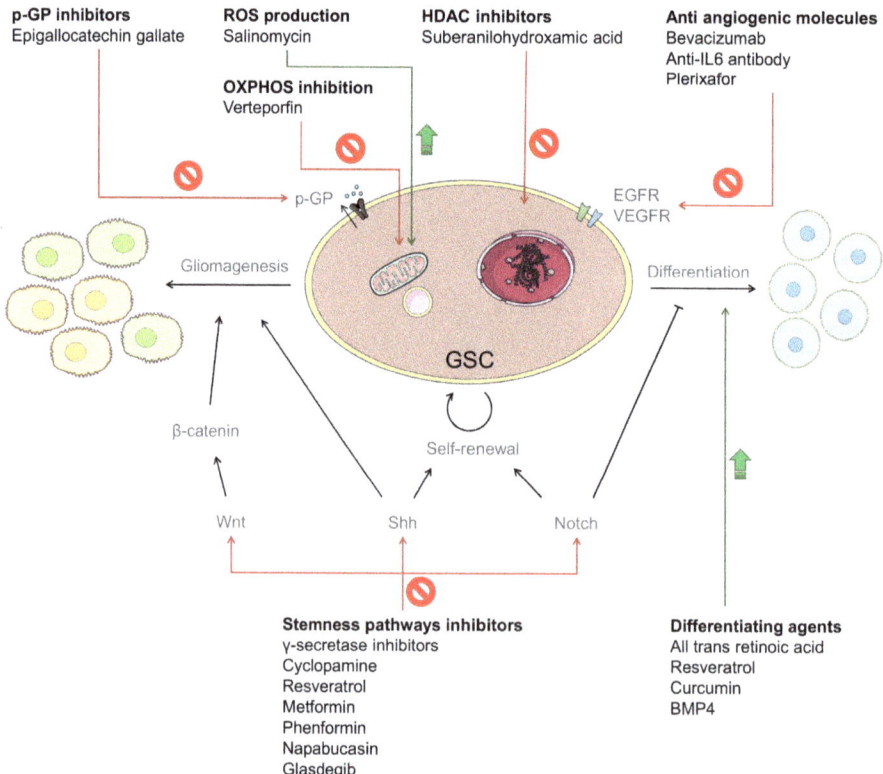

Figure 2. Anti-GSC molecules and their mechanisms of action.

One of the strategies that has been explored to attack the GSC population is to inhibit specific GSC pathways, such as Notch, Wnt, and Shh. For example, the inhibition of Notch activation through γ-secretase inhibitors is reported to reduce the CD133-positive GBM cell population in vitro and to reduce tumorigenicity of pretreated brain tumor cells subcutaneously injected in athymic mice [37]. Cyclopamine, a Shh inhibitor, was able to reduce neurosphere formation and block the tumor formation of intracranially injected GSC cells [38]. Resveratrol can modulate the Wnt pathway and decrease the proliferation and mobility of GSCs [39]. Metformin can inhibit AKT signaling, which is involved in the response to stress conditions to promote GSC growth and survival [40]. Its analog Phenformin is also able to inhibit the self-renewal of GSCs, thus reducing the growth of xenograft tumors and prolonging mice survival [41]. Napabucasin, a STAT3 inhibitor, can inhibit the expression of stemness-associated genes and the growth of GBM spheroids in vitro [42], and has led to the loss of GSCs associated genes, induction of apoptosis, and inhibition of in vivo tumor growth of GSCs derived from recurrent GBM [43]. This drug has also been used in a phase I/II clinical trial in combination with TMZ [44]. Glasdegib and RO4929097, a Shh pathway inhibitor and a γ-secretase inhibitor, respectively, are also being used in combination with TMZ in two different ongoing clinical studies [45,46].

GSCs are also implied in therapy resistance, and they can actively participate to this process though mechanisms like DNA repair, pro-surviving signaling, and most importantly, drug efflux [47]. Therefore, another approach is to employ P-gp (permeability glycoprotein) or to induce the differentiation in normal GBM cells, in order to sensitize them to conventional chemotherapy. It has been demonstrated that CD133 contributes to the regulation of MDR1 through the phosphoinositide 3-kinase (PI3K)- or Akt–NF-κB signal pathway [48]. Moreover, the invasive margin of GBM displays an increased expression of ABCG2 [49], which is another efflux pump belonging to the ABC transporters superfamily. It has been shown that reduction in ABCG2 expression can decrease the cell migration and invasion of GSCs [50]. An example of P-gp inhibitor is epigallocatechin gallate, which was able to reduce the P-gp expression and neurosphere formation of GSCs obtained from the U87 cell line, and increase the sensitivity of these cells to TMZ [51]. The differentiating agent transretinoic acid was able to deplete GSC markers and reduce the formation of neurospheres, and the effect on cell migration was improved in combination with rapamycin [52]. Resveratrol can induce the degradation of Nanog, which is essential for stemness maintenance, thus leading to the loss of GSC markers and decreased tumorigenicity [53]. Curcumin was demonstrated to activate autophagy, thus triggering the differentiation cascade of GSCs and causing a decrease in its self-renewal and clonogenic abilities [54]. Finally, bone morphogenetic protein 4 (BMP4) is commonly used to reduce the number of GSCs by inducing their differentiation, and therefore increasing the response to conventional therapies [55]. BMP4 is also currently being administered through convection-enhanced delivery (CED) in a phase I clinical trial [56].

Additionally, tackling the tumor microenvironment through antiangiogenic or antivasculogenic molecules can also decrease the number of GSCs. The treatment with bevacizumab was able to reduce the number of CD133$^+$/Nestin$^+$ cells, along with reducing the microvasculature density and tumor growth in U87 glioma xenografts [57]. Moreover, the administration of antibodies against a proangiogenic factor like IL-6 could delay the growth of tumors obtained by the injection of GSCs in a xenograft model [58]. Another antivasculogenic molecule, the biciclame compound plerixafor (AMD3100), was able to inhibit irradiation-induced vasculogenesis in vivo by preventing the binding of the chemokine stromal cell-derived factor 1 (SDF-1, involved in the migratory process of GBM) to its receptor C-X-C chemokine receptor type 4 (CXCR4) [59].

Targeting the DNA methylation of GSCs through histone deacetylase inhibitors (HDAC) inhibitors is another strategy that has been described in the literature. In fact, suberanilohydroxamic acid (SAHA) is able to induce autophagy in GSCs, thus leading to decreased cell viability in vitro and reduced tumor growth in vivo [60].

Finally, salinomycin has been used on GBM cells in combination with HDAC inhibitors, such as valproate and vorinostat [61], and it has also shown anti-CSC activity in other cancer types [62]. Even though its mechanism of action needs to be elucidated, it has been reported that it can induce ROS production in GSCs, thus leading to endoplasmic reticulum stress and cell death via regulated necrosis [63]. Additionally, verteporfin can target the mitochondria of GSCs and inhibit OXPHOS without any toxicity to normal cells [64].

In many cases, the elimination or impairment of GSCs has led to decreased tumor growth and increased survival in preclinical in vivo models, highlighting once again the importance of tackling GSCs in the treatment of GBM. However, only a few of the above-mentioned molecules are being tested in clinical trials (mostly GSC pathway inhibitors), and the results are not yet available.

4. Nanomedicine against GSCs

4.1. Nanomedicine for GBM Treatment

The intrinsic limits of chemotherapy are the lack of specificity, harmful side effects, low therapeutic index, and transport limitations [65]. Indeed, many drugs, including those cited in the previous chapter, have poor solubility, high toxicity due to the uncontrolled drug biodistribution, or poor stability in the physiological environment. Moreover, when administered systemically, they need to cross the blood–brain barrier (BBB) to reach the GBM tumor site at therapeutic concentrations, often leading to severe, dose-related systemic side effects. Some drugs are not stable in biological fluids and have a very short half-life; therefore, multiple administrations are required to achieve the therapeutic concentration at the tumor site, reducing patient compliance.

Nanomedicine can help provide a solution for these problems. The encapsulation of drugs in nanosized carriers can protect them from degradation, increase the amount of drug reaching the tumor site, and decrease the intensity of the side effects, thus increasing the safety of the treatment. The maintenance of a correct therapeutic level can be facilitated by the controlled release of the drug over time. Moreover, the surface of the nanocarrier can be suitably modified with targeting moieties in order to actively and specifically recognize GBM cells and GSCs, or to cross the BBB more easily. This can further increase the uptake of the nanoparticles (NPs) by GSCs and enhance their residence time in the tumor.

The BBB is a natural barrier that protects the central nervous system from exogenous compounds or macromolecules. Even though in GBM the patients' BBB parts are disrupted and leaky [66,67], the crossing of the BBB still represents a challenge for GBM treatment, due to the poor blood perfusion and the high interstitial pressure. The BBB can be bypassed by administering drugs locally, through implants or CED. A local delivery has the advantage of increasing the drug concentration in its site of action while minimizing the side effects. However, systemic delivery is still the preferred strategy for inoperable tumors, and thanks to its being less invasive, also allows for the administration of multiple doses.

Herein, we review the nanomedicine approaches that have been developed in the last 5 years against GSCs, dividing them by nontargeted and targeted systems (Tables 1 and 2, respectively).

Table 1. Nontargeted nanosystems for the treatment of preclinical glioblastoma (GBM).

Molecule(s)	Nanoparticle	Cell Line(s)	Preclinical Model	Outcome	References
Etoposide	Layered double hydroxide nanocomposites	U87 MG U87 MG-derived GSCs	Nude mice, hypodermically injected GSCs, treated by i.p. injection	GSC elimination Downregulation of pluripotency genes Decreased tumor growth Increased drug accumulation	[68]

Table 1. Cont.

Molecule(s)	Nanoparticle	Cell Line(s)	Preclinical Model	Outcome	References
miR-148a miR-296-5p	Cationic polymeric NPs	GBM1A	Orthotopic human GBM xenografts, treated by intracranial infusion	Lower expression of GSC-correlated genes ~70% animal survival	[69]
Curcumin Epicatechin gallate Resveratrol	Liposomes	GL261	Orthotopic syngenic mice, treated by i.p. injection	Decrease of CD133+ and SOX2+ cells Constant plasma concentration Increased mice survival	[70]
HOTAIR-siRNA	SPIONs	SHG44	Subcutaneous injection of pretreated human GSCs in nude mice	Inhibition of CD133+ cell proliferation	[71]
miR-182	Gold NPs	Patient-derived cells U87 MG	Orthotopic xenograft model, treated by i.v. injection	Higher animal survival	[72]
siRNA	Lipopolymeric NPs	Patient-derived cells	Orthotopic xenografts, treated by intracranial injection or intracranial infusion	Knock-down of CSC-related markers Extension of the median survival	[73]
GLUT3 siRNA	PEG–PLA NPs	U87 MG U251	Subcutaneous human glioma xenograft, treated by i.v. injection	Increased the internalization Reduction of tumor growth and CSC markers	[74]
Zinc-doped copper oxide nanocomposites TMZ *	Zinc-doped copper oxide nanocomposites	C6 U87 U251 A172	Subcutaneous GBM xenografts, treated by i.t. injection	Higher cytotoxic effect Reduction of sphere and colony formation	[75]
microRNA-374a overexpression plasmid	SPIONs	Patient-derived CD133+ GBM cells	Subcutaneous injection of pretreated human GSCs in nude mice	Decreased proliferation rate and invasiveness of CD133+ cells Tumorigenicity inhibition	[76]
Iguratimod	PLGA NPs	U87 U118 U251	Subcutaneous xenograft model, treatment by i.v. injection	Cell growth inhibition Sphere formation inhibition Decreased tumor growth	[77]

Legend: * free drug. Abbreviations: HOTAIR: HOX transcript antisense RNA; TMZ: Temozolomide; NPs: nanoparticles; SPION: superparamagnetic iron oxide NPs; GSCs: glioma stem cells; CSCs: cancer stem cells; i.p.: intraperitoneal; i.v.: intravenous.

Table 2. Targeted nanosystems for the treatment of preclinical glioblastoma.

Molecule(s)	Nanoparticle	Targeting	Cell Line(s)	Preclinical Model	Outcome	References
Antisense oligonucleotides targeting laminin-411	Polymeric nanoconjugate	anti-TfR receptor antibodies	U87 MG LN229 Patient-derived cells	Orthotopic xenograft model, treatment by i.v. injection	Reduced protein expression Prolonged mouse survival	[78]
Antisense oligonucleotides targeting CK2α and EGFR/EGFRvIII	Polymeric nanoconjugate	anti-TfR mAb anti-EGFR mAb cetuximab	U87 MG LN229	Orthotopic xenograft model, treatment by i.v. injection	Lower CSC marker expression Improved survival	[79]

Table 2. Cont.

Molecule(s)	Nanoparticle	Targeting	Cell Line(s)	Preclinical Model	Outcome	References
p53encoding plasmid TMZ *	Cationic liposomes	anti-TfR antibody	U87 T98G LN-18 U87–luc2 U251	Subcutaneous and orthotopic xenograft models, treatment by i.v. injection	Cell sensitization to TMZ Tumor growth reduction Mean survival increase	[80,81]
Bevacizumab Chloroquine	Bevacizumab	Bevacizumab	U87 Primary GBM specimens	Orthotopic injection of GSCs, treatment by i.p. injection	Decreased tumor growth Improved overall survival	[82]
Paclitaxel Survivin siRNA	Cationic liposomes	Angiopep-2 A15	U251–CD133- U251–CD133+	Orthotopic xenograft model, treatment by i.v. injection	Improved uptake of CSCs Decreased CD133+ cell viability Tumor growth reduction Prolonged mouse survival	[83]
IR700	Anti-CD133 antibody	Anti-CD133 antibody	CD133–OE U251 NCH421k GBM-SC	Subcutaneous and orthotopic xenograft models, treatment by i.v. injection	Extended overall survival	[84]
Paclitaxel	Liposomes	Octa-arginine-conjugated cyclic RGD	C6	Orthotopic injection of C6 cells, treatment by i.v. injection	Induction of apoptosis on C6 stem cells Improved mice survival Better safety profile	[85]
Vinorelbine Tetrandrine	Liposomes	Polyethylenimine Vapreotide	C6 GSCs	Orthotopic injection of GSCs, treatment by i.v. injection	Higher cytotoxic effect Higher antitumor efficacy	[86]
Cetuximab	Iron oxide NPs	Cetuximab (anti-EGFR antibody)	U87 MG U87 MGwtEGFR LN229wtEGFR Patient-derived cells	Orthotopic xenograft model, treatment by CED infusion	Enhanced cytotoxicity Improved animal survival	[87]
Mercaptoundeca-hydrododecaborate	polyamido amine dendrimers	Anti-CD133 antibody	SU2 U87	Orthotopic xenograft model, treatment by i.t and/or i.v. injection	Increased uptake Decreased clonogenic survival Prolonged survival	[88]

Table 2. Cont.

Molecule(s)	Nanoparticle	Targeting	Cell Line(s)	Preclinical Model	Outcome	References
Curcumin Quinacrine	Liposomes	p-aminophenyl-α-d-mannopyranoside	C6	Orthotopic injection of GSCs, treatment by i.v. injection	Higher growth inhibition for CSCs Higher efficacy of the combination	[89]
TMZ	Liposomes	Angiopep-2 Anti-CD133 antibody	U87 MG	Orthotopic xenograft model, treated by i.v. injection	Increased cytotoxicity Decreased tumor size Prolonged mice survival	[90]
Antisense oligonucleotides	Polymeric micelles	Cyclic RGD	Patient-derived GSCs	Orthotopic xenograft model, treated by i.v. injection	Induction of apoptosis Accumulation in the tumor site Enhanced TUG1 silencing	[91]

Legend: * free drug. Abbreviations: CK2α: protein kinase CK2 catalytic α subunit; EGFR: epidermal growth factor receptor; TMZ: Temozolomide; NPs: nanoparticles; TfR: transferrin receptor; RGD: Arginyl-glycyl-aspartic acid peptide; GSCs: glioma stem cells; CSCs: cancer stem cells; i.p.: intraperitoneal; i.v.: intravenous.

4.2. Non-Targeted Nanomedicines

NPs can exploit the enhanced permeation and retention (EPR) effect to accumulate and increase their residency time at the tumor site [92,93]. The EPR effect consists of the preferential accumulation of NPs in the tumor site caused by two components: (i) due to their rapid growth, blood vessels in the tumor present a leaky and less organized structure than normal blood vessels; and (ii) inefficient lymphatic drainage. However, in the past few years, due to its intratumor and intertumor variability, together with the differences between animal models and patients, the EPR effect has been questioned [94,95]. Despite this controversial topic, in order to eliminate GSCs, nanomedicine can still offer many advantages when compared to conventional chemotherapy (Table 1, Figure 3).

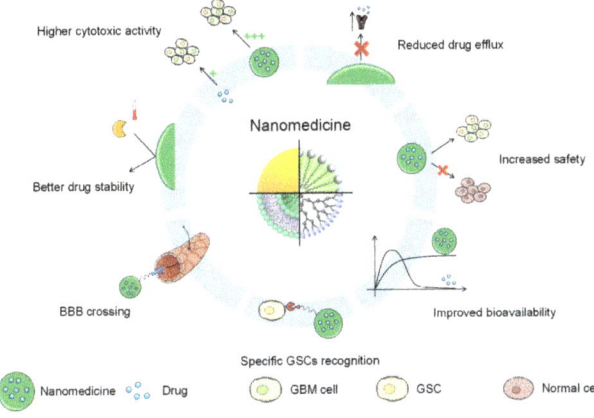

Figure 3. Potential advantages of nanomedicine against GSCs.

One of the advantages of using a drug delivery system is the increase in safety compared to the free drug. For example, paclitaxel-loaded chitosan NPs covered with

1,3β-glucan were demonstrated to have a lower half maximal inhibitory concentration (IC50) value than the free drug on C6-derived stem-like cells, and significantly lower hemolytic activity than the drug suspension [96], thus showing an increased safety profile. Cytarabine-loaded liposomes showed an increased safety profile compared to the free drug [97]. This formulation is currently being examined in a phase I/II clinical trial [98], and is reported to tackle the subventricular zone, which is one of the proposed sites of origin for GSCs [99].

Another advantage of nanomedicine is the increased stability. The encapsulated molecule can be protected from degradation processes, such as hydrolysis, enzymatic degradation, or metabolism. This is usually the case for nucleic acids, such as miRNAs and siRNAs, as their blood half-life is very low. Various types of nucleic acids have been encapsulated in polymeric NPs [69,74], lipid–polymer NPs [73], superparamagnetic iron oxide NPs [71,76], and gold NPs [72,100]. These formulations were able to increase the internalization of the nucleic acid by passive targeting, inducing an efficient silencing of GSC-related genes, reducing GSC proliferation and invasion, and prolonging animal survival in vivo.

Moreover, encapsulation in a drug delivery system can also reduce the efflux of the drug. Unlike free drugs, which enter the cells through diffusion and locate near the efflux pumps, nanomedicines enter the cells through endocytosis and are transported into the cell via endo-lysosomal trafficking, preventing them from being a substrate for drug efflux pumps [101]. Etoposide, which is an efflux pump substrate, was loaded in layered double-hydroxide nanocomposites, thus prolonging its retention time in the cells and increasing its accumulation in the tumor site. This brought about the elimination of GSCs in vitro and decreased tumor growth in the xenograft mouse model [68].

Nanomedicine can also improve the bioavailability of molecules like curcumin. Curcumin was formulated in liposomes in combination with epicatechin gallate and resveratrol, and after intraperitoneal injection, it obtained an almost constant plasma concentration, which led to increased mouse survival in the in vivo experiment. Furthermore, this liposomal formulation was able to decrease the GSC subpopulation of GL261 cells [70].

Additionally, even though this advantage is less common than others, drug delivery systems can in some cases increase the activity of the drugs. Atorvastatine-loaded polymeric micelles were indeed able to inhibit the growth of CSC spheroids compared to the single drug [102]. In the case of zinc-doped copper oxide nanocomposites, the NPs have an intrinsic inhibitory effect, decreasing the colony formation of TMZ-resistant GSCs, but at the same time exerting lower toxicity on normal cells [75].

4.3. Targeted Nanomedicines

The design of nanosystems can be implemented by the addition of a targeting agent, usually an antibody or a ligand, that selectively recognizes cell surface markers overexpressed in a certain population. This has the aim of making the carrier interact with the cell surface, and thanks to the interaction, induce its cellular uptake by endocytosis, ultimately acting as a Trojan horse and releasing its cargo directly inside the cell. Therefore, targeted nanomedicines have the advantage of increasing the amount of cytotoxic agent inside the target cell, reducing the proportion of drug that is delivered to healthy tissues.

Different strategies have been employed to specifically target GSCs (Table 2, Figure 4), and the most common and straightforward is the use of antibodies against CD133, which is the most described GSC marker in the literature. The conjugation of anti-CD133 antibodies to polymeric dendrimers loaded with mercaptoundecahydrododecaborate, a substance employed in boron neutron capture therapy, has led to significantly increased drug uptake and the decreased clonogenic survival of CD133+ cells after neutron radiation. This also produced significantly prolonged mouse survival in an orthotopic xenograft model [88]. Anti-CD133 antibodies were also used as carriers and targeting agents at the same time. IR700, an agent employed in near-infrared photoimmunotherapy, was conjugated to the antibody with a theranostic application. The authors successfully detected CD133+ cells following intravenous administration and laser irradiation in mice bearing orthotopic brain tumors initiated from patient-derived GSCs, and at the same time observed extended overall survival [84].

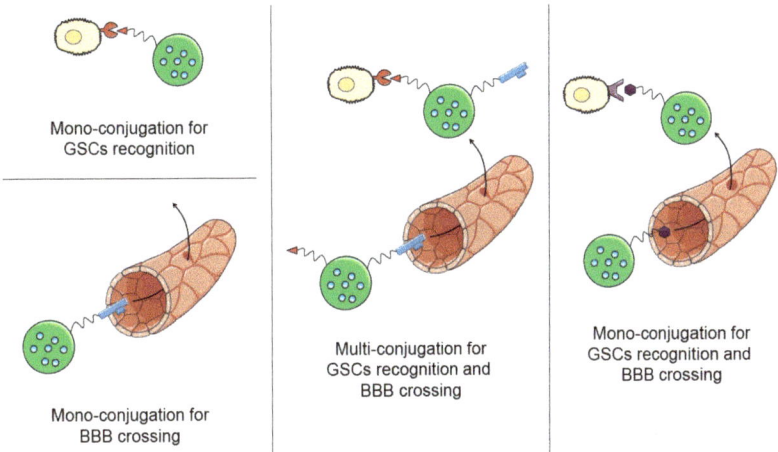

Figure 4. Targeting strategies employed to reach GSCs.

Another common strategy that has been adopted is the conjugation of anti-transferrin receptor (anti-TfR) antibodies. Resveratrol-loaded targeted liposomes are capable of reducing the growth of glioma neurospheres. Moreover, the targeted formulation has shown a significantly increased association with glioma neurospheres compared to the nontargeted liposomes [103]. In addition, targeted polymeric NPs were conjugated to antisense oligonucleotides against laminin-411, which is correlated to GSC marker expression. This nanosystem was able to reduce the protein expression and prolong the survival of mice intracranially transplanted with LN229 and U87 MG cells [78].

Another approach that has been applied is the use of the anti-EGFR antibody. Cetuximab was bound to iron NPs, and showed enhanced uptake by EGFR- and EGFRvIII-expressing GSCs and neurospheres, as well as a significantly increased animal survival in vivo [87].

One of the main obstacles that nanomedicine encounters in the treatment of GBM is the crossing of the BBB, whose natural function is to prevent exogenous structures from reaching the brain. Consequently, nanocarriers for GBM must be designed to cross the BBB and reach the tumor site in higher amounts. The cyclic RDG peptide was linked to micelles loaded with an antisense nucleotide against TUG1, a gene participating in Notch signaling. The formulation in a targeted micellar delivery system allowed the crossing of the BBB and the accumulation in the tumor site, thus enhancing TUG1 silencing in a mouse xenograft model [91].

Several authors developed multifunctional nanocarriers by combining the targeting of GSCs and the crossing of the BBB. TMZ-loaded liposomes were conjugated with an anti-CD133 antibody for targeting GSCs and angiopep-2 for BBB crossing. Angiopep-2 can bind to the low-density lipoprotein (LDL) receptor-related protein, which is highly expressed on the endothelium of the BBB. This system was able to bind to GSCs more efficiently than the nontargeted system, and showed an increased permeability of the BBB in vitro. Moreover, the dual-targeted liposomes were able to decrease the tumor size and prolong the mice survival in the orthotopic, in vivo GSC model [90]. Paclitaxel and surviving siRNA-loaded liposomes were also conjugated with an anti-CD133 aptamer for targeting GSCs and Angiopep-2 for crossing the BBB. Targeted liposomes had an improved uptake in cancer stem cells compared to the nontargeted ones. Moreover, while Taxol and nontargeted liposomes had almost the same effect, targeted liposomes produced a significant decrease in the cell viability of CD133+ cells. The formulation was also able to significantly reduce tumor growth and prolong mouse survival in vivo [83].

Finally, the same targeting moiety can be employed for both targeting GSCs and crossing the BBB. A mannose derivative, p-aminophenyl-α-d-mannopyranoside, was used to functionalize curcumin- and quinacrine-loaded liposomes. Compared to the nontargeted one, this nanocarrier was able to cross a BBB in vitro model more efficiently and significantly increase the uptake in GSCs. Moreover, the targeted liposomes could increase the median survival and inhibit the tumor growth of tumor-bearing mice [89]. Surprisingly, the anti-TfR antibody has also been demonstrated to exert both functions in p53-loaded liposomes. This formulation was also capable of crossing the BBB and targeting GSCs in vivo. Moreover, the delivery of a p53-encoding plasmid was able to decrease the expression of O^6-methylguanine-DNA methyltransferase (MGMT), thus increasing the sensitivity of the cells to TMZ. Due to the promising preclinical results, this formulation is currently under investigation in a phase II clinical study; however, no results have been released yet [80,81,104].

5. Conclusions

Despite extensive research, the need for an efficient, long-term treatment against GBM remains high. As GSCs play a major role in GBM recurrence and resistance to treatment, it is important to take them into account and include anti-GSC molecules in combination regimens to increase their therapeutic benefit. In this review, we have examined the nanosystems that have been developed and used against GSCs in the past 5 years (Tables 1 and 2), trying to highlight their advantages compared to conventional chemotherapeutic treatments. Surprisingly, most of the delivery systems reported in the literature have been developed for systemic administration, while the use of local delivery systems, which have the advantage of bypassing the BBB and delivering high drug concentrations at the tumor site, are poorly represented. In our opinion, a suitable delivery system should be adaptable to the resection cavity to ensure adhesion to the brain tissue, thus delivering the drug(s) in the regions where recurrence is more probable. In fact, most of the recurrences arise nearby the resection cavity [105]. Moreover, this delivery system should include multiple drugs, at least one directed against normal GBM cells and at least one directed against GSCs, as the combination therapy approach is considered promising and is being tested in various clinical trials [106]. Finally, the drug(s) should preferentially be released from the delivery system in a sustained way, in order to maintain a therapeutic drug concentration at least until the beginning of the conventional radio- and chemotherapy (or even beyond, provided that none of the drugs interact with TMZ in an antagonistic manner). However, only a few of the nanomedicine systems included in this review have reached the clinical stage up to now, and therefore, there is still considerable research to be performed in order to explore new potential routes or consolidate established nanomedicine strategies. However, nanomedicine can be a promising strategy for adjuvant GBM therapies, in order to eliminate the GSC population and eradicate these deadly tumors.

Author Contributions: Literature search, manuscript writing, figures, and tables, E.B.; critical revision of manuscript and supervision, C.B.; supervision and critical revision of manuscript, V.P. All authors have read and agreed to the published version of the manuscript.

Funding: The authors thank the EuroNanoMed III found Gliogel, the Fondation ARC pour la Recherce sur le Cancer, the Fondation contre le cancer (Belgium: FAC-C:2016/830), and the Fonds De La Recherche Scientifique (FNRS: Research Credit 33669945) for their financial support.

Conflicts of Interest: The authors declare no conflict of interest.

References

1. Stupp, R.; Hegi, M.E.; Mason, W.P.; van den Bent, M.J.; Taphoorn, M.J.; Janzer, R.C.; Ludwin, S.K.; Allgeier, A.; Fisher, B.; Belanger, K.; et al. Effects of radiotherapy with concomitant and adjuvant temozolomide versus radiotherapy alone on survival in glioblastoma in a randomised phase III study: 5-year analysis of the EORTC-NCIC trial. *Lancet Oncol.* **2009**, *10*, 459–466. [CrossRef]
2. Stupp, R.; Taillibert, S.; Kanner, A.; Read, W.; Steinberg, D.; Lhermitte, B.; Toms, S.; Idbaih, A.; Ahluwalia, M.S.; Fink, K.; et al. Effect of Tumor-Treating Fields Plus Maintenance Temozolomide vs Maintenance Temozolomide Alone on Survival in Patients With Glioblastoma: A Randomized Clinical Trial. *JAMA* **2017**, *318*, 2306–2316. [CrossRef] [PubMed]
3. Perrin, S.L.; Samuel, M.S.; Koszyca, B.; Brown, M.P.; Ebert, L.M.; Oksdath, M.; Gomez, G.A. Glioblastoma heterogeneity and the tumour microenvironment: Implications for preclinical research and development of new treatments. *Biochem. Soc. Trans.* **2019**, *47*, 625–638. [CrossRef] [PubMed]
4. Meyer, M.; Reimand, J.; Lan, X.; Head, R.; Zhu, X.; Kushida, M.; Bayani, J.; Pressey, J.C.; Lionel, A.C.; Clarke, I.D.; et al. Single cell-derived clonal analysis of human glioblastoma links functional and genomic heterogeneity. *Proc. Natl. Acad. Sci. USA* **2015**, *112*, 851–856. [CrossRef] [PubMed]
5. Patel, A.P.; Tirosh, I.; Trombetta, J.J.; Shalek, A.K.; Gillespie, S.M.; Wakimoto, H.; Cahill, D.P.; Nahed, B.V.; Curry, W.T.; Martuza, R.L.; et al. Single-cell RNA-seq highlights intratumoral heterogeneity in primary glioblastoma. *Science* **2014**, *344*, 1396–1401. [CrossRef]
6. Sottoriva, A.; Spiteri, I.; Piccirillo, S.G.; Touloumis, A.; Collins, V.P.; Marioni, J.C.; Curtis, C.; Watts, C.; Tavare, S. Intra-tumor heterogeneity in human glioblastoma reflects cancer evolutionary dynamics. *Proc. Natl. Acad. Sci. USA* **2013**, *110*, 4009–4014. [CrossRef]
7. Galli, R.; Binda, E.; Orfanelli, U.; Cipelletti, B.; Gritti, A.; De Vitis, S.; Fiocco, R.; Foroni, C.; Dimeco, F.; Vescovi, A. Isolation and characterization of tumorigenic, stem-like neural precursors from human glioblastoma. *Cancer Res.* **2004**, *64*, 7011–7021. [CrossRef]
8. Gimple, R.C.; Bhargava, S.; Dixit, D.; Rich, J.N. Glioblastoma stem cells: Lessons from the tumor hierarchy in a lethal cancer. *Genes Dev.* **2019**, *33*, 591–609. [CrossRef]
9. Wang, X.; Prager, B.C.; Wu, Q.; Kim, L.J.Y.; Gimple, R.C.; Shi, Y.; Yang, K.; Morton, A.R.; Zhou, W.; Zhu, Z.; et al. Reciprocal Signaling between Glioblastoma Stem Cells and Differentiated Tumor Cells Promotes Malignant Progression. *Cell Stem Cell* **2018**, *22*, 514–528. [CrossRef]
10. Badr, C.E.; Silver, D.J.; Siebzehnrubl, F.A.; Deleyrolle, L.P. Metabolic heterogeneity and adaptability in brain tumors. *Cell Mol. Life Sci.* **2020**, *77*, 5101–5119. [CrossRef]
11. Prager, B.C.; Bhargava, S.; Mahadev, V.; Hubert, C.G.; Rich, J.N. Glioblastoma Stem Cells: Driving Resilience through Chaos. *Trends Cancer* **2020**, *6*, 223–235. [CrossRef] [PubMed]
12. Liu, J.M.; Mao, B.Y.; Hong, S.; Liu, Y.H.; Wang, X.J. The postoperative brain tumour stem cell (BTSC) niche and cancer recurrence. *Adv. Ther.* **2008**, *25*, 389–398. [CrossRef] [PubMed]
13. Haar, C.P.; Hebbar, P.; Wallace, G.C.; Das, A.; Vandergrift, W.A., 3rd; Smith, J.A.; Giglio, P.; Patel, S.J.; Ray, S.K.; Banik, N.L. Drug resistance in glioblastoma: A mini review. *Neurochem. Res.* **2012**, *37*, 1192–1200. [CrossRef] [PubMed]
14. Smith, A.G.; Macleod, K.F. Autophagy, cancer stem cells and drug resistance. *J. Pathol.* **2019**, *247*, 708–718. [CrossRef] [PubMed]
15. Lin, J.; Zhang, X.M.; Yang, J.C.; Ye, Y.B.; Luo, S.Q. gamma-secretase inhibitor-I enhances radiosensitivity of glioblastoma cell lines by depleting CD133+ tumor cells. *Arch. Med. Res.* **2010**, *41*, 519–529. [CrossRef] [PubMed]
16. Liebelt, B.D.; Shingu, T.; Zhou, X.; Ren, J.; Shin, S.A.; Hu, J. Glioma Stem Cells: Signaling, Microenvironment, and Therapy. *Stem Cells Int.* **2016**, *2016*, 7849890. [CrossRef]
17. Hu, Y.Y.; Zheng, M.H.; Cheng, G.; Li, L.; Liang, L.; Gao, F.; Wei, Y.N.; Fu, L.A.; Han, H. Notch signaling contributes to the maintenance of both normal neural stem cells and patient-derived glioma stem cells. *BMC Cancer* **2011**, *11*, 82. [CrossRef]
18. Saito, N.; Aoki, K.; Hirai, N.; Fujita, S.; Iwama, J.; Hiramoto, Y.; Ishii, M.; Sato, K.; Nakayama, H.; Harashina, J.; et al. Effect of Notch expression in glioma stem cells on therapeutic response to chemo-radiotherapy in recurrent glioblastoma. *Brain Tumor Pathol.* **2015**, *32*, 176–183. [CrossRef]
19. Wang, J.; Xu, S.L.; Duan, J.J.; Yi, L.; Guo, Y.F.; Shi, Y.; Li, L.; Yang, Z.Y.; Liao, X.M.; Cai, J.; et al. Invasion of white matter tracts by glioma stem cells is regulated by a NOTCH1-SOX2 positive-feedback loop. *Nat. Neurosci.* **2019**, *22*, 91–105. [CrossRef]
20. Zhang, N.; Wei, P.; Gong, A.; Chiu, W.T.; Lee, H.T.; Colman, H.; Huang, H.; Xue, J.; Liu, M.; Wang, Y.; et al. FoxM1 promotes beta-catenin nuclear localization and controls Wnt target-gene expression and glioma tumorigenesis. *Cancer Cell* **2011**, *20*, 427–442. [CrossRef]
21. Zheng, H.; Ying, H.; Wiedemeyer, R.; Yan, H.; Quayle, S.N.; Ivanova, E.V.; Paik, J.H.; Zhang, H.; Xiao, Y.; Perry, S.R.; et al. PLAGL2 regulates Wnt signaling to impede differentiation in neural stem cells and gliomas. *Cancer Cell* **2010**, *17*, 497–509. [CrossRef] [PubMed]
22. Clement, V.; Sanchez, P.; de Tribolet, N.; Radovanovic, I.; Ruiz i Altaba, A. HEDGEHOG-GLI1 signaling regulates human glioma growth, cancer stem cell self-renewal, and tumorigenicity. *Curr. Biol.* **2007**, *17*, 165–172. [CrossRef] [PubMed]
23. Shmelkov, S.V.; St Clair, R.; Lyden, D.; Rafii, S. AC133/CD133/Prominin-1. *Int. J. Biochem. Cell Biol.* **2005**, *37*, 715–719. [CrossRef] [PubMed]
24. Wang, J.; Sakariassen, P.O.; Tsinkalovsky, O.; Immervoll, H.; Boe, S.O.; Svendsen, A.; Prestegarden, L.; Rosland, G.; Thorsen, F.; Stuhr, L.; et al. CD133 negative glioma cells form tumors in nude rats and give rise to CD133 positive cells. *Int. J. Cancer* **2008**, *122*, 761–768. [CrossRef]

25. Ludwig, K.; Kornblum, H.I. Molecular markers in glioma. *J. Neurooncol.* **2017**, *134*, 505–512. [CrossRef]
26. Lathia, J.D.; Mack, S.C.; Mulkearns-Hubert, E.E.; Valentim, C.L.L.; Rich, J.N. Cancer stem cells in glioblastoma. *Genes Dev.* **2015**, *29*, 1203–1217. [CrossRef]
27. Hoang-Minh, L.B.; Siebzehnrubl, F.A.; Yang, C.; Suzuki-Hatano, S.; Dajac, K.; Loche, T.; Andrews, N.; Schmoll Massari, M.; Patel, J.; Amin, K.; et al. Infiltrative and drug-resistant slow-cycling cells support metabolic heterogeneity in glioblastoma. *EMBO J.* **2018**, *37*. [CrossRef]
28. Teng, J.; da Hora, C.C.; Kantar, R.S.; Nakano, I.; Wakimoto, H.; Batchelor, T.T.; Chiocca, E.A.; Badr, C.E.; Tannous, B.A. Dissecting inherent intratumor heterogeneity in patient-derived glioblastoma culture models. *Neuro. Oncol.* **2017**, *19*, 820–832. [CrossRef]
29. Di Tomaso, T.; Mazzoleni, S.; Wang, E.; Sovena, G.; Clavenna, D.; Franzin, A.; Mortini, P.; Ferrone, S.; Doglioni, C.; Marincola, F.M.; et al. Immunobiological characterization of cancer stem cells isolated from glioblastoma patients. *Clin. Cancer Res.* **2010**, *16*, 800–813. [CrossRef]
30. Wei, J.; Barr, J.; Kong, L.Y.; Wang, Y.; Wu, A.; Sharma, A.K.; Gumin, J.; Henry, V.; Colman, H.; Priebe, W.; et al. Glioblastoma cancer-initiating cells inhibit T-cell proliferation and effector responses by the signal transducers and activators of transcription 3 pathway. *Mol. Cancer Ther.* **2010**, *9*, 67–78. [CrossRef]
31. Iwadate, Y. Plasticity in Glioma Stem Cell Phenotype and Its Therapeutic Implication. *Neurol. Med. Chir.* **2018**, *58*, 61–70. [CrossRef] [PubMed]
32. Chow, K.H.; Park, H.J.; George, J.; Yamamoto, K.; Gallup, A.D.; Graber, J.H.; Chen, Y.; Jiang, W.; Steindler, D.A.; Neilson, E.G.; et al. S100A4 Is a Biomarker and Regulator of Glioma Stem Cells That Is Critical for Mesenchymal Transition in Glioblastoma. *Cancer Res.* **2017**, *77*, 5360–5373. [CrossRef] [PubMed]
33. Velpula, K.K.; Dasari, V.R.; Tsung, A.J.; Dinh, D.H.; Rao, J.S. Cord blood stem cells revert glioma stem cell EMT by down regulating transcriptional activation of Sox2 and Twist1. *Oncotarget* **2011**, *2*, 1028–1042. [CrossRef] [PubMed]
34. Zhang, J.; Cai, H.; Sun, L.; Zhan, P.; Chen, M.; Zhang, F.; Ran, Y.; Wan, J. LGR5, a novel functional glioma stem cell marker, promotes EMT by activating the Wnt/beta-catenin pathway and predicts poor survival of glioma patients. *J. Exp. Clin. Cancer Res.* **2018**, *37*, 225. [CrossRef] [PubMed]
35. Bianco, J.; Bastiancich, C.; Jankovski, A.; des Rieux, A.; Preat, V.; Danhier, F. On glioblastoma and the search for a cure: Where do we stand? *Cell Mol. Life Sci.* **2017**, *74*, 2451–2466. [CrossRef] [PubMed]
36. Ranjan, T.; Howard, C.M.; Yu, A.; Xu, L.; Aziz, K.; Jho, D.; Leonardo, J.; Hameed, M.A.; Karlovits, S.M.; Wegner, R.E.; et al. Cancer Stem Cell Chemotherapeutics Assay for Prospective Treatment of Recurrent Glioblastoma and Progressive Anaplastic Glioma: A Single-Institution Case Series. *Transl. Oncol.* **2020**, *13*, 100755. [CrossRef]
37. Fan, X.; Matsui, W.; Khaki, L.; Stearns, D.; Chun, J.; Li, Y.M.; Eberhart, C.G. Notch pathway inhibition depletes stem-like cells and blocks engraftment in embryonal brain tumors. *Cancer Res.* **2006**, *66*, 7445–7452. [CrossRef]
38. Bar, E.E.; Chaudhry, A.; Lin, A.; Fan, X.; Schreck, K.; Matsui, W.; Piccirillo, S.; Vescovi, A.L.; DiMeco, F.; Olivi, A.; et al. Cyclopamine-mediated hedgehog pathway inhibition depletes stem-like cancer cells in glioblastoma. *Stem Cells* **2007**, *25*, 2524–2533. [CrossRef]
39. Cilibrasi, C.; Riva, G.; Romano, G.; Cadamuro, M.; Bazzoni, R.; Butta, V.; Paoletta, L.; Dalpra, L.; Strazzabosco, M.; Lavitrano, M.; et al. Resveratrol Impairs Glioma Stem Cells Proliferation and Motility by Modulating the Wnt Signaling Pathway. *PLoS ONE* **2017**, *12*, e0169854. [CrossRef]
40. Yu, Z.; Zhao, G.; Xie, G.; Zhao, L.; Chen, Y.; Yu, H.; Zhang, Z.; Li, C.; Li, Y. Metformin and temozolomide act synergistically to inhibit growth of glioma cells and glioma stem cells in vitro and in vivo. *Oncotarget* **2015**, *6*, 32930–32943. [CrossRef]
41. Jiang, W.; Finniss, S.; Cazacu, S.; Xiang, C.; Brodie, Z.; Mikkelsen, T.; Poisson, L.; Shackelford, D.B.; Brodie, C. Repurposing phenformin for the targeting of glioma stem cells and the treatment of glioblastoma. *Oncotarget* **2016**, *7*, 56456–56470. [CrossRef] [PubMed]
42. Han, D.; Yu, T.; Dong, N.; Wang, B.; Sun, F.; Jiang, D. Napabucasin, a novel STAT3 inhibitor suppresses proliferation, invasion and stemness of glioblastoma cells. *J. Exp. Clin. Cancer Res.* **2019**, *38*, 289. [CrossRef] [PubMed]
43. Ashizawa, T.; Miyata, H.; Iizuka, A.; Komiyama, M.; Oshita, C.; Kume, A.; Nogami, M.; Yagoto, M.; Ito, I.; Oishi, T.; et al. Effect of the STAT3 inhibitor STX-0119 on the proliferation of cancer stem-like cells derived from recurrent glioblastoma. *Int. J. Oncol.* **2013**, *43*, 219–227. [CrossRef] [PubMed]
44. NCT02315534. A Study of BBI608 in Combination with Temozolomide in Adult Patients with Recurrent or Progressed Glioblastoma. Available online: https://ClinicalTrials.gov/show/NCT02315534 (accessed on 15 September 2020).
45. NCT03466450. Glasdegib (PF-04449913) With Temozolomide Newly Diagnosed Glioblastoma. Available online: https://ClinicalTrials.gov/show/NCT03466450 (accessed on 15 September 2020).
46. NCT01119599. RO4929097, Temozolomide, and Radiation Therapy in Treating Patients with Newly Diagnosed Malignant Glioma. Available online: https://ClinicalTrials.gov/show/NCT01119599 (accessed on 15 September 2020).
47. Auffinger, B.; Spencer, D.; Pytel, P.; Ahmed, A.U.; Lesniak, M.S. The role of glioma stem cells in chemotherapy resistance and glioblastoma multiforme recurrence. *Expert Rev. Neurother.* **2015**, *15*, 741–752. [CrossRef]
48. Xi, G.; Li, Y.D.; Grahovac, G.; Rajaram, V.; Wadhwani, N.; Pundy, T.; Mania-Farnell, B.; James, C.D.; Tomita, T. Targeting CD133 improves chemotherapeutic efficacy of recurrent pediatric pilocytic astrocytoma following prolonged chemotherapy. *Mol Cancer.* **2017**, *16*, 21. [CrossRef]

49. Smith, S.J.; Diksin, M.; Chhaya, S.; Sairam, S.; Estevez-Cebrero, M.A.; Rahman, R. The Invasive Region of Glioblastoma Defined by 5ALA Guided Surgery Has an Altered Cancer Stem Cell Marker Profile Compared to Central Tumour. *Int. J. Mol. Sci.* **2017**, *18*, 2452. [CrossRef]
50. Shi, L.; Wang, Z.; Sun, G.; Wan, Y.; Guo, J.; Fu, X. miR-145 inhibits migration and invasion of glioma stem cells by targeting ABCG2. *Neuromol. Med.* **2014**, *16*, 517–528. [CrossRef]
51. Zhang, Y.; Wang, S.X.; Ma, J.W.; Li, H.Y.; Ye, J.C.; Xie, S.M.; Du, B.; Zhong, X.Y. EGCG inhibits properties of glioma stem-like cells and synergizes with temozolomide through downregulation of P-glycoprotein inhibition. *J. Neurooncol.* **2015**, *121*, 41–52. [CrossRef]
52. Friedman, M.D.; Jeevan, D.S.; Tobias, M.; Murali, R.; Jhanwar-Uniyal, M. Targeting cancer stem cells in glioblastoma multiforme using mTOR inhibitors and the differentiating agent all-trans retinoic acid. *Oncol. Rep.* **2013**, *30*, 1645–1650. [CrossRef]
53. Sato, A.; Okada, M.; Shibuya, K.; Watanabe, E.; Seino, S.; Suzuki, K.; Narita, Y.; Shibui, S.; Kayama, T.; Kitanaka, C. Resveratrol promotes proteasome-dependent degradation of Nanog via p53 activation and induces differentiation of glioma stem cells. *Stem Cell Res.* **2013**, *11*, 601–610. [CrossRef]
54. Zhuang, W.; Long, L.; Zheng, B.; Ji, W.; Yang, N.; Zhang, Q.; Liang, Z. Curcumin promotes differentiation of glioma-initiating cells by inducing autophagy. *Cancer Sci.* **2012**, *103*, 684–690. [CrossRef] [PubMed]
55. Nayak, S.; Mahenthiran, A.; Yang, Y.; McClendon, M.; Mania-Farnell, B.; James, C.D.; Kessler, J.A.; Tomita, T.; Cheng, S.Y.; Stupp, S.I.; et al. Bone Morphogenetic Protein 4 Targeting Glioma Stem-Like Cells for Malignant Glioma Treatment: Latest Advances and Implications for Clinical Application. *Cancers* **2020**, *12*, 516. [CrossRef] [PubMed]
56. NCT02869243. A Dose Escalation Phase I Study Of Human-Recombinant Bone Morphogenetic Protein 4 Administrated Via CED In GBM Patients. Available online: https://ClinicalTrials.gov/show/NCT02869243 (accessed on 15 September 2020).
57. Calabrese, C.; Poppleton, H.; Kocak, M.; Hogg, T.L.; Fuller, C.; Hamner, B.; Oh, E.Y.; Gaber, M.W.; Finklestein, D.; Allen, M.; et al. A perivascular niche for brain tumor stem cells. *Cancer Cell* **2007**, *11*, 69–82. [CrossRef] [PubMed]
58. Wang, H.; Lathia, J.D.; Wu, Q.; Wang, J.; Li, Z.; Heddleston, J.M.; Eyler, C.E.; Elderbroom, J.; Gallagher, J.; Schuschu, J.; et al. Targeting interleukin 6 signaling suppresses glioma stem cell survival and tumor growth. *Stem Cells* **2009**, *27*, 2393–2404. [CrossRef] [PubMed]
59. Kioi, M.; Vogel, H.; Schultz, G.; Hoffman, R.M.; Harsh, G.R.; Brown, J.M. Inhibition of vasculogenesis, but not angiogenesis, prevents the recurrence of glioblastoma after irradiation in mice. *J. Clin. Investig.* **2010**, *120*, 694–705. [CrossRef]
60. Chiao, M.T.; Cheng, W.Y.; Yang, Y.C.; Shen, C.C.; Ko, J.L. Suberoylanilide hydroxamic acid (SAHA) causes tumor growth slowdown and triggers autophagy in glioblastoma stem cells. *Autophagy* **2013**, *9*, 1509–1526. [CrossRef]
61. Booth, L.; Roberts, J.L.; Conley, A.; Cruickshanks, N.; Ridder, T.; Grant, S.; Poklepovic, A.; Dent, P. HDAC inhibitors enhance the lethality of low dose salinomycin in parental and stem-like GBM cells. *Cancer Biol. Ther.* **2014**, *15*, 305–316. [CrossRef]
62. Naujokat, C.; Steinhart, R. Salinomycin as a drug for targeting human cancer stem cells. *J. Biomed. Biotechnol.* **2012**, *2012*, 950658. [CrossRef]
63. Xipell, E.; Gonzalez-Huarriz, M.; Martinez de Irujo, J.J.; Garcia-Garzon, A.; Lang, F.F.; Jiang, H.; Fueyo, J.; Gomez-Manzano, C.; Alonso, M.M. Salinomycin induced ROS results in abortive autophagy and leads to regulated necrosis in glioblastoma. *Oncotarget* **2016**, *7*, 30626–30641. [CrossRef]
64. Kuramoto, K.; Yamamoto, M.; Suzuki, S.; Sanomachi, T.; Togashi, K.; Seino, S.; Kitanaka, C.; Okada, M. Verteporfin inhibits oxidative phosphorylation and induces cell death specifically in glioma stem cells. *FEBS J* **2020**, *287*, 2023–2036. [CrossRef]
65. Nichols, J.W.; Bae, Y.H. EPR: Evidence and fallacy. *J. Control. Release* **2014**, *190*, 451–464. [CrossRef] [PubMed]
66. Ganipineni, L.P.; Danhier, F.; Preat, V. Drug delivery challenges and future of chemotherapeutic nanomedicine for glioblastoma treatment. *J. Control. Release* **2018**, *281*, 42–57. [CrossRef] [PubMed]
67. Watkins, S.; Robel, S.; Kimbrough, I.F.; Robert, S.M.; Ellis-Davies, G.; Sontheimer, H. Disruption of astrocyte-vascular coupling and the blood-brain barrier by invading glioma cells. *Nat. Commun.* **2014**, *5*, 4196. [CrossRef] [PubMed]
68. Wang, Z.; Liang, P.; He, X.; Wu, B.; Liu, Q.; Xu, Z.; Wu, H.; Liu, Z.; Qian, Y.; Wang, S.; et al. Etoposide loaded layered double hydroxide nanoparticles reversing chemoresistance and eradicating human glioma stem cells in vitro and in vivo. *Nanoscale* **2018**, *10*, 13106–13121. [CrossRef]
69. Lopez-Bertoni, H.; Kozielski, K.L.; Rui, Y.; Lal, B.; Vaughan, H.; Wilson, D.R.; Mihelson, N.; Eberhart, C.G.; Laterra, J.; Green, J.J. Bioreducible Polymeric Nanoparticles Containing Multiplexed Cancer Stem Cell Regulating miRNAs Inhibit Glioblastoma Growth and Prolong Survival. *Nano. Lett.* **2018**, *18*, 4086–4094. [CrossRef]
70. Mukherjee, S.; Baidoo, J.N.E.; Sampat, S.; Mancuso, A.; David, L.; Cohen, L.S.; Zhou, S.; Banerjee, P. Liposomal TriCurin, A Synergistic Combination of Curcumin, Epicatechin Gallate and Resveratrol, Repolarizes Tumor-Associated Microglia/Macrophages, and Eliminates Glioblastoma (GBM) and GBM Stem Cells. *Molecules* **2018**, *23*, 201. [CrossRef]
71. Fang, K.; Liu, P.; Dong, S.; Guo, Y.; Cui, X.; Zhu, X.; Li, X.; Jiang, L.; Liu, T.; Wu, Y. Magnetofection based on superparamagnetic iron oxide nanoparticle-mediated low lncRNA HOTAIR expression decreases the proliferation and invasion of glioma stem cells. *Int. J. Oncol.* **2016**, *49*, 509–518. [CrossRef]
72. Kouri, F.M.; Hurley, L.A.; Daniel, W.L.; Day, E.S.; Hua, Y.; Hao, L.; Peng, C.Y.; Merkel, T.J.; Queisser, M.A.; Ritner, C.; et al. miR-182 integrates apoptosis, growth, and differentiation programs in glioblastoma. *Genes Dev.* **2015**, *29*, 732–745. [CrossRef]

73. Yu, D.; Khan, O.F.; Suva, M.L.; Dong, B.; Panek, W.K.; Xiao, T.; Wu, M.; Han, Y.; Ahmed, A.U.; Balyasnikova, I.V.; et al. Multiplexed RNAi therapy against brain tumor-initiating cells via lipopolymeric nanoparticle infusion delays glioblastoma progression. *Proc. Natl. Acad. Sci. USA* **2017**, *114*, E6147–E6156. [CrossRef]
74. Xu, C.F.; Liu, Y.; Shen, S.; Zhu, Y.H.; Wang, J. Targeting glucose uptake with siRNA-based nanomedicine for cancer therapy. *Biomaterials* **2015**, *51*, 1–11. [CrossRef]
75. Wu, N.; Zhang, C.; Wang, C.; Song, L.; Yao, W.; Gedanken, A.; Lin, X.; Shi, D. Zinc-doped copper oxide nanocomposites reverse temozolomide resistance in glioblastoma by inhibiting AKT and ERK1/2. *Nanomedicine* **2018**, *13*, 1303–1318. [CrossRef] [PubMed]
76. Pan, Z.; Shi, Z.; Wei, H.; Sun, F.; Song, J.; Huang, Y.; Liu, T.; Mao, Y. Magnetofection Based on Superparamagnetic Iron Oxide Nanoparticles Weakens Glioma Stem Cell Proliferation and Invasion by Mediating High Expression of MicroRNA-374a. *J. Cancer* **2016**, *7*, 1487–1496. [CrossRef] [PubMed]
77. Younis, M.; Faming, W.; Hongyan, Z.; Mengmeng, T.; Hang, S.; Liudi, Y. Iguratimod encapsulated PLGA-NPs improves therapeutic outcome in glioma, glioma stem-like cells and temozolomide resistant glioma cells. *Nanomedicine* **2019**, *22*, 102101. [CrossRef] [PubMed]
78. Sun, T.; Patil, R.; Galstyan, A.; Klymyshyn, D.; Ding, H.; Chesnokova, A.; Cavenee, W.K.; Furnari, F.B.; Ljubimov, V.A.; Shatalova, E.S.; et al. Blockade of a Laminin-411-Notch Axis with CRISPR/Cas9 or a Nanobioconjugate Inhibits Glioblastoma Growth through Tumor-Microenvironment Cross-talk. *Cancer Res.* **2019**, *79*, 1239–1251. [CrossRef]
79. Chou, S.T.; Patil, R.; Galstyan, A.; Gangalum, P.R.; Cavenee, W.K.; Furnari, F.B.; Ljubimov, V.A.; Chesnokova, A.; Kramerov, A.A.; Ding, H.; et al. Simultaneous blockade of interacting CK2 and EGFR pathways by tumor-targeting nanobioconjugates increases therapeutic efficacy against glioblastoma multiforme. *J. Control. Release* **2016**, *244*, 14–23. [CrossRef]
80. Kim, S.S.; Rait, A.; Kim, E.; Pirollo, K.F.; Chang, E.H. A tumor-targeting p53 nanodelivery system limits chemoresistance to temozolomide prolonging survival in a mouse model of glioblastoma multiforme. *Nanomedicine* **2015**, *11*, 301–311. [CrossRef]
81. Kim, S.S.; Rait, A.; Kim, E.; Pirollo, K.F.; Nishida, M.; Farkas, N.; Dagata, J.A.; Chang, E.H. A nanoparticle carrying the p53 gene targets tumors including cancer stem cells, sensitizes glioblastoma to chemotherapy and improves survival. *ACS Nano* **2014**, *8*, 5494–5514. [CrossRef]
82. Wu, H.B.; Yang, S.; Weng, H.Y.; Chen, Q.; Zhao, X.L.; Fu, W.J.; Niu, Q.; Ping, Y.F.; Wang, J.M.; Zhang, X.; et al. Autophagy-induced KDR/VEGFR-2 activation promotes the formation of vasculogenic mimicry by glioma stem cells. *Autophagy* **2017**, *13*, 1528–1542. [CrossRef]
83. Sun, X.; Chen, Y.; Zhao, H.; Qiao, G.; Liu, M.; Zhang, C.; Cui, D.; Ma, L. Dual-modified cationic liposomes loaded with paclitaxel and survivin siRNA for targeted imaging and therapy of cancer stem cells in brain glioma. *Drug Deliv.* **2018**, *25*, 1718–1727. [CrossRef]
84. Jing, H.; Weidensteiner, C.; Reichardt, W.; Gaedicke, S.; Zhu, X.; Grosu, A.L.; Kobayashi, H.; Niedermann, G. Imaging and Selective Elimination of Glioblastoma Stem Cells with Theranostic Near-Infrared-Labeled CD133-Specific Antibodies. *Theranostics* **2016**, *6*, 862–874. [CrossRef]
85. Liu, Y.; Mei, L.; Yu, Q.; Xu, C.; Qiu, Y.; Yang, Y.; Shi, K.; Zhang, Q.; Gao, H.; Zhang, Z.; et al. Multifunctional Tandem Peptide Modified Paclitaxel-Loaded Liposomes for the Treatment of Vasculogenic Mimicry and Cancer Stem Cells in Malignant Glioma. *ACS Appl. Mater. Interfaces* **2015**, *7*, 16792–16801. [CrossRef] [PubMed]
86. Li, X.T.; Tang, W.; Jiang, Y.; Wang, X.M.; Wang, Y.H.; Cheng, L.; Meng, X.S. Multifunctional targeting vinorelbine plus tetrandrine liposomes for treating brain glioma along with eliminating glioma stem cells. *Oncotarget* **2016**, *7*, 24604–24622. [CrossRef] [PubMed]
87. Kaluzova, M.; Bouras, A.; Machaidze, R.; Hadjipanayis, C.G. Targeted therapy of glioblastoma stem-like cells and tumor non-stem cells using cetuximab-conjugated iron-oxide nanoparticles. *Oncotarget* **2015**, *6*, 8788–8806. [CrossRef] [PubMed]
88. Sun, T.; Li, Y.; Huang, Y.; Zhang, Z.; Yang, W.; Du, Z.; Zhou, Y. Targeting glioma stem cells enhances anti-tumor effect of boron neutron capture therapy. *Oncotarget* **2016**, *7*, 43095–43108. [CrossRef] [PubMed]
89. Wang, Y.; Ying, X.; Xu, H.; Yan, H.; Li, X.; Tang, H. The functional curcumin liposomes induce apoptosis in C6 glioblastoma cells and C6 glioblastoma stem cells in vitro and in animals. *Int. J. Nanomedicine* **2017**, *12*, 1369–1384. [CrossRef] [PubMed]
90. Kim, J.S.; Shin, D.H.; Kim, J.S. Dual-targeting immunoliposomes using angiopep-2 and CD133 antibody for glioblastoma stem cells. *J. Control. Release* **2018**, *269*, 245–257. [CrossRef] [PubMed]
91. Katsushima, K.; Natsume, A.; Ohka, F.; Shinjo, K.; Hatanaka, A.; Ichimura, N.; Sato, S.; Takahashi, S.; Kimura, H.; Totoki, Y.; et al. Targeting the Notch-regulated non-coding RNA TUG1 for glioma treatment. *Nat. Commun.* **2016**, *7*, 13616. [CrossRef]
92. Maeda, H.; Nakamura, H.; Fang, J. The EPR effect for macromolecular drug delivery to solid tumors: Improvement of tumor uptake, lowering of systemic toxicity, and distinct tumor imaging in vivo. *Adv. Drug Deliv. Rev.* **2013**, *65*, 71–79. [CrossRef]
93. Torchilin, V. Tumor delivery of macromolecular drugs based on the EPR effect. *Adv. Drug Deliv. Rev.* **2011**, *63*, 131–135. [CrossRef]
94. Danhier, F. To exploit the tumor microenvironment: Since the EPR effect fails in the clinic, what is the future of nanomedicine? *J. Control. Release* **2016**, *244*, 108–121. [CrossRef]
95. Lammers, T.; Kiessling, F.; Hennink, W.E.; Storm, G. Drug targeting to tumors: Principles, pitfalls and (pre-) clinical progress. *J. Control. Release* **2012**, *161*, 175–187. [CrossRef] [PubMed]
96. Singh, P.K.; Srivastava, A.K.; Dev, A.; Kaundal, B.; Choudhury, S.R.; Karmakar, S. 1, 3beta-Glucan anchored, paclitaxel loaded chitosan nanocarrier endows enhanced hemocompatibility with efficient anti-glioblastoma stem cells therapy. *Carbohydr. Polym.* **2018**, *180*, 365–375. [CrossRef] [PubMed]

97. Salehi, B.; Selamoglu, Z.; S Mileski, K.; Pezzani, R.; Redaelli, M.; Cho, W.C.; Kobarfard, F.; Rajabi, S.; Martorell, M.; Kumar, P.; et al. Liposomal Cytarabine as Cancer Therapy: From Chemistry to Medicine. *Biomolecules* **2019**, *9*, 773. [CrossRef] [PubMed]
98. NCT01044966. A Study of Intraventricular Liposomal Encapsulated Ara-C (DepoCyt) in Patients With Recurrent Glioblastoma. Available online: https://ClinicalTrials.gov/show/NCT01044966 (accessed on 15 September 2020).
99. Frankel, B.M.; Cachia, D.; Patel, S.J.; Das, A. Targeting Subventricular Zone Progenitor Cells with Intraventricular Liposomal Encapsulated Cytarabine in Patients with Secondary Glioblastoma: A Report of Two Cases. *SN Compr. Clin. Med.* **2020**, *2*, 836–843. [CrossRef]
100. Kunoh, T.; Shimura, T.; Kasai, T.; Matsumoto, S.; Mahmud, H.; Khayrani, A.C.; Seno, M.; Kunoh, H.; Takada, J. Use of DNA-generated gold nanoparticles to radiosensitize and eradicate radioresistant glioma stem cells. *Nanotechnology* **2019**, *30*, 055101. [CrossRef]
101. Kunjachan, S.; Rychlik, B.; Storm, G.; Kiessling, F.; Lammers, T. Multidrug resistance: Physiological principles and nanomedical solutions. *Adv. Drug Deliv. Rev.* **2013**, *65*, 1852–1865. [CrossRef]
102. Lubtow, M.M.; Oerter, S.; Quader, S.; Jeanclos, E.; Cubukova, A.; Krafft, M.; Haider, M.S.; Schulte, C.; Meier, L.; Rist, M.; et al. In Vitro Blood-Brain Barrier Permeability and Cytotoxicity of an Atorvastatin-Loaded Nanoformulation Against Glioblastoma in 2D and 3D Models. *Mol. Pharm.* **2020**, *17*, 1835–1847. [CrossRef]
103. Jhaveri, A.; Luther, E.; Torchilin, V. The effect of transferrin-targeted, resveratrol-loaded liposomes on neurosphere cultures of glioblastoma: Implications for targeting tumour-initiating cells. *J. Drug Target* **2019**, *27*, 601–613. [CrossRef]
104. NCT02340156. Phase II Study of Combined Temozolomide and SGT-53 for Treatment of Recurrent Glioblastoma. Available online: https://ClinicalTrials.gov/show/NCT02340156 (accessed on 15 September 2020).
105. Westphal, M.; Hilt, D.C.; Bortey, E.; Delavault, P.; Olivares, R.; Warnke, P.C.; Whittle, I.R.; Jaaskelainen, J.; Ram, Z. A phase 3 trial of local chemotherapy with biodegradable carmustine (BCNU) wafers (Gliadel wafers) in patients with primary malignant glioma. *Neuro. Oncol.* **2003**, *5*, 79–88. [CrossRef]
106. Ghosh, D.; Nandi, S.; Bhattacharjee, S. Combination therapy to checkmate Glioblastoma: Clinical challenges and advances. *Clin. Transl. Med.* **2018**, *7*, 33. [CrossRef]

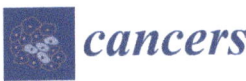

Review

One-Carbon Metabolism Associated Vulnerabilities in Glioblastoma: A Review

Kimia Ghannad-Zadeh [1,2] and Sunit Das [1,2,3,*]

1. The Arthur and Sonia Labatt Brain Tumour Research Centre, The Hospital for Sick Children, Toronto, ON M5G 0A4, Canada; Kimia.ghannad.zadeh@mail.utoronto.ca
2. Institute of Medical Science, University of Toronto, Toronto, ON M5S 1A8, Canada
3. Division of Neurosurgery, St. Michael's Hospital, Toronto, ON M5B 1W8, Canada
* Correspondence: sunit.das@utoronto.ca; Tel.: +1-(416)-864-5548

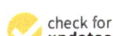

Citation: Ghannad-Zadeh, K.; Das, S. One-Carbon Metabolism Associated Vulnerabilities in Glioblastoma: A Review. *Cancers* **2021**, *13*, 3067. https://doi.org/10.3390/cancers13123067

Academic Editor: Stanley Stylli

Received: 30 May 2021
Accepted: 17 June 2021
Published: 19 June 2021

Publisher's Note: MDPI stays neutral with regard to jurisdictional claims in published maps and institutional affiliations.

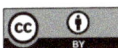

Copyright: © 2021 by the authors. Licensee MDPI, Basel, Switzerland. This article is an open access article distributed under the terms and conditions of the Creative Commons Attribution (CC BY) license (https://creativecommons.org/licenses/by/4.0/).

Simple Summary: Glioblastoma tumours are the most malignant and common type of central nervous system tumours. Despite aggressive treatment measures, disease recurrence in patients with glioblastoma is inevitable and survival rates remain low. Glioblastoma cells, like other cancer cells, can leverage metabolic pathways to increase their rate of proliferation, maintain self-renewal, and develop treatment resistance. Furthermore, many of the metabolic strategies employed by cancer cells are similar to those employed by stem cells in order to maintain self-renewal and proliferation. One-carbon metabolism and de novo purine synthesis are metabolic pathways that are essential for biosynthesis of macromolecules and have been found to be essential for tumourigenesis. In this review, we summarize the evidence showing the significance of 1-C-mediated de novo purine synthesis in glioblastoma cell proliferation and tumourigenesis, as well as evidence suggesting the effectiveness of targeting this metabolic pathway as a therapeutic modality.

Abstract: Altered cell metabolism is a hallmark of cancer cell biology, and the adaptive metabolic strategies of cancer cells have been of recent interest to many groups. Metabolic reprogramming has been identified as a critical step in glial cell transformation, and the use of antimetabolites against glioblastoma has been investigated. One-carbon (1-C) metabolism and its associated biosynthetic pathways, particularly purine nucleotide synthesis, are critical for rapid proliferation and are altered in many cancers. Purine metabolism has also been identified as essential for glioma tumourigenesis. Additionally, alterations of 1-C-mediated purine synthesis have been identified as commonly present in brain tumour initiating cells (BTICs) and could serve as a phenotypic marker of cells responsible for tumour recurrence. Further research is required to elucidate mechanisms through which metabolic vulnerabilities may arise in BTICs and potential ways to therapeutically target these metabolic processes. This review aims to summarize the role of 1-C metabolism-associated vulnerabilities in glioblastoma tumourigenesis and progression and investigate the therapeutic potential of targeting this pathway in conjunction with other treatment strategies.

Keywords: glioblastoma; glioma; one-carbon metabolism; de novo purine synthesis; metabolic reprogramming; metabolic treatment

1. Introduction

Altered cell metabolism is a hallmark of cancer cell biology [1]. Many groups have identified ways in which cancer cells use adaptive metabolic strategies to facilitate the process of tumourigenesis. Folate-mediated one-carbon (1-C) metabolism is a metabolic process in which 1-C unit carriers are produced for use in biosynthetic pathways [2]. Recently, there has been great interest in the role of 1-C metabolism in cancer cell proliferation with many genomic and metabolomic studies showing upregulation of this metabolic process in various cancers, including glioblastoma [2,3].

Glioblastoma is the most common primary brain tumour in adults [4]. Despite aggressive treatment, including resective surgery followed by concomitant radiotherapy and chemotherapy, treatment failure and disease recurrence remain universal [4,5]. The constant nature of recurrence in glioblastoma and general ineffectiveness of second line therapies highlight the need for improved understanding of the molecular characteristics of this disease and the development of novel approaches to its treatment.

Reprogramming of cellular metabolism has been identified as a critical step in glial cell transformation during glioblastoma tumourigenesis [6]. Metabolic reprogramming in glioma cells has been studied in the context of a variety of mechanisms, including increased Warburg effect and aerobic glycolysis [7–10], the pentose phosphate pathway (PPP) [11–15], amino acid metabolism [16–19], oxidative phosphorylation [14,20–24], and lipid metabolism [25–30]. Many of these metabolic pathways manifest in synthesis of macromolecules needed for proliferation.

Among the various metabolic strategies used by glioma cells, the folate-methionine pathway and 1-C metabolism remain understudied [7]. These metabolic pathways are critical for nucleotide synthesis and DNA methylation [2,7,11,31]. Additionally, de novo purine synthesis and upregulation of the related 1-C metabolism pathway have been noted as characteristics of less differentiated stem and progenitor cells as well as brain tumour initiating cells (BTICs) responsible for tumorigenesis [31–34]. In the following sections, we aim to summarize the role of 1-C metabolism-associated vulnerabilities in cancer, and particularly in glioma cells. Additionally, we will evaluate whether this altered metabolic program can serve as a phenotypic identifier of BTICs and as a potential therapeutic target in glioblastoma. Further elucidation of the role of 1-C metabolism-related vulnerabilities in glioblastoma might uncover novel mechanisms that mediate and control cell proliferation and reveal effective novel treatment strategies.

2. Metabolic Reprogramming in Cancer and Cancer Initiating Cells

Tumourigenic cells alter their metabolic processes to meet the increased substrate demands required to sustain rapid proliferation, self-replication, and invasion. Since the identification of the Warburg effect, many groups have identified a variety of ways in which cancer cells reprogram metabolic pathways. In fact, metabolic reprogramming has been established as one of the hallmarks of cancer [1,9]. Metabolic programs play a significant role in balancing proliferation and cell-fate regulation. This role becomes particularly important in stem cells, which need to retain self-renewal capacity and the ability to differentiate [35]. Interestingly, cancer cells and normal stem cells share a number of similarities in their signalling pathways regulating metabolic phenotypes, which are conducive to increased proliferation, enhanced self-renewal, and improved adaptability to differing environmental conditions [35].

The first metabolic alteration in cancer cells was observed to be an upregulation in glucose uptake and a preference for glycolysis in oxygen-rich environments, a phenomenon referred to as aerobic glycolysis, or the Warburg effect [9]. Cancer cells and stem cells both engage in increased levels of aerobic glycolysis [36,37]. Additionally, both cancer cells and stem cells are heavily reliant on exogenous glucose and glutamine supplies [38–40].

Upstream of the mentioned metabolic changes, cancer cells and stem cells share a number of growth signalling pathways involved in metabolic regulation. In normal cells, growth factor-mediated activation of receptor tyrosine kinases engages signalling pathways such as PI3K, Ras, MEK/ERK, and mTOR to increase anabolic pathways and macromolecule synthesis [41]. These pathways are often overactivated in cancer cells, and many have also been shown to regulate pluripotent cell growth [35].

A number of the discussed metabolic alterations have been reported in connection with pro-oncogenic signalling in glioma cells [7]. In glioblastoma cell lines, activation of ERK1/2 by epithelial growth factor (EGF) leads to the nuclear translocation of pyruvate kinase M2 (PKM2), a critical enzyme involved in the production of pyruvate in the glycolysis pathway, leading to a positive feedback loop that ultimately results in an increase in aerobic glycolysis [42]. The PPP, which is necessary for the maintenance of a constant supply of nucleotides, has been shown to be upregulated in actively dividing cells within gliomas [43]. Mutations in Krebs cycle enzymes isocitrate dehydrogenase 1/2 (IDH1/2) are present in a subset of glioblastoma cases, affecting amino acid metabolism and glucose oxidation [16]. Our group has shown that the reduction in glioblastoma tumour formation after inhibition of inhibitor of DNA-binding 1 (ID1) is mediated by downregulation of EGF and downstream ERK1/2 signalling [44]. ERK1/2 activation induces transcriptional regulators of glycolysis, the tricarboxylic acid cycle, and macromolecular biosynthesis, as well as cell proliferation programs [8]. Furthermore, ID1 is a marker of relatively quiescent glioma stem-like cells that are required for tumourigenesis, are resistant to chemotherapy, and can be responsible for initiating tumour recurrence [44,45]. These data suggest that metabolic reprogramming may play a role in mediation of the stem-like phenotype in glioma cells.

Cancer stem cells are a class of cells that exhibit the features of both normal stem cells and cancer cells; however, the metabolic characteristics of these cells, especially BTICs, have been poorly understood [35,46]. It has been suggested that BTICs are less glycolytic than more differentiated glioma cell populations [47]. Additionally, BTICs are known to have increased glucose uptake and upregulation of the de novo purine synthesis pathway, metabolic pathways which allow maintenance of rapid proliferation and growth [32]. Further, BTICs have a higher mitochondrial reserve than differentiated glioma cells, suggesting that these cells use adaptive metabolic strategies to resist therapeutic stress [47]. These data suggest that metabolic alterations, particularly in certain pathways such as nucleotide synthesis, may be a characteristic of the stem-like phenotype in glioma and may thus be critical to treatment resistance.

3. 1-C-Mediated de Novo Purine Synthesis: A Brief Overview

The abundance of the nucleotide pool, as well as the level and activity of different rate-limiting enzymes of the nucleotide synthesis pathway, significantly affects the proliferative capacity of cells as well as their capacity for DNA replication and repair [15]. 1-C metabolism and the closely related purine synthesis pathway are critical to these issues [7].

1-C metabolism provides carbon units for biosynthesis through folate intermediates. Tetrahydrofolate (THF), after entering the 1-C cycle, can bind methyl groups and act as a carbon donor. 10-Formyl-THF is produced in the mitochondria from the reduction of 5,10-methyl-THF by methylenetetrahydrofolate dehydrogenase 2-like protein (MTHFD2/L), and is primarily involved in de novo purine synthesis [2,48]. Cells require a steady supply of nucleotides to complete the processes of DNA replication and cell division. Nucleotides can be produced either through salvage pathways recycling existing nucleobases or through de novo synthesis pathways [49]. De novo purine synthesis has the largest demand for 1-C units [2]. De novo purine synthesis results in the production of inosine monophosphate (IMP) from phosphoribosyl pyrophosphate (PRPP), which is further converted into guanosine monophosphate (GMP) or adenosine monophosphate (AMP). De novo purine synthesis is preferentially activated in conditions with higher requirement for purine nucleotides, such as in rapidly dividing cells [49–52]. The reactions of de novo purine synthesis are mediated in the cytosol by enzymes working in a metabolic complex named the purinosome, increasing the efficiency of this anabolic process [53,54].

THF, and subsequently 10-formyl-THF, are essential to the synthesis of purine nucleotides [52,53]. Due to the dependency of de novo purine synthesis on 1-C metabolism, deficiencies in 1-C metabolism leading to reduction in its products would result in a lower availability of essential intermediates for purine synthesis. 1-C metabolism also produces other metabolically significant compounds, including glycine and serine. Glycine is a substrate for glutathione and purine synthesis, and serine can be used to synthesize glycine in the absence of an exogenous supply [2,55,56]. 1-C metabolism is compartmentalized between the cytosol and mitochondria. The compartmentalization of these reactions allows for the existence of parallel metabolic processes, increasing the metabolic adaptability of cells [48]. Figure 1 shows a schematic of 1-C-mediated purine synthesis and the enzymes involved in this process.

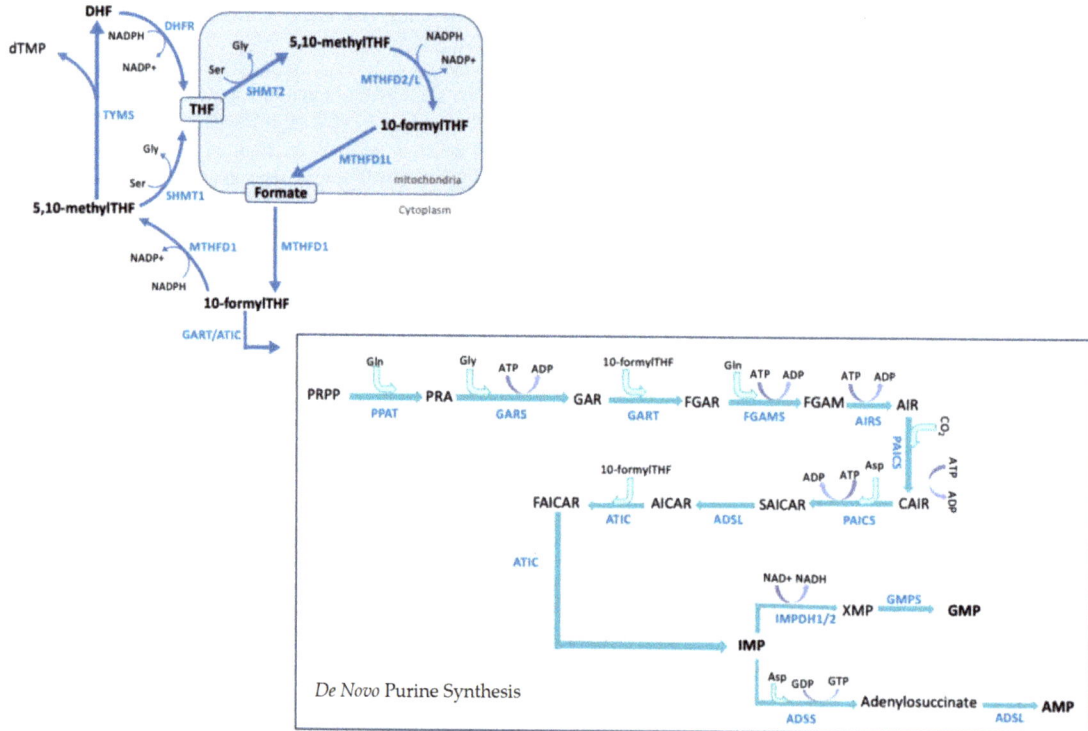

Figure 1. One-carbon-mediated de novo purine synthesis. Dietary folate is reduced to dihydrofolate (DHF) and subsequently tetrahydrofolate (THF) by dihydrofolate reductase (DHFR). THF is acted on by a series of enzymes in the mitochondria, which add methyl groups to THF, allowing it to act as the initial 1-C carrier required for a variety of biosynthesis processes. 10-Formyl-THF is produced in the mitochondria from the reduction of 5,10-methyl-THF by methylene tetrahydrofolate dehydrogenase 2 (MHFD2/L). 10-Formyl-THF is then used in de novo purine synthesis as a carbon donor. The purine ring is built directly onto the 5-phosphoribose-1-pyrophosphate (PRPP) backbone during de novo purine synthesis, and requires the substrates glutamine, glycine, bicarbonate and 10-formyl-THF. De novo purine synthesis is a 10-step cytosolic reaction that results in the production of inosine monophosphate (IMP). IMP is further converted into guanosine monophosphate (GMP) via the activity of the enzymes inosine monophosphate dehydrogenase (IMPDH1) and guanosine monosphosphate synthetase (GMPS), or adenosine monophosphate (AMP) via the activity of the enzyme adenylosuccinate synthase (ADSS) and adenylosuccinate lyase (ADSL). TYMS: thymidylate synthase; dTMP: deoxythymidine monophosphate; SHMT1/2: serine hydroxymethyltrasnferase 1/2; PPAT: phosphoribosyl pyrophosphate amidotransferase; GART: glycinamide ribonucleotide transformylase; MTHFD1L: Methylenetetrahydrofolate Dehydrogenase (NADP+-Dependent) 1 Like; FGAMS: formylglycinamidine ribonucleotide synthase (FGAMS); PAICS: phosphoribosylaminoimidazole carboxylase; AICAR: 5-Aminoimidazole carboxamide ribonucleotide; ATIC: 5-aminoimidazole-4-carboxamide ribonucleotide formyltransferase/IMP cyclohydrolase; XMP: xanthosine monophosphate.

4. 1-C-Mediated de Novo Purine Synthesis: Relevance in Cancer and Glioblastoma

Differential expression of metabolic enzymes, for example, those of glycolysis and the PPP, has been found to be a source of intratumoural heterogeneity in glioblastoma [13], and often results in differential rates of nucleotide synthesis within glioma cells [13]. The enzymes of the mitochondrial folate cycle, including MTHFD2/L and serine hydroxymethyltrasnferase (SHMT), have been found to be expressed at markedly higher levels in cancer cells, including hepatocellular carcinoma, colorectal cancer, breast cancer, and glioblastoma [55–59]. BTICs show increased expression of 1-C metabolism enzymes, and it has been hypothesized that folate cycle reprogramming is associated with acquisition of the stem-like phenotype in glioblastoma tumour cells [31,60]. Alterations in 1-C metabolism have been shown to influence overall survival in some cancers, including head and neck squamous cell carcinomas, colorectal cancer, pancreatic cancer, breast cancer, lung adenocarcinoma, and paediatric medulloblastoma [59,61–65]. Knockdown of MTHFD2/L has been shown to result in reduced cell growth and Ki67 staining, reduced in vivo tumourigenesis, and G0/G1 cell cycle arrest in lung adenocarcinoma [50,66]. Deficiency of MTHFD2/L and alteration of mitochondrial 1-C metabolism result in defects in other metabolic pathways, particularly de novo purine synthesis. Additionally, accumulation of glutaminolysis, glycolysis, and PPP intermediates has been observed after MTHFD2/L knockdown [66]. The inhibition of MTHFD2/L from 1-C metabolism results in purine nucleotide deficiency and reduced cell proliferative capacity, which can be restored by external supplementation of hypoxanthine and the purine salvage pathway [67–69]. Studies have shown that knockdown of MTHFD2/L results in reduced rates of IMP, AMP, and GMP—i.e., of the products of de novo purine synthesis [50].

As mentioned previously, purine synthesis is a limiting factor for the growth, proliferation, and maintenance of BTICs [32,70]. Deficiencies in purine synthesis enzymes such as 5-aminoimidazole-4-carboxamide ribonucleotide formyltransferase/IMP cyclohydrolase (ATIC), formylglycinamidine ribonucleotide synthase (FGAMS), adenylosuccinate lyase (ADSL), phosphoribosylaminoimidazole carboxylase (PAICS), guanosine monophosphate (GMPS) and inosine monophosphate dehydrogenase (IMPDH2) have been found to result in altered purinosome assembly and reduced purine synthesis rates [71,72]. Purine synthesis enzymes are found to be overexpressed in patient populations across a variety of tumour types, including glioblastomas [33,61,73]. Goswami et al. report increased expression of PAICS and PPAT in lung cancer [74]. Expression of PPAT and PAICS was independently associated with patient survival in lung adenocarcinomas; further, a subset of adenocarcinoma patients harbour aneuploidy and amplification in divergently transcribed loci of PPAT and PAICS [74].

Mutations in ADSL are known to abrogate purinosome formation, limiting purine synthesis [50,71]. Purinosome formation is significantly affected in patients with ADSL deficiency, an autosomal recessive disorder of purine metabolism [71]. Skin fibroblasts derived from patients with ADSL deficiency show reduced spatial overlap between the purine synthesis enzymes ADSL, ATIC, GART, and phosphoribosyl pyrophosphate amidotransferase (PPAT), suggesting reduced purinosome formation and reduced purine synthesis [71]. Disruption of purinosome assembly has also been shown to enhance sensitivity to chemotherapy agents such as methotrexate [73]. shRNA-mediated knockdown of ADSL and GMPS in BTICs results in abrogation of self-renewal and tumourigenesis in xenografts [32]. IMPDH2 expression has also been found to be necessary for glioblastoma tumourigenesis in vivo [75]. Knockdown of ADSL and GMPS results in increased levels of cleaved caspase-3 and reduced levels of Ki-67 and SOX2 in BTICs [32]. Additionally, data from The Cancer Genome Atlas (TCGA) show increased expression of PRPS1, GMPS, and ADSL protein in BTICs compared to normal brain tissues [32,76]. Wang et al. show that BTICs have an upregulation of H3K27ac at purine synthesis pathway genes, suggesting priming of purine pathway genes in glioblastoma compared to normal brain tissue [32]. Increased levels of ADSL, adenylosuccinate synthase (ADSS), IMPDH1, and PPAT are associated with poor prognosis in glioblastoma patients [32]. Additionally, overexpression of PPAT, IMPDH1, and ADSS correlate with worse survival among glioblastoma patients [32].

In addition to proliferation of BTICs, purine nucleotide synthesis has been shown to regulate DNA repair and therapeutic resistance in glioblastoma [77]. Overexpression of IMPHD2 in glioblastoma tumour cells results in a high turnover of GTP, which is required for DNA replication and proliferation, rRNA and tRNA synthesis, as well as certain signalling pathways [75,78]. In addition to GTP, extracellular ATP and ADP show extremely low degradation rates in glioma cell lines compared to normal astrocytes, which speaks to the importance of adenosine for glioma cell proliferation [79]. Furthermore, adenosine has neuroprotective abilities that can induce angiogenesis, which makes high adenosine levels even more beneficial to glioma cells [79–81]. Downregulation of inosinates and guanilates correlates positively with sensitivity to radiotherapy [77]; while nucleotide availability did not prevent DNA damage induction, exogenous supplementation of purines following treatment with radiation did reduce DNA damage, suggesting that purine nucleotides enhance the ability of glioblastoma cells to repair DNA lesions [77]. Inhibition of GTP synthesis resulted in a reversal of radiotherapy resistance in a patient-derived xenograft (PDX) model of glioblastoma [77]. Other groups suggest that purine synthesis may also be a driver for chemoresistance in glioblastoma cells [78]. TMZ therapy has been shown to results in epigenetic modifications that cause glioblastoma cells to rely on de novo purine synthesis [78]. Increased rates of de novo nucleotide synthesis provide tumour cells with enhanced ability to repair DNA damage caused by alkylating agents, such as TMZ, in addition to preventing cells from recycling damaged nucleotides from the extracellular environment through the purine salvage pathway [78].

The expression of purine synthesis enzymes in glioma initiating cells has been shown to be regulated in a concerted manner, which suggests the influence of upstream transcriptional regulators or programs [32]. Although alteration of purine metabolism has not been exclusively associated with specific oncogenic events in cancer, many oncogenic alterations that drive glioblastoma formation, including of PTEN, EGFR, and PI3CA, can cause similar alternations in nucleotide synthesis and metabolism [67,77,82–84]. Table 1 provides a summary of the discussed 1-C metabolism and purine synthesis associated vulnerabilities.

Table 1. Summary of described 1-C metabolism and purine synthesis associated vulnerabilities in cancer.

Metabolic Enzyme	Implication	Cancer Type/Cell Type	Reference
MTHFD2	Cell growth and tumourigenesis; knockdown of MTHFD2 resulted in reduced cell growth and Ki-67 staining	Lung adenocarcinoma	[66]
MTHFD2	Cell migration and invasion; overexpression associated with poor prognosis and increased metastasis	Breast cancer	[85]
MTHFD2	Cell growth and survival; metabolic adaptation to glutamine starvation	Glioblastoma	[86]
DHFR, SHMT1, MTHFD1	Tumour sphere formation, methionine dependency, and stem-like phenotype	Glioblastoma	[31]
MTHFD2	Highly overexpressed; overexpression associated with poor prognosis	Various cancer types	[58]
SHMT2	Polymorphisms associated with increased risk of cancer	Squamous cell carcinoma of the head and neck	[61]
SHMT2, MTHFD2, MTHFD1	Overexpressed and associated with increased proliferation; associated with increased mortality in breast cancer	Various cancer types	[56]

Table 1. *Cont.*

Metabolic Enzyme	Implication	Cancer Type/Cell Type	Reference
MTHFD2, SHMT2, ALDH1L2 [1]	Overexpressed; overexpression associated with poor prognosis	Colorectal cancer	[59]
MTHFD2 and SHMT2, ALDH1L2	High expression associated with lower overall survival and shorter progression free survival	Pancreatic cancer	[62]
DHFR, TYMS, MTHFD2	Overexpression associated with poor prognosis	Group 4 Medulloblastoma	[63]
PPAT, PAICS	Overexpressed; overexpression associated with aneuploidy and gene amplification in subgroup of patients	Lung adenocarcinoma	[74]
DHFR, TYMS, MTHFD2	Tumourigenesis; overexpression associated with poor prognosis	Brain tumour initiating cells	[32]
IMPDH2	Cell proliferation and tumourigenesis; overexpression associated with poor prognosis	Glioblastoma	[75]
IMPDH2	Chemoresistance	Glioblastoma	[78]
IMPDH2	Resistant to radiotherapy	Glioblastoma	[77]

[1] ALDH12L: aldehyde dehydrogenase 1 family member L 2.

5. Signalling Pathways Upstream of Metabolic Reprogramming

A number of signalling pathways have been proposed to be upstream of the metabolic changes described above. The activation of the PI3K/Akt pathway induces excessive glucose uptake and dependency on aerobic glycolysis, while overexpression of Myc can induce uptake of glutamine in excess of bioenergetic needs [15]. The PI3K-Akt and Myc pathways have been associated with increased proliferation and metabolic reprogramming in cancer cells [8,58], as well as regulation of purine synthesis in glioblastoma cells [32]. PI3K-Akt activation has been shown to lead to excessive glucose uptake by cancer cells, increasing their dependence on aerobic glycolysis, and as a consequence increasing the availability of glycolysis intermediates required for biosynthetic pathways [15].

As a master regulator of metabolism, mTORC1 has been studied extensively in the context of cancer cell metabolism, and mTORC inhibitors such as rapamycin have been used to delay tumourigenesis [49]. Activation of the mTORC1-ATF4 axis by growth signals has been shown to lead to an increase in the transcription of MTHFD2/L [2]. Ben-Sahara et al. show that rapamycin-mediated mTORC inhibition results in the depletion of MTHFD2/L, as well as the downstream de novo purine synthesis pathway [67]. Nucleotide metabolism has been reported to be regulated both by oncogenes and tumour suppressors [87]. For example, Mtp53 regulates nucleotide pools by transcriptionally upregulating nucleotide biosynthesis pathways and has been shown to support invasion and proliferation in cancer cell lines [87]. It has also been shown that p53 silencing results in the reduced expression of nucleotide metabolism enzymes, including DHFR, TYMS, and IMPDH1/2 [87].

One of the pathways most extensively studied in relation to purine synthesis regulation is the AMPK signalling pathway. AMPK acts as a metabolic checkpoint regulator of cell growth [6,88]. AMPK is known to be highly active in high-grade gliomas, regardless of their genetic background, and AMPK-mediated transcriptional regulation of bioergenetics has been found to be essential for tumour growth [89–91]. While AMPK is more classically known as a suppressor of cell growth due to its inhibitory effects on anabolism, some studies have shown that AMPK-deficient cells are at a growth disadvantage [90,92]. The differential effects of AMPK activation on metabolic reprogramming and growth may be due to the differential environmental stressors impacting cancer cells and the need to adapt to these conditions for survival. For example, AMPK activation can lead to the reduced activity of phosphoribosylpyrophosphate synthetase (PRPS), which is required for the production of the phosphoribosyl backbone of nucleotides via the PPP, a critical substrate for cell replication [50,86,93,94]. Furthermore, AMPK activation has been shown to lead to the sequestration of the de novo purine synthesis enzyme FGAMS [95], which can impair purinosome assembly [52–54,71].

While growth signalling pathways can result in metabolic reprogramming of cancer cells, metabolic changes can consequently alter cell signalling pathways. As an example, decreased rate of de novo purine synthesis has been shown to result in accumulation of 5-aminoimidazole carboxamide ribonucleotide (AICAR), the final purine synthesis intermediate before IMP in the de novo purine synthesis pathway [32,66]. AICAR is an activator of AMPK signalling and hence can inhibit cell growth. AICAR treatment results in reduced cell growth in a dose-dependent manner and, combined with gefitinib, has resulted in enhanced sensitivity to the EGFR inhibitor in lung cancer cells [66]. Guo et al. show that AICAR-mediated AMPK activation also leads to negative regulation of glioblastoma cell growth, particularly in EGFR-activated cells [6]. This growth inhibitory effect seems to be mediated through metabolic reprograming, as AICAR treatment resulted in AMPK-mediated inhibition of lipogenesis in EGFR-activated tumours, which could be reversed by exogenous supplementation of malonate and palmitate [6].

6. Treatments Targeting 1-C Metabolism and Purine Synthesis in Cancer

Although 1-C-mediated purine synthesis has received significant attention as a regulator of cancer cell proliferation and treatment resistance, the importance of this process as a viable target for anticancer therapy remains understudied [96]. Drugs targeting cytosolic 1-C metabolism, such as methotrexate (MTX) and pemetrexed, have been used as anticancer agents [96]. MTX is a competitive inhibitor of DHFR, while pemetrexed targets multiple enzymes involved in nucleotide synthesis, including DHFR, thymidylate synthase (TYMS), and glycinamide ribonucleotide transformylase (GART) [93,94,97,98]. Walling provides a thorough review of antifolates and their use as therapeutic agents [99]. While these compounds are inhibitors of 1-C metabolism, physiologically relevant concentrations of extracellular hypoxanthine inhibit the toxic effect of MTX, which suggests that MTX-mediated DHFR inhibition also results in downstream inhibition of the purine synthesis pathway [68]. This finding suggests that purine synthesis may also be a viable therapeutic target in cancer.

Drugs that directly inhibit de novo purine synthesis, such as L-alanosine and thiopurines, have also been studied in cancer. The toxicity of these chemicals can be influenced by the expression of other metabolic enzymes or the selective reliance of cancer cells on certain metabolic pathways. For example, sensitivity to thiopurines such as 6-mercaptopurine (6-MP) and 6-thioguanine (6-TG)—compounds extensively used for the treatment of leukaemias—has been shown to be dependent on the expression of methyladenosine phosphorylase (MTAP) [69]. The deletion of the MTAP gene is a frequent event in many cancers, and results in the dependence of cancer cells on de novo purine synthesis or exogenous purine salvage [69,100–105]. In the event of limited exogenous purine availability, MTAP-deficient cancer cells are more sensitive to inhibitors of de novo purine synthesis [69,106]. Loss of MTAP in glioblastoma cells promotes stemness as well as susceptibility to purine starvation and inhibition of de novo purine synthesis using L-alanosine [106]. Direct inhibition of purine synthesis in glioblastoma has gained recent therapeutic interest with studies showing the correlation between treatment resistance and purine metabolism in glioblastoma [77,78]. Mycophenolate mofetil (MMF), an inhibitor of IMPDH1 and GTP synthesis, was found to sensitize glioblastoma cells to radiation therapy and significantly improve survival in combination with TMZ in a PDX model of glioblastoma [77,78]. There is currently an ongoing phase 0/I trial of MMF in recurrent and primary glioblastomas (NCT04477200) [107].

One of the major downfalls of targeting metabolic programs in cancer treatments is the possibility of adverse effects that may rise due to disturbance of normal cell metabolism. For example, combination of high-dose MTX with other therapeutic strategies, such as radiotherapy, has shown to result in neurotoxic adverse events [99]. Studies have shown that the same antiproliferative effects observed in cancer cells are not observed in normal cells with the inhibition of mitochondrial 1-C metabolism enzymes [58]. This effect may be due to the existence of parallel 1-C metabolism pathways in the cytoplasm [65] or some toxic event that is unrelated to normal cell metabolism, perhaps related pathways that are further upregulated in highly proliferative cancer cells, such as de novo purine synthesis. Asai et al. have identified chemical compounds, MTHFD2 Inhibitor for THF pocket (MIT) and MTHFD2 Inhibitor for NAD pocket (MIN), that can effectively target and inhibit MTHFD2 in colorectal cancer cells [108]. Additionally, small-molecule inhibitors of SHMT1/2 have been demonstrated to be effective at exerting cytotoxic effects against diffuse B-cell lymphoma progression in vitro [109]. Although both cytosolic and mitochondrial processes are significant for 1-C metabolism, it has been indicated that mitochondrial folate metabolism affects the prognosis of patients more significantly [58,108]. Inhibitors of mitochondrial 1-C metabolism have not been studied in clinical settings; however, pre-clinical studies highlight them as attractive therapeutic targets. This warrants further research into the metabolic reprogramming of 1-C metabolism in cancer cells. Zhou et al. also show that GTP synthesis is preferentially upregulated in glioblastoma cells and not normal brain tissue, resulting in minimal toxic effects of GTP synthesis inhibition in normal cells [77]. In addition to selective targeting of cancer cells, inhibitors of purine synthesis do not require a specific oncogenic event for activity; this means that even genetically heterogeneous tumours can potentially benefit from purine synthesis inhibition [70,78,85]. Table 2 provides a summary of recent studies showing the efficacy of targeting 1-C-mediated purine synthesis enzymes in inhibition of glioblastoma cell growth and tumourigenesis.

Table 2. Summary of recent studies targeting 1-C metabolism and purine synthesis-related metabolic pathways in glioblastoma.

Chemical Compound/Drug	Metabolic Target	Reference
Mycophenolate Mofetil	IMPDH2	[107]
Mycophenolate Mofetil	IMPDH2; Purine synthesis	[78]
Mycophenolate Mofetil	IMPDH2; Purine synthesis	[77]
Methotrexate	DHFR; Folate-mediated 1-C metabolism	[60]
Pemetrexed	DHFR, TYMS; Folate-mediated 1-C metabolism, nucleotide synthesis	[110]
siRNA-mediated knockdown SERBP1 [1]	SERBP1 Methionine synthesis and 1-C metabolism	[111]
siRNA-mediated knockdown of MTHFD2	MTHFD2; Purine synthesis	[86]
L-Alanosine	ADSS; Purine synthesis	[106]
Adenosine Deaminase	Adenosine synthesis	[112]
shRNA-mediated knockdown of PRPS1 [2], GMPS and ADSL	De novo purine synthesis enzymes	[32]

[1] SERBP1: Serpine1 mRNA-binding protein; [2] PRPS1: phosphoribosyl pyrophosphate synthetase.

7. Conclusions

Macromolecules, including nucleic acids, lipids, and proteins, are fundamental requisite substrates for proliferation in all mammalian cells. Cancer cells and stem cells rely on diverse metabolic strategies to maintain macromolecule synthesis. As discussed in this review, a number of 1-C metabolism and purine synthesis-related vulnerabilities exist in glioblastoma cells that can be leveraged to inhibit tumour cell proliferation and tumour growth. To sustain proliferation, glioblastoma cells, and particularly BTICs, upregulate and rely on anabolic pathways such as 1-C-mediated purine synthesis. Multiple studies have suggested that these metabolic vulnerabilities are not associated with specific oncogenic events or specific genetic subtypes in glioblastoma, yet are specific to tumour cells. As a result, tumour-specific 1-C-mediated purine synthesis vulnerabilities may be effective therapeutic targets to inhibit tumour growth with minimal adverse effects on normal cells. The importance of nucleotide synthesis pathways for maintenance of BTICs also suggests that these metabolic pathways may offer an attractive strategy to overcome treatment resistance and prevent tumour recurrence. Further research is required to understand the underlying mechanisms through which these vulnerabilities may arise in BTICs. Such studies can elucidate more concrete ways to target the metabolic processes that underly the glioma proliferation and resistance.

Author Contributions: K.G.-Z. and S.D. wrote this manuscript. All authors have read and agreed to the published version of the manuscript.

Funding: K.G.-Z. is supported by the Ontario Graduate Scholarship. S.D. is supported by an operating grant from the Canadian Institutes of Health Research (CIHR-OG-341329) and a Province of Ontario Young Investigator Award.

Institutional Review Board Statement: Not applicable.

Informed Consent Statement: Not applicable.

Data Availability Statement: Not applicable.

Conflicts of Interest: The authors declare no conflict of interest.

References

1. NHanahan, D.; Weinberg, R.A. Hallmarks of cancer: The next generation. *Cell* **2011**, *144*, 646–674. [CrossRef]
2. Ducker, G.S.; Rabinowitz, J.D. One-Carbon Metabolism in Health and Disease. *Cell Metab.* **2017**, *25*, 27–42. [CrossRef] [PubMed]
3. Amelio, I.; Cutruzzolá, F.; Antonov, A.; Agostini, M.; Melino, G. Serine and glycine metabolism in cancer. *Trends Biochem. Sci.* **2014**, *39*, 191–198. [CrossRef] [PubMed]
4. Wirsching, H.-G.; Galanis, E.; Weller, M. Chapter 23—Glioblastoma. In *Handbook of Clinical Neurology*; Berger, M.S., Weller, M., Eds.; Elsevier: Amsterdam, The Netherlands, 2016; Volume 134, pp. 381–397. ISBN 9780128029978.
5. Stupp, R.; Mason, W.P.; van den Bent, M.J.; Weller, M.; Fisher, B.; Taphoorn, M.J.B.; Belanger, K.; Brandes, A.A.; Marosi, C.; Bogdahn, U.; et al. Radiotherapy plus Concomitant and Adjuvant Temozolomide for Glioblastoma. *N. Engl. J. Med.* **2005**, *352*, 987–996. [CrossRef] [PubMed]
6. Guo, D.; Hildebrandt, I.J.; Prins, R.M.; Soto, H.; Mazzotta, M.M.; Dang, J.; Czernin, J.; Shyy, J.Y.J.; Watson, A.D.; Phelps, M.; et al. The AMPK agonist AICAR inhibits the growth of EGFRvIII-expressing glioblastomas by inhibiting lipogenesis. *Proc. Natl. Acad. Sci. USA* **2009**, *106*, 12932–12937. [CrossRef]
7. Strickland, M.; Stoll, E.A. Metabolic reprogramming in glioma. *Front. Cell Dev. Biol.* **2017**, *5*, 43. [CrossRef] [PubMed]
8. Papa, S.; Choy, P.M.; Bubici, C. The ERK and JNK pathways in the regulation of metabolic reprogramming. *Oncogene* **2019**, *38*, 2223–2240. [CrossRef] [PubMed]
9. Warburg, O.; Wind, F.; Negelein, E. The metabolism of tumors in the body. *J. Gen. Physiol.* **1927**, *8*, 519–530. [CrossRef]
10. Poteet, E.; Choudhury, G.R.; Winters, A.; Li, W.; Ryou, M.G.; Liu, R.; Tang, L.; Ghorpade, A.; Wen, Y.; Yuan, F.; et al. Reversing the Warburg effect as a treatment for glioblastoma. *J. Biol. Chem.* **2013**, *288*, 9153–9164. [CrossRef]
11. De Santis, M.C.; Porporato, P.E.; Martini, M.; Morandi, A. Signaling pathways regulating redox balance in cancer metabolism. *Front. Oncol.* **2018**, *8*, 126. [CrossRef] [PubMed]
12. Liu, R.; Li, W.; Tao, B.; Wang, X.; Yang, Z.; Zhang, Y.; Wang, C.; Liu, R.; Gao, H.; Liang, J.; et al. Tyrosine phosphorylation activates 6-phosphogluconate dehydrogenase and promotes tumor growth and radiation resistance. *Nat. Commun.* **2019**, *10*, 991. [CrossRef]
13. Kathagen-Buhmann, A.; Schulte, A.; Weller, J.; Holz, M.; Herold-Mende, C.; Glass, R.; Lamszus, K. Glycolysis and the Pentose Phosphate Pathway Are Differentially Associated with the Dichotomous Regulation of Glioblastoma Cell Migration versus Proliferation. Available online: https://www.ncbi.nlm.nih.gov/pmc/articles/PMC4998991/ (accessed on 23 March 2020).
14. Marin-Valencia, I.; Cho, S.K.; Rakheja, D.; Hatanpaa, K.J.; Kapur, P.; Mashimo, T.; Jindal, A.; Vemireddy, V.; Good, L.B.; Raisanen, J.; et al. Glucose metabolism via the pentose phosphate pathway, glycolysis and Krebs cycle in an orthotopic mouse model of human brain tumors. *NMR Biomed.* **2012**, *25*, 1177–1186. [CrossRef] [PubMed]
15. Tong, X.; Zhao, F.; Thompson, C.B. The molecular determinants of de novo nucleotide biosynthesis in cancer cells. *Curr. Opin. Genet. Dev.* **2009**, *19*, 32–37. [CrossRef]
16. Izquierdo-Garcia, J.L.; Cai, L.M.; Chaumeil, M.M.; Eriksson, P.; Robinson, A.E.; Pieper, R.O.; Phillips, J.J.; Ronen, S.M. Glioma cells with the IDH1 mutation modulate metabolic fractional flux through pyruvate carboxylase. *PLoS ONE* **2014**, *9*, e108289. [CrossRef] [PubMed]
17. Goji, T.; Takahara, K.; Negishi, M.; Katoh, H. Cystine uptake through the cystine/glutamate antiporter xCT triggers glioblastoma cell death under glucose deprivation. *J. Biol. Chem.* **2017**, *292*, 19721–19732. [CrossRef]

18. Suh, E.H.; Hackett, E.P.; Wynn, R.M.; Chuang, D.T.; Zhang, B.; Luo, W.; Sherry, A.D.; Park, J.M. In vivo assessment of increased oxidation of branched-chain amino acids in glioblastoma. *Sci. Rep.* **2019**, *9*, 340. [CrossRef] [PubMed]
19. Tönjes, M.; Barbus, S.; Park, Y.J.; Wang, W.; Schlotter, M.; Lindroth, A.M.; Pleier, S.V.; Bai, A.H.C.; Karra, D.; Piro, R.M.; et al. BCAT1 promotes cell proliferation through amino acid catabolism in gliomas carrying wild-type IDH1. *Nat. Med.* **2013**, *19*, 901–908. [CrossRef] [PubMed]
20. Park, J.; Shim, J.K.; Kang, J.H.; Choi, J.; Chang, J.H.; Kim, S.Y.; Kang, S.G. Regulation of bioenergetics through dual inhibition of aldehyde dehydrogenase and mitochondrial complex i suppresses glioblastoma tumorspheres. *Neuro. Oncol.* **2018**, *20*, 954–965. [CrossRef] [PubMed]
21. Izquierdo-Garcia, J.L.; Viswanath, P.; Eriksson, P.; Cai, L.; Radoul, M.; Chaumeil, M.M.; Blough, M.; Luchman, H.A.; Weiss, S.; Cairncross, J.G.; et al. IDH1 mutation induces reprogramming of pyruvate metabolism. *Cancer Res.* **2015**, *75*, 2999–3009. [CrossRef]
22. Miska, J.; Lee-Chang, C.; Rashidi, A.; Muroski, M.E.; Chang, A.L.; Lopez-Rosas, A.; Zhang, P.; Panek, W.K.; Cordero, A.; Han, Y.; et al. HIF-1α Is a Metabolic Switch between Glycolytic-Driven Migration and Oxidative Phosphorylation-Driven Immunosuppression of Tregs in Glioblastoma. *Cell Rep.* **2019**, *27*, 226–237.e4. [CrossRef]
23. Lu, C.-L.; Qin, L.; Liu, H.-C.; Candas, D.; Fan, M.; Li, J.J. Tumor Cells Switch to Mitochondrial Oxidative Phosphorylation under Radiation via mTOR-Mediated Hexokinase II Inhibition - A Warburg-Reversing Effect. *PLoS ONE* **2015**, *10*, e0121046. [CrossRef] [PubMed]
24. Altman, B.J.; Stine, Z.E.; Dang, C.V. From Krebs to clinic: Glutamine metabolism to cancer therapy. *Nat. Rev. Cancer* **2016**, *16*, 619–634. [CrossRef] [PubMed]
25. Lewis, C.A.; Brault, C.; Peck, B.; Bensaad, K.; Griffiths, B.; Mitter, R.; Chakravarty, P.; East, P.; Dankworth, B.; Alibhai, D.; et al. SREBP maintains lipid biosynthesis and viability of cancer cells under lipid- and oxygen-deprived conditions and defines a gene signature associated with poor survival in glioblastoma multiforme. *Oncogene* **2015**, *34*, 5128–5140. [CrossRef]
26. Geng, F.; Cheng, X.; Wu, X.; Yoo, J.Y.; Cheng, C.; Guo, J.Y.; Mo, X.; Ru, P.; Hurwitz, B.; Kim, S.H.; et al. Inhibition of SOAT1 suppresses glioblastoma growth via blocking SREBP-1-mediated lipogenesis. *Clin. Cancer Res.* **2016**, *22*, 5337–5348. [CrossRef] [PubMed]
27. Pirmoradi, L.; Seyfizadeh, N.; Ghavami, S.; Zeki, A.A.; Shojaei, S. Targeting cholesterol metabolism in glioblastoma: A new therapeutic approach in cancer therapy. *J. Investig. Med.* **2019**, *67*, 715–719. [CrossRef] [PubMed]
28. Wu, F.; Zhao, Z.; Chai, R.C.; Liu, Y.Q.; Li, G.Z.; Jiang, H.Y.; Jiang, T. Prognostic power of a lipid metabolism gene panel for diffuse gliomas. *J. Cell. Mol. Med.* **2019**, *23*, 7741–7748. [CrossRef]
29. Guo, D. SCAP links glucose to lipid metabolism in cancer cells. *Mol. Cell. Oncol.* **2016**, *3*, e1132120. [CrossRef] [PubMed]
30. Rusu, P.; Shao, C.; Neuerburg, A.; Acikgöz, A.A.; Wu, Y.; Zou, P.; Phapale, P.; Shankar, T.S.; Döring, K.; Dettling, S.; et al. GPD1 Specifically Marks Dormant Glioma Stem Cells with a Distinct Metabolic Profile. *Cell Stem Cell* **2019**, *25*, 241–257. [CrossRef] [PubMed]
31. Zgheib, R.; Battaglia-Hsu, S.F.; Hergalant, S.; Quéré, M.; Alberto, J.M.; Chéry, C.; Rouyer, P.; Gauchotte, G.; Guéant, J.L.; Namour, F. Folate can promote the methionine-dependent reprogramming of glioblastoma cells towards pluripotency. *Cell Death Dis.* **2019**, *10*, 1–12. [CrossRef]
32. Wang, X.; Yang, K.; Xie, Q.; Wu, Q.; Mack, S.C.; Shi, Y.; Kim, L.J.Y.Y.; Prager, B.C.; Flavahan, W.A.; Liu, X.; et al. Purine synthesis promotes maintenance of brain tumor initiating cells in glioma. *Nat. Neurosci.* **2017**, *20*, 661–673. [CrossRef]
33. Lamb, R.; Harrison, H.; Smith, D.L.; Townsend, P.A.; Jackson, T.; Ozsvari, B.; Martinez-Outschoorn, U.E.; Pestell, R.G.; Howell, A.; Lisanti, M.P.; et al. Targeting tumor-initiating cells: Eliminating anabolic cancer stem cells with inhibitors of protein synthesis or by mimicking caloric restriction. *Oncotarget* **2015**, *6*, 4585–4601. [CrossRef]
34. Zhang, J.; Nuebel, E.; Daley, G.Q.; Koehler, C.M.; Teitell, M.A. Metabolic regulation in pluripotent stem cells during reprogramming and self-renewal. *Cell Stem Cell* **2012**, *11*, 589–595. [CrossRef]
35. Intlekofer, A.M.; Finley, L.W.S. Metabolic signatures of cancer cells and stem cells. *Nat. Metab.* **2019**, *1*, 177–188. [CrossRef] [PubMed]
36. Chung, S.; Dzeja, P.P.; Faustino, R.S.; Perez-Terzic, C.; Behfar, A.; Terzic, A. Mitochondrial oxidative metabolism is required for the cardiac differentiation of stem cells. *Nat. Clin. Pract. Cardiovasc. Med.* **2007**, *4*. [CrossRef]
37. Zhou, W.; Choi, M.; Margineantu, D.; Margaretha, L.; Hesson, J.; Cavanaugh, C.; Blau, C.A.; Horwitz, M.S.; Hockenbery, D.; Ware, C.; et al. HIF1α induced switch from bivalent to exclusively glycolytic metabolism during ESC-to-EpiSC/hESC transition. *EMBO J.* **2012**, *31*, 2103–2116. [CrossRef] [PubMed]
38. Vander Heiden, M.G.; DeBerardinis, R.J. Understanding the Intersections between Metabolism and Cancer Biology. *Cell* **2017**, *168*, 657–669. [CrossRef] [PubMed]
39. Fan, J.; Kamphorst, J.J.; Mathew, R.; Chung, M.K.; White, E.; Shlomi, T.; Rabinowitz, J.D. Glutamine-driven oxidative phosphorylation is a major ATP source in transformed mammalian cells in both normoxia and hypoxia. *Mol. Syst. Biol.* **2013**, *9*. [CrossRef] [PubMed]
40. Tohyama, S.; Fujita, J.; Hishiki, T.; Matsuura, T.; Hattori, F.; Ohno, R.; Kanazawa, H.; Seki, T.; Nakajima, K.; Kishino, Y.; et al. Glutamine Oxidation Is Indispensable for Survival of Human Pluripotent Stem Cells. *Cell Metab.* **2016**, *23*, 663–674. [CrossRef] [PubMed]
41. Palm, W.; Thompson, C.B. Nutrient acquisition strategies of mammalian cells. *Nature* **2017**, *546*, 234–242. [CrossRef] [PubMed]

42. Yang, W.; Zheng, Y.; Xia, Y.; Ji, H.; Chen, X.; Guo, F.; Lyssiotis, C.A.; Aldape, K.; Cantley, L.C.; Lu, Z. ERK1/2-dependent phosphorylation and nuclear translocation of PKM2 promotes the Warburg effect. *Nat. Cell Biol.* **2012**, *14*, 1295–1304. [CrossRef]
43. Ahmad, F.; Dixit, D.; Sharma, V.; Kumar, A.; Joshi, S.D.; Sarkar, C.; Sen, E. Nrf2-driven TERT regulates pentose phosphate pathway in glioblastoma. *Cell Death Dis.* **2016**, *7*. [CrossRef] [PubMed]
44. Sachdeva, R.; Wu, M.; Smiljanic, S.; Kaskun, O.; Ghannad-Zadeh, K.; Celebre, A.; Isaev, K.; Morrissy, A.S.; Guan, J.; Tong, J.; et al. ID1 is critical for tumorigenesis and regulates chemoresistance in glioblastoma. *Cancer Res.* **2019**, *79*, 4057–4071. [CrossRef]
45. Sachdeva, R.; Wu, M.; Johnson, K.; Kim, H.; Celebre, A.; Shahzad, U.; Graham, M.S.; Kessler, J.A.; Chuang, J.H.; Karamchandani, J.; et al. BMP signaling mediates glioma stem cell quiescence and confers treatment resistance in glioblastoma. *Sci. Rep.* **2019**, *9*. [CrossRef]
46. Batlle, E.; Clevers, H. Cancer stem cells revisited. *Nat. Med.* **2017**, *23*, 1124–1134. [CrossRef]
47. Vlashi, E.; Lagadec, C.; Vergnes, L.; Matsutani, T.; Masui, K.; Poulou, M.; Popescu, R.; Della Donna, L.; Evers, P.; Dekmezian, C.; et al. Metabolic state of glioma stem cells and nontumorigenic cells. *Proc. Natl. Acad. Sci. USA* **2011**, *108*, 16062–16067. [CrossRef]
48. Tibbetts, A.S.; Appling, D.R. Compartmentalization of Mammalian Folate-Mediated One-Carbon Metabolism. *Annu. Rev. Nutr.* **2010**, *30*, 57–81. [CrossRef]
49. Villa, E.; Ali, E.S.; Sahu, U.; Ben-Sahra, I. Cancer cells tune the signaling pathways to empower de novo synthesis of nucleotides. *Cancers* **2019**, *11*, 688. [CrossRef]
50. Yin, J.; Ren, W.; Huang, X.; Deng, J.; Li, T.; Yin, Y. Potential Mechanisms Connecting Purine Metabolism and Cancer Therapy. *Front. Immunol.* **2018**, *9*, 1697. [CrossRef] [PubMed]
51. Di Virgilio, F.; Adinolfi, E. Extracellular purines, purinergic receptors and tumor growth. *Oncogene* **2017**, *36*, 293–303. [CrossRef] [PubMed]
52. Chan, C.Y.; Zhao, H.; Pugh, R.J.; Pedley, A.M.; French, J.; Jones, S.A.; Zhuang, X.; Jinnah, H.; Huan, T.J.; Benkovic, S.J. Purinosome formation as a function of the cell cycle. *Proc. Natl. Acad. Sci. USA* **2015**, *112*, 1368–1373. [CrossRef]
53. An, S.; Kumar, R.; Sheets, E.D.; Benkovic, S.J. Reversible compartmentalization of de novo purine biosynthetic complexes in living cells. *Science* **2008**, *320*, 103–106. [CrossRef]
54. Pedley, A.M.; Benkovic, S.J. A New View into the Regulation of Purine Metabolism: The Purinosome. *Trends Biochem. Sci.* **2017**, *42*, 141–154. [CrossRef] [PubMed]
55. Hatefi, Y.; Huennekens, F.M.; Kay, L.D. Manometric assay and cofactor requirements for serine hydroxymethylase. *J. Biol. Chem.* **1957**, *224*, 435–444. [PubMed]
56. Jain, M.; Nilsson, R.; Sharma, S.; Madhusudhan, N.; Kitami, T.; Souza, A.L.; Kafri, R.; Kirschner, M.W.; Clish, C.B.; Mootha, V.K. Metabolite profiling identifies a key role for glycine in rapid cancer cell proliferation. *Science* **2012**, *336*, 1040–1044. [CrossRef]
57. Hatefi, Y.; Osborn, M.J.; Kay, L.D.; Huennekens, F.M. Hydroxymethyl tetrahydrofolic dehydrogenase. *J. Biol. Chem.* **1957**, *227*, 637–647. [CrossRef]
58. Nilsson, R.; Jain, M.; Madhusudhan, N.; Sheppard, N.G.; Strittmatter, L.; Kampf, C.; Huang, J.; Asplund, A.; Mootha, V.K. Metabolic enzyme expression highlights a key role for MTHFD2 and the mitochondrial folate pathway in cancer. *Nat. Commun.* **2014**, *5*, 3128. [CrossRef]
59. Miyo, M.; Konno, M.; Colvin, H.; Nishida, N.; Koseki, J.; Kawamoto, K.; Tsunekuni, K.; Nishimura, J.; Hata, T.; Takemasa, I.; et al. The importance of mitochondrial folate enzymes in human colorectal cancer. *Oncol. Rep.* **2017**, *37*, 417–425. [CrossRef]
60. Fawal, M.A.; Jungas, T.; Davy, A. Inhibition of DHFR targets the self-renewing potential of brain tumor initiating cells. *Cancer Lett.* **2021**, *503*, 129–137. [CrossRef]
61. Zhang, Z.; Shi, Q.; Sturgis, E.M.; Spitz, M.R.; Wei, Q. Polymorphisms and haplotypes of serine hydroxymethyltransferase and risk of squamous cell carcinoma of the head and neck: A case-control analysis. *Pharmacogenet. Genom.* **2005**, *15*, 557–564. [CrossRef]
62. Noguchi, K.; Konno, M.; Koseki, J.; Nishida, N.; Kawamoto, K.; Yamada, D.; Asaoka, T.; Noda, T.; Wada, H.; Gotoh, K.; et al. The mitochondrial one-carbon metabolic pathway is associated with patient survival in pancreatic cancer. *Oncol. Lett.* **2018**, *16*, 1827–1834. [CrossRef]
63. Park, A.K.; Lee, J.Y.; Cheong, H.; Ramaswamy, V.; Park, S.-H.; Kool, M.; Phi, J.H.; Choi, S.A.; Cavalli, F.; Taylor, M.D.; et al. Subgroup-specific prognostic signaling and metabolic pathways in pediatric medulloblastoma. *BMC Cancer* **2019**, *19*, 571. [CrossRef]
64. Liu, F.; Liu, Y.; He, C.; Tao, L.; He, X.; Song, H.; Zhang, G. Increased MTHFD2 expression is associated with poor prognosis in breast cancer. *Tumor Biol.* **2014**, *35*, 8685–8690. [CrossRef]
65. Koseki, J.; Konno, M.; Asai, A.; Colvin, H.; Kawamoto, K.; Nishida, N.; Sakai, D.; Kudo, T.; Satoh, T.; Doki, Y.; et al. Enzymes of the one-carbon folate metabolism as anticancer targets predicted by survival rate analysis. *Sci. Rep.* **2018**, *8*, 1–7. [CrossRef] [PubMed]
66. Nishimura, T.; Nakata, A.; Chen, X.; Nishi, K.; Meguro-Horike, M.; Sasaki, S.; Kita, K.; Horike, S.-i.; Saitoh, K.; Kato, K.; et al. Cancer stem-like properties and gefitinib resistance are dependent on purine synthetic metabolism mediated by the mitochondrial enzyme MTHFD2. *Oncogene* **2019**, *38*, 2464–2481. [CrossRef]
67. Ben-Sahra, I.; Hoxhaj, G.; Ricoult, S.J.H.; Asara, J.M.; Manning, B.D. mTORC1 induces purine synthesis through control of the mitochondrial tetrahydrofolate cycle. *Science* **2016**, *351*, 728–733. [CrossRef]
68. Kong, W.; Wang, J. Hypoxanthine Transport in Human Glioblastoma Cells and Effect on Cell Susceptibility to Methotrexate. *Pharm. Res.* **2003**, *20*, 1804–1811. [CrossRef]

69. Coulthard, S.A.; Redfern, C.P.F.; Vikingsson, S.; Lindqvist-Appell, M.; Skoglund, K.; Jakobsen-Falk, I.; Hall, A.G.; Taylor, G.A.; Hogarth, L.A. Increased sensitivity to thiopurines in methylthioadenosine phosphorylase-deleted cancers. *Mol. Cancer Ther.* **2011**, *10*, 495–504. [CrossRef] [PubMed]
70. Tardito, S.; Oudin, A.; Ahmed, S.U.; Fack, F.; Keunen, O.; Zheng, L.; Miletic, H.; Sakariassen, P.Ø.; Weinstock, A.; Wagner, A.; et al. Glutamine synthetase activity fuels nucleotide biosynthesis and supports growth of glutamine-restricted glioblastoma. *Nat. Cell Biol.* **2015**, *17*, 1556–1568. [CrossRef] [PubMed]
71. Baresova, V.; Skopova, V.; Sikora, J.; Patterson, D.; Sovova, J.; Zikanova, M.; Kmoch, S. Mutations of ATIC and ADSL affect purinosome assembly in cultured skin fibroblasts from patients with AICA-ribosiduria and ADSL deficiency. *Hum. Mol. Genet.* **2012**, *21*, 1534–1543. [CrossRef]
72. Mazzarino, R.C.; Baresova, V.; Zikánová, M.; Duval, N.; Wilkinson, T.G.; Patterson, D.; Vacano, G.N. The CRISPR-Cas9 crADSL HeLa transcriptome: A first step in establishing a model for ADSL deficiency and SAICAR accumulation. *Mol. Genet. Metab. Rep.* **2019**, *21*, 100512. [CrossRef]
73. French, J.B.; Zhao, H.; An, S.; Niessen, S.; Deng, Y.; Cravatt, B.F.; Benkovic, S.J. Hsp70/Hsp90 chaperone machinery is involved in the assembly of the purinosome. *Proc. Natl. Acad. Sci. USA* **2013**, *110*, 2528–2533. [CrossRef]
74. Goswami, M.T.; Chen, G.; Chakravarthi, B.V.S.K.; Pathi, S.S.; Anand, S.K.; Carskadon, S.L.; Giordano, T.J.; Chinnaiyan, A.M.; Thomas, D.G.; Palanisamy, N.; et al. Role and regulation of coordinately expressed de novo purine biosynthetic enzymes PPAT and PAICS in lung cancer. *Oncotarget* **2015**, *6*, 23445–23461. [CrossRef]
75. Kofuji, S.; Hirayama, A.; Eberhardt, A.O.; Kawaguchi, R.; Sugiura, Y.; Sampetrean, O.; Ikeda, Y.; Warren, M.; Sakamoto, N.; Kitahara, S.; et al. IMP dehydrogenase-2 drives aberrant nucleolar activity and promotes tumorigenesis in glioblastoma. *Nat. Cell Biol.* **2019**, *21*, 1003–1014. [CrossRef]
76. Brennan, C.W.; Verhaak, R.G.W.; McKenna, A.; Campos, B.; Noushmehr, H.; Salama, S.R.; Zheng, S.; Chakravarty, D.; Sanborn, J.Z.; Berman, S.H.; et al. The somatic genomic landscape of glioblastoma. *Cell* **2013**, *155*, 462. [CrossRef] [PubMed]
77. Zhou, W.; Yao, Y.; Scott, A.J.; Wilder-Romans, K.; Dresser, J.J.; Werner, C.K.; Sun, H.; Pratt, D.; Sajjakulnukit, P.; Zhao, S.G.; et al. Purine metabolism regulates DNA repair and therapy resistance in glioblastoma. *Nat. Commun.* **2020**, *11*, 1–14. [CrossRef]
78. Shireman, J.M.; Atashi, F.; Lee, G.; Ali, E.S.; Saathoff, M.R.; Park, C.H.; Savchuk, S.; Baisiwala, S.; Miska, J.; Lesniak, M.S.; et al. De novo purine biosynthesis is a major driver of chemoresistance in glioblastoma. *Brain* **2021**. [CrossRef]
79. Wink, M.R.; Lenz, G.; Braganhol, E.; Tamajusuku, A.S.K.; Schwartsmann, G.; Sarkis, J.J.F.; Battastini, A.M.O. Altered extracellular ATP, ADP and AMP catabolism in glioma cell lines. *Cancer Lett.* **2003**, *198*, 211–218. [CrossRef]
80. Conti, C.R. Adenosine: Clinical pharmacology and applications. *Clin. Cardiol.* **1991**, *14*, 91–93.
81. Allard, B.; Longhi, M.S.; Robson, S.C.; Stagg, J. The ectonucleotidases CD39 and CD73: Novel checkpoint inhibitor targets. *Immunol. Rev.* **2017**, *276*, 121–144. [CrossRef] [PubMed]
82. Wang, W.; Fridman, A.; Blackledge, W.; Connely, S.; Wilson, I.A.; Pilz, R.; Boss, G.R. The phosphatidylinositol 3-kinase/Akt cassette regulates purine nucleotide synthesis. *J. Biol. Chem.* **2009**, *284*, 3521–3528. [CrossRef] [PubMed]
83. Saha, A.; Connelly, S.; Jiang, J.; Zhuang, S.; Amador, D.T.; Phan, T.; Pilz, R.B.; Boss, G.R. Akt phosphorylation and regulation of transketolase is a nodal point for amino acid control of purine synthesis. *Mol. Cell* **2014**, *55*, 264–276. [CrossRef]
84. Jin, N.; Bi, A.; Lan, X.; Xu, J.; Wang, X.; Liu, Y.; Wang, T.; Tang, S.; Zeng, H.; Chen, Z.; et al. Identification of metabolic vulnerabilities of receptor tyrosine kinases-driven cancer. *Nat. Commun.* **2019**, *10*, 1–15. [CrossRef]
85. Lehtinen, L.; Ketola, K.; Mäkelä, R.; Mpindi, J.P.; Viitala, M.; Kallioniemi, O.; Iljin, K. High-throughput RNAi screening for novel modulators of vimentin expression identifies MTHFD2 as a regulator of breast cancer cell migration and invasion. *Oncotarget* **2013**, *4*, 48–63. [CrossRef]
86. Tanaka, K.; Sasayama, T.; Nagashima, H.; Irino, Y.; Takahashi, M.; Izumi, Y.; Uno, T.; Satoh, N.; Kitta, A.; Kyotani, K.; et al. Glioma cells require one-carbon metabolism to survive glutamine starvation. *Acta Neuropathol. Commun.* **2021**, *9*, 16. [CrossRef]
87. Kollareddy, M.; Dimitrova, E.; Vallabhaneni, K.C.; Chan, A.; Le, T.; Chauhan, K.M.; Carrero, Z.I.; Ramakrishnan, G.; Watabe, K.; Haupt, Y.; et al. Regulation of nucleotide metabolism by mutant p53 contributes to its gain-of-function activities. *Nat. Commun.* **2015**, *6*. [CrossRef] [PubMed]
88. Racanelli, A.C.; Rothbart, S.B.; Heyer, C.L.; Moran, R.G. Therapeutics by cytotoxic metabolite accumulation: Pemetrexed causes ZMP accumulation, AMPK activation, and mammalian target of rapamycin inhibition. *Cancer Res.* **2009**, *69*, 5467–5474. [CrossRef]
89. Liu, X.; Chhipa, R.R.; Pooya, S.; Wortman, M.; Yachyshin, S.; Chow, L.M.L.; Kumar, A.; Zhou, X.; Sun, Y.; Quinn, B.; et al. Discrete mechanisms of mTOR and cell cycle regulation by AMPK agonists independent of AMPK. *Proc. Natl. Acad. Sci. USA* **2014**, *111*, E435–E444. [CrossRef] [PubMed]
90. Dasgupta, B.; Hirota, Y.; Fujii, Y.; Osaka, N.; Ito, D.; Plas, D.R.; Sasaki, A.T. Targeting Energy Metabolism to Overcome Therapeutic Resistance of Glioblastoma and Tumor-associated Edema. In *Gliomas*; Exon Publications: Brisbane, Australia, 2021; pp. 121–138.
91. Chhipa, R.R.; Fan, Q.; Anderson, J.; Muraleedharan, R.; Huang, Y.; Ciraolo, G.; Chen, X.; Waclaw, R.; Chow, L.M.; Khuchua, Z.; et al. AMP kinase promotes glioblastoma bioenergetics and tumour growth. *Nat. Cell Biol.* **2018**, *20*, 823–835. [CrossRef]
92. Laderoute, K.R.; Amin, K.; Calaoagan, J.M.; Knapp, M.; Le, T.; Orduna, J.; Foretz, M.; Viollet, B. 5′-AMP-Activated Protein Kinase (AMPK) Is Induced by Low-Oxygen and Glucose Deprivation Conditions Found in Solid-Tumor Microenvironments. *Mol. Cell. Biol.* **2006**, *26*, 5336–5347. [CrossRef] [PubMed]
93. Adjei, A.A. Pharmacology and mechanism of action of pemetrexed. *Clin. Lung Cancer* **2004**, *5*, S51–S55. [CrossRef]

94. Chattopadhyay, S.; Moran, R.G.; Goldman, I.D. Pemetrexed: Biochemical and cellular pharmacology, mechanisms, and clinical applications. *Mol. Cancer Ther.* **2007**, *6*, 404–417. [CrossRef] [PubMed]
95. Schmitt, D.L.; Cheng, Y.; Park, J.; An, S. Sequestration-Mediated Downregulation of *de Novo* Purine Biosynthesis by AMPK. *ACS Chem. Biol.* **2016**, *11*, 1917–1924. [CrossRef] [PubMed]
96. Asai, A.; Konno, M.; Koseki, J.; Taniguchi, M.; Vecchione, A.; Ishii, H. One-carbon metabolism for cancer diagnostic and therapeutic approaches. *Cancer Lett.* **2020**, *470*, 141–148. [CrossRef]
97. Puig, L. Methotrexate: New Therapeutic Approaches. *Actas Dermo-Sifiliográficas English Ed.* **2014**, *105*, 583–589. [CrossRef]
98. Maksimovic, V.; Pavlovic-Popovic, Z.; Vukmirovic, S.; Cvejic, J.; Mooranian, A.; Al-Salami, H.; Mikov, M.; Golocorbin-Kon, S. Molecular mechanism of action and pharmacokinetic properties of methotrexate. *Mol. Biol. Rep.* **2020**, *47*, 4699–4708. [CrossRef]
99. Walling, J. From methotrexate to pemetrexed and beyond. A review of the pharmacodynamic and clinical properties of antifolates. *Invest. New Drugs* **2006**, *24*, 37–77. [CrossRef]
100. Palanichamy, K.; Thirumoorthy, K.; Kanji, S.; Gordon, N.; Singh, R.; Jacob, J.R.; Sebastian, N.; Litzenberg, K.T.; Patel, D.; Bassett, E.; et al. Methionine and kynurenine activate oncogenic kinases in glioblastoma, and methionine deprivation compromises proliferation. *Clin. Cancer Res.* **2016**, *22*, 3513–3523. [CrossRef]
101. Hori, H.; Tran, P.; Carrera, C.J.; Hori, Y.; Rosenbach, M.D.; Carson, D.A.; Nobori, T. Methylthioadenosine phosphorylase cDNA transfection alters sensitivity to depletion of purine and methionine in A549 lung cancer cells. *Cancer Res.* **1996**, *56*, 5653–5658.
102. de Menezes, W.P.; Silva, V.A.O.; Gomes, I.N.F.; Rosa, M.N.; Spina, M.L.C.; Carloni, A.C.; Alves, A.L.V.; Melendez, M.; Almeida, G.C.; da Silva, L.S.; et al. Loss of 5′-Methylthioadenosine Phosphorylase (MTAP) is Frequent in High-Grade Gliomas; Nevertheless, it is Not Associated with Higher Tumor Aggressiveness. *Cells* **2020**, *9*, 492. [CrossRef] [PubMed]
103. Li, W.W.; Su, D.; Mizobuchi, H.; Martin, D.S.; Gu, B.; Gorlick, R.; Cole, P.; Bertino, J.R. Status of methylthioadenosine phosphorylase and its impact on cellular response to L-alanosine and methylmercaptopurine riboside in human soft tissue sarcoma cells. *Oncol. Res.* **2004**, *14*, 373–379. [CrossRef]
104. Karikari, C.A.; Mullendore, M.; Eshleman, J.R.; Argani, P.; Leoni, L.M.; Chattopadhyay, S.; Hidalgo, M.; Maitra, A. Homozygous deletions of methylthioadenosine phosphorylase in human biliary tract cancers. *Mol. Cancer Ther.* **2005**, *4*, 1860–1866. [CrossRef]
105. Batova, A.; Cottam, H.; Yu, J.; Diccianni, M.B.; Carrera, C.J.; Yu, A.L. EFA(9-β-D-erythrofuranosyladenine) is an effective salvage agent for methylthioadenosine phosphorylase-selective therapy of T-cell acute lymphoblastic leukemia with L-alanosine. *Blood* **2006**, *107*, 898–903. [CrossRef]
106. Hansen, L.J.; Sun, R.; Yang, R.; Singh, S.X.; Chen, L.H.; Pirozzi, C.J.; Moure, C.J.; Hemphill, C.; Carpenter, A.B.; Healy, P.; et al. MTAP loss promotes stemness in glioblastoma and confers unique susceptibility to purine starvation. *Cancer Res.* **2019**, *79*, 3383–3394. [CrossRef] [PubMed]
107. National Library of Medicine (U.S.) Mycophenolate Mofetil Combined With Radiation Therapy in Recurrent Glioblastoma. Available online: https://www.clinicaltrials.gov/ct2/show/NCT04477200 (accessed on 10 May 2021).
108. Asai, A.; Koseki, J.; Konno, M.; Nishimura, T.; Gotoh, N.; Satoh, T.; Doki, Y.; Mori, M.; Ishii, H. Drug discovery of anticancer drugs targeting methylenetetrahydrofolate dehydrogenase 2. *Heliyon* **2018**, *4*, e01021. [CrossRef] [PubMed]
109. Ducker, G.S.; Ghergurovich, J.M.; Mainolfi, N.; Suri, V.; Jeong, S.K.; Hsin-Jung Li, S.; Friedman, A.; Manfredi, M.G.; Gitai, Z.; Kim, H.; et al. Human SHMT inhibitors reveal defective glycine import as a targetable metabolic vulnerability of diffuse large B-cell lymphoma. *Proc. Natl. Acad. Sci. USA* **2017**, *114*, 11404–11409. [CrossRef] [PubMed]
110. Zhao, M.; Tan, B.; Dai, X.; Shao, Y.; He, Q.; Yang, B.; Wang, J.; Weng, Q. DHFR/TYMS are positive regulators of glioma cell growth and modulate chemo-sensitivity to temozolomide. *Eur. J. Pharmacol.* **2019**, *863*. [CrossRef] [PubMed]
111. Kosti, A.; De Araujo, P.R.; Li, W.Q.; Guardia, G.D.A.; Chiou, J.; Yi, C.; Ray, D.; Meliso, F.; Li, Y.M.; Delambre, T.; et al. The RNA-binding protein SERBP1 functions as a novel oncogenic factor in glioblastoma by bridging cancer metabolism and epigenetic regulation. *Genome Biol.* **2020**, *21*. [CrossRef] [PubMed]
112. Niechi, I.; Uribe-Ojeda, A.; Erices, J.I.; Torres, Á.; Uribe, D.; Rocha, J.D.; Silva, P.; Richter, H.G.; San Martín, R.; Quezada, C. Adenosine Depletion as A New Strategy to Decrease Glioblastoma Stem-Like Cells Aggressiveness. *Cells* **2019**, *8*, 1353. [CrossRef]

MDPI
St. Alban-Anlage 66
4052 Basel
Switzerland
Tel. +41 61 683 77 34
Fax +41 61 302 89 18
www.mdpi.com

Cancers Editorial Office
E-mail: cancers@mdpi.com
www.mdpi.com/journal/cancers

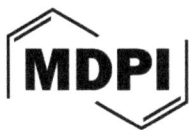

www.ingramcontent.com/pod-product-compliance
Lightning Source LLC
LaVergne TN
LVHW070140100526
838202LV00015B/1860

9 7 8 3 0 3 6 5 2 5 9 9 0